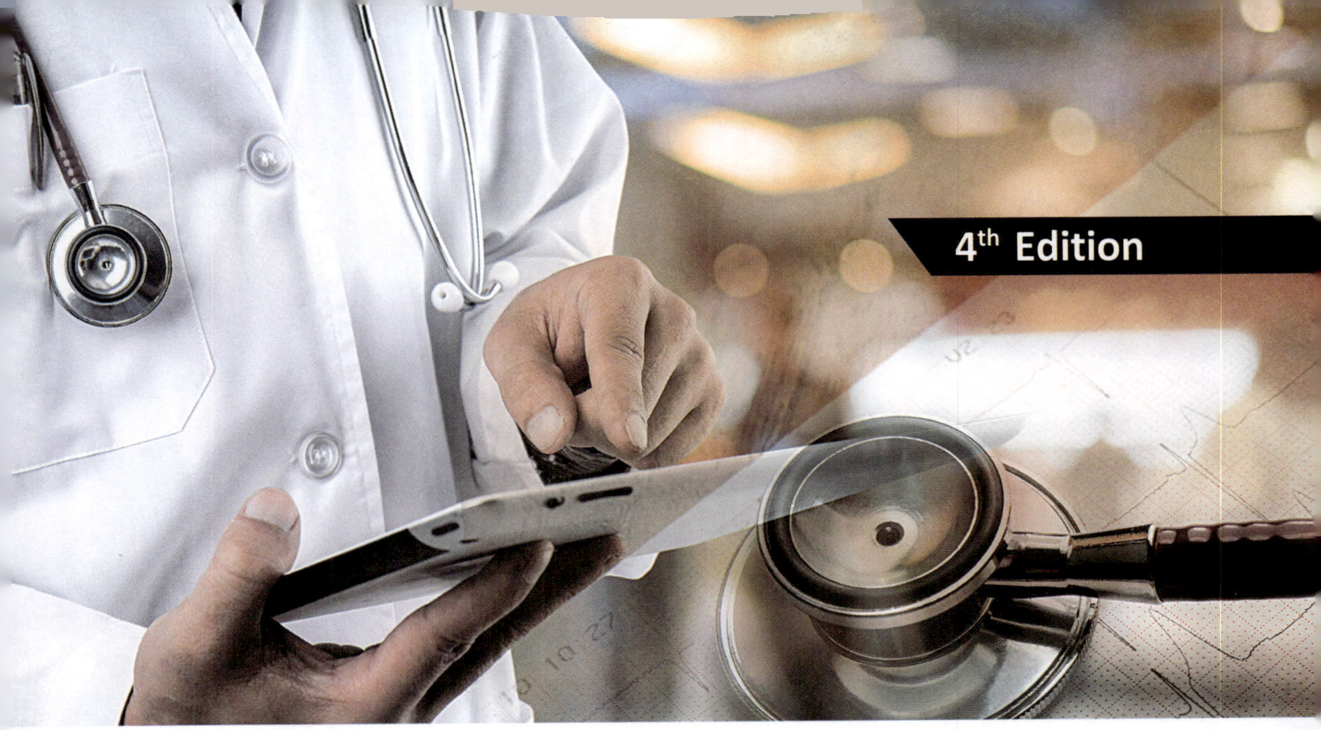

4th Edition

GENERAL PRACTICE AS SPECIALITY

Includes Comprehensive Guide to Basic General Practice

Prakash Mahajan

MBBS, DDV, FCGP
Mahajan Clinic, Chinar Heights
Deep Bunglow Chowk, Model Colony
Pune, Maharashtra, India

Editor

Madhu Oswal

Paras Medical Publisher
Hyderabad ▪ New Delhi, India

GENERAL PRACTICE AS SPECIALITY

PARAS

Empowering Healthcare Professionals

Paras Medical Publisher
5-1-475, First Floor, Putlibowli
Hyderabad—500095, India
parasmedpub@hotmail.com
www.parasmedicalpublisher.com

Branch Office:
2/25, Ground Floor
Daryaganj, Ansari Road,
New Delhi-110002, India

1Ed 2003, 2Ed 2006, 3Ed 2013
Reprint 2015, 4Ed 2023, 1st Reprint 2025

ISBN: 978-81-8191-547-4

Note: Medicine is an ever-changing science. As new research and clinical experience broaden our knowledge, changes in the diagnosis and treatment occur. The authors and the publisher of this work have checked with sources believed to be reliable in their efforts to provide information that is complete and generally in accord with the standards accepted at the time of publication. Exhaustive efforts have been made to ensure accuracy and correctness of contents of the book at the time of going to press. However, in view of possibility of human error or changes in medical science, the author, publisher or any other person who has been involved in preparation of this work accepts no responsibility for any errors or omissions or results obtained from use of information given in the book. Every effort has been made to put reference to tables and figures. If any table and figure has been taken from a source, which has not been quoted it is an oversight and will be corrected at the earliest possible opportunity. The authors have made every effort to trace the copyright holders for borrowed material. If they have inadvertently overlooked any, they will be pleased to make the necessary arrangements at the first opportunity. This book is being published with the understanding that the material provided by the author(s) is original. This book is for sale in India only and cannot be exported without the permission of the publisher in writing. Any disputes and legal matters to be settled under Hyderabad jurisdiction only. *Printed in Hyderabad, Telangana, India*.

PREFACE TO THE FOURTH EDITION

The first edition of this book "***General Practice as Specialty***" was published in 2005. Over these many years, the field of specialist medical practice in India has evolved greatly and specialists are constantly going into more and more super specialized practice in their own domain. Keeping pace with these developments, the Indian general practitioner has to constantly evolve and upgrade his practice. This book has evolved simultaneously with each edition to include in a general practitioner's armamentarium a vast array of subspecialities he/she can develop in his clinic while at the same time polishing the art of medicine, maintaining ethical practice, with the ultimate objective of giving optimal care to the sick patient.

Our ultimate endeavour is to make this book more and more practice oriented and useful for the general practitioner in his day-to-day practice.

I have made the following additions and changes in shaping and revising the fourth edition of this book:

- All the chapters have been evaluated and upgraded.
- It is clearly necessary to upgrade our knowledge about pharmacology periodically. Hence, the whole first section of book on prescriber has been thoroughly reviewed by **Dr Bhagyashri D Rajopadhye**, MD (Pharmacology), Associate Professor of Pharmacology, Bharati Vidyapeeth Medical College, Pune.
- A new chapter on "**Hair loss treatment clinic**" has been added. This is a speciality which can be easily included in the general practitioners' armamentarium as it does not require costly investments, and given patience and perseverance can be easily managed by a general practitioner.
- A new topic on "**How to digitalize your clinic**": As a part of '**Digital Transformation**' going all over the world, it is high time for all individual medical practitioners to digitalise their clinics also. All big hospitals have digitalized their processes to provide better service to their patients. Why shouldn't we? Hence this chapter. This has been written by **Mr Chittaranjan Deo**, MSc (Physics), IT Consultant, Pune.
- A new chapter on "**Generic drugs**": With the Government of India insisting on the use of generic drugs so that medicines are available to all citizens at affordable cost, the knowledge about generic drugs and branded drugs is of prime importance.
- The previous chapter on Administering IV fluids in clinic has been totally replaced by a new one under the guidance of a senior physician.
- A new 4th section has been created which includes in addition to the formulary, tables on best guess approach to antibiotics. Admittedly, due to practice constraints, general

practitioners in the Indian subcontinent prescribe antibiotics by guessing the possible pathogen in the particular case at hand and prescribe the best possible antibiotics. This chapter will be immensely useful for general practitioners to do this more in a scientifically correct manner.

- 3 tables on Cardiac Arrhythmias have been added which will serve as a ready reference for diagnosis of a cardiac arrythmia on ECG in a physician's busy OPD.
- The chapter on ECG has been exhaustively evaluated by a senior cardiologist and relevant changes suggested have been made.
- The chapter on "**The De-addiction Centre**" has been fortified with addition of a section explaining the true nature of addictions that it is universally accepted as a disease and treated as such. This understanding is of utmost importance in treating addictions.

From the stand point of physical appearance, the following striking changes have been made:

1. A completely new format with professional new design and layout.
2. Text is well organised for ease of reading.
3. Old figures and cartoons have been replaced with new improved ones.

Finally, I continue to be highly indebted to Paras Medical Publishers in general and Mr Divyesh Arvind Kothari in particular for giving me constant encouragement and guiding me in the many changes instated in this fourth edition of this book. I hope you will enjoy reading this book as much as I have enjoyed writing this book!

Prakash Mahajan
drpmahajan51@gmail.com

WHY THE SECOND EDITION?

I once asked a senior and a highly respected general practitioner from Pune, Dr Anand Gokhale, as to how this book should be modified so that it becomes more useful for a GP? "Well", he said in his characteristic aplomb, "No. 1 - the book should be comprehensive enough for the average GP. A generalist cannot afford to buy books on every speciality of medicine and surgery. And No. 2 - the book should serve as a constant companion in his clinic. Like it or not, very few GPs have time and inclination to go home and read."

Keeping the same advice in mind and complying with the several suggestions given by well meaning colleagues, I have made the following modifications in this edition.

All the chapters have been reviewed and revised as needed.

In order to make it more comprehensive for an average GP, I have added a lot many more conditions and their treatment in section I of the book. In the second section, most common topics of diabetes and hypertension have been added. In the third section dealing with surgery, I have included the chapters on injections in general practice, suturing techniques of wounds, intralesional injections. Dr Madhu Oswal, my colleague in my clinical practice, has been kind enough to contribute a "formulary of drugs" for ready reference, making the book a constant companion in your clinic.

All in all, this makes this book grow in utility but (unfortunately) also in size. But then, we have to respond to what the great Sir William Osler noted a century ago: "*It is astonishing how with only a little reading a doctor can practice medicine. But it is not astonishing how badly he may do it.*"

Despite my best efforts, there might be several lacunae in the book and suggestions are most welcome from readers.

WHY THIS BOOK?

Twenty-five years ago, I started my medical practice and I regret to say that "day one" was an absolute disaster for me. I had passed my MBBS examination fairly well and was on top of the world, oozing with confidence, till my first patient walked into my newly furnished empty clinic.

A middle-aged man came to me complaining that he has been having hiccups for the last two days and had tried all home remedies without benefit. Frankly, I did not know how to treat him. In the college, I was taught how to treat acute diarrhoea, but not the method to treat acute hiccups. What was I supposed to do? I opened a standard textbook of medicine, but could not find even a remote reference of hiccups. "Practice of Surgery" said that persistent hiccups are due to irritation of the phrenic nerve on the undersurface of the diaphragm, but skipped the treatment part. Another reputed textbook of medicine said, if simple measures fail (which had failed in my patient), give IV chlorpromazine or a phrenic nerve block! Not knowing what to do, I dispensed a few antacid and metoclopramide tablets and sent back the patient. Needless to add, the patient has never come back to me for the past 25 years!

It was then, I realized the need of the fresh general practitioners—to have a book at hand in the clinic itself, which tells him what to do in such situations, not big fat textbooks neatly placed in a cozy cupboard. Criticizing textbooks? No, far from it. The fascinating range of textbooks that we use give us a lot of information, very much essential to pass various examinations. But what we require is information on how to tackle an ailing patient standing right in front of you, waving aside many theoretical considerations, e.g., a genital ulcer, according to textbooks, has to be diagnosed first as syphilis, chancroid etc., and then treated accordingly. This is quite demanding of an inexperienced GP. Hence, in this book the syndromic approach in the management of STDs is given, which does not stipulate an exact diagnosis requiring refined clinical judgement and sophisticated instruments. It is simple and practical. Moreover, it enables the GP to eat, drink, and survive!

The first section of this book is a "compact guide" for you, if you are a budding and aspiring GP. If you are an established and experienced GP and after going through the first few pages, you feel that the information is too basic, don't throw away this book. Move on confidently to the second or the third section. There is definitely something in store for you.

The second and the third sections cover a few topics in medicine and surgery, which are useful for a general practitioner when he wants to open up his horizons and aspires to become a 'Master in General Practice,' and is not satisfied with just remaining 'Bachelor in Medicine and Bachelor in Surgery.' This is just to begin with. There are many more areas in which a GP may want to specialize. The opportunities are endless.

Coming back to the point, "Was a book on general practice needed?" Well, I felt the necessity a few years back and went to a reputed library in search of a book for general practitioners. To my amazement, the library had only 3 books on general practice but 42 books on psychiatry! I also noticed to my amusement that it had 8 books on lizards, almost 3 times as many books than on general practice!! This was one of the many reasons why this book was written.

I do sincerely hope that medical students and interns (including allopathy, ayurveda, and homoeopathy), budding general practitioners, as well as established practitioners will find this book informative and beneficial.

ACKNOWLEDGEMENTS

It is indeed a daunting task for a practising doctor to write a book of this size without the active guidance and help from teachers, friends and colleagues. This help was showered upon me and I am deeply grateful to all those who have given me their time, energy, materials, advice, opinions, etc.

Each and every chapter of the book has been reviewed by the relevant specialist. My profuse thanks to all of them for their time spent in reviewing, correcting and suggesting modifications. My sincere thanks to Dr Arvind Ghodekar for taking photographs of the patients which were to be included in this book. My profuse thanks to Dr Sham Mhadekar for providing the "*GP tips*."

My wife Sheetal deserves to be thanked profusely. She was probably worst hit by my decision to write a book. Throughout the year, she managed to take care of the household and the children resolutely without even a murmur, letting me fully concentrate on writing this book.

At times, I felt depressed thinking how my lovely and obedient daughters, Kashmira, Asmani, Shalmali and my affectionate mother, must have missed my company. They never complained and in fact were so encouraging by enquiring every now and then about the progress of this book. I am indeed fortunate to have blessings from my mother, support from my wife, and love from my delightful daughters.

I also want to thank Mr Divyesh Arvind Kothari, Paras Medical Publisher, the publisher of this book for his timely assistance, exemplary guidance, and generous cooperation throughout the writing of this book, many times giving me a feeling that I was indeed fortunate to get 'Paras' as publishers.

I specifically want to thank the partner in my clinic Dr Madhu from the deepest corner of my left ventricle for all that she has done to help me in writing this book. Without her help, this book was virtually impossible. Apart from contributing the sections on Gynaecology, Acupuncture, Homoeopathy, and Immunization, she has been largely responsible for proofreading the manuscript of this book. But her most important contribution was her infectious belief and optimism that such a book was needed and could be written.

Finally I thank God, as all went well during the making of this book.

CONTENTS

SECTION 1 | BASIC GENERAL PRACTICE |

SECTION 2 | SPECIALITY MEDICAL GENERAL PRACTICE |

SECTION 3 | SPECIALITY SURGICAL GENERAL PRACTICE |

SECTION 4 | DRUG FORMULARY |

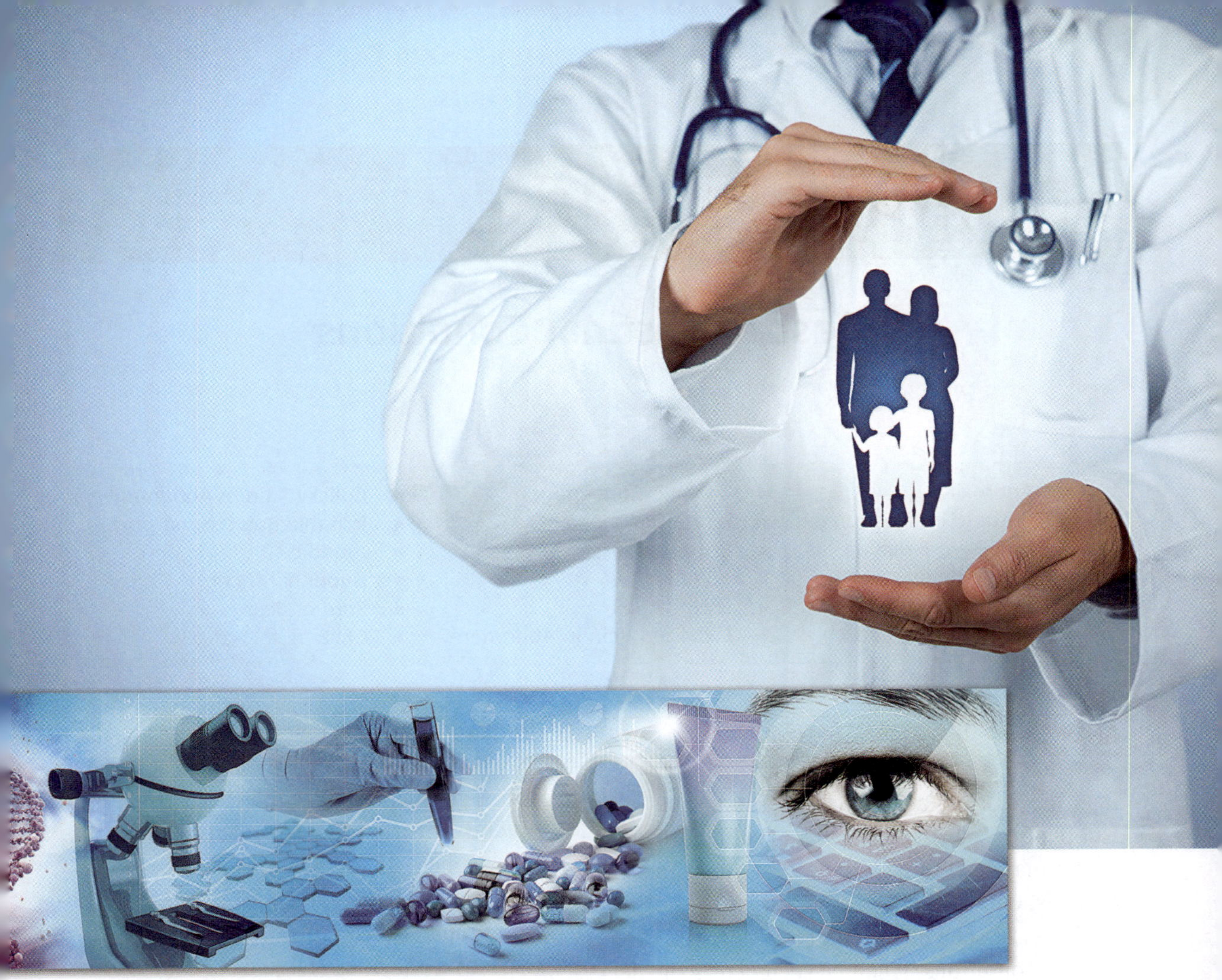

SECTION 1

BASIC GENERAL PRACTICE

CHAPTER 1

Gastrointestinal Conditions

- Anorexia
- Chronic Indigestion
- Excessive Belching
- Sore Tongue
- Hiccoughs (Hiccups)
- Acute Constipation
- Chronic Constipation
- Acute Diarrhoea
- Chronic Diarrhoea
- Vomiting
- Dysphagia
- Localized Pain in Abdomen
- Colicky Pain in Abdomen
- Irritable Bowel Syndrome
- Jaundice
- Duodenal Ulcer
- Peptic Ulcer
- GERD

ANOREXIA

It is the loss of desire to eat. First, rule out 'sitophobia', which means fear of eating because eating may lead to pain, e.g., oral ulcers, acute gastritis, etc.

1. It can be seen in any full blown disease. In a few conditions, it can be seen *before* the development of other manifestations of the disease, e.g., viral hepatitis, alcoholic hepatitis, anaemia, uraemia, pulmonary TB and stomach cancer.
2. Drugs like metronidazole, digitalis, etc., can cause anorexia.
3. Psychogenic causes include depression (seen especially in females because of domestic problems or in children because of demanding parents).

Empirical Treatment

1. Take proper history to find out if anorexia is functional.
2. Withdraw offending drugs if any.
3. Tonics—do have a placebo effect.
4. Any B-complex tablet of a standard company.
5. Tab. Cyproheptadine (Ciplactin, Periactin) 4 mg bd before food (**or**) Tab. Buclizine (Longiphen) 25 mg bd before food.
6. Tab. Liv 52, 2 tds.
7. Iron preparations (Autrin, Fefol, etc.)
8. Digestive enzymes (Digeplex, Unienzyme, etc.)
9. IV Dextrose saline if severe anorexia has led to dehydration.
10. Adequate exercises—very important.

Specific Treatment

If the patient does not respond to the above treatment, try to find out the cause and treat accordingly.

1. Haemogram → for anaemia
2. Urine-routine → for silent UTI
3. S. bilirubin → for jaundice
4. Blood urea, S. creatinine → for uraemia
5. X-ray chest → for pulmonary Koch's

6. Gastroscopy and USG abdomen → for Ca. stomach

CHRONIC INDIGESTION

Indigestion is a non-specific term used by patients and means different symptoms to different patients and different doctors, e.g., abdominal fullness, belching, water brash, heart burn, diarrhoea and even headache or failure to gain weight.

Causes

1. No apparent cause in half the patients.
2. Upper GI problems like gastritis, hiatus hernia, etc.
3. Lower GI problems like amoebiasis, giardiasis, worms, etc.
4. Biliary tract problems like cholecystitis, gall bladder calculus.
5. Chronic pancreatitis.
6. Intolerance to foods containing lactose in milk or wheat. Allergy to certain foods as suggested by associated urticaria.
7. Irritable bowel syndrome.
8. Extra-intestinal diseases like uraemia, CCF, etc.

Empirical Treatment

1. First evaluate the exact nature of the complaint.
2. Lifestyle management
   a) Avoid overeating. Prefer undereating with multiple small feeds.
   b) Weight reduction if overweight.
   c) Cessation of smoking and alcohol.
   d) Avoidance of fatty foods and aerated drinks.
   e) Brisk walk after each meal.
3. Tab. Domperidone (Domstal) 10 mg bd (or) Tab. Cisapride (Ciza MPS) 10 mg bd before food.
4. Oral enzyme preparations (Unienzyme or Liquid Lupizyme) after food.
5. Tab. Albendazole (Zentel) 400 mg single dose.
6. Tab. Metronidazole (Flagyl) 400 mg tds × 5 days.
7. Antacids (Gelusil or Digene) 30 mL after food, preferably containing methyl polysiloxane or simethicone.
8. Omeprazole capsule (Omez) 20 mg bd or od.
9. Avoidance of intolerant or allergic foods if implicated.

Specific Treatment

Most of the patients respond to above treatment. In those rare cases who do not, investigate and treat accordingly.

1. Stool examination → Giardiasis, amoebiasis, worms
2. USG abdomen → Gall bladder, pancreatic problems
3. Gastroscopy, sigmoidoscopy → Rarely required

EXCESSIVE BELCHING

Patient swallows air (without admitting it!) and even demonstrates to the doctor.

- Make patient aware that he is swallowing air while eating (aerophagia).
- Ask patient to eat slowly and chew food thoroughly before swallowing.
- Avoid aerated soft drinks like Thums-up and Coca-cola.
- Ask patient to eat with his mouth closed and even belch with his mouth closed.

If belching persists:

Prescribe antacid preparations with methyl polysiloxane or simethicone (e.g., Gelusil MPS).

If it still persists:
Ask the patient to place a cork or an eraser in between the molars after each meal for half an hour. Warn him not to swallow it accidentally!

SORE TONGUE (Stomatitis)

When the patient c/o burning in the mouth, first see whether there is diffuse inflammation or localized ulcerations. If there are ulcers, ask if these are recurrent. If the answer is yes, then these are aphthous ulcers, the commonest cause of stomatitis.

Causes

1. **Diffuse inflammation**
   - A fiery red tongue is usually due to '*B-complex deficiency*'.
   - A white depapillated and smooth tongue is usually due to '*iron deficiency*'.
   - White exudates which can be easily removed are due to '*oral candidiasis*' (thrush) associated with HIV/AIDS or diabetes.
   - White patches which cannot be removed, are '*leucoplakia*', which is a premalignant condition.
   - A white palate associated with difficulty in opening the mouth is '*submucous fibrosis*' caused by Manikchand or beetle-nut chewing.
2. **Recurrent stomal ulcers**
   Recurrent stomal ulcers which come and go spontaneously for no reason at all are virtually always due to *aphthous stomatitis*. Lay people in India usually associate the relapse due to 'heat' produced by non-vegetarian food or alcohol.
3. **Non-recurrent ulcers**
   Non-recurrent ulcers can be due to:
   - Infections such as herpangina, syphilis, etc.
   - Traumatic ulcer due to sharp tooth.
   - Chemical burns with aspirin used locally to stop toothache.
   - Skin diseases like lichen planus, pemphigus and drug reaction.
   - Finally, carcinoma of tongue or cheek, which should never be missed.

Treatment of Aphthous Ulcers

1. Avoid spicy food, hot drinks and tobacco chewing.
2. ***Local application***: Glycerine borax (or Gelora cream) three times a day for its soothing effect.
   Or
   Tantum liquid or Betadine oral wash should be used to rinse mouth.
   Or
   2% xylocaine if applied before food will facilitate eating without pain.
   Or
   Triamcinolone oral paste (Kenacort) if applied without rubbing will reduce inflammation and give good symptomatic relief.
   Or
   Beclomethasone (Beclate) inhaler used by asthmatics can be used to spray the ulcers with good effect.
3. Traditionally, B-complex orally is used by one and all without scientific basis. Aphthous ulcers heal spontaneously within a week. (With B-complex "treatment", they heal within 7 days!) Recurrences are common and unpredictable.

Treatment of other causes of stomatitis

- Red magenta tongue → High doses of B-complex
- White depapillated tongue → Oral iron preparations

- Oral thrush → Clotrimazole (Candid) oral paint tds and Fluconazole (Zocon) 150 mg single dose stat
- Submucous fibrosis → No simple effective treatment available Refer to ENT specialist
- Non-recurrent ulcers → Treatment of the cause

Any ulcer which is single, large, hard to feel and nontender should be thought of being malignant and biopsied without delay.

HICCOUGHS (Hiccups)

Hiccups are due to involuntary spasms of the inspiratory muscles followed by abrupt closure of the glottis. They are usually precipitated by irritation of the diaphragm usually caused by distension of the stomach.

For Simple Brief Episodes

Advice

- Valsalva manoeuvre.
- Breathing in and out in a plastic bag.
- Breath holding for as long as possible.
- Pressure on the eyeballs.
- Drink ice cold water.

Prescribe

- Antacid gel with xylocaine (e.g., mucaine) 2 tsf tds.
- Antispasmodic tablet (Cyclopam or Spasmoproxyvon) stat and repeat after 2 hrs sos.
- Tab. Chlorpromazine (Largactil) 50 mg stat. Repeat after 6 hrs sos.
- Tab. Metoclorpramide (Reglan) 10 mg tds
- Tab. Baclofen (Leofen, Lioresal) 25 mg bd, muscle relaxant.

If Persistent

Pass a nasogastric tube in the stomach. This relieves distension and also prevents abrupt closure of the glottis.

If still Persistent

Advise

a) X-ray chest → For pleurisy or mediastinal mass
b) Blood urea and S. creatinine → For uraemia
c) USG abdomen → For sub-diaphragmatic abscess
d) Gastroscopy → For gastritis or ulcer

ACUTE CONSTIPATION

If this is due to Pain at the Anus

The cause is either a perianal abscess or fissure in ano.

- *For perianal abscess*, incision and drainage has to be done urgently. This can be done by the GP in his clinic (please see chapter on minor surgery) or referred to a surgeon.
- *For fissure in ano*:
  - Xylocaine ointment locally.
  - Amoxicillin (Mox) 500 tds.
  - Metronidazole (Metrogyl) 400 tds.
  - Diclofenac (Voveran) 100 bd.
  - Liquid paraffin (Cremaffin or Agarol) 3 tsf hs.
  - **If no response, refer to a surgeon.**

If not Associated with Pain at the Anus (Idiopathic Functional Constipation)

- Tab. Bisacodyl (Dulcolax) 3 hs **(or)**
- Soap water enema **(or)**
- Neotonic enema **(or)**
- Castor oil 15–20 mL in morning.
- In elderly patients, manual removal of hard faecal masses with gloved fingers.

If associated with severe pain in abdomen and vomiting

The cause could be intestinal obstruction (hyperperistalsis) or paralytic ileus (no peristalsis) or a case of acute abdomen. Admit immediately.

CHRONIC CONSTIPATION (HABITUAL CONSTIPATION)

Advice

1. At least 8–10 glasses of water per day.
2. High roughage diet, plenty of green vegetables, green salads, bananas, potato and fresh fruits with skin left on whenever possible.
3. Regular exercises, including abdominal muscles exercises.
4. Establish regular bowel habit. Avoid suppressing natural reflex.
5. Avoid drugs like iron or antacids which can cause constipation.
6. Use drugs as a last resort to achieve regularity.
   a) First try Isabgol (Naturolax, Isogel or Softovac) two spoons in a glass of water to be taken freshly prepared.
   b) If constipation is not relieved, try stronger preparations like bisacodyl (Dulcolax), cremaffin or castor oil.
   c) If still not relieved, use Dulcolax or glycerin suppository or neotonic enema.

Remember

In an elderly individual with alternate constipation and diarrhoea or with constipation associated with PR bleeding, refer the patient to a surgeon to r/o rectal or colonic cancer.

ACUTE DIARRHOEA

1. *Advice regarding oral intake*: Initially only fluids for 24 hrs. Plenty of water, butter milk, black tea, coconut water, fruit juices, etc. Once the frequency of loose motions has decreased, allow over-ripe bananas, curd, soft rice, dal, ganji, etc. Avoid milk and its products initially because of secondary lactate deficiency.
2. Cap. Loperamide (Imosec) 2 caps stat. Then, 1 cap after each loose motion till they stop. Do not exceed 8 caps in a day. Avoid in children below 4 years.
3. If associated with abdominal pain, give cap Spasmoproxyvon or Tab. Cyclopam 1 tds.
4. If vomiting is present, give Inj. Metoclopramide 2 mL IM stat. Watch for extra-pyramidal reaction. Do not use metoclopramide and loperamide together. Instead, codeine 30 mg tds can be used.
5. If fever, it is infective diarrhoea. Use one of the following antibiotics:
   a) Ciprofloxacin (Ciplox) 500 mg bd, **or** Norfloxacin (Norflox) 400 mg bd, **or** Nalidixic acid (Gramoneg) 500 mg tds.
   b) Metronidazole (Flagyl) 400 mg tds or Tinidazole (Tini) 500 mg bd.
6. If you suspect it is drug-induced diarrhoea, stop the drug. Commonly used drugs which cause diarrhoea are antibiotics like amoxicillin, iron preparations, magnesium containing antacids, etc.

If there is hypotension or dehydration

Shift the patient to a hospital or if this is not immediately feasible, tide over the crisis by the following measures:

- Start a fast IV drip using Ringer lactate and DNS.
- Inj. Mephentin 1–2 mL iv stat.

- Inj. Efcorlin 100–200 mg iv stat.
- Inj. Gentamicin 80 mg iv stat.

Then shift the patient to a hospital for further management, as this could be a septicaemic shock.

CHRONIC DIARRHOEA

Causes

Causes are many. A few important ones are: ulcerative colitis, opportunistic infections associated with HIV/AIDS, chronic pancreatitis, sprue, laxative abuse, lactase deficiency, hyperthyroidism, diabetes, irritable bowel syndrome (IBS), drugs and intestinal TB.

Empirical Treatment

- Avoid fatty foods, raw vegetables, uncooked meat.
- Cap. Loperamide (Imosec) tds.
- Tab. Metronidazole (Metrogyl) 400 mg tds.
- Tab. Albendazole (Zentel) 400 mg single dose.
- Tab. TMP-SMX (Ciplin DS) tds × 7 days, for HIV associated diarrhoea.
- Cap. Doxycycline (Doxy 1) 100 mg bd × 10 days, for sprue.
- Cap. Neutrolin B tds × 1 week.
- Tab. Alprazolam 0.25 mg bd, if IBS is suspected.
- Tab. Folic acid (Folvite) 5 mg bd × 10 days.

If there is no response to the above measures, refer to a gastroenterologist for an extensive work up.

Do not go on treating chronic diarrhoea empirically, if the patient clinically worsens with anorexia, loss of weight, low grade fever, malaise, etc. In such cases, intestinal TB is a distinct possibility and is emminently treatable.

VOMITING

- For *symptomatic treatment* of vomiting in an adult, give Inj. Metoclopramide (Reglan, Perinorm) 10 mg stat, if severe. If mild, give Tab. Reglan 10 mg tds or Tab. Domperidone (Domstal) tds; Cap. Omeprazole (Omez) 20 mg stat can be added empirically.
- For *hyperemesis gravidarum* (vomiting in pregnancy) give Tab. Doxylamine succinate (Doxynate) 2 hs × 2–3 weeks or Tab. Meclizine HCl (Pregnidoxin) 12.5 mg tds or 2 tds till asymptomatic.
- For *severe vomiting with dehydration*, give Inj. Ondansetron 4 mg IM stat and correct the dehydration by giving IV DNS and Ringer lactate.

Most important: Find out the cause and treat (see Chapter 22).

DYSPHAGIA

1. *Dysphagia* means difficulty in swallowing. *Odynophagia* means painful swallowing. These terms usually refer to problems in the oesophagus. But in general practice, these subtle differences should be laid aside because the cause of difficult or painful swallowing is more commonly seen in the pharynx, e.g., acute severe pharyngitis, exudative tonsillitis or peritonsillar abscess (quinsy). We will call this '*pseudodysphagia*'.
   a) Inj. Procaine penicillin 8 lakhs IM od × 7 days AST (**or**)
      Tab. Roxithromycin (Roxibid) 150 mg bd on empty stomach (**or**)
      Tab. Azithromycin (Azithral) 500 mg od × 3 days.

b) Gargle with betadine oral solution. Simply putting 2–3 granules of potassium permanganate in warm water and using this solution for gargling is equally effective.
c) Pain-killers like aspirin or diclofenac.

2. If the throat is clear, it is '*true dysphagia*'. The most common cause is oesophagitis.
   a) Bland, semisolid diet.
   b) Antacid gel preferably with a local anaesthetic (Mucaine gel) 3 tsf – 3 hourly.
   c) Cap. Omeprazole (Omez) 20 mg bd.
   d) Tab. Cisapride (Ciza) 10 mg tds to treat reflux oesophagitis.
   e) Tab. Fluconazole (Forcan) 150 mg × 10 days in HIV +ve patients.
3. '*Mechanical dysphagia*': If the patient gives a history that there is obstruction to the passage of solid food in the chest, this is mostly a cancer of the oesophagus unless proved otherwise. Refer immediately.

LOCALISED PAIN IN ABDOMEN

In general practice, pain in abdomen is commonly seen in three quadrants out of the standard nine quadrants described in textbooks.

Epigastric Pain

The common causes are gastritis (drug induced or alcohol induced), gastric ulcer, duodenal ulcer, enlarged left lobe of liver, hook worm and amoebiasis affecting the transverse colon. Pancreatitis or gastric malignancies are rarely seen in general practice.

a) Cap. Omeprazole (Omez) 20 mg bd.
b) Tab. Cyclopam or Spasmoproxyvon tds.
c) Antacid gel (e.g., Gelusil) 2 tds qid.
d) Metronidazole (Flagyl) 400 mg tds, if associated with altered bowel movements.
e) Tab. Albendazole (Zentel) 400 mg stat.

If no response, investigate:

a) USG abdomen → for hepatitis, CCF and amoebic liver abscess.
b) Gastroscopy → for DU, GU, gastric malignancy.
c) Stool examination → for worms, occult blood.

Pain in Right Hypochondrium

The common diseases causing pain in this region are infective hepatitis, amoebic hepatitis, alcoholic hepatitis, tender liver because of CCF, duodenal ulcer and cholecystitis. The diagnosis can be suspected by the associated symptoms and signs:

a) Yellow sclera and high coloured urine is s/o infective hepatitis.
b) H/o alcohol abuse is s/o alcoholic hepatitis.
c) H/o recurrent amoebic dysentery is s/o amoebic liver abscess.
d) Signs of right ventricular failure, i.e., hepatomegaly, oedema over legs, engorged neck veins are s/o CCF.
e) Palpable gallbladder is s/o cholecystitis.

The diagnosis can be confirmed by:

a) USG abdomen
b) Liver function tests
c) ECG/2D-Echo

The treatment has to be individualized.

Pain in Right Iliac Fossa

The common causes are amoebic colitis, acute appendicitis and right ureteric colic. *Amoebic colitis* is usually associated with mucus in stools. *Acute appendicitis* is usually associated with vomiting, fever and severe tenderness in right iliac fossa (Mc Burney's point). *Ureteric colic* is usually associated with dysuria, there is no tenderness and the pain is colicky.

Initially, treat all the three possibilities:

a) Inj. Voveran or inj. Cyclopam 2 mL IM

b) Tab. Ciprofloxacin 500 mg bd or IV Ciprofloxacin, if vomiting is very severe.
c) Tab. Metronidazole 400 mg tds.
d) Inj. Gentamicin 80 mg bd IV

If there is no response within 48 hrs, then investigate:

1. USG abdomen → for ureteric stone. It is difficult to diagnose appendicitis on USG.
2. WBC count → more than 11,000 is s/o appendicitis.
3. Urine examination → RBC in urine is s/o calculi.
4. Stool examination → *E. histolytica* in stools is s/o amoebic colitis.

COLICKY PAIN IN ABDOMEN

Six types of colics are commonly seen. A colic is a pain in abdomen, which comes suddenly, increases in severity and stops suddenly only to come back again. Renal and biliary colics are not true colics in the real sense, because the pain is by and large constant.

Renal Colic

Renal colic is usually caused by stone in the pelvis of the kidney. There is a pain in the right or left renal angle. It may be associated with vomiting.

a) Inj. Voveran 2 mL IM stat.
b) Inj. Reglan 2 mL IM stat, if vomiting.
c) Tab. Cyclopam 1 tds.
d) IV fluids, if vomiting is severe.
e) Advise urine examination for the presence of RBCs.
f) Advise USG abdomen for the presence of kidney stone.

If the stone is found and is large, refer to a urologist.

Ureteric Colic

Severe spasmodic pain on one side of abdomen, coming suddenly and travelling from loin to groin, i.e., from the back to the front. The pain is so severe that the patient refuses to lie down. There is no tenderness, and dysuria may be present.

a) Inj. Pentazocin (Fortwin) 1 mL IM stat, if available (or)
b) Inj. Declofenac (Dynapar) im stat
c) Inj. Phenargan IM stat as a sedative and also to treat associated vomiting. Make the patient lie down and rest after the injections.
d) Tamsulosin 0.4 mg bd (alpha blocker) od to accelerate stone passage.
e) Send for USG abdomen. This may locate the calculus and exclude other causes of pain.
f) Plain X-ray abdomen on empty stomach after bowel preparation with three Dulcolax and three Gasex tablets on the night before, may confirm the calculus. If the stone is less than 6 mm in size, try '*hydrotherapy*'. Give IV 5% dextrose 3 pints fast using a 20 no. needle, to be completed in 1½ hrs. Give IV Lasix and IV Cyclopam in the third pint. Repeat this procedure daily for 3 days. Again repeat USG abdomen to see, if the stone has passed. If it has not, refer to a urologist for further treatment. If the stone is more than 6 mm, do not give hydrotherapy. Such stones cause partial obstruction and this procedure may cause hydronephrosis. Refer to a urologist for lithotripsy.

Small Intestinal Colic

Severe colicky pain in central abdomen commonly caused by amoebiasis, worms or intestinal obstruction.

a) First, r/o intestinal obstruction. There is severe central abdominal pain with colic occurring every 3–10 min lasting for a minute or so. It is associated with vomiting, distension and absolute constipation. If so, admit immediately.

b) If not s/o obstruction,
- Tab. Flagyl 400 mg tds.
- Tab. Zentel 400 mg stat.
- Inj. Cyclopam 2 mL IM stat.

Large Intestinal Colic

Severe colic away from the centre of the abdomen usually on the left or right side. It may or may not be associated with dysentery caused by *E. histolytica*, *Shigella* or *E. coli*.

a) Inj. Cyclopam 2 mL IM stat.
b) Tab. Norfloxacin (Norflox) 400 mg bd.
c) Tab. Metronidazole (Flagyl) 400 mg tds.

Biliary Colic

Acute onset pain in right hypochondrium, which may or may not be associated with jaundice. It is usually caused by stone in the gallbladder or infection of the gallbladder (cholecystitis).

a) Inj. Cyclopam as above.
b) Inj. Amoxicillin (Mox) 500 mg IV stat followed by oral amoxicillin 500 mg tds.
c) Tab. Flagyl as above.
d) Investigate: Urine examination, USG abdomen and S. bilirubin.
e) Admit, if diagnosis confirmed.

Spasmodic Dysmenorrhoea

Severe lower abdominal pain, especially in young unmarried girls on the first or second day of menses.

a) Tab. Mefenamic acid (Meftal spas) 500 mg tds.
b) Inj. Voveran 2 mL IM stat, if pain is severe.
c) Hot fomentation of lower abdomen.
d) Bed rest for 2 days.

IRRITABLE BOWEL SYNDROME (IBS)

The patient usually presents to his family doctor with vague abdominal complaints which have been going on for many years. He has visited many doctors in the past, done many investigations, all of which have been normal. IBS is a clinical diagnosis and a diagnosis of exclusion. It is associated with mental stress and depression. Explain the nature of the illness to the patient and reassure that it is not a serious condition.

Rome criteria for diagnosis of IBS

Symptoms of at least 3 months duration:

1) Abdominal pain or discomfort which is:
   - Relieved with defaecation.
   - Associated with change in frequency of stools.
   - Associated with change in consistency of stools.

   AND

2) Two or more of the following:
   - Altered stool frequency
   - Altered stool form
   - Altered stool passage
   - Passage of mucus
   - Bloating

Treatment

1. If stools are hard and constipation is present:
   a) High fibre diet.
   b) Isogel or Softovac 1 tsf bd along with plenty of water.
2. If the patient has to go to the toilet more than 4–5 times a day and has soft stools:
   a) Cap. Loperamide (Imosec) bd (**or**)
   b) Tab. Dephenoxylate (Lomotil) 2.5 mg bd.
3. If there is a pain in abdomen and fullness:
   a) Tab. Merbeverin (Colospa) 100 mg tds.
   b) Tab. Dicyclomine (Cyclopam) bd.

c) Tab. Drotaverine (Dotavine) 40 mg, 80 mg tds (**or**)

d) Tab. Propanthaline (Peplevor Spastheline) 15 mg tds.

Finally, whatever the abdominal symptoms, add an antidepressant whether symptoms of depression are present or not:

1. Cap. Fluoxetine (Fludac) 20 mg od (**or**)
2. Tab. Imipramine (Depsonil) 25 mg tds.

JAUNDICE

The patient usually presents to a general practitioner with anorexia, low grade fever, weakness and high coloured urine. O/e the liver may or may not be palpable or tender. Sclera is yellow. Under the circumstances, advise urine examination (for bile salts and bile pigments) and serum bilirubin. If bile salts and pigments are present and S. bilirubin is raised, your diagnosis is confirmed. Further work up is done by requesting Australia antigen (for hepatitis B) and S. alkaline phosphatase (for obstructive jaundice). Both these types of jaundice are better dealt with by a gastroenterologist. Having ruled out both these conditions, your diagnosis is viral hepatitis A, which is treated as follows:

- Bed rest is essential initially when S. bilirubin is high. Advise gradual return to work.
- Diet: High carbohydrate and adequate proteins are advocated. Usually a fat free diet is prescribed. This is not necessary. Advise good normal healthy food. Glucon-D powder can be given additionally.
- In case of fever, Low dose Paracetamol (Crocin) 250–500 mg. High dose paracetamol can increase liver damage.
- In case of severe vomiting, IV 10% dextrose with Inj. Reglan daily till vomiting stops. IV 25% Dextrose can be given in addition.
- Tab. Silymarin (Silybon) 140 mg bd or Cap. Phospholipids (Essentiate) 175 mg cap 1 tds is prescribed to help in regeneration of the damaged liver cells.
- Ayurvedic brands such as Tab. Liv 52, 2 tds or Arogyavardhini 2 tsf tds are very popular and can be given empirically.
- Steroids prescribed commonly to 'white wash' the jaundice should be avoided as it leads to chronicity.

While treating jaundice always keep a watch on:

1. **Deepening of jaundice**: Repeat S. bilirubin after every 3–4 days. If it goes on increasing, it could be obstructive jaundice. This can be confirmed by repeating S. alkaline phosphatase and by USG abdomen. Refer.
2. **Sensorium of the patient**: If the patient starts becoming drowsy and the sensorium is disturbed, admit immediately as this could be hepatic precoma.

DUODENAL ULCER

The patient presents to a general practitioner with epigastric pain of some duration and some severity. Treatment with antacids and ranitidine is usually done. When the patient fails to respond, a gastroduodenoscopy is advised and a diagnosis of duodenal ulcer is made. Now what is to be done?

1. Advise *strict dietary discipline*. Bland diet. Frequent small feeds. Limit hot tea and hot coffee. Strictly no smoking, no alcohol, no NSAIDs orally.
2. Advise easy going *lifestyle* at work. Avoid mental and physical stress, late nights, etc.
3. Prescribe enthusiastic *drug treatment*.
   a) Gelusil liquid 2 tsf 2 hourly.
   b) Eradicate *H. pylori* by using one of the many '*H. pylori* kits'. Various combinations are available. A popular combination is Omeprazole + Amoxicillin + Tinidazole (Helibact) bd × 1 week.

c) Follow this with Cap. Omeprazole 20 mg bd × 2 months or any other drug given in the box.
d) Tab. Buscopan 10 mg sos when pain is severe.

Repeat gastroduodenoscopy after 2 months. See if the ulcer has healed, which is usually the case. If so, give maintenance therapy with Cap. Omeprazole or Pantoprazole for 6 more months. If not, refer to a surgeon.

Drugs which reduce the gastric acid secretions

1. Ranitidine (Zinetac) 150 mg bd.
2. Famotidine (Famocid) 20 mg bd.
3. Roxatidine (Rotane) 75 mg bd.
4. Omeprazole (Omez) 20 mg od or bd.
5. Lansoprazole (Lan) 30 mg od.
6. Pantoprazole (Pantacid) 40 mg od.
7. Rabiprazole (Rabifast) 20 mg od.

PEPTIC ULCER

Presence of an ulcer either in the stomach and duodenum. Gastric ulcer pain increases with food intake. Therefore, patients have loss of weight. Duodenal ulcer pain decreases with food intake. Therefore, patients put on weight. If not treated, life-threatening haematemesis or perforation can occur. In 75% of patients the ulcer is due to *H. pylori* infection. Another important cause is analgesic abuse.

Treatment

1. Stop smoking completely.
2. Nimesulide, Paracetamol, Ibuprofen cause less gastric irritation and should be used when analgesic is required.
3. *H. pylori* kit—daily one kit × 7 days. A single kit contains:
   a) Omeprazole 20 mg + Amoxicillin 750 mg + Tinidazole 500 mg (Helibact) **(Or)**
   b) Lansoprazole 30 mg + Clarithromycin 250 mg + Tinidazole 500 mg (Pylokit) 1 kit daily, 7 days, in 2 divided doses.
4. Report immediately if haematemesis, melaena, severe pain in abdomen.
5. Cap. Omeprazole (Omez) 20 mg bd (**Or**) Tab Pantoprazole (Pantocid) 40 mg bd × 6 weeks.
6. Repeat endoscopy after 6 weeks.

GERD

Heartburn, water-brash, retrosternal discomfort experienced after meals. This is because of regurgitation of gastric contents into the oesophagus through an incompetent gastro-oesophageal os. Rarely, GERD is implicated in chronic cough, laryngitis or recurrent lower respiratory tract in children, thought to be because of reflux of gastric acids into these areas.

Treatment

1. Reduction of weight, avoid fatty foods, alcohol, excessive tea/coffee, etc.
2. Stop smoking completely.
3. Antacid gel (Gelusil MPS) 3 tsf QID before meals.
4. Tab Domperidone (Domstal) 10 mg tds **or** Tab Mosapride (Moza) 5 mg tds.
5. Cap Omeprazole (Omez) 20 mg bd **or** Tab Pantoprazole 40 mg bd before meals × 15 days.

If inadequate response, do endoscopy. If endoscopy shows severe ulceration of lower end of oesophagus—repeat above course for 3 months. If it reveals a peptic ulcer, treat as given above.

GP Tip

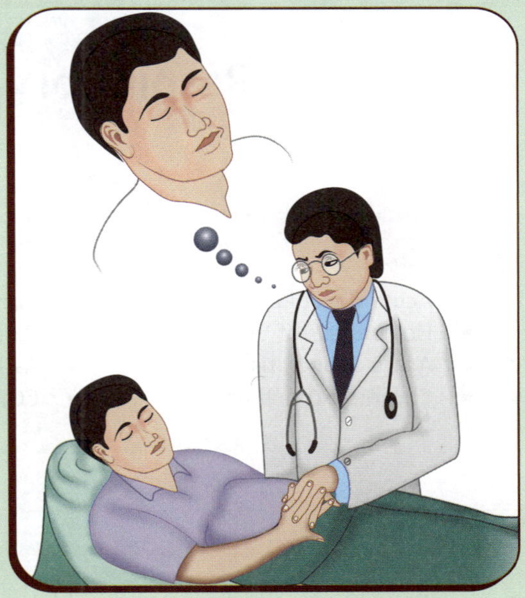

Problem: A ticklish, giggly patient won't let you examine his belly.

Solution: Give a broad smile, ask the patient to place *his* hand on his abdomen, place *your* fingers in between the patient's fingers and then examine!

This chapter has been reviewed by ***Dr Atchut Joshi****, MD, Consultant Physician, Pune.*

CHAPTER 2

Respiratory Conditions

- Acute Chest Pain
- Hoarseness of Voice
- Acute Bronchitis
- Chronic Bronchitis
- Pneumonia
- Pulmonary Tuberculosis
- Asthma
- COPD

ACUTE CHEST PAIN

Chest pain of recent onset is a symptom, which alarms the patient (as well as the doctor attending on him). The patient equates all chest pain with "heart attack" and death. Probably, he is justified and the first job of the attending physician is to know whether it is a cardiac chest pain or a non-cardiac chest pain. This can be largely achieved by taking an ECG. Hence, every GP should possess an ECG machine or at least have an access to one at short notice.

> The typical chest pain of cardiac origin is retrosternal. The patient often uses the clenched fist to demonstrate the type of pain.
>
> Chest pain = Cardiac pain, unless proved otherwise.

Please refer to topic on "Myocardial infarction" in Chapter 22.

Having ascertained that the chest pain is not of cardiac origin, the chest pain can originate from four other sources.

Respiratory

Three causes are commonly seen in general practice, viz., pleurisy, lobar pneumonia and acute tracheitis. In *pleurisy*, pain increases with inspiration, there is a pleural rub and air entry is decreased if there is an effusion. In *pneumonia*, there is high grade fever, severe unilateral chest pain and cough. In acute *tracheitis*, there is mild central chest pain with associated respiratory symptoms and fever. One more type of chest pain not commonly encountered in general practice but has disastrous consequences if missed is spontaneous *pneumothorax*. Here, we get acute chest pain with severe dyspnoea in a known asthmatic. Admit immediately.

Oesophageal-Gastric

Pain during deglutition is due to *oesophagitis*. Spasm of the lower end of the oesophagus can give rise to retrosternal chest pain radiating upwards towards the jaw. Occasionally, *upper abdominal diseases* like cholecystitis, pancreatitis or gastric ulcer can cause retrosternal chest pain and dilemma!

Chest wall

Costochondritis of the second, third or fourth costochondral junction is a common cause of chest pain (Tietz's disease). Elicit by *light* pressure on these sites. Pain due to *fracture ribs* is quite obvious because of h/o trauma. Similarly, *postherpetic neuralgia* can be diagnosed by h/o herpes zoster. Preherpetic neuralgia, i.e., pain in chest preceding the eruption of herpes zoster is virtually impossible to diagnose. Cardiologist diagnoses it as angina and orthopaedic surgeons diagnose it as fibromyalgia, only to get a surprise when the vesicular eruption is seen! Do not make a diagnosis of "*myalgia chest*" just because you do not have any other diagnosis. Do not be misled by h/o lifting weights. Lifting of weights should give rise to pain in biceps and not chest pain. *Cervical spondylosis* commonly leads to pain radiating to the arm but only occasionally to chest pain. Remember the golden rule: *If in doubt, do an ECG.*

Functional

Diagnose with confidence when patient gives a h/o recurrent chest pain with multiple ECGs, which have always been normal. Acute chest pain following severe mental stress should be diagnosed as angina, unless proved otherwise. For treatment, refer to the relevant chapters.

HOARSENESS OF VOICE

Causes of hoarseness may range from innocent acute infective laryngitis to traumatic laryngitis because of misuse and overuse of voice, to malignancy. Hence, if hoarseness persists for more than 2 weeks despite conservative treatment given below, always refer to an ENT specialist for laryngoscopy.

Treatment

- The patient should restrict speaking to the minimum and preferably communicate with a notebook and a pen. Whispering is more traumatic to the vocal cords than normal speaking and should not be done.
- Steam inhalation is very soothing and also loosens the sticky secretions on the vocal cords.
- Tincture Benzoin or Vicks may be added to boiling water for better effect.
- Tab. Roxithromycin (Roxid) 150 mg bd on empty stomach × 7 days.
- Smoking should be stopped.
- Tab. Betamethasone (Betnelan) tds × 7 days is very useful to reduce the inflammation.

> If after the above treatment the voice still remains hoarse, the patient should be referred for laryngoscopy. In an old man, where there is no evidence of upper respiratory tract infection, no h/o overuse of voice, the patient should be directly referred before giving any treatment.

ACUTE BRONCHITIS

The patient presents with fever, cough with expectoration and retrosternal chest pain. O/e there are few rhonchi and crepitations, which are bilateral.

Treatment

- Bed rest, cessation of smoking.
- Steam inhalation with tinc. Benzoin or Vicks.
- Benadryl expectorant 2 tsf tds.
- Tab. Bromhexine 8 mg tds × 7 days.
- Antipyretics for fever and pain.

- Cap. Amoxicillin (Novamox) 500 tds × 7 days is usually given, though most cases are of viral origin.
- Bronchodilators, e.g., Tab. Deriphylline, only if the patient complains of dyspnoea.

CHRONIC BRONCHITIS

Any patient who has cough with expectoration of long duration (at least 2 years) and on auscultation has wide-spread rhonchi, basal crepitations and prolonged expiration is diagnosed clinically as having chronic bronchitis. Fever is usually absent except during an exacerbation. Usually the patient has already taken an X-ray chest which has shown prominent bronchovascular markings.

If the patient comes in acute exacerbation

- Steam inhalation with tinc. Benzoin or Vicks, three times a day.
- Tab. Bromhexine 8 mg tds × 1 week.
- If there is dyspnoea, Tab. Salbutamol (Asthalin) 2–4 mg tds × 1 week (**or**) Tab. Terbutaline (Bricanyl) 2.5 mg tds × 1 week.
- Cap. Amoxicillin 500 tds × 7 days. If the patient does not respond (which is many times the case as the patient has already taken many antibiotics many times) try alternative antibiotics.
  - Cap. Cephelexin (Phexin) 500 mg qid (**or**)
  - Tab. Cefuroxime (Ceftum) 250 mg bd (**or**)
  - Tab. Azithromycin (Azithral) 500 mg od.
- Tab. Prednisolone 10 mg tds, if bronchospasm is persistent.

Once the acute episode is over

- Avoid possible irritants and allergens in the atmosphere.
- No smoking. Reducing smoking by a few cigarettes is useless.
- Tab. Doxycycline (Doxy-1) 100 mg 1 daily from first to the fifth of every month.
- Educated patients can be given 15 caps of amoxicillin 500 mg to be used whenever the sputum becomes purulent or yellow.

PNEUMONIA

The patient presents to the general practitioner with high grade fever and chills, cough with expectoration, unilateral chest pain and looking toxic. On auscultation, there may be localized crepitations, bronchial breathing or the chest may be clear. Request for an X-ray chest. If the X-ray shows pneumonia:

First decide, if hospitalization is required.

Treatment

Admit, if

- Age is over 60 years.
- There is co-existing illness like diabetes.
- High fever, dehydrated, looking toxic, etc.
- X-ray shows involvement of more than one lobe.
- Patient refuses/unable to take oral treatment.

If the above features are not present, give:

- Tab. Azithromycin (Azithral) 500 mg od. for 3–5 days
- Tab. Gatifloxacin (Gatiquin) 400 od × 1 week.
- Benadryl cough expectorant 2 tsf tds.
- Tab. Brufen + Paracetamol (Combiflam) tds.

Note: Azithromycin covers most of the pathogens causing community acquired pneumonia like *S. pneumoniae*, *H. influenzae* and *Mycoplasma*.

PULMONARY TUBERCULOSIS

An early diagnosis of pulmonary TB can be made, if the doctor has high index of suspicion for TB. Advise an X-ray chest under the following situations, even if there are no detectable clinical signs:

- Cough > 3 weeks, not responding to antibiotics.
- Cough with haemoptysis.
- Cough with chest pain.
- Prolonged cough in HIV+ve patients.
- F/H/O pulmonary tuberculosis.
- Fever not responding to antibiotics (FUO).
- Unexplained loss of weight.

If X-ray is doubtful, additional investigations will be required. Advise:

- WBC count: It is raised in pneumonitis and normal in TB.
- ESR is raised in TB.
- Sputum if +ve for AFB, is diagnostic. Consecutive 3 days sputum should be tested.
- Tuberculin test—if strongly +ve, gives additional evidence.

If the diagnosis still cannot be made, refer the patient to a chest physician because other sophisticated tests will be required, e.g., bronchoscopy, PCR test, sputum culture, etc.

If the diagnosis of pulmonary TB is confirmed—treat.

Treatment

It is useful to place the patient in one of the following categories suggested by WHO in 1993:

Category I	Sputum +ve new patients	HRZE × 2 mths + HR × 4 mths
Category II	Treatment failures or relapsed cases	SHRZE × 2 mths HRZE × 1 mth + HRE × 5 mths

Category I patients can be easily managed by a general practitioner with a basic knowledge of four antitubercular drugs. The dosage and the main side effects are given below. Category II patients are difficult to treat, failure rate is high and may require second line drugs, which are very costly. These patients are better managed by a chest physician.

The above drugs can be given independently or as is the recent trend, in a combination pack.

Examples

Category I → AKT-4 1 kit daily for 2 months. Then Cap. Rcinex 1 tab daily for 4 months.

Personally, I feel that DOTS (directly observed treatment with short course chemotherapy) where the patient is asked to take medicines in front of the health worker at weekly intervals and then weekly medicines supplied, is not convenient in general practice.

According to new Revised National Tuberculosis guidelines (RNTCP), due to

Drug	Daily dose		Side effects
	Child (mg/kg/day)	Adult (day)	
1. Isoniazid (H)	10–20	300 mg	Neuritis, rashes
2. Rifampicin (R)	10–15	450 mg	Hepatitis, rashes
3. Pyrazinamide (Z)	20–30	1.5 g	Arthralgia, hepatitis
4. Ethambutol (E)	15–25	800 mg	Optic neuritis
5. Streptomycin (S)	20–40	1 g	Ototoxicity, nephrotoxicity

increase in cases of MDR tuberculosis, geneXpert/CBNAAT test to detect resistance to Rifamycin and /or INH, has to be done before initiating treatment.

ASTHMA

Treatment of Acute, Severe Attack

Hospitalize the patient if:

1. Patient is too breathless to talk
2. Pulse > 120/min.
3. RR > 30 breaths/min.
4. Cyanosis present.

If not

Step 1

1. Nebulise with salbutamol (Asthalin) plus ipratropium bromide (Ipravent) solution.
2. Inj. hydrocortisone hemisuccinate (Efcorlin) 200 mg IV stat. If no response, then

Step II

1. Inj. Terbutaline (Bricanyl) 1 mL SC **or**
2. Inj. Aminophylline 250 mg diluted in 20 mL of 5% dextrose IV very slowly.
3. If still no response after 15–20 min, then

Step III

1. Inj. Adrenaline 0.5 mL SC (use in patients below 40 years).
2. If still no response—admit.

Maintenance Treatment

Depends on severity and frequency of attacks.

1. **Mild intermittent asthma**: Attacks occur <1 week and are mild:
   a) Salbutamol (Asthalin) 2 puffs stat and 2–3 times/day with inhaler or rotahaler, **or**
   b) Tab. Salbutamol (Asthalin) 4 mg bd, **or**
   c) Tab. Terbutaline (Bricanyl) 5 mg bd, **or**
   d) Tab. Theophylline (Deriphylin) tds, till attack stops.
2. **Mild persistent asthma**: Attacks occur more than 2 times a week but not daily.
   a) Beclomethasone diproprionate (Beclate) 500 mg bd to be inhaled with inhaler or rotahaler daily, to prevent attacks (or) budesonide (Budecort).
   b) Salbutamol (Asthalin) 2–3 puffs sos if attacks occur.
3. **Severe persistent asthma**: Patient gets attack almost daily.
   a) Beclomethasone (Beclate) 500 mg bd to be inhaled as above.
   b) Salmetrol (Serobid) to be inhaled bd daily.
   c) Salbutamol to be inhaled 2–3 puffs sos.
   d) Tab. Prednisolone 5 mg tds sos.

CHRONIC OBSTRUCTIVE PULMONARY DISEASE (COPD)

Treatment

- Tiova 9 µg inhaler (Tiotropium Bromide) 2 puffs od with zerostat VT spacer.
- Foracort 200 mg inhaler (Formeteral + Budesonide) 2 puffs bd with zerostat VT spacer.
- Cap. Abphylline 100 mg bd (Acebrophylline).
- Good chest physiotherapy under guidance of physiotherapist.
- High protein diet.

Pleural effusion—See Chapter 22.

Haemoptysis—See Chapter 22.

*This chapter has been reviewed by **Dr Himanshu Pophale**, MD, Chest Physician, Pune.*

CHAPTER 3

Cardiovascular Conditions

- Hypertension
- Palpitations
- Ischaemic Heart Disease
- Congestive Cardiac Failure

HYPERTENSION

For adults, hypertension is:
Diastolic pressure > 90 mm Hg
Systolic pressure > 140 mm Hg

- Isolated systolic hypertension is systolic pressure > 140 in the presence of normal diastolic pressure.
- Mild hypertension is diastolic pressure between 90 and 110, moderate between 110 and 130, severe is 130 and above.
- Essential hypertension is a term used when the cause is not known.

Management of Essential Hypertension

Mild Hypertension (Stage 1)

The plan should be to put the patient on '*non-drug therapy*'. Record the blood pressure every week for 1 month and if after this period the blood pressure has not come down, start a low-dose single-drug treatment.

- Increased walking exercises. "Stop smoking and start walking".
- Reduction in stress and change in lifestyle.
- Reduction in weight.
- Cessation of smoking, reduction of alcohol intake.
- Low salt diet. No extra salt in food. Use 'Losalt'.
- Low fat diet: Use polyunsaturated oil like sunflower oil. No deep fried foods.
- If blood pressure has not reduced in spite of the above measures, add Tab. Atenolol (Aten) 25 mg od or Tab. Amlodipine (Stamlo) 2.5 mg od.

Moderate Hypertension (Stage 2)

The plan should be to start with a single drug (monotherapy) and if the BP does not come down in 1 month, the dose of the drug is increased to the maximum or one more drug is added (combination therapy).

- Start with an ACE inhibitor, e.g., Tab. Enalapril (Enam) 5 mg od (**or**)
  - Tab. Telmisartan 40 or 80 mg od

  If the patient does not respond then add a calcium channel blocker, e.g.,
  - Tab. Amlodipine (Stamlo) 5 mg od (**Plus**)
  - A diuretic like Hydrochlorothiazide 12.5 mg od

  If the patient does not respond, add a beta-blocker like
  - Atenolol (Aten) 50 od.

Severe Hypertension (Stage 3)

If the patient has diastolic BP > 130 mm Hg and also has severe headache, vomiting, visual disturbances, convulsions, transient paralysis or coma, it is a case of "malignant hypertension". This is a life-threatening medical emergency. Admit immediately.

If the diastolic BP > 130 mm Hg but the patient does not have any of the above symptoms, it is a case of "*accelerated hypertension*". This is a "*hypertensive urgency*".

Treatment

- Absolute bed rest.
  - Tab. Labetalol 100–200 mg Stat and bd (acts within 2–4 min).
  - Tab. Amlodipine (Stamlo) 10 mg stat and repeat after 12 hrs.
  - Nefidepine sublingual stat now not advocated as hypotension can result.

If the diastolic BP does not come down below 110 mm Hg within 24 hrs, refer to a physician.

PALPITATIONS

Palpitation is awareness of the beating of one's own heart. A normal person experiences this during exercise. Otherwise, it can be caused by:

1. Acute anxiety and cardiac neurosis (panic attack).
2. Cardiac causes like paroxysmal ventricular tachycardia or extrasystoles.
3. Noncardiac causes like hyperthyroidism or hypoglycaemia.

The most common cause of palpitation is anxiety state and cardiac neurosis where the patient comes to the clinic with severe palpitation and a fear of death. Anxiety causes palpitations and palpitations in turn lead to more anxiety.

- First, rule out a cardiac cause. This can be simply done by a proper history, presence of a regular pulse and by auscultating the heart.

If no abnormality is noted:

- Rule out hypoglycaemia. This is almost always seen in insulin dependent diabetics who have missed a meal.
- Hyperthyroidism can be ruled out clinically by absence of tachycardia.
- The diagnosis then is severe anxiety. Reassure the patient that he has no heart disease. But unless an ECG is taken the patient is unlikely to be satisfied.

Treatment

1. Tab. Lorazepam (Ativan) 1 mg stat and bd for 3–4 days.
2. Tab. Propranolol (Inderal) 10–40 mg tds is the drug of choice as it will control the somatic symptoms of anxiety and by virtue of its anti-arrhythmic action, control cardiac arrhythmias.

If the palpitations still persist, refer for:

- T_3, T_4, TSH, for hyperthyroidism.
- Holter monitor testing, for cardiac causes.

ISCHAEMIC HEART DISEASE

This is a group of heart diseases where the myocardium suddenly gets less than normal blood supply because of atherosclerosis, coronary artery spasm or coronary artery thrombosis. Depending on the degree of obstruction, a spectrum of IHD is seen.

Stable Angina Pectoris

There is transient ischaemia without necrosis of myocardium. Typically, a middle-aged person c/o sudden chest pain, which may radiate to left arm, neck or jaw. Pain is relieved by rest or by giving tablet of nitroglycerine.

During Attack

- Take ECG to r/o myocardial infarction.
- Tab. Isosorbide dinitrate (Sorbitrate) 5 mg **Or** Tab. Nitroglycerine (Angised) 0.5 mg given sublingually. The dose may be repeated sos but not more than 3 tabs in 15 min.

To Prevent Attack

- Tab. Isosorbide mononitrate (Ismo-20) 20 mg bd orally.
- Tab. Atenolol (Aten) 50 mg od OR Tab. Diltiazem (Dilgard) 30 mg tds, if beta-blocker is contraindicated.
- Tab. Aspirin (Colosprin) 150 mg od.
- Tab. Clopidogrel (Clopiget) 300 mg stat followed by 75 mg bd.
- Tab. Nicorandil (Nicoran) 5 mg tds, if attacks still continue.

Unstable Angina (Pre-infarction Syndrome)

Entity midway between stable angina and MI. Pain more severe, lasts longer, occurs at rest, not completely relieved by nitroglycerine.

Myocardial Infarction (MI)

There is necrosis of myocardium. For both unstable angina and MI:

- Take ECG to confirm diagnosis.

Even if ECG is normal, but clinically suspected:

- Call ambulance. In the meantime—
- Tab. Aspirin (Dispirin) 300 mg to be chewed stat.
- Tab. Nitroglycerine (Angised) 0.5 mg sublingually stat.
- Inj. Atropine 0.6 mg IV stat, if bradyca-rdia.
- Inj. Frusemide (Lasix) 40 mg IV stat, if patient has dyspnoea. When ambulance arrives—admit.

Follow up Treatment after Discharge

- Take drugs regularly.
- Stop smoking.
- Weight reduction if obese.
- Adequate rest, moderate exercise.
- Low fat diet.
- Advise angiography, if patient can afford.

CONGESTIVE CARDIAC FAILURE (CCF)

A general practitioner is occasionally called upon to manage a patient of CCF. He has been diagnosed and treated in a hospital and sent back home for domiciliary management. They are virtually bed-ridden and cannot visit the hospital frequently because of dyspnoea.

Management

- Rest in bed. Patient is allowed to sit on an arm chair near the bed. He can visit the toilet with help.
- Diet should be salt free. Fluid intake should be limited. Small feeds at a time.
- Tab. Digitalis 0.25 mg (Lanoxin) 1 daily for 6 days in a week (Sunday off).
- Tab. Lasix 40 mg od. Adjust the dose depending on the oedema.
- Liquid Kesol 1 tsf tds with a glass of water.
- Instead of Lasix-Kesol combination, Tab. Amifru or Tab. Lasilactone can be given when potassium supplement is not needed.
- Tab. Enalepril 2.5 mg.
- Tab. Metoprolol 25 mg od.
- In case of sudden increase in breathlessness, give Inj. Aminophylline, 10 mL diluted in 20 mL of 25% dextrose, slowly over a period of 5 min.
- Cap. Moxclav (Clavum) 625 mg tds, if respiratory tract infection, which is common.
- For severe failure, add Tab. Telmisartan 40 mg od or bd.

If no response, then hospitalize.

*This chapter has been reviewed by **Dr Parag Vaste**, MD, Consultant Physician, Pune.*

GP Tip

*Cannot hear the **Korotkoff's sounds** through your stethoscope? Here's a trick.*

Raise the pressure in the BP instrument cuff above 200 mm Hg. Ask the patient to alternately open and close the fist for 5–6 times. Now the sounds will be distinctly audible!

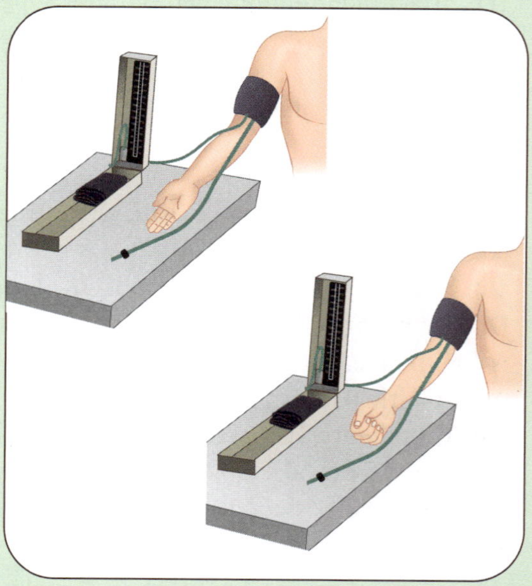

GP Tip

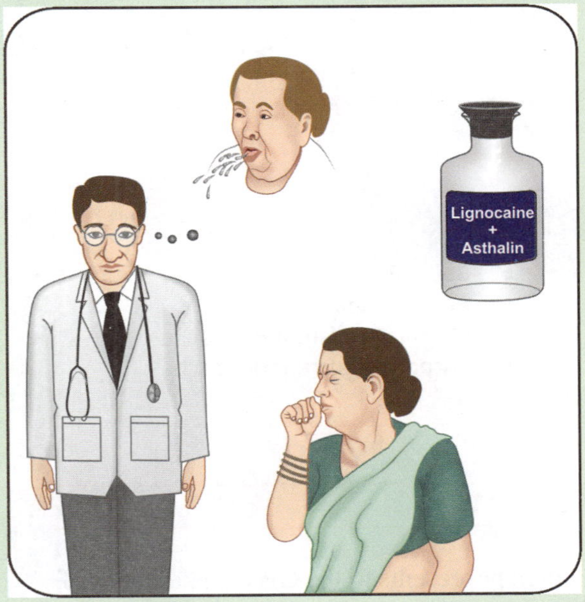

Intractable continuous cough*?*

Try this*: Mix 1 mL of Lignocaine with 1 mL of Salbutamol respiratory solution and nebulise the patient with this solution.*

CHAPTER 4

Central Nervous System

- Bell's Palsy
- Acute Headache
- Chronic Persistent Headache
- Chronic Recurrent Headache
- Hangover due to Alcohol
- Tremors
- Peripheral Neuropathy

BELL'S PALSY

The patient presents to the GP with paralysis of the whole one side of the face which has occurred suddenly during sleep. O/e the forehead cannot wrinkle on the affected side. The eye on the affected side also cannot be closed due to which tears roll down. The angle of the mouth is pulled towards the normal side while talking. Drinking and chewing is difficult. On closing the eyes, the eyeball rotates upwards.

Treatment

- Tab. Prednisolone (Wysolone) 1 mg/kg/day × 5 days, provided patient presents within 24 hrs of onset.
- Cap. Omeprazole (Omez) 20 mg od × 8 days.
- Inj. Neurobion IM, alternate days × 5.
- Moisol eye drops—2 drops qid.
- Dark glasses to protect the eyes.
- Massage of the affected side of the face with olive oil at least 3 times a day, or refer to a physiotherapist.

- Before starting treatment make sure that you are not dealing with other facial palsies, i.e., that may be caused by a cerebral tumour. Here, the forehead can be wrinkled on the affected side.
- About 80% of the patients recover spontaneously within 1 month; 10% within the next 6 months; the rest will have some residual damage. Refer them to a plastic surgeon.
- Prednisolone works only if started early.

ACUTE HEADACHE

This means that the headache is of a few hours to a few days in duration and is not recurrent. This presents to a GP in one of the following ways:

Headache as the only Symptom

Sometimes, it is difficult to ascertain the cause. Give symptomatic relief:

- Tab. Aspirin (Disprin) 300 mg tds.
- Inj. Diclofenac 3 mL IM stat, if no relief.

- Apply 'Amrutanjan' as a counter irritant.
- Rest in a dark quiet room.
- Observe for development of other associated symptoms, when specific treatment can be given.

Headaches as part of Other Infections

For example, URTI, viral fever or malaria.

- Give treatment as above.
- Treat specific infections.

Headaches which can cause Loss of Vision

Example, glaucoma (as diagnosed by red eye and firm hard eyeball) or temporal arteritis (severe unilateral temporal headache seen in elderly individuals). *Refer immediately.*

Headaches which can be Life-threatening

Though rare in general practice, all GPs should be aware of these two conditions:

- ***Meningitis*** **(*Brain fever*)**: There is severe headache with high-grade fever and vomiting. O/e neck stiffness is present.
- ***Subarachnoid haemorrhage*** **(*SAH*) (*Brain haemorrhage*)**: There is sudden onset splitting headache described as the worst headache in the life-time. Vomiting is present and fever is absent. Loss of consciousness usually follows. Neck stiffness is present. About 40% die before treatment can be given. *Hospitalize immediately.*

CHRONIC PERSISTENT HEADACHE

This means headache of a few days or a few months in duration without headache-free intervals in-between.

First, examine the patient for e/o raised intracranial tension or brain tumour. Here, there is vomiting, fever, disturbance of vision or paralysis—if so, refer for MRI scan.

Chronic persistent headache is usually due to one of these three causes mentioned below.

Sinus Headache

Usually unilateral, associated symptoms of URTI, tenderness over frontal and maxillary sinuses, maximum in the mornings.

- Steam inhalation with Vicks Vaporub, tinc. Benzoin.
- Cap. Amoxicillin (Mox) 500 mg tds (**Or**)
- Tab. Cefadroxil (Cefadur) 500 mg bd × 7 days.
- Analgesics.
- X-ray skull, if no response. If haziness is seen in the sinuses on the X-ray, refer to ENT specialist for draining the sinus.

Tension Headache (Muscular Contraction Headache)

Maximum over the vertex. Increases in the evenings.

- Advise regarding stress reduction (not easy).
- Reassure that headache is harmless.
- Mild analgesics like paracetamol, aspirin.
- Avoid tranquillizers and antidepressants, if possible.
- Tab. Amitriptyline (Tryptomer) 10 mg hs. But, if headache does not subside, increase dose till 75 mg daily × 3 months.

Eye Strain Headache

Headache is severe in the evenings and after straining the eyes as after reading, sewing, etc. Refer to an ophthalmologist.

CHRONIC RECURRENT HEADACHE (Migraine)

For all practical purposes, migraine is the only cause of recurrent headache seen in the general practice. There are two types of migrainous headaches. One is the uncommon but 'classical' variety where the patient gets an aura, followed by a throbbing unilateral headache, which is terminated by vomiting. The other type is common, called the "common migraine", where the patient does not get an aura and the headache is mild and generalised but recurrent. Hence, the patient does not approach the doctor unless the headache is severe, but goes on taking 'Disprin' or 'Crocin' from the market whenever required.

Treatment

1. ***When the attack is mild***:
   a) Tab. Paracetamol 500 mg + Metoclopramide (Paramet) 1–2 tds till the headache subsides.
   b) Rest in a quiet and dark room.
   c) 'Amrutanjan' should be rubbed on the forehead.
   d) Tab. Paracetamol + Ibuprofen (Ibugesic plus), if the pain does not stop in 2 hrs.
   e) Inj. Analgin 2 mL IM, sos.
2. ***When attack is severe***:
   a) Tab. Ergotamine (Migranil or Vasograin) 1 mg 2 tabs stat and 1 tab every 30 min till the attack stops. Maximum 6 tabs in a day (**or**) Tab. Sumatriptan (Suminat) 50 mg stat and repeated after 2 hrs till the headache subsides.
   b) Tab. Ibugesic plus can be used in addition.
   c) Give these medicines at the earliest.
   d) Rest in a quiet and dark room.
3. ***When the attacks are very frequent***:
   a) Tab. Propranolol (Ciplar) 40 mg tds × 3 months (**or**)
   Tab. Amytriptyline (Tryptomer) 10–25 mg hs × 3 months (**or**)
   Tab. Flunarizine (Sibelium) 10–20 mg od × 3 months.
   b) Try to avoid known precipitating factors.

Remember

- Most of the headaches seen during general practice can be diagnosed by a proper history alone.
- Most common cause of headache seen in GP is tension headache (which many doctors get during off season!)
- Always be on alert for dangerous headaches like meningitis or SAH.
- The common cause of headache is 'common migraine' seen commonly in general practice. 'Classical migraine' is seen commonly in textbooks!
- The longer the duration of the headaches, safer is the headache.
- Do not blame impacted molars, cervical spondylosis, constipation as a cause of the headache.
- Hypertension causes headaches only when diastolic pressure is >120 mm Hg.
- Small refractory error with cylindrical numbers usually is responsible for eye strain headache rather than large refractory errors. Myopia is never a cause of headache.

HANGOVER DUE TO ALCOHOL

A very common cause of headache experienced by the patient the next day after heavy alcohol consumption.

Prevention

- Drink alcohol on a full stomach.
- Do not exceed more than 2 standard pegs.
- Avoid drinking too fast.
- Be fastidious about the choice of drink.
- Avoid 'cocktails'.
- Take 2 tablets of 'Aspirin' before going to sleep.
- Avoid alcohol!

Treatment

- Alcohol causes dehydration. Take plenty of fluids.

- Take aspirin 600 mg or any other analgesic.
- Have a good full meal.
- *Home remedies*: Honey in lemon juice or black coffee with roasted toast.

TREMORS

The common types of tremors seen in regular practice and their treatment is given below:

1. **Alcohol withdrawal tremors**
   a) Tab. Chlordiazepoxide (Librium) 10 mg 2 tds
   b) Tab. Diazepam (Valium) 10 mg 1 hs × 5 days.
   c) Inj. Vit $B_1 + B_6 + B_{12}$ (Neurobion) 3 mL IM × 5 days
   d) Cap. Becosule 1 bd × 5 days.
2. **Salbutamol-induced tremors**
   Stop salbutamol, try theophylline or inhalation therapy for asthma.
3. **Stress-induced tremors**
   a) Tab. Propranolol (Inderal) 40 mg tds.
   b) Tab. Alprazolam (Restyl) 0.25 mg tds.
   c) Deal with the stress.
4. **Tremors due to hyperthyroidism**
   a) Suspect if tachycardia and other signs of the disease are present.
   b) Start Tab. Propranolol 40 mg tds and order for T_3, T_4, TSH.
   c) If confirmed, add Tab. Neomercazole 5 mg tds.
5. **Tremors due to parkinsonism**
   a) Tab. Syndopa (levodopa + carbidopa) tds.
   b) Tab. Pacitane 2 mg ½ bd.
6. **Senile tremors**
   No treatment available.

- Diagnosis of alcohol withdrawal and salbutamol-induced tremors is very obvious.
- Confusion can arise in diagnosis of stress and hyperthyroidism-tremors. When in doubt, do T_3, T_4, TSH.

- Parkinsons has a resting tremor, most marked when hands are supported on the lap. The others are action tremors, easily seen on outstretched arms.

PERIPHERAL NEUROPATHY (Tingling numbness)

Bilateral

If present in both arm and legs.

Causes

- Diabetes
- Alcohol abuse
- Vitamin deficiency
- Anaemia
- Renal failure
- HIV infection

Treatment

a) Tab. Multivitamin (Supradyn) bd.
b) Cap. Autrin bd.
c) Tab. Carbamazepine (Tegretol) 200 mg. Initially ½ bd × 5 days, then 1 tds × 5 days.
   (Or)
   Tab. Phenytoin (Dilantin) 100 mg tds.
d) Tab. Amitriptyline (Tryptomer) 25 mg hs.
e) Stop alcohol.

If no response within 10 days, advise:
a) BSL
b) Haemogram
c) S. creatinine
d) HIV test

Localized

If present in one arm, hand, leg or foot.

Causes

a) Cervical spondylosis with radiculopathy (pain in neck radiating to one arm).
b) Median nerve compression in wrist (carpal-tunnel syndrome—tingling numbness in hand especially at night).

c) Sciatica (pain and tingling numbness in one leg).
d) Leprosy (hypopigmented anaesthetic patches along with tender nerves).

Treatment

a) Inj. $B_1 + B_6 + B_{12}$ (Neurobion) IM daily empirically.
b) Tab. Diclofenac (Voveran) 100 mg bd.
c) Tab. Prednisolone (Wysolone) 5 mg bd, if severe.

- In case of cervical spondylosis—cervical traction and short wave diathermy.
- In case of carpal tunnel syndrome, Inj. Kenacort in the wrist joint near median nerve.
- In case of sciatica, bed rest & lumbar traction.
- In case of leprosy, refer to dermatologist.

- Do not go on treating tingling numbness with Inj. $B_1 + B_6 + B_{12}$ indefinitely without ascertaining the cause. Vitamin deficiency does not come spontaneously without any reason.
- Although alcoholism is the commonest cause, the causes which should never be missed are diabetes, leprosy and HIV infection.
- In case of alcoholism, stop alcohol completely. In case of diabetes, use insulin instead of oral drugs for control of blood sugar.
- It is worth learning the technique of intra-articular steroid injections (see Chapter 41).

*This chapter has been reviewed by **Dr Parag Vaste**, MD, Consultant Physician, Pune.*

GP Tip

***Migraine** or **Sinusitis**? A day-to-day dilemma for a GP.*

Give a supraorbital nerve block and wait for 5 min. The headache due to sinusitis will disappear temporarily, as the nerve supply to the frontal sinus will be blocked, while the vascular headache of migraine will persist.

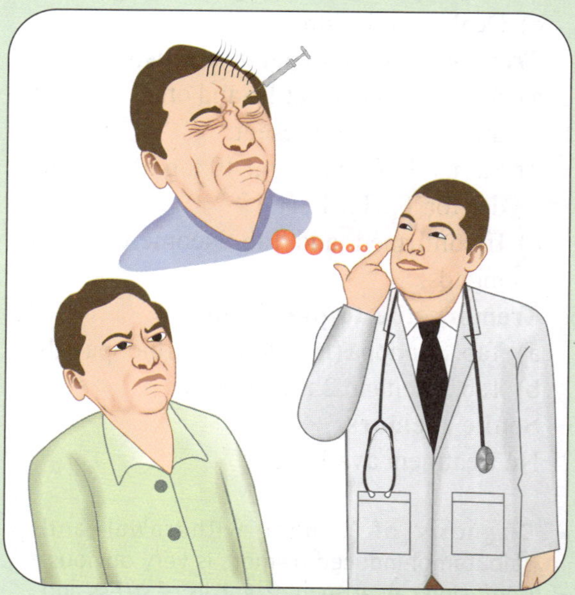

GENERAL PRACTICE AS SPECIALITY

CHAPTER 5

Orthopaedic Conditions

- Ankle Sprain
- Fractures
- Acute Neck Stiffness
- Nocturnal Cramps in Calf
- Cervical Spondylosis
- Osteoporosis
- Osteomalacia
- Shoulder Pain
- Osteoarthritis
- Low Backache
- Chronic Polyarthritis

ANKLE SPRAIN

Severe Pain and Swelling

This could be complete ankle ligament tear or an underlying fracture. Advise X-ray (AP and lateral). Even if there is no fracture, refer for total immobilization with a plaster of Paris cast or surgery for torn ligament.

Moderate to Mild Pain

In the First 48 hrs

- Tab. Diclofenac (Voveran) 100 mg bd after food.
- Tab. Chymoral forte qid before food.
- Volini ointment for local application.
- Advise **RICE**.

  R: Rest, depending on the severity. Use crutches if necessary.

  I: Ice packs every 3–4 hrs.

  C: Crepe bandage from the midfoot to the midcalf.

  E: Elevate the leg to reduce swelling.

After 48 hrs

- Encourage patient to gradually start walking.
- Stop ice packs. Start hot fomentations.
- Passive exercises, isometric exercises and finally full normal activity within 2 weeks.

FRACTURES

Big fractures resulting from road accidents like fracture spine, femur, tibia, etc., are always directly rushed to a hospital. Patients with moderate injury are brought to a GP's clinic and then it is his job to suspect and diagnose the fracture and give primary aid (see Chapter 42).

Symptoms and Signs

- Pain at affected site, which increases with movements. Therefore, movements are restricted.
- Swelling at site.
- Local tenderness.
- Deformity, abnormal mobility.

If the above features are present, request for an X-ray. If an X-ray confirms the diagnosis, immediately immobilize the part, give pain killers and refer.

How to immobilize ?

- **The shoulder**—apply a sling made of roller bandage around the neck and the wrist to elevate the arm.
- **Proximal part of the upper arm**—apply sticking plaster or Dynaplast across the chest, upper limb and back.
- **Distal part of the forearm**—use a straight wooden stick or even a thick rolled up newspaper will do. Make sure to immobilize the wrist and the elbow also.
- **The hip**—to prevent external rotation, lie down the patient and place a pillow on the lateral part of the leg or apply Thomas Splint if available.

If pain persists

- Inj. Pentazocine (Fortwin) IM stat
- Inj. Promethazine (Phenargan) IM stat.
- Refer to orthopaedic surgeon.
- Keep NBM

The following fractures can be easily missed clinically as well as radiologically, giving a bad reputation to the GP:

- Impacted fractured humerus. The displaced one may compress on the radial artery. Watch the pulse.
- Impacted fractured hip.
- Fractured metatarsal or metacarpal bones.
- Green stick fracture of the forearm in children.
- Fracture scaphoid in the wrist. Initial X-ray is normal. If there is scaphoid tenderness, repeat X-ray after 2 weeks. If missed and not treated, permanent stiffness will result.
- Rib fracture.

ACUTE NECK STIFFNESS (Wry neck, Torticollis)

Patient comes with pain and inability to move the neck. Starts suddenly, usually lasts for a day or two and disappears spontaneously.

- Gentle mobilization.
- Hot fomentation to the neck.
- Gentle massage with Voveran gel.
- Tab. Diclofenac plus Paracetamol tds.
- Tab. Tizanidine (Sirdalud) 2 mg tds, till pain subsides.
- Neck collar if pain is recurrent or persistent.

NOCTURNAL CRAMPS IN CALF

Treat the cause, if it is known.

- Electrolyte disturbance following diarrhoea.
- Occupational, e.g., tailors, telephone operators and typist who sit for prolonged periods or overuse calf muscles.
- Unaccustomed overexertion, e.g., trekkers, tennis players, etc.
- Calcium deficiency.
- Uncontrolled diabetes.
- Unfortunately, most of the time the cause is not known (idiopathic).

Treat Empirically

Physical treatment

- Alternate muscle stretching and relaxation exercises of calf muscles at bed time for 5 min daily. This can be done by standing against a wall for support and alternately standing on the toes and heels.
- Massage with oil while retiring to bed.
- Plenty of oral fluids with electral powder.

Drug treatment

- Tab. Shellcal 500 mg bd.
- Tab. Neurobion bd.

- Tab. Evion 400 mg bd.
- Tab. Quinine sulphate 300 mg hs. If not available, use Tab. Anacin.
- Tab. Voveran 100 mg sos during pain.

CERVICAL SPONDYLOSIS

Usually, an elderly patient presents with subacute pain and stiffness in the neck, which radiates to one arm. There is also tingling numbness in the same arm (root pain or radiculitis). It is an aging process, where osteophytes formed on the vertebra compress the nerves, producing the symptoms. Rarely, the osteophytes will compress the vertebral artery, causing giddiness or syncope (basovertebral insufficiency). X-ray is not diagnostic, as osteophytes are seen commonly on X-rays at this age.

Treatment

- Local heat and analgesic ointment, e.g., Felini ointment to be applied 3–4 times a day to the neck.
- Physiotherapy—either short wave diathermy (SWD) or cervical traction.
- Inj. Diclofenac IM plus Inj. Decadron IM, if pain is severe.
- Tab. Ibuprofen (Brufen) 400 mg tds.
- Tab. Tizanidine (Sirdalud) 2 mg tds, till pain subsides.
- Tab. Diazepam (Valium) 5 mg hs.

Prevention of Attacks

- Use a thin pillow.
- Use cervical collar during day time.
- Neck exercises daily. Head bending forwards, backwards, to the left and to the right for 15–20 times a day. Then static movements against resistance, e.g., place left hand on left cheek and prevent the head bending on that side. Repeat the procedure for other movements also.
- Shoulder exercises, movements in all direction, first active and then static against resistance.

OSTEOPOROSIS

Usually, elderly subjects especially ladies present to a GP with fractures following minimal trauma. The most common fractures seen are Colles fracture following a fall on the road or fracture neck femur after slipping in the bathroom or multiple old vertebral fractures seen in X-ray spine taken for low backache. Osteoporosis is evident on the X-ray. Osteoporosis means a porous bone where the calcium content of the bone is less.

Treatment

- Tab. Calcium with Vitamin D (Ossopan) 500 mg bd × 6 months.
- Inj. Arachitol (Vitamin D) 6 lakh units IM at weekly intervals × 6 injections.
- Inj. Decaneurabol (Anabolic steroid) 25 mg IM monthly × 3 months.
- Treatment of individual fractures.
- Tab. Alendronate 35 or 70 mg/week (Osteophos) (or) Tab. Ibandronate (Idrofos) 150 mg/month.

Prevention

- Regular physical exercises, e.g., brisk walk for 2–3 km daily. Spinal extension exercises.
- Avoid smoking completely.
- Exposure to sunlight from noon to 5 pm.
- Restrict alcohol intake.
- Tab. Shellcal 500 mg bd × 6 months.
- Hormone replacement therapy (HRT) in postmenopausal women. Give Tab. Premarin 0.625 mg od (Controversial).

OSTEOMALACIA

These patients present with persistent backache, muscular weakness and with bone pains. The patient finds it difficult to get out of a chair or climb up the stairs. Spontaneous fractures may also occur. Osteomalacia means softening of the bone and is due to Vitamin D deficiency.

Treatment

- Inj. Arachitol (Vitamin D) 6 lakh units IM at weekly intervals × 6 injections (**or**)
  Calcirol granules (6 lakh units) available in sachets. One sachet in milk every month × 6 months.
- Tab. Shellcal 500 mg bd × 6 months.
- Diet should include plenty of milk, cheese and proteins, green vegetables, eggs, fish, etc.

SHOULDER PAIN

The first job on hand is to r/o referred pain to the shoulder from other structures, e.g., pain referred on the right side from the gallbladder or anginal pain to the left shoulder or to either shoulder due to cervical spondylosis. This can be easily done by moving the shoulder through all its movements. If the pain is referred, then the pain will not increase with these movements.

Young Individual

The cause is usually an inflammation of the tendon surrounding the joint (supraspinatus, infraspinatus or bicipital tendonitis). There is pain and restriction of movements.

Elderly Individual

The cause is usually frozen shoulder. Initially, there is severe pain. Then, gradually in a month or so the pain decreases, but the stiffness increases. Finally, there is no pain but the shoulder is stiff (frozen).

Treatment

This will depend on the symptoms:

1. ***Severe pain without stiffness***
   a) Tab. Diclofenac (Voveran) 100 mg bd.
   b) Volini ointment for local application.
   c) Inj. Methylprednisolone or Triamcinolone with xylocaine to be infiltrated, as described in Chapter 41.
   d) No active exercises during this phase.
2. ***Moderate pain with moderate stiffness***
   Same treatment as above, except:
   Allow active and passive exercises to the affected shoulder, preferably under the guidance of a physiotherapist.
3. ***No pain, only stiffness (frozen shoulder)***
   a) No drug therapy works.
   b) Active exercises with the help of a physiotherapist.
   c) Refer for homeopathic treatment.

OSTEOARTHRITIS

Degeneration of joints is mainly seen in weight bearing joints like knee, hip and spine. The most common is knee joint arthritis seen in postmenopausal women. There is pain which is gradual in onset. There are intermittent exacerbations with repeated effusions following minor trauma.

Advice

- Avoid excessive walking, sitting on floor, Indian toilet and climbing stairs.
- Weight reduction.
- Walking stick if necessary to avoid strain on the knee.
- Hot fomentation.
- Local analgesic ointments.
- Quadriceps exercises: Tie sand bags on the ankle. Extend the knee after sitting on a chair, for at least 15–20 times a day. Gradually increase the weight of the sand bags.
- Physiotherapy—SWD, wax bath, etc.

Drug Treatment

- Simple analgesics like paracetamol or diclofenac.
- Cap. Rejoint 2 od × 1 year. Costly treatment, effectiveness doubtful. Supposed to help regeneration of the damaged cartilage.
- If severe pain, give intra-articular steroid injection.
- If severe pain with deformity, refer to orthopaedic surgeon for surgery.

LOW BACKACHE (LBA)

Acute Lumbago (Mechanical LBA)

The pain comes suddenly usually following lifting of heavy weight, bending, etc. Pain does *not* radiate to the legs and is *not* aggravated by coughing, sneezing or straining at stools. There is *no* anaesthesia in the legs and *no* loss of power like thigh muscle weakness or foot drop. The straight leg-raising (SLR) test is *negative*. Spasm in the back muscles may or may not be present. If present, the back movements are difficult and painful.

Treatment

Acute LBA without spasm

- No bed rest, normal daily activities.
- Simple analgesics like paracetamol, aspirin or ibuprofen × 10–12 days.
- Back exercises (like raising legs with knees extended 20–25 times a day with the patient in recumbent position) once the pain has reduced.

Acute LBA with spasm

- Absolute bed rest × 2–3 days.
- Inj. Voveran 3 mL IM stat.
- Tab. Voveran SR 100 mg bd.
- Tab. Sirdalud 2 mg bd.
- Tab. Valium 5 mg bd.
- Felini ointment to be applied locally 3–4 times a day.
- Short wave diathermy (SWD).

When the acute attack is over, treat as LBA without spasm.

Acute LBA with Nerve Pain (Sciatica or Prolapsed Disc)

Severe sudden pain in back radiating to one leg along with tingling numbness. Here all the features which were *absent* in acute lumbago are present (see above).

Treatment

- Absolute bed rest × 3–4 days.
- Inj. Voveran 3 mL IM stat.
- Tab. Voveran SR 100 mg bd.
- SWD, lumbar traction.

Admit the patient if:

- No response to the above treatment for 3 days.
- Retention of urine.
- Motor involvement, e.g., foot drop.

In such cases a CT scan or MRI, epidural anaesthesia or surgery may be required.

Chronic LBA (More than 3 Months Duration)

This is usually seen in males > 50 years or in postmenopausal women where the cause is degeneration of the spine (lumbar spondylosis). The pain is dull nagging type, which is increased by prolonged sitting, bending, etc. Stiffness especially in the mornings, is an important feature. Advise an X-ray of lumbosacral spine, which usually shows a lot of changes like osteoporosis, osteophytes, compression fractures, all of which usually do not correlate with the clinical picture. In women with LBA due to depression, the X-ray is normal.

Treatment

- Simple analgesics.
- Tab. Shellcal 500 mg bd × 3 months.
- Adequate rest combined with light back exercises.
- SWD/lumbosacral belt.
- Physiotherapy.

CHRONIC POLYARTHRITIS

Most of the cases seen in general practice are of *rheumatoid arthritis*. The patient is usually a middle aged woman who c/o pain and swelling in many peripheral large joints like wrist, elbows, fingers, knees, ankles, etc. There is early morning stiffness and hence the patient finds it difficult to get up from the bed. The ESR is raised and the rheumatoid arthritis factor (RA) test is usually positive.

Treatment

- Explain chronicity of the disease to the patient. "*It is not curable, but it is treatable.*"
- Stress the importance of regular exercise.
- The affected joints should be moved through their full range of movements daily to prevent stiffness and contractures.
- NSAIDs given in the box should be used interchangeably.
- Cap. Omeprazole (Omez) 20 mg bd.
- In case of acute exacerbation, Tab. Prednisolone (Wysolone) 5 mg.
  - 2 tds × 5 days, then
  - 1 tds × 5 days, then
  - 1 bd × 5 days.
- Intra-articular Inj. Kenacort, if intractable pain in one or two joints.
- Cap. Indomethacin sustained release (Indocap SR) at bedtime to reduce morning stiffness.
- Remission inducing drugs like methotrexate, chloroquine, gold salts, etc., should be reserved for the specialists.

NSAIDs

- Tab. Diclofenac 100 mg (Voveran) 1 bd.
- Tab. Piroxicam 20 mg (Pirox) 1 od.
- Tab. Mefenamic acid 500 mg (Meftal) 1 tds
- Tab. Ibuprofen 400 mg (Brufen) 1 tds.
- Tab. Naproxen 250 mg (Naprosyn) 2 bd.
- Tab. Nimesulide 100 mg (Nise) 1 bd.
- Tab. Meloxicam 15 mg (Mel-OD) 1 od.
- Tab. Indomethacin 25 mg (Indocid) 1 tds.
- Tab. Valdecoxib (Valcox) 10 mg od.

*This chapter has been reviewed by **Dr Rahul Shinde**, MS Orthopaedics, Consultant Orthopaedic Surgeon, Pune.*

CHAPTER 6

Psychiatric Conditions

- Generalised Anxiety State
- Reactive Depression
- Mixed Anxiety Depression (MAD)
- Acute Conversion Reaction (Hysteria)
- Psychosomatic Illness (Somatization)
- Mild Schizophrenia
- Drug Treatment for Transient Insomnia

The role of a general practitioner in treating psychiatric illness is, I suppose, fairly well defined.

1. ***To identify patients of psychiatric illness***: It is easy to diagnose a severe case of psychiatric illness (i.e., psychosis), if hallucinations, illusions and delusions are present (see below). In case of a minor psychiatric illness (i.e., neurosis), again, if the patient has classical symptoms, the diagnosis is easy. The problem comes, if the patient presents with a physical complaint because of anxiety or depression, e.g., headache. If the GP knows only two causes of headache, e.g., sinusitis and migraine and if the patient does not fulfill the classical picture of any of these diseases, he will usually label the headache as 'functional'. If the GP knows 10 causes of headache, he will make the diagnosis of 'functional headache' after ruling out these 10 causes. It should be remembered that a psychiatric illness is not a diagnosis of exclusion. Rather, it should be made on specific symptoms of specific psychiatric illness.
2. ***To identify 'psychotic' patients and separate them from neurotic patients***: In *neurosis*, the patient has symptoms caused by stimulation of the sympathetic nervous system like palpitations, tremors, sweating, etc. He is aware of these symptoms and wishes to get rid of them. In *psychosis* on the other hand, the patient is unaware that he is ill and is brought forcibly by the relatives to your clinic. He has in addition, illusions, delusions and hallucinations, e.g., he is convinced that somebody is plotting to kill him or he hears voices talking to him to which he replies loudly (muttering to himself). In short, lay people call him 'mad'. Psychosis is a serious disorder, which is best managed by a psychiatrist, who will probably give him high doses of antipsychotic drugs or electroconvulsive therapy (electric shock treatment). Once the diagnosis of neurosis is made, it is for the GP to decide whether the patient should be managed by a physician or by himself.

3. ***To manage patients of functional overlay***: This means that on a physical illness, e.g., heart attack, neurotic symptoms like repeated chest pain, palpitations, etc., get superimposed because of the fear of death. A GP is in a better position to manage these patients than either a psychiatrist or a physician because of the better rapport he has with the patient's family.
4. ***To manage patients with mild psychiatric disorders like***:
   a) Generalised anxiety state
   b) Reactive depression
   c) Mixed anxiety depression
   d) Conversion reaction
   e) Psychosomatic illness
   f) Mild schizophrenia
   g) Transient insomnia

GENERALISED ANXIETY STATE

Low level anxiety persists throughout the day. The patient is unusually anxious and tense. He or she will complain of palpitations. Vertex headache, tingling numbness, sweating of palms and soles, tremors, shortness of breath, dryness of mouth, increased sensitivity to sound, etc. The sleep is disturbed and there is 'initial insomnia' i.e., on going to bed the patient lies awake worrying about his problems. Finally, when he falls asleep, he wakes up intermittently.

Treatment

- Be a good listener and allow the patient to 'release' himself by talking.
- Investigate appropriately depending on the symptoms (e.g., ECG for chest pain) to reassure the patient.
- Tab. Alprazolam (Trika, Restyl) 0.25 tds (**or**) Tab. Chlordiazepoxide (Librium) 10 mg tds (**or**)
  Tab. Diazepam (Valium, Calmpose) 5 mg ½–½–1 (**or**)
  Tab. Lorazepam (Ativan) 1 mg tds (**or**)
  Tab. Clonazepam (Rivotril) 0.5 mg tds.
- Tab. Propranolol (Inderal, Ciplar) 10–40 mg tds, if excessive tremors, palpitations or sweating are present.
- Add antidepressants, if depression is also present (see below).
- Use antipsychotics in small doses if anxiety symptoms are severe, e.g., Tab. Chlorpromazine (Largactil) 25 mg tds or Tab. Trifluoperazine (Eskazine) 1 mg bd or hs.

> Anti-anxiety drugs should be given for a short time only to tide over the crises. These drugs may cause addiction. Hence, they should be given for 2–3 weeks and then gradually tapered off in the next 2–3 weeks. For long-term maintenance, give antidepressants, which also have anti-anxiety action.

REACTIVE DEPRESSION

This is one of the most common illnesses seen in GP. This usually follows some bad events such as failure in examinations, death in the family or financial loss in the business, etc. Hence, it is called 'reactive'. But, this need not be necessarily so. A patient can get mild depression without any reason whatsoever. The patient is gloomy, sad, not interested in his work, not interested even in pleasurable activities like sex. His thoughts are pessimistic, i.e., he sees only the unhappy side of every event in his life.

The sleep is disturbed and there is early morning waking. He gets up 2–3 hrs before his usual waking time, cannot go to sleep and feels restless and frustrated in the mornings. As the day progresses, he is slightly better off. The patient will have many other complaints like headache, weakness, anorexia, constipation, etc. (somatisation). He wishes he was dead and will tell you so, but will not actually make an attempt to commit suicide. If he does or even plans to make an attempt, it is 'major depression'.

Treatment

- Cap. Fluoxetine (Fludac, Prodep) 20 mg od (**or**)
  Tab. Sertraline (Serta, Serlift) 50 mg od (**or**)
  Tab. Imipramine (Depsonil) 25 mg tds (**or**)
  Tab. Amitriptyline (Tryptomer) 10 mg tds (**or**)
  Tab. Doxepin (Spectra) 10 mg tds.
- Inj. Beplex forte 2 mL alternate days X 5 days.
- Santivini tonic 2 tsf bd.
- Symptomatic treatment of physical symptoms.

If depression is severe, i.e., there is marked weight loss, the patient talks in slow motion, there is excessive feeling of guilt and worthlessness and the patient has thoughts of suicide—refer immediately.

MIXED ANXIETY DEPRESSION (MAD)

Although anxiety and depression have been described separately, in practice we usually see symptoms of both the diseases in the same patient. You should then use a combination of an antidepressant drug and an anti-anxiety drug. The anti-anxiety drug should be withdrawn within 2 weeks because of its addictive potential.

All antidepressants have anxiolytic properties in addition to antidepressant effects but the action starts after about 2 weeks. Hence after this period, the patient should be put on an optimum dose of an antidepressant alone. Fixed dose combination (Libotryp, Depranil plus, etc.) should be as far as possible avoided as dosage adjustments in the long run become difficult.

Treatment

- Tab. Amitriptyline (Tryptomer) 10 mg tds plus Tab. Chlordiazepoxide (Librium) 10 mg tds (**or**)
- Tab. Imipramine (Depsonil) 25 mg tds plus Diazepam (Valium) 5 mg ½–½–1 (**or**)
- Cap. Fluoxetine (Fludac) 20 mg od plus Alprazolam (Restyl) 0.25 mg tds (**or**)
- Tab. Sertraline (Serta, Serlift) 50 mg od plus Tab. Clonazepam (Rivotryl) 0.5 mg tds.

> - The old antidepressants like amitriptyline and imipramine have marked sedative effects and many side effects. The new antidepressants like fluoxetine and sertraline are less sedating and have less side effects. Their therapeutic effects are almost the same.
> - Many 'new' antidepressants are introduced into the market by drug companies, mainly for commercial reasons. The general practitioner should master only 2 or 3 of these and use these frequently till he feels 'confident'.

ACUTE CONVERSION REACTION (Hysteria)

The most common type of hysteria seen in general practice is '*hysterical fit*'. Here, the fit usually occurs after severe mental strain, e.g., a housewife has an argument with the mother-in-law and suddenly gets a 'fit' with clenching of teeth, unconsciousness, etc. It always occurs in front of many people, never in sleep, there is no tongue biting or passage of urine during the episode. This has to be differentiated from epilepsy (see Chapter 22).

Treatment

- Clear the people watching 'the show'.
- Display confidence and take charge of the situation.
- Take dramatic measures like making the patient breathe through a plastic bag or putting cotton soaked in 'smelling salt' on the nostrils, etc.
- Give placebo Inj. B complex or even placebo IV DNS drip.
- Inj. Chlorpromazine (Largactil) 2 mL IM stat or Inj. Haloperidol (Serenase) 5 mg IM stat, if the patient does not wake up with the above measures (**or**) Inj phenargan 25 ms IM.
- Once the acute episode is over, try and deal with the cause of the fit. Never tell the patient that she is 'acting' and does not have any illness.

PSYCHOSOMATIC ILLNESS (Somatization)

The patient will repeatedly approach the GP with a large number of physical complaints which are not related to each other, e.g., headache, weakness, backache, polyarthralgia, epigastric pain, constipation, insomnia, low backache, chronic leucorrhoea in females, loss of sexual drive in males, etc. These are called the *hypochondriac or the polysomatic patients*.

- Listen to all the symptoms with active interest.
- Make sure that you are not missing any physical disease by conducting the relevant investigations, e.g., ECG for chest pain. Even if these investigations are normal, it may not satisfy him that there is no disease.
- Better to ask ready questionnaire which will lead to diagnosis of depression.
- Low dose antidepressant and anti-anxiety drugs:
  - Tab. Sertraline (Serlift) 50 mg od × 2 mths
  - Tab. Lorazepam (Ativan) 1 mg bd × 1 wk.

MILD SCHIZOPHRENIA

A healthy 20-year-old boy starts behaving in an odd way. Sometimes, he laughs and talks to himself for no reason. At times, he becomes withdrawn and lost in his own thoughts. He has gradually become poor in his studies. He tells his friends that the police have told his teacher to poison him (paranoid delusions). He describes hearing voices (auditory hallucinations). In short, his friends and family members say that he is behaving like a 'mad person'.

If the illness is mild and the GP is confident, these patients can be managed by him. If not, an initial referral to a psychiatrist should be made. The old antipsychotic drugs like chlopromazine should be used in large doses without fear by the GP. The new antipsychotic drugs like risperidone or olanzapine can be used in small doses.

Treatment

- Tab. Chlorpromazine (Largactil) 50 mg tds plus
  Tab. Trifluoperazine (Eskazine) 5 mg tds plus
  Tab. Pacitane 2 mg bd (**or**)
- Tab. Haloperidol (Serenase) 10 mg tds plus
  Tab. Trifluoperazine (Eskazine) 5 mg tds plus
  Tab. Pacitane bd (**or**)
- Tab. Risperidone (Risdone) 1 mg bd (**or**)
- Tab. Olanzapine (Oliza) 2.5 mg bd.

If good response

- Tab. Fluphenazine deconate (Anatensol) 12.5 mg IM every 15 days × many years.

If no response

- Refer to a psychiatrist, as electric shock treatment may be required.

DRUG TREATMENT FOR TRANSIENT INSOMNIA

The following drugs are to be used for short time only, in case of temporary loss of sleep. This can result from severe mental trauma like death in family, postoperative insomnia or in case of severe painful conditions like cancer pain.

- Tab. Diazepam (Calmpose) 5–10 mg (**or**)
- Tab. Nitrazepam (Nitravet) 5–10 mg (**or**)
- Tab. Lorazepam (Ativan) 1–2 mg (**or**)
- Tab. Zolpidem (Nitrest) 10–20 mg (**or**)
- Tab. Zopiclone (Zonap) 7.5–15 mg.

This chapter has been reviewed by ***Dr Shailesh Chougule****, MD Psychiatry, Practising Psychiatrist, Pune.*

CHAPTER 7

Dermatological Conditions

- Acne Vulgaris
- Herpes Zoster
- Herpes Simplex
- Urticaria
- Leprosy
- Scabies
- Fungal Infections
- Bacterial Infections
- Eczema
- Psoriasis
- Vitiligo
- Alopecia
- Dandruff
- STD
- Maggots
- Miliaria Rubra
- Pityriasis Alba
- Melasma
- Molluscum Contagiosum

ACNE VULGARIS (Pimples) (Fig. 7.1)

Patients will present to a general practitioner with any of the three types of acne:

Mainly Blackheads

a) Apply Tretinoin (Retino-A or Eudyna cream) 0.025% at bedtime only. Do not expose to sun after applying this cream. Apply gently; do not rub as this would cause irritation and erythema.

b) Benzoyl peroxide (Persol gel or Benzac AC gel) 2.5% during day time. Watch for irritation. If irritation is severe, discontinue for 2 days.

c) Express blackheads with an 'acne-expressor' available in any surgical shop. It is cheap and very useful.

Mainly Pustules

a) Apply Erythromycin (Eryacne) cream or Clindamycin (Clindac A) gel on face bd.

b) Cap. Doxycycline (Doxy 1) 100 mg od × 3 months (**or**)
Cap. Cynomycin (Minocycline) 100 mg od 3 months (**or**)
Tab. Erythromycin (Althrocin) 500 mg bd (**or**)
Tab. Azithromycin (Azee) 500 mg once a week × 3–6 months

Both Pustules and Blackheads

a) Apply Erytop cream in the morning and Eudyna cream at bed time.

b) Oral antibiotics—doxycycline or cynomycin or erythromycin as above.

Instructions to the Patient

a) Wash the face 4–5 times a day. (You may prescribe 'Acnil soap'.)

b) Avoid cosmetics.

c) Do not prick the acne as this may leave bad scars.

d) No hair oil application.

HERPES ZOSTER (HZ) (Fig. 23.7)

It presents as groups of vesicles along a nerve route, associated with severe burning pain. It is common in elderly age. If seen in a young sexually active individual, offer an HIV test after giving detailed explanation of the nature of the disease to the patient. There is a misconception that

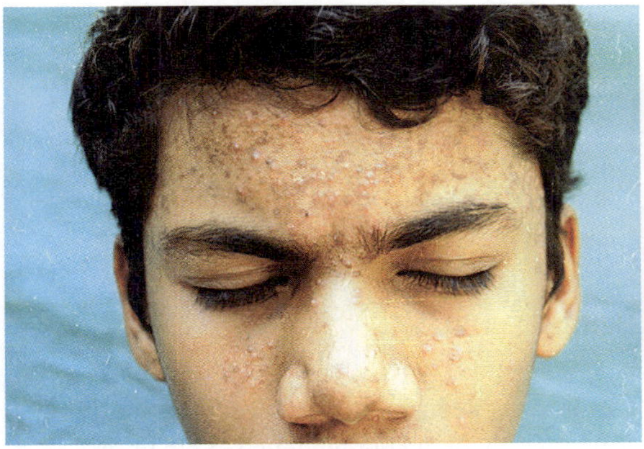

| Fig. 7.1 Acne vulgaris |

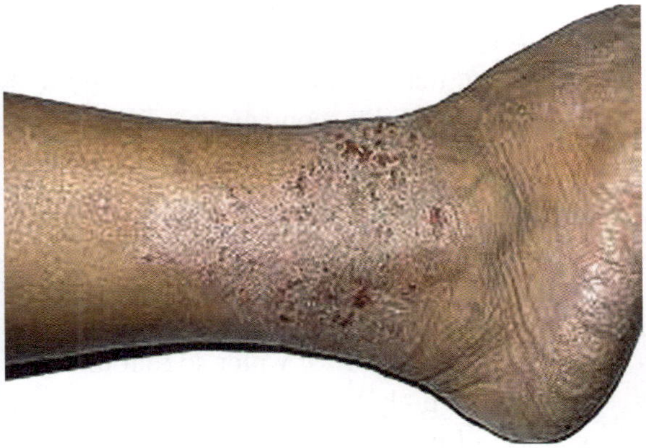

| Fig. 7.2 Eczema ankle |

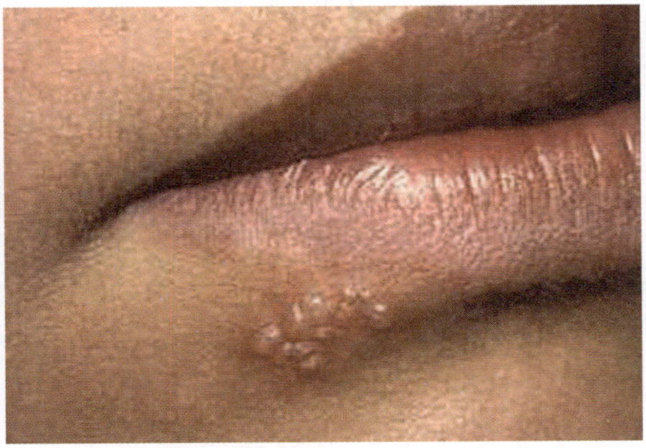

| Fig. 7.3 Herpes labialis |

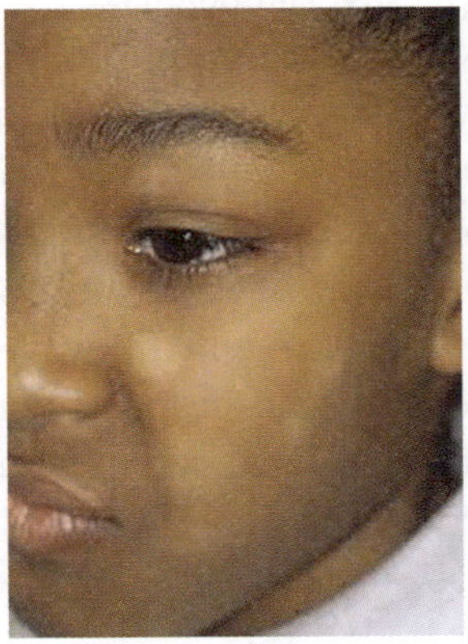

| Fig. 7.4 Pitysiasis alba |

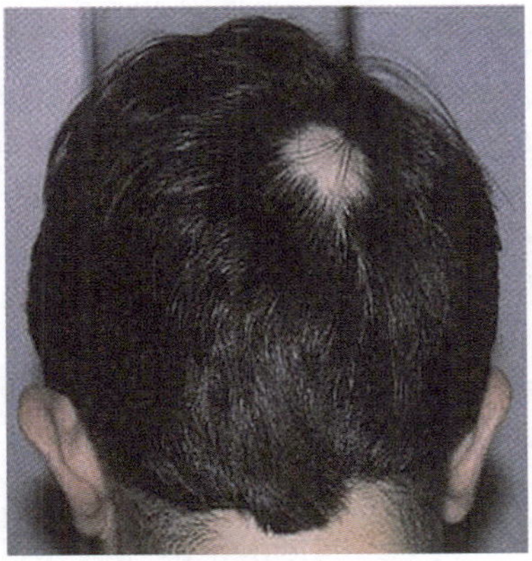

| Fig. 7.5 Alopecia areata |

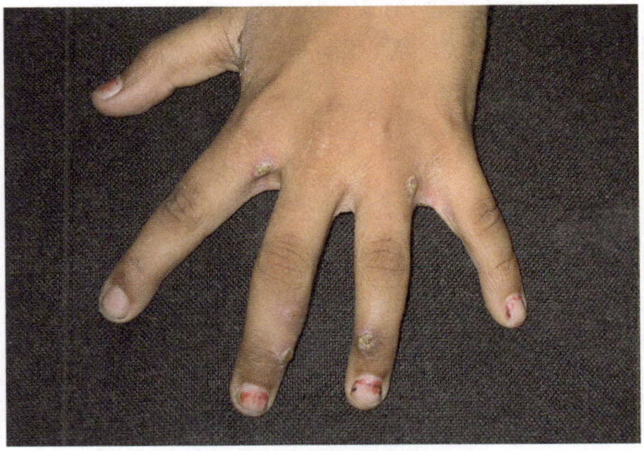

| Fig. 7.6 Scabies |

if the rash spreads on both the sides of the body and encircles it completely the person is going to die. Reassure that the disease is not dangerous or fatal. It is only mildly contagious. Children can acquire chicken pox, after contact with a patient of HZ.

Local Treatment

- Give potassium permanganate soaks. Put 3–4 crystals in a bowl of water so that the colour is faint pink. Soak a cotton towel in this water and put it on the rash for 5–10 min. Remove the towel. Mop the water with a dry cloth.
- Then apply silver sulphadiazine cream locally, which is non-irritating and does not give rise to allergic dermatitis. Do not use furacin, soframycin or neomycin creams as these can give rise to allergic dermatitis and worsen the picture. Acyclovir cream is of little use as an antiviral agent, is very costly and causes stinging pain on application. Calamine lotion, though used for its cooling effect causes caking on the lesions and is difficult to remove after drying.

Systemic Treatment

- Tab. Paracetamol, if the pain is mild. Inj. Tramadol or Inj. Fortagesic, if pain is severe.
- Tab. Ciprofloxacin (Cifran) 500 mg bd, if there is secondary infection.
- Tab. Acyclovir (Zovirax, Herpex) 800 mg 3–5 times a day × 7 days in selected cases (see Box) (**or**) Tab. Valacyclovir (Valcivir) 1000 mg tds × 7–10 days.
- Take ophthalmic opinion in HZ ophthalmicus, especially if there are vesicles on the tip of the nose.

Indications for the use of acyclovir in HZ

1. Immunocompromised patients.
2. Ophthalmic zoster.
3. Any extensive zoster.

It is effective only if started within 72 hrs of the onset of the rash. Do not prescribe, if new vesicles have stopped erupting.

HERPES SIMPLEX

Commonly seen as group of vesicles on the lips following fever or spontaneously. Self-limiting but recurrent (Fig. 7.3)

- Apply Soframycin cream locally (**or**)
- Acyclovir cream (Herpex, Zovirax) 5%—5 times a day × 5–6 days.
- Tab. Acyclovir (Acivir) 400 mg tds × 5 days (**or**) Tab.Valacyclovir (Valcivir) 500 mg bd × 5 days.

URTICARIA (Fig. 23.4)

It can be either acute or chronic and recurrent.

- Give antihistaminics like Tab. Avil 25 mg or Tab. Atarax 25 mg stat and then bd. These cause sedation.
- Alternatively, give non-sedating antihistaminics.
  - Cetrizine (Cetzine) 10 mg od (**or**)
  - Loratidine (Lorfast) 10 mg od (**or**)
  - Fexofenadine (Allegra) 180 mg od (**or**)
  - Levocetrizine (Xyzal) 5 mg od

  Best combination would be a non-sedating antihistaminic in the morning with a sedating one at bedtime.
- Oral steroid can be added. Prednisolone 5 mg tds, to be gradually tapered off.

If the urticaria is severe and mucous membranes are involved, as indicated by lip swelling or hoarseness of voice (*angioneurotic oedema*), give:

- In. Phenargan 2 mL IV bd.
- Inj. Hydrocortisone (Efcorlin) 100 mg IV stat.
- Inj. Adrenaline 0.5 mL SC, if extensive and associated with hypotension.

Chronic Urticaria

- Take careful history to find out the allergen like food or drugs.
- Tab. Cetrizine 10 mg od × 2–3 months.
- Tab. Ranitidine (Zinetac) 150 mg od × 2–3 months.
- Do differential WBC count. If eosinophil percentage is high, give Tab. Hetrazan 1 tds × 21 days.
- Tab. Zentel 400 mg single dose.

> Do not waste patient's time and money in too many investigations to detect the allergen. Do not go for allergy testing. They usually do not help. Most of the patients sooner or later get desensitized spontaneously to the unknown allergen and the urticaria subsides permanently.
>
> In acute urticaria, always take a h/o drug intake. If present, keep a proper record, so that the drug can be avoided in future.

LEPROSY (Hansen's Disease) (Fig. 23.8)

Suspect if the patient presents with hypopigmented patches, which are anaesthetic to touch and pinprick. Examine the ulnar, greater auricular and lateral popliteal nerves. These may be enlarged and tender. If there are contractures of the fingers and 'lion like' face, the diagnosis is almost certain. In case of doubt, take a biopsy (see Chapter 38). This will confirm the diagnosis and also tell you, if the disease is of tuberculoid or lepromatous type.

Tuberculoid Type

- Tab. Dapsone 100 mg od × 1 year
- Tab. Rifampicin (R-cin) 600 mg, if wt. > 50 kg and 450 mg, if wt. < 50 kg, once a month for at least 1 year.

Lepromatous Type

- Tab. Dapsone 100 mg od × 3 years
- Cap. R-cin 600 mg once a month for 3 years
- Cap. Clofazimine (Hansepran) 50 mg daily and 300 mg once a month × 3 years.

Lepra Reaction

Always watch for lepra reactions. In case of a lepra reaction, where the patches suddenly increase in size and number and the nerves become more painful:

- Tab. Prednisolone 10 mg qid daily for 8–10 days. Then, gradually taper it till reaction subsides.
- Cap. Clofazimine 100 mg tds × 1 month.
- Do not stop dapsone or rifampicin.
- Once the reaction has subsided, start the original doses.

SCABIES (Fig. 7.6)

- Treat all family members and contacts simultaneously, even if asymptomatic.
- Treat secondary infection with ciprofloxacin (Cifran) 500 mg bd × 5–7 days before you start antiscabetic treatment.
- To control itching, give Tab. Levocetrizine 5 mg od and Tab. Betnesol 0.5 mg tds for 7–10 days.
- Tab. Ivermectin (Scarista) 6 mg 2 stat. Repeat after 2 weeks, in children 200 μg/kg.
- ***Antiscabetic lotions and how to use them***:
  Benzyl benzoate (Ascabiol) 25% **(or)**
  Gama-benzene HCL (Gamascab) 1% **(or)**
  Permethrin (Permite) cream 5% **(or)**
  Crotomiton (Crotorax)

Lotion is to be applied all over the body except face, after bath and kept for 24 hrs. Apply for 2 consecutive days. During bath, the whole body should be scrubbed to open up the burrows. After the completion of the treatment, the clothes, towel and bed linen should be boiled in soap water and dried in the sun.

The itching may last for 2 weeks. Apply crotorax lotion daily after bath for its anti-pruritic and antiscabetic action. In children, dilute the lotion to 50% with water.

For pediculosis of the body, the same treatment can be given. For head lice, use Permethrin (Perlice) 1% lotion at bed time for 3 days and wash off in the morning.

FUNGAL INFECTIONS

Tinea Versicolour

Multiple hypopigmented, hyperpigmented and brownish (variety of colours = versi-colour) patches seen on the trunk. Asymptomatic.

1. Selenium sulphide (Selsun) shampoo or Candid TV lotion to be applied 1 hr before bath (**or**)
   Tolnaftate lotion (Tinaderm) to be applied after bath and at bed time (**or**)
   Hypo(sodium thiosulphate) solution available in photography shops is also effective. To be applied after bath.
2. Tab. Fluconazole (Forcan, Zocon) 200 mg 2 tablets stat per week for 3 weeks (**or**)
   Tab. Ketoconazole (Nizral) 200 mg od for 4 weeks. It is a costly option without added benefits.

Ringworm of the Skin

Starts as a small patch, which spreads peripherally with an elevated border and central clearing. Depending on the sites, it is called tinea corporis (body), t. cruris (groins), t. pedis (feet), t. capitis (scalp), t. manum (hands), etc. (Fig.7.7)

Topically

- Candid powder after bath, in groins.
- Candid/Terbinafine/Zole/Nizral cream bd.

Systemically

- Tab. Griseofulvin (Grisactin forte) 250 mg bd × 3 weeks (**or**)
- Tab. Fluconazole (Zocon) 150 mg/week for 3 weeks.

In case of failure of treatment or severe forms

- Do HIV test and BSL.
- Tab. Ketoconazole (Nizral, Phytoral) 200 mg od for 14 days (**or**)
- Tab. Itraconazole (Sporonox) 100 mg bd for 7 days.

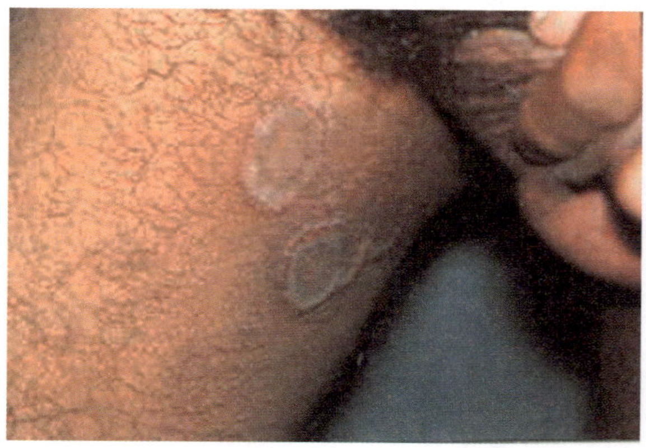

| Fig. 7.7 Fungal infection: groin |

Ringworm of Nails

- Tab. Griseofulvin as above for 6 months (**or**)
  Tab. Fluconazole as above for 12 weeks (**or**)
  Cap. Itraconazole 100 mg bd × 7 days followed by a drug free interval of 3 weeks. This is one pulse. Prescribe three such pulses. A costly treatment.
- Consider surgical removal of nails in resistant cases.

Monilial Intertrigo

Erythematous itchy lesions seen in between toes, especially in women who keep their feet soaked in water. Also seen in diabetics.

- For all candidial infections, Griseofulvin does not work.
- Tab. Fluconazole 150 mg/week × 4 weeks.
- Candid powder or Absorb powder during day time.
- Nizral ointment during night.
- R/O diabetes. Avoid prolonged soaking in water. Keep feet dry.

BACTERIAL INFECTIONS

Impetigo

Impetigo is a bacterial infection of the skin seen mainly in children. Usually starts around the nose and the mouth and if untreated, spreads to the trunk and the extremities. Initial lesion is a pustule, which bursts and discharges the fluid on the skin. This fluid dries to form a heavy crust, which is the hallmark of the disease. As the infection is beneath the crust, the removal of crust is of utmost importance in addition to local and systemic antibiotics. Caused by Streptococci and Staphylococci.

Ecthyma

Ecthyma looks similar to impetigo but the crusting is heavier, which when removed leaves a deep ulcer. Commonly seen on the legs.

Folliculitis or Furunculosis (Boils)

This is an infection of the hair follicles. Multiple indurated nodular lesions are seen here and there on the skin, which ripen in 2–3 days to form pus. Some lesions might get resolved without forming pus. Staphylococci are usually implicated.

Carbuncles (Fig. 7.5)

Carbuncles are a group of furuncles combining to form a large indurated lesion with multiple openings. They are commonly seen on the neck and back especially in diabetics. Usually caused by Staphylococci.

Erysipelas

It is a superficial lymphangitis of the skin involving the upper dermis. It is caused by Streptococci. The face and the lower extremities are the common sites. Diagnosis is made clinically by the typical large red patch with a sharp border.

Cellulitis

This involves the deeper subcutaneous layers and is usually seen on the legs. Systemic manifestations with severe pain and high grade fever is common. It can spread to deeper layers and then requires I & D under GA. Both Streptococci and Staphylococci are causative agents.

Treatment

As you can see the organisms responsible for skin infection are either Staphylococci or Streptococci.

For Staphylococci

Cloxacillin (Klox) 500 mg tds qid × 7–10 days is the drug of choice followed by cefadroxil (Odoxil) 500 mg bd or cefixime (Taxim-O) 200 mg bd.

For Streptococci

Inj. Procaine penicillin 8 lakhs IU IM AST × 1 week is the drug of choice. Azithromycin 500 mg od × 6 days is also effective. Ampicillin 500 mg qid is a time tested antibiotic against streptococci. When in doubt give a combination of ampicillin + cloxacillin (Baxin) qid, which will cover both the organisms.

Locally, fucidic acid (Fucidin) or mupirocin ointments (Bactroban) are very effective.

ECZEMA

The treatment of eczema will depend on whether the eczema is acute or chronic. Acute eczema is characterized by erythema and oozing while the chronic variety by thickening and lichenification.

Acute Oozing Eczema

a) Potassium permanganate soaks as described for Herpes zoster. This is followed by the application of:
b) Mild to moderately potent steroid ointment like clobetasol butyrate (Eumosone) or hydrocortisone acetate (Wycort).
c) Antibiotics, if secondary infection.
d) Antihistaminics have doubtful role.
e) Prednisolone (Wysolone) 5 mg bd × 7 days.

Chronic Lichenified Eczema

a) Potent steroid with salicylic acid, e.g., Dipsalic oint.
b) Tab. Prednisolone 5 mg tds × 7 days followed by 5 mg bd × 7 days.
c) If no response, give Inj. Kenacort intralesionally. 5–10 mg of Inj. Kenacort should be diluted with 2–3 mL of xylocaine and injected into the eczema. Multiple injections are given at 1 cm distances, finally to cover the whole eczema. This can be repeated after 1½ months. Make sure that there is no infection present before injecting Kenacort.

PSORIASIS

A chronic recurrent skin disease where we see well circumscribed erythematous raised plaques of various sizes, which are covered by thick silvery scales. These scales come off after scratching exposing a few bleeding points. Commonly seen on the scalp, elbows, knees, palms and soles. The disease is characterized by exacerbations and remissions.

- Tab. Prednisolone 5 mg tds for 8–10 days during acute exacerbations only.
- A potent steroid with Salicylic acid ointment, e.g., Dipsalic ointment, morning and bed time.
- Tar ointment in the afternoon, e.g., Exora ointment or Dithranol (Derobin) ointment.

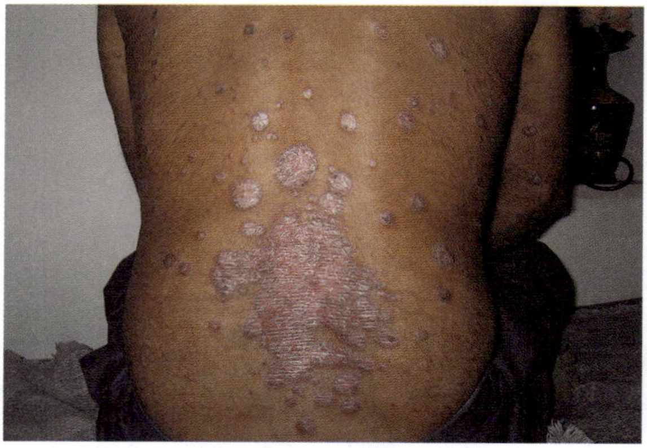

| **Fig. 7.8** Psoriasis |

In case there is no response:

- PUVA therapy can be tried. Give Tab. Neosoralen (Trioxsalen)—two tablets in the morning followed by exposure to sunlight for 15–20 min after 2 hrs.
- Tab. Methotrexate (Neotrexate) 2.5 mg od × 2–3 weeks. A potentially dangerous drug as it can cause sudden bone marrow depression; to be used by specialists only.

VITILIGO (Leucoderma)

The only effective treatment is PUVA therapy (Psoralens + UVA) which involves exposing the patches to sunlight after giving psoralen group of drugs. These drugs sensitize the skin to sunlight, which then induces erythema, inflammation and finally pigmentation.

Systemic Treatment

- Tab. Neosoralen 5 mg 2 tablets should be taken orally in the morning. The patches should be exposed to sunlight after 2 hrs, initially for 15 min and gradually increasing to 30 min over weeks.

Local Treatment

- Local Melanocyl ointment (or Neosoralen lotion diluted in equal amounts of rose water or spirit) should be used in addition in the afternoon.
- The surrounding normal skin is covered by paraminol cream, to prevent hyperpigmentation in the adjoining area.
- Tenovate cream (a potent steroid) should be applied at bed time, which also induces pigmentation.
- Eyes should be protected by using dark glasses during exposure.
- Good erythema results on the patches. If it does not, increase the exposure to sunlight by 5 min.
- Over a period of months, pigmentation should develop in the patches.

Severe erythema and bleb formation can take place in the patches. If so, stop PUVA treatment, apply Tenovate ointment 2–3 times a day till the reaction subsides. Then again restart the treatment using less exposure time with only one tablet of Neosoralen.

ALOPECIA (Loss of Hair)

This can be either localized, when the most common cause is *alopecia areata* or generalized, when it is called *diffuse alopecia.*

Alopecia Areata

There are two or three oval patches on the scalp or in the beard area. These are totally bald areas, have come all of a sudden and are asymptomatic.

First r/o tinea capitis, i.e., fungal infection of the scalp. Here the patches are not totally bald and broken hair are seen. There is intense itching. If so, treat with Tab. Grisiovin 250 mg bd × 3 weeks and Candid lotion to be applied locally bd.

- Betnovate or Dipsalic scalp lotion to be applied at bed time.
- Neosoralen lotion to be applied in the morning with cotton attached to a match-stick. Irritation caused by this medicine leads to stimulation of the hair roots and growth of hair.
- Minoxidil 2% or 5% solution (Gromane, Hebald) to be applied two times a day, can be used as an alternative to the above combination, if there is no response within 1½ months.
- Inj. Kenacort 1–2 mg diluted in about 1ml of Xylocaine can be injected directly into the patches in resistant cases.

Diffuse Alopecia

- Loss of few hair daily is quite normal and there is nothing to get alarmed. Explain this to the patient.
- Loss of hair after severe illness, e.g., typhoid fever, is to be expected and usually lasts for about 3 months. Loss of hair after pregnancy is physiological and lasts for a similar duration. The hair loss stops spontaneously. Take advantage of this fact, give placebo and take the credit!
- Few diseases are known to cause alopecia, e.g., excessive dandruff, hyperthyroidism, HIV infection, severe anaemia and hypoproteinaemia. Treat them, if present.
- The rest of the cases are idiopathic.

Male Pattern Baldness

- This is hereditary baldness seen in males. Loss of hair is maximum from the vertex and there is forehead recession on both sides.
- Apply Minoxidil solution 2% or 5% (Hebald or Gromane) on the affected area, 1 mL 2 times a day for at least 6 months for the growth of hair to be seen. Inform the patient that this treatment is life-long.
- Tab. Finasteride (Finpecia) 1 mg od × 6 months for the growth of hair to be seen. May be required life-long.
- Minoxidil locally and oral finasteride can be usefully combined.
- If this fails even after 1 year of proper treatment, the only alternative is hair transplant surgery. Hence, it is better to accept baldness gracefully as a sign of maturity and learn to live with it!

DANDRUFF

***For mild dandruff*:**

- Selenium sulphide (Selsun shampoo) to be applied biweekly (**or**)
- Endruff lotion biweekly.

For severe dandruff and those cases who have not responded:

- Ketoconazole (Nizral) shampoo biweekly.
- Tab. Nizral 200 mg od × 2 weeks.
- Betnovate scalp lotion to be applied at bedtime daily.

SEXUALLY TRANSMITTED DISEASES

The syndromic management of STDs is given here. This means that the general practitioner does not waste time in diagnosing specific venereal diseases like syphilis, chancroid, LGV, herpes, gonorrhoea, etc., but gives treatment as the patient presents to him. The patient can present to the doctor in one of the following ways:

1. Genital ulcer syndrome
2. Urethral discharge syndrome
3. Inguinal bubo syndrome

This approach is justified now because of the HIV epidemic. The priority is to cure the patient as fast as possible so that transmission of HIV is not facilitated through these ulcers or discharge. Always insist on an HIV test.

Genital Ulcer Syndrome

- Inj. Ceftriaxone (C-Tri, Monocef) 250 mg single dose stat IM. This is a painful injection, so mix with 2 mL Xylocaine, plus
- Tab. Doxycycline (Doxy 1) 100 mg bd × 10 days.

This should cure both syphilis and chancroid, which are the commonest causes of a genital ulcer. The other common cause of a genital ulcer is herpes genitalis, which is a viral infection and does not require treatment. Granuloma inguinale is one more cause of a genital ulcer but is very very rare in India.

Urethral Discharge Syndrome

- Inj. Ceftriaxone 250 mg stat single dose as above, plus
- Tab. Doxy 1 as above.

This should cover both gonococcal and non-gonococcal urethritis, which are the commonest causes of a urethral discharge.

Inguinal Bubo Syndrome

- The same above combination of single dose of Inj. Ceftriaxone followed by Tab. Doxycycline.

- Aspirate the buboes from a nondependent area, approaching from a healthy skin. Multiple aspirations may be required. Avoid the temptation to incise the bubo as a nonhealing sinus will result.

This same combination will cure syphilitic lymphadenopathy, chancroidal bubo and bubo of LGV.

Summary: So in any case of STD, treat with an injection of Ceftriaxone 250 mg IM stat followed by Doxy 1 bd ´ 10 days. Insist on an HIV test. Always treat the sexual partner.

MAGGOTS (Myiasis)

It is the infestation of infected wounds or foul smelling discharge in the nose or ear by the larvae of flies. Larvae can be seen if skin overlying the wound is removed.

a) Remove debris and enlarge opening of wound by multiple small incisions.
b) Pour turpentine oil over the wound.
c) As the maggots come out, remove them manually by toothed forceps.

MILIARIA RUBRA (Prickly Heat)

Common in the hot humid climate of summer. Excessive sweating during this period leads to blockage of sweat pores and rupture of sweat ducts into the epidermis. There are severely itchy erythematous papules on areas which sweat a lot, e.g., back, shoulders or face.

a) Keep skin cool by cold baths, fans, plenty of fresh air, etc.
b) Prickly heat powder (Dermicool) or any talcum powder—sprinkle liberally bd.
c) Tab. Azithromycin (Azee) 500 mg 1 hs before food × 3 days, if secondary infection is present.
d) Tab. Levocetrizine (Elriz) 5 mg hs × 1 week.

PITYRIASIS ALBA (Fig. 7.4)

These are asymptomatic oval hypopigmented patches on the face, especially on cheeks of children. The patches spontaneously disappear and reappear till child attains adulthood. Cause is not known but lay people and even doctors blame worms and calcium deficiency. R/o vitiligo where lesions are totally depigmented and patches are seen elsewhere on the body.

Treatment

- Mometasone (Elocon) cream, **or**
- Hydrocortisone (Lacticare) cream, **or**
- Prednicarbate (Dermatop) cream, **or**
- Clobetasone butarate (Eumosone) cream.

These are all mild steroids, safe on face. Apply thin layer bd, till patches disappear. Explain to parents that the condition is harmless and will disappear with time.

MELASMA (Chloasma)

Common condition seen mostly in females. Hyperpigmented patches seen on face mostly on cheeks, nose, forehead and around mouth. It usually follows pregnancy or OC pills. Sunlight increases pigmentation.

Treatment

a) Sunscreen agents (Shade or Sunban lotion) to be applied before exposure to sun.
b) Depigmentary ointments to be applied at bed time:
    - Hydroquinone (**or**)
    - Glycolic acid (**or**)
    - Azelic acid (**or**)
    - Combination ointment like Melacare (mometaone + tretinoin + hydroquinone)

Note: Continue local applications for at least 3 months. Educate patient about partial and temporary response.

MOLLUSCUM CONTAGIOSUM

These are flesh-coloured dome-shaped papules with central umbilication. The central core contains a cheesy material called "*molluscum body*." It is a viral infection. Multiple lesions are seen on the face in children and are transmitted via towels, in swimming pool, etc. In adults, they are present on genitalia and are transmitted sexually. They involute spontaneously within 6–24 months. Treated either by chemical or electric cautery.

Treatment

a) ***Chemical cautery***: Preferred in children.
   - Remove molluscum body with tip of needle.
   - Stop bleeding by pressure with wet gauze piece.
   - Touch raw area with 10–20% phenol or with tinc. iodine.
   - Small lesions can be pierced with tip of needle dipped in phenol without removing molluscum body.

b) ***Electric cautery***: Preferred when multiple lesions are present in genital area in adults. Molluscum body electrically burnt by a diathermy machine. Refer to a dermatologist. Always advise an HIV test in sexually active adults.

CHAPTER 8

Ophthalmic Conditions

- Stye
- Blepharitis
- Acute Conjunctivitis
- Xerosis of Conjunctiva
- Acute Dacryocystitis
- Angular Conjunctivitis
- Spring Catarrh
- Corneal Ulcer
- Chalazion
- Senile Cataract

STYE

It is an infection of the hair follicle of the eyelid. A red painful nodular swelling is seen at the eyelid margin, of 4–5 days duration, along with a diffuse swelling of the eyelid. The swelling may ripen and drain spontaneously. Recurrence is common.

- Hot compresses hasten ripening.
- Ciprofloxacin (Ciplox) eye drops qid (or) Tobramycin eyedrops qid.
- Cap. Cephelexin (Phexin) 500 mg qid.
- If pus points at lid margin, pull out a hair to drain.
- If pus points on the skin of the lid, incise using a horizontal incision. A small pus pocket will drain spontaneously.

BLEPHARITIS

The margins of the eyelids are red and swollen and there are many scales at the base of the eye lashes. It is a chronic condition.

- Ask the patient to remove scales with a wet handkerchief before applying ointment.
- Rub Neosporin H eye ointment on the lid margins.
- Repeat above procedure tds × 10–15 days.
- Treat dandruff of scalp if present. This will prevent recurrence (see p. 48).

ACUTE CONJUNCTIVITIS

There is redness, watering and foreign body sensation in the eye. In bacterial conjunctivitis, there is a mucopurulent discharge due to which the eyelids stick together on waking. In viral conjunctivitis, discharge is mucoid or serous.

- Keep patient's towel separate, not to be used by family members.
- If only one eye is affected, prevent infection to the other by lying on the affected side.
- Dark goggles, if photophobia.
- Wash with boiled and cooled water before instillation of eye drops.
- Antibiotic eye drops 2 hourly (Genticyn, Ciplox, Norflox etc.).
- Avoid antibiotic + steroid eye drops.

- Antibiotic eye ointment at bed time (Chloromycetin applicaps).
- In severe cases, Cap. Amoxicillin (Novamox) 500 tds × 5 days.

In an epidemic, it is easy to diagnose conjunctivitis. Otherwise, always rule out iridocyclitis.

XEROSIS OF THE CONJUNCTIVA AND BITOT'S SPOTS

These are signs of Vitamin A deficiency. The eye looks dry and lustreless. Bitot's spots are seen as rough triangular white patches in the conjunctiva, on the side of the cornea.

- Moisol (Methyl cellulose eye drops)
- Inj. Aquasol A 2 mL IM every week × 3 weeks.
- Tab. Multivit FM od × 1 month.
- Sunglasses
- Diet rich in vit A (milk, milk products, egg, green vegetables, carrot, etc.)

ACUTE DACRYOCYSTITIS

Infection of the lacrimal sac results in erythema and swelling on the lateral side of the nose unilaterally, just below the medial side of the lower eye lid. In severe cases, the cheek and the lower eyelid is also swollen. If not treated properly, pus points below the medial part of the eye and bursts leaving a permanent fistula.

- Genticyn eye drops 5–6 times a day.
- Cap. Cephalexin (Sporidex) 500 mg qid × 7 days.
- Tab. Voveran 100 mg bd × 7 days.
- If pus points, a small incision is made into the skin and the pus is drained.

Once the infection has subsided, refer to ophthalmologist for surgical treatment.

ANGULAR CONJUNCTIVITIS

There is erythema of the conjunctiva at the angle of the eye along with eczematous condition of the skin near the canthi. It is a subacute infection caused by bacteria and is contagious.

- Zincosulpha eye drops qid.
- Neosporin H eye ointment bd. Apply inside the eye as well as to the affected skin near the angle of the eyelids.
- If no response, Pyrimon eye drops (antibiotic + steroid) qid × 1 week.

SPRING CATARRH

It is a chronic allergic conjunctivitis seen commonly in young individuals and comes in summer and disappears in winter. Lasts for several years and then subsides spontaneously. The patient c/o burning sensation in the eyes with intense itching and profuse lacrimation. Absolute eosinophilic count confirms the diagnosis. Treatment is symptomatic.

- Steroid + antibiotic eye drops 4 times a day. (Pyrimon, Sofracort, Dexaber-C, etc.).
- Cromolyn (Fintal) 2% eye drops, 1 drop 4 times a day to prevent recurrences.
- Tab. Loratidine (Lorfast) 10 mg od (or) Tab. Levocetrizine (Xyzal) 5 mg od.

Do not prescribe steroid eye drops continuously for more than 3 weeks without review by an ophthalmologist.

CORNEAL ULCER

The patient presents with severe pain and photophobia and profuse lacrimation of the affected eye. O/e there is a small ulcer on the cornea. The area surrounding the cornea has bluish blood vessels radiating outwards from the limbus. Most of these ulcers are caused by bacterial infections; a few are due to viruses and fungi. Treat as bacterial at least initially.

- Ciplox eye drops 2 hourly (plus) Tobramycin eye drops 2 hrly.
- Homatropine or atropine eye drops tds.
- Chloromycetin applicaps at bed time.
- Oral analgesics, e.g., Diclofenac.
- Cap. Amoxicillin 500 mg qid × 5 days.

If after 2 days there is no response—refer, as late referral can lead to perforation.

CHALAZION

Painless, hard swelling on the eyelid at some distance from the lid margin may be confused with a stye. It is due to chronic inflammation of *Meibomian* glands.

- For small chalazion of short duration (a few days) warm compresses followed by gentle massage and antibiotic eye drops.
- For moderate size chalazion, try intralesional steroid injection.
- Large size chalazion of long duration requires incision and curettage (refer Chapter 38).

Local triamcinolone injection for chalazion—method

First give Inj. Xylocaine on the skin surface in the area surrounding the chalazion. Wait for 2 min. Then, give Inj. Triamcinolone (Kenacort) 10 mg/mL vial, 0.2 mL inside the chalazion from the conjunctiva surface with an insulin syringe.

SENILE CATARACT

Gradually progressive painless opacities, resulting in diminution of vision, occur in old age. Examination with torch light reveals white opacities in the lens.

- No drug available to prevent or treat cataract.
- Only treatment is surgical, i.e., lens extraction and replacement with artificial lens. Refer to an ophthalmologist.
- If surgery not immediately possible, correct refractory error by prescribing spectacles and control diabetes and hypertension, if present.
- It is not necessary to wait for immature cataract to mature with time for surgery.
- Delay in surgery may lead to complications such as lens-induced glaucoma, iritis or displacement of lens. Refer on diagnosis.

*This chapter has been reviewed by **Dr Mrudula Patil**, MD Ophthalmology, Deenanath Hospital, Pune.*

GP Tip

Easily instilling eye drops in children
- Force is useless.
- Preferably, instill when the child is asleep.
- When awake, instill a drop at the inner canthus of the closed eye. The child will open the eye and the medicine will then spread smoothly.

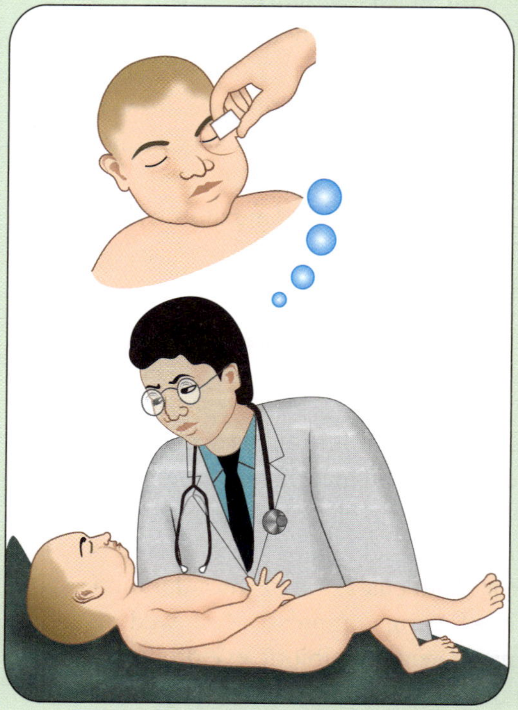

CHAPTER 9

ENT Conditions

- Pain in Throat
- Nasal Obstruction
- Common Cold
- Acute Sinusitis
- Chronic Otorrhoea
- Earache
- Tinnitus
- Traumatic Perforation of the Ear Drum
- Furuncle in the Nose
- Allergic Rhinitis
- Bleeding through Nose
- ASOM
- Wax in Ear
- Halitosis

PAIN IN THROAT

Acute Pharyngitis

It is a viral or a bacterial infection. There is burning sensation in the throat. Pain is increased while swallowing. It may be associated with headache, fever and rhinitis.

a) Steam inhalation with Tinc. Benzoin or Vicks.
b) Azithromycin 500 mg od × 3 days.
c) Ibuprofen + Paracetamol (Ibugesic plus), if fever or headache.
d) Tab. Zyrtec-D bd, if rhinitis.

Chronic Pharyngitis

Chronic irritation in the throat often with a foreign body sensation. O/e the posterior pharyngeal wall is full of pink or red granules. Usually, it is a part of some pathology in the nasal sinuses. The common causes are:

a) Smoking (smoker's throat).
b) Chronic nasal block forces the patient to be a 'mouth breather', leading to chronic pharyngitis.
c) Chronic infection in the respiratory tract, e.g., tonsillitis, sinusitis, bronchitis.
d) Air pollution.

Treatment

a) Steam inhalation.
b) Treat the pathology in the sinus or bronchus.
c) Mandl's paint applied to the throat is soothing.
d) Remove the cause like smoking and treat the associated respiratory infection.

Acute Tonsillitis

Exudates are seen in the crypts of the tonsils with surrounding inflammation. Lymph nodes below the angle of the mandible (jugulo-digastric) are enlarged and tender. Severe pain while swallowing. Fever is usually present.

- Inj. Procaine penicillin 8 lakhs IM. AST × 5 days (**or**)
- Tab. Azithromycin (Aziwok) 500 mg od × 3 days (**or**)

- Tab. Cefadroxil (Odoxil) 500 mg bd × 5 days.
- Symptomatic treatment.

Quinsy (Peritonsillar Abscess)

There is severe one sided pain in the throat, which radiates to the ear. Swallowing is painful and there is difficulty in opening the mouth (trismus). O/e swelling and redness is seen near the tonsil and the uvula may be pushed to opposite side.

a) Inj. Procaine penicillin or Azithromycin as above.
b) Analgesics
c) Incision and drainage is required if abscess forms. Refer to ENT surgeon.

Diphtheria

Diphtheria is seen rarely these days because of immunisation. If a white patch is seen on the throat, which cannot be removed with the tongue depressor without bleeding—refer immediately.

> Tonsillitis or pharyngitis in children are usually due to Streptococci. If not treated with proper antibiotics, rheumatic heart disease or glomerulonephritis may result.

NASAL OBSTRUCTION

Two sets of patients are seen in practice. A few have permanent blockage of one nostril. The majority have intermittent blockage of both the nostrils. If the block is unilateral and permanent, the patient should be referred to an ENT surgeon.

Causes of Unilateral & Permanent Obstruction

a) Severe deviated nasal septum (DNS).
b) Nasal polyps: These are seen as smooth pearly white swellings in the nostril.
c) Foreign body in children.
e) A malignant tumour in old patients.

These conditions cannot be managed by a GP.

Causes of Bilateral & Intermittent Obstruction

a) Mild DNS
b) Hypertrophy of the inferior turbinates
c) Chronic sinusitis
d) Chronic allergic rhinitis

These conditions can be managed by a GP.

Treatment

a) Nasivion or Otrivin nasal drops, 2 drops sos. Use infrequently as far as possible as it is habit forming and causes rebound nasal blockage.
b) Tab. Cetrizine (Cetzine) 10 mg od.
c) Rhinocort nasal spray (Budesonide) in each nostril 2 times a day.
d) Tab. Wysolone 5 mg tds for short courses.

COMMON COLD

It is caused by virus infecting the nasal mucosa. It is a self-limiting condition and resolves spontaneously within a week. Hence only symptomatic treatment is needed unless secondary bacterial infection has taken place.

- Decongestant nasal drops (like Nasivion) 2–3 times a day.
- Steam inhalation with tinc. Benzoin is comforting.
- Tab. Cetrizine + Pseudoephedrine (Zyrtec D) bd × 5 days.
- Cap. Amoxicillin (Mox) 500 mg tds, if the discharge becomes thick, yellow or purulent.

ACUTE SINUSITIS

Either the maxillary or the frontal sinuses or both may get infected. In *maxillary sinusitis*, the pain in the maxillary region is aggravated on bending down, coughing or sneezing.

In *frontal sinusitis*, the pain in the frontal region is severe in the morning due to collection of secretions in the night in the lying down position. It gradually subsides during the day due to drainage in the vertical position.

X-ray of the paranasal sinus (Water's view) will show haziness or fluid level in these sinuses.

- Cap. Amoxclav (Augmentin) 625 mg tds × 7 days
- Tab. Actifed bd × 7 days.
- Tab. Ibuprofen 400 + Paracetamol 500 mg (Ibugesic plus) tds.
- Otrivin nasal drops.
- Steam inhalation with tinc. Benzoin.

CHRONIC OTORRHOEA

Discharge from the ear. First note the type of the discharge:

- *Serous* discharge may be due to otitis externa.
- *Purulent* discharge may come from middle ear infection with perforation of the drum.
- *Foul smelling* discharge may be due to cholesteatoma.
- *Bloody* discharge may be due to trauma, tumour or polyp.
- Black discharge may be due to fungal infection.

Treatment

- Keep the ear dry by cleaning with Johnson's ear buds each time before instilling ear drops.
- Genticyn or Chloromycetin or Ciprofloxacin ear drops 3–4 times/day.
- Cap. Cephalexin (Phexin) 500 mg qid × 7 days **(or)**
  Cap. Amoxclav (Augmentin) 625 mg tds × 7 days **(or)**
  Tab. Azithromycin 500 mg od × 6 days.
- Tab. Zyrtec D bd × 7 days.
- Otrivin or Nasivion nasal drops tds.
- Tab. Bromhexine 8 mg tds × 7 days.

If the discharge persists, refer to ENT specialist for further treatment, possibly tympanoplasty.

EARACHE

An otoscope is a very useful, economical and basic instrument which all GPs should keep in their clinics. The external auditory canal and the tympanic membrane can be visualized very clearly and the diagnosis made easily. The first step when the patient c/o pain in the ear is to examine the external ear with an otoscope or at least with a powerful torch to find out the cause of the pain.

Examination may Reveal

1. ***Impacted wax***: This is the most common condition.
   - First try to remove it by a wax hook or a vectis. Pass the hook beyond the wax and pull it out by gentle traction. If it causes pain because the wax is very hard, abandon the procedure.
   - Prescribe Soliwax or Waxolve ear drops to be instilled 5–6 times a day.
   - Remove the softened wax after 5–6 days using an aural syringe (see procedures). If the syringe is not available, remove it by a vectis or wax-hook.
   - Do not use hydrogen peroxide or ear buds.
2. ***Furuncle***: Furuncle in the ear canal can be easily diagnosed as it is very tender to touch.
   - Hot fomentation to ear.
   - Tab. Azithromycin 500 mg od × 6 days.
   - Cap. Amoxclav (Augmentin) 625 mg tds × 7 days.
   - Tab. Voveran 100 mg bd.
   - Otogesic ear drops 3–4 times a day.
   - Local dressing with glycerine.
3. ***Otomycosis***: This is a fungal infection of the external auditory canal. It can be seen as a

white cotton like mass with black spores in the mass. There is itching and pain.

- Remove the debris with a wax hook or a cotton bud.
- Instill Candid ear drops 3–4 drops tds.
- Tab. Cetrizine (Cetzine) 10 mg od, if itching is severe.
- Cap. Amoxclav (Augmentin) 625 mg tds × 7 days, if secondary infection.
- Remove the debris again after 5 days.
- Avoid antibiotic plus steroid ear drops.
- Treatment to be given at least for 6 weeks.

If Examination does not Reveal Any Abnormality

The pain could be due to:

1. ***Acute otitis media or blockage of the eustachian tube***
   - Cap. Baxin 500 mg qid × 5 days.
   - Tab. Voveran 100 mg bd × 5 days.
   - Otrivin nasal drops to keep the tube patent.
   - Tab. Zyrtec-D bd × 5 days.
2. ***Referred pain from***
   - Tonsil (quinsy)
   - Tooth (impacted wisdom tooth)
   - Temporomandibular joint (arthritis)
   - Examine and treat accordingly.
3. ***Mastoiditis***: It is a complication of otitis media. Diagnosis is made by the h/o otitis media and by severe tenderness on the mastoid bone behind the pinna.
   - Tab. Cefuroxime (Ceftum) 250 mg bd × 7 days.
   - Tab. Voveron 100 mg bd.
   - Tab. Chymoral forte qid.
   - Refer to ENT specialist. Patients with mastoiditis are better managed by ENT specialists.

TINNITUS (Ringing in the Ears)

It is very common but annoying symptom and at the same time very difficult to treat. Hence if the treatment given below does not help the patient, then refer to ENT specialist.

- Remove local cause, e.g., wax or otitis media.
- Tab. Complamina retard bd.
- Tab. Carbamazepine (Tegretol) 100 mg tds.
- Tab. Alprazolam (Restyl) 0.25 mg bd.
- Masking the tinnitus by background noise, e.g., music. If no response, refer.

TRAUMATIC PERFORATION OF EAR DRUM

Usually, the trauma is caused by a slap or accidental injury. Otoscope is essential for diagnosis.

- No local antibiotic or any other ear drops.
- Keep ear absolutely dry.
- Tab. Cephalexin (Phexin) 500 mg qid (**or**) Cap. Amoxclav (Augmentin) 625 mg tds × 7 days.
- Tab. Ciprofloxacin 500 mg bd × 7 days.
- Tab. Diclofenac (Voveran) 100 mg bd.

If after 6 weeks, the perforation does not heal, refer to ENT specialist.

FURUNCLE IN THE NOSE (Vestibulitis)

The boil can be seen easily in the nose. It is very painful and tender to touch. Cellulitis of the skin of the nose may develop.

- Fucidin ointment locally two times a day.
- Cap. Cephalexin (Phexin) 500 mg qid × 5 days (**or**)
  Cap. Amoxclav (Augmentin) 625 mg tds × 7 days.
- Tab. Diclofenac 100 mg bd.

- Do not squeeze the boil.
- If recurrent in an old patient, do blood sugar.

ALLERGIC RHINITIS

This condition is due to hypersensitivity of mucous membrane of nose to allergens. The allergens are usually difficult to recognize. Hence, permanent cure is difficult. But, symptoms can be controlled with treatment. Two types of patients are seen:

1. **Seasonal allergic rhinitis (SAR)**: The patient has attacks of sneezing, watery discharge and itching in the nose only during particular seasons.
2. **Perennial allergic rhinitis (PAR)**: The patient has symptoms almost throughout the year. Discharge is thick, there is post nasal discharge and nasal block.

Treatment

1. Tab. Levocetrizine (Xyzal) 5 mg hs **(or)**
   Tab. Cetrizine (Zyrtec) 10 mg hs **(or)**
   Tab. Loratidine (Lorfast) 10 mg hs.
   To be taken till symptoms continue.
2. *If blocking of nose*
   Normal saline nasal drops (Nasomist) **(or)**
   Xylometazoline nasal drops (Otrivin) **(or)**
   Oxymetazoline nasal drops (Nasivion)
   1–2 drops in each nostril 2–3 times/day.
3. *If symptoms continue*
   Rhinocort nasal spray (Budesonide) in each nostril 2 times a day.
4. *If symptoms still persist*
   Tab. Prednisolone (Wysolone) 5 mg tds 7 days.

BLEEDING THROUGH NOSE (Epistaxis)

1. Make the patient sit up and pinch the nostrils firmly below the nasal bones. Wait for 10 min. Ask the patient to breathe through the mouth and spit out the blood collected in the throat. In the mean time, monitor pulse and BP.
2. Remove the pinch after 10 min and check, if fresh bleeding occurs.
3. If fresh bleeding does occur, break an ampoule of adrenaline. Dilute it in 5–10 mL of normal saline or water for injection. Soak two gauze pieces in this solution and pack both the nostrils tightly with these gauze pieces.
4. Remove the packs after 10 min and watch again for fresh bleeding. If bleeding has not stopped, refer to ENT specialist for posterior nasal pack or cautery or arterial ligation, etc.

ACUTE SUPPURATIVE OTITIS MEDIA (ASOM)

Acute infection of middle ear cavity following upper respiratory tract infection. There is severe throbbing pain. The ear drum finally perforates and pus is discharged through the ear.

1. Tab. Ibuprofen (400 mg) + Paracetamol (500 mg) (Ibugesic plus) sos.
2. Cap. Amoxicillin (Mox) 500 mg tds × 7 days, **(or)**
   Cap. Cephalexin (Phexin) 500 mg qid × 7 days.
3. Xylometazoline (Otrivin) nasal drops in each nostril 2–3 times/day. If there is severe pain and pus is not drained through spontaneous perforation, refer to ENT specialist for myringotomy.

WAX IN EAR

Wax in small quantities does not cause any symptoms and should be left alone. If impacted however, it can cause pain, deafness, tinnitus, reflex cough, vertigo, etc., and then has to be removed.

1. Tab. Diclofenac (Voveran) 100 mg bd.

2. Soliwax ear drops to be instilled in the ear for 5 days to soften the wax.
3. This is followed by removal by syringing or by a hook.

Removal of wax

- ***Syringing***—Take lukewarm water in aural syringe. To dislodge the wax, water is directed with force on the posterior wall of the meatus. Mop the external canal dry with cotton after the wax has come out. Before syringing, ensure that there is no perforation in the ear drum by asking H/o discharge through the ear.
- ***Removal with hook***—Use good light to make wax fully visible. Put hook behind the wax and pull out with firm and steady force. Take care not to injure the ear drum by ensuring that the hook does not go more than 2.5 cm deep into the external auditory canal.
- Do not use ear buds as they can push the wax deeper.

HALITOSIS

Halitosis means unpleasant smelling breath. It is sensed by the patient as well as the observer. The ammoniacal smelling breath of renal failure, fishy odour of hepatic failure and fruity odour of ketoacidosis are seen in indoor patients.

Halitophobia is a condition where patient perceives his or her breath as unpleasant, which is actually not.

Common Causes

- Transient—due to strong smelling substances like garlic, onion, alcohol, etc.
- Periodontal disease, caries, gingivitis, gum abscess, Vincent's angina, etc.
- Sinusitis
- Atrophic rhinitis
- Lung abscess, Bronchiectasis
- Renal failure
- Hepatic failure
- Ketoacidosis

Management

- Treat the cause.
- For oral infective conditions like gum abscess, gingivitis, etc., give Chlorhexidine (Hexidine) mouthwash and refer to a dentist.
- Oral hygiene.

*This chapter has been reviewed by **Dr Naina Karodpati**, ENT Specialist, Pune.*

CHAPTER 10

Dental Conditions

TOOTHACHE

A. ***If inspection of the painful tooth reveals caries with a cavity*** (which is the commonest cause).
   - Soak a cotton bud in clove oil and pack it firmly in the carious cavity. This gives instant pain relief for a few hours.
   - Tab. Ibuprofen and Paracetamol (Ibuflam plus) sos. This can be taken every 3–4 hrs.
   - Refer to dentist for filling the cavity or extraction.

B. ***If jaw is swollen***, this could be periodontal or alveolar abscess.
   - Cap. Amoxicillin (Novamox) 500 mg tds × 5–7 days.
   - Tab. Metronidazole (Flagyl) 400 mg tds × 5–7 days.
   - Tab. Diclofenac (Voveran) 100 mg bd × 5–7 days.
   - Tab. Chymoral forte qid × 5–7 days.
   - Refer to dentist for further management.

C. Then, examine the gums for signs of inflammation. If present, it is ***gingivitis*** or ***gum abscess***.
   - Amoxicillin + Metronidazole + Diclofenac as above.
   - Betadine mouthwash 10 mL bd, held in mouth for at least 2 min.
   - Gum massage with fingers, tds.
   - Use dental floss, bd.
   - Brush carefully at gum line with Sensodyne toothpaste.
   - Take dental opinion, if there is no response or if there is a relapse.

D. If gingivitis or apical abscess are absent, examine the **3rd molar** to see if there is a partially erupted (***pericoronitis***) or impacted wisdom tooth, which is a common cause of pain. Pericoronitis causes trismus, pain while swallowing, pain radiating to the temporal region, headache and mild fever.
   - Amoxicillin + Metronidazole + Diclofenac as above.

- Refer to dentist for X-ray and corrective treatment.

E. ***If the teeth look normal***:
- Examine closely for impacted *vegetable matter*, e.g., guava seed in-between the teeth. If present, remove it with a hypodermic needle.
- Try to identify the offending tooth by tapping teeth vertically in the area of suspicion with a hard instrument like a forceps. The patient will feel sharp pain in the offending tooth if there is infection below the tooth, i.e., *apical abscess*.
  i) Amoxicillin + Metronidazole + Diclofenac as above.
  ii) Refer to dentist for draining of the abscess.
- Finally, if none of the above are present, is it a *non-dental pain?* Consider:
  i) Referred pain from sinuses, ears, nose or pharynx.
  ii) Migraine.
  iii) Trigeminal or postherpetic neuralgia.
  iv) Angina pectoris.

  If any of the above is present, treat accordingly.

HYPERSENSITIVE TEETH

This is a common condition seen in middle age and old age. Because of the recession of the gums, the root may be exposed, which is highly sensitive to hot, cold, sweet or sour food or drink. Also the enamel may be worn out because of physiological wear and tear, forceful brushing and habit of daily drinking of lime juice or regurgitation of gastric acid in the mouth, which erodes the enamel, exposing the more sensitive dentine.

- Advise proper dental hygiene.
- Use a soft toothbrush, which should be changed every 3 months or so.
- Avoid hard toothbrushes, harsh tooth powders, burnt tobacco or charcoal for brushing teeth.
- Advise use of medicated de-sensitizing tooth paste like Senolin (contains Strontium chloride) or Sensoform (contains formalin) or Sensicure–K (contains Potassium nitrate).
- If a single tooth is hypersensitive, this could be due to unsatisfactory filling, etc. Refer to a dentist.

INFECTIONS OF THE GUMS

1. Generalized (gingivitis) when there are pus pockets in the gums. There is pain, foul smell and the gums bleed to touch.
   - Amoxicillin + Metronidazole + Diclofenac as above.
   - Tab. Vit. C (Celin) 500 mg bd × 15 days.
   - Betadine mouthwash bd.
   - Regular brushing with soft toothbrush.
   - Gum massage.
   - Advise use of dental floss, to clean spaces in between teeth.
   - Avoid tobacco, Manikchand and chocolates.
   - Refer to dentist for scaling (removal of tartar).
2. Localized to one tooth (gum boil).
   Usually due to infection coming from the apex of a tooth (apical or periapical abscess). There is toothache, pain in the gums and a gumboil.
   - Amoxicillin + Diclofenac + Metronidazole as above.
   - Refer to a dentist.
3. Localized inflammation of a part of a gum on a partially erupted or an unerupted tooth (pericoronitis).
   - Refer to a dentist for X-rays and possibly minor surgical intervention.

BLEEDING GUMS

The most common cause of bleeding gums is gingival infection (gingivitis or periodontitis).

If the gums are normal and not inflamed or ulcerated, one should always think of systemic cause like platelet disorder or blood dyscrasias (acute leukaemia or aplastic anaemia). Contrary to the popular belief, scurvy is a rare cause of bleeding gums these days as Vit. C deficiency is rare. Coagulation defects rarely cause gum bleeding except in very severe cases.

Management

- Always rule out systemic causes if gums look normal. Advice haemogram, platelet count and if normal, advise coagulation factor studies.
- ***If gingivitis***:
  - Cap. Amoxicillin (Mox) 500 mg tds × 5–7 days.
  - Tab. Metrogyl (Flagyl) 400 ml bd × 5–7 days.
  - Good oral hygiene.
  - Gargle with Listerine mouthwash or dilute hydrogen peroxide solution.
  - Gentle gum massage.
  - Dental gloss usage.

This is What Patients Usually Say...

1. "Extraction of the upper teeth results in refractory errors making it necessary to wear spectacles".
   Wrong.
2. "I did not bring my baby for treatment because I thought the diarrhoea was because of teething".
   Teething is seen during weaning when diarrhoea is common. Hence the common man's association. There is nothing called "physiological diarrhoea."
3. "Don't refer me to a dentist. It's such a painful treatment".
   Wrong. That was true 2–3 decades ago, not now.
4. "Anyway, my teeth are going to be shed off in a few years. Why bother?"
   Unlike milk teeth, the permanent teeth do not have a specific age for shedding. With proper dental care, the life of the teeth can be prolonged indefinitely.
5. "Wisdom teeth should never be extracted".
   If a wisdom tooth erupts in a wayward direction causing problem to the adjoining bone or tooth, it is wise to remove it.
6. My friend says "Regular professional cleaning (scaling) weakens the teeth."
   No. Removing tartar regularly is essential to prevent periodontal disease.
7. "I apply *burnt* tobacco (*mishri*). This does not cause oral cancer".
   Tobacco is tobacco (raw or burnt) and cancer is cancer.
8. "Shall I remove my teeth for my arthritis?"
   Four to five decades ago even doctors believed this and advised extraction. Not today.
9. "Pregnant women should not be advised extraction of teeth".
   False. Tooth extraction cannot cause foetal anomalies.
10. "Dental treatment is very costly".
    Very true. Hence prevention is better than cure.

Don't Refer to a Dentist...

1. All cases of *bleeding gums* without gingivitis should be given Tab. Vit. C (Celin) 500 mg bd (for treatment of scurvy, which is rare) but simultaneously investigated for blood dyscrasias and leukaemias. Order haemo-

gram, BT/CT/PT. In case of abnormal reports (presence of blast cells or abnormal WBC count), refer to a *physician* for opinion.

2. An ulcer on the cheek, lips or palate not healing for more than 2 weeks—think of *oral cancer* and refer to a *surgeon*.
3. If a diffuse dense white patch is seen on the soft palate or pharynx associated with difficulty in opening the mouth (trismus), this is *submucus fibrosis*. It is caused by eating tobacco, pan-masala and betel-nuts. It is a precancerous condition. Refer to an *ENT specialist*.

*This chapter has been reviewed by **Dr Milind Desai**, Dentist, Pune.*

GP Tip

Want to examine a child's throat without a struggle?

- Keep the tongue depressor away and ask the child to put out his tongue and pant like a dog!

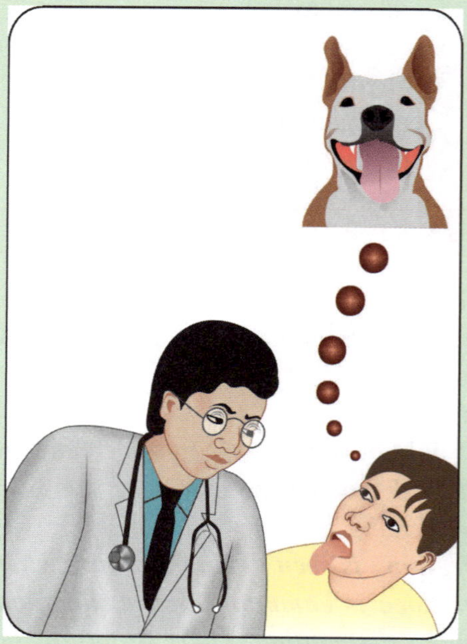

CHAPTER 11

Renal Conditions

- Lower Urinary Tract Infection
- Haematuria
- Management of Urinary Calculi
- Bed-wetting
- Benign Enlargement of Prostate
- Acute Glomerulonephritis
- Acute Pyelonephritis
- Chronic Pyelonephritis

LOWER URINARY TRACT INFECTION

The patient presents to a GP in various ways:

- With burning micturition.
- As an STD, when he has pus per urethra.
- As fever with chills with or without burning micturition.
- As a scrotal swelling, when urine examination reveals pus cells.
- During routine investigation.

Management

1. ***Request for urine examination***:
   If urine shows pus cells > 5 per high power field, the diagnosis is confirmed. Request for a urine culture sensitivity test, before starting antibiotics.
2. ***Start one of the following antibiotics***:
   - Tab. Norfloxacin (Norflox) 400 mg bd.
   - Tab. Ciprofloxacin (Cifran) 500 mg bd.
   - Tab. Sparfloxacin (Sparta) 200 mg od.
   - Tab. Cotrimoxazole (Cilplin DS) bd.
   - Tab. Nalidixic acid (Gramoneg) 500 mg qid.
   - Tab. Nitrofurantion (Furadantin) 100 mg qid.
   - Fosfomycin sachet (Monurol) 3 g single dose (Dissolve in a cup of water and drink 1 hr before meal).
3. ***Give in addition, symptomatic treatment***:
   - Cital liquid 1 tsf in a glass of water tds.
   - Plenty of oral fluids.
   - Tab. Pyridium 200 mg 2 tds, if burning is severe.
4. ***Await the culture report, meanwhile do relevant investigation***:
   - USG abdomen, if there is pain in loin or abdomen.
   - Scrotal USG, if there is swelling of the scrotum.
   - Urethral swab for gonococci, if there is h/o exposure.
5. ***Repeat urine examination after 5 days***:
   - If no pus cells in urine—continue the treatment for 5 more days.

- If pus cells still present, select appropriate antibiotic depending on culture-sensitivity report.
- If symptomatically not better after 10 days and urine still shows pus cells—refer.

- Pain in loin with UTI could be acute pyelonephritis.
- Scrotal swelling is usually acute epididymoorchitis.
- Both patients are better managed in a hospital.
- Always collect urine in a sterile bottle before giving antibiotics. A single tablet can affect the culture-sensitivity report.

HAEMATURIA

When the patient c/o of haematuria, he usually comes to the clinic with the urine sample to show to the doctor. The urine is reddish brown in colour. Is it blood in the urine? Is it jaundice? Is it due to B-complex tablet? Ask the patient to get the urine examination (routine) and USG abdomen done.

If the urine shows RBCs and pus cells, treat as UTI. Most common cause for haematuria is cystitis in females and prostatitis in males.

USG abdomen may show calculi, another common cause of haematuria. Treat as given below.

If no calculi in USG abdomen and haematuria persists after 5 days of antibiotics—refer to a urologist for further work up.

Haematuria is a symptom and not a disease. It is a serious symptom and even a single episode of haematuria has to be investigated till the diagnosis is made.

MANAGEMENT OF URINARY CALCULI

The role of a GP in treating urinary calculi is four-fold.

1. Treatment of an acute attack (see ureteric colic).
2. Give hydrotherapy, if stones are small (<6 mm) and there is no associated hydronephrosis.
3. Establish the location, number and size of each stone by means of KUB, USG or IVU. All calcium containing stones are visible on plain X-ray of kidney-ureter-bladder (KUB), but uric acid or cystine stones are usually not visualised. Hence, also advise an ultra sonography (USG) of the abdomen. All stones are visualised in a USG though very small stones and ureteric stones lying behind intestinal gas can be missed. Intravenous urography (IVU) demonstrates them as 'filling defects'. This is a costly and a risky procedure and is really not needed in general practice.
4. Educate the patient about the treatment-options available. This question is usually put to the family doctor. Treatment depends on the location and size of the stone.
   - **Kidney**: Small stones may pass. Large stones (up to 3 cm) can be fragmented by shock waves generated under water. The fragments are then passed in the urine. This is called **extra corporal shock wave lithotripsy (ESWL)** or **simply lithotripsy**, costing about Rs.10,000/-. ESWL is a noninvasive procedure, no incisions and no passage of scopes. Staghorn stones or stones larger than 3 cm are removed by percutaneous nephrolithotomy (PCNL). Here, through a small key hole incision in the loin, the stone is fragmented and removed.

- **Ureters**: Around 90% of stones of <8 mm in size pass spontaneously. Stones of <1 cm in size and lying in the lower third of the ureter can be removed by an ureteroscope either intact or after fragmentation with a lithoclast. Stones larger than 1 cm and lying in the upper 2/3rd of the ureter have to be removed surgically.
- **Bladder**: Stones can be crushed endoscopically with a lithoclast and the fragments washed out of the bladder. Usually bladder stones are secondary to obstruction of the bladder neck or urethra, which should also be corrected by surgery.

BED-WETTING (Nocturnal Enuresis)

Passing of urine involuntarily in bed at night is considered significant, if this continues in a child after the age of 6 years. After this age, investigate with USG abdomen for urinary tract abnormalities and a blood sugar test for juvenile diabetes. If normal, give the following advice to the parents:

- Do not stop the child from drinking water after dinner, but explain to him the benefits of not drinking.
- Remind him to pass urine before going to sleep.
- If possible, wake him up at night to pass urine.
- Tell the child to hold urine as long as possible during the day.
- Praise the child in the morning, if he does not pass urine in the bed at night. Do not scold, if he does.

If the above measures fail, give:

- Tab. Imipramine (Dapsonil) 25 mg 2 hs × 3 months.
- Desmopressin (D-void) nasal spray in lower part of each nostril at night. It is a synthetic antidiuretic hormone.

BENIGN ENLARGEMENT OF PROSTATE

This condition seen in elderly males, may present to a GP in any of the following ways:

1. Increased frequency of urination, initially only at night and gradually both at night and day.
2. *Urgency*: The patient complains that he is unable to control the act of micturition.
3. The patient complains that there is difficulty in starting micturition, the stream of urine is weak and there is terminal dribbling. Hence, urination takes a longer time.
4. *Acute retention of urine*: O/e the patient has a full bladder.
5. *Chronic retention*, urination is incomplete and the bladder gradually but progressively distends.
6. *Haematuria*—rare, suspect carcinoma of prostate in such cases.

Diagnosis

Once suspected, the diagnosis can be confirmed at a GP level by a PR examination or a USG.

Management

Refer for surgery, as only surgery can offer permanent relief. If the surgery is not immediately possible for some reason, temporary relief can be obtained in mild cases with the following measures:

- Avoid coffee, alcohol, water before bedtime.
- Wait for ½ min after urination to ensure that the bladder is empty.
- Tab. Prazosin (Prazopress) 2 mg ½ hs × 3 days. Watch BP for postural hypotension. If normal, increase dose gradually to ½ bd 14 days, then 1 bd till operation is possible **(or)**

Tab. Doxazosin (Doxacard) (**or**) Tab. Terazosin as above (**or**)
Tab. Finasteride (Finast) 5 mg hs (**or**)
Tamsulosin (Urimax) 0.4 mg 30 mg after meal.

ACUTE GLOMERULONEPHRITIS

A school-going child is brought by parents with the following features:

1. Puffiness of face especially in the mornings, which gradually involves the whole body.
2. Smoky urine. Urine examination reveals plenty of RBCs, albumin + pus cells are few. RBC casts—present.
3. Hypertension is present.
4. H/o sore throat 10–12 days back.

Refer to a paediatrician. If this is not possible, the child can be managed by a GP under close supervision. Usually complete recovery occurs in 95% of children spontaneously within 2–3 weeks. In adults, the prognosis is not so good. Always refer.

Treatment

- Bed rest till BP is normal and oedema has reduced.
- Low salt diet, restricted water intake.
- Tab. Hydrochlorthiazide (Esidrex) 2–4 mg/day × 10 days.
- Record BP daily. Adjust dosage to keep it under control.
- Inj. Procaine penicillin 50,000 IU/kg/day × 10 days.

Admit immediately, if convulsions (hypertensive encephalopathy) or signs of acute renal failure. No long-term prophylactic penicillin is necessary.

ACUTE PYELONEPHRITIS

The patient, usually a female, presents to a GP with:

- Sudden onset pain in one or both loins, radiating to the iliac fossa. There is tenderness at the renal angle.
- High-grade fever with rigors and vomiting.
- Burning micturition and frequency of urination, because of associated urethritis and cystitis.
- Cloudy urine. Microscopic urine examination will show "numerous" pus cells. If pus cells are "occasional", revise your diagnosis. Also there will be few RBCs, bacteria and casts.

Treatment

- Rest in bed. If possible, hospitalize.
- Send urine for culture sensitivity before giving antibiotics.
- Inj. Diclofenac, if pain severe.
- Inj. Metoclopramide (Reglan), if vomiting.
- IV fluids, if dehydration.
- Tab. Ciprofloxacin (Ciplox) 500 mg bd (**or**)
  Tab. Norfloxacin (Norflox) 400 mg bd (**or**)
  Cap. Amoxicillin (Mox) 500 mg tds (**or**)
  Cap. Cephalexin (Phexin) 500 mg qid (**or**)
  Tab. Cotrimoxazole (Ciplin DS) bd.

1. After culture-sensitivity report is available, change antibiotics, if clinical response is not adequate.
2. After the acute attack is over, the patient should always be investigated for urinary stones, stricture urethra or other abnormalities of the urinary tract.

CHRONIC PYELONEPHRITIS

A general practitioner should suspect this diagnosis if in a patient with unexplained tiredness and vague ill-health, routine investigations reveal the following:

- Plenty of pus cells in the urine (without high-grade fever or severe urinary symptoms).
- Albumin is present in urine.
- Raised blood urea.
- Hypertension.

Always refer these patients to a urologist because:

- It is difficult to establish the diagnosis, as there are no uniform diagnostic criteria.
- It is difficult to eradicate the chronic infections, antibiotics might be required life-long.
- It is a chronic disease with frequent acute exacerbation.
- Complication like pyonephrosis (pus in the kidney) or renal failure may develop.

A GP's job is to suspect these patients, make a probable diagnosis and refer them to a urologist for further management.

*This chapter has been reviewed by **Dr Amol Talaulikar**, MD, Urologist, Pune.*

CHAPTER 12

Obstetrics & Gynaecology Conditions

- Delayed Menarche
- Abnormal and Excessive Uterine Bleeding
- Dysmenorrhoea
- Preponement and Postponement of Menses
- Vaginal Discharge
- Pruritus Vulvae
- Climacteric Symptoms
- Advice for Contraception
- Lump in Breast
- Screening for Breast Cancer
- Screening for Ca Cervix
- Antenatal Care
- Problems in Pregnancy
- Drugs for Lactational Control
- Infertility and Sterility
- Drugs in Pregnancy
- Breast Pain

— Madhu Oswal

DELAYED MENARCHE

Menstrual cycle usually establishes by the age of 16 years, but may be delayed up to 18 years of age. But, a girl is usually brought for investigations at a much earlier age. We can make two broad categories:

1. **Primary amenorrhoea with secondary sex characters not developed**
   Refer, as cause is most probably endocrinal or developmental.
2. **Primary amenorrhoea with secondary sex characters developed**
   a) **Girl with normal built**: The cause is most probably imperforate hymen, absent or underdeveloped uterus.
   Do USG. If *uterus is underdeveloped*, needs hormonal treatment.
   - Tab. Oestrogen + Progesterone (Ovral) for 21 days (**or**)
   - Tab. Ethinyl oestradiol (Lynoral) 0.05 mg tds for 21 days.

   Try for not more than 3 cycles. Refer if regular menses fails to get established. If *imperforate hymen*, refer for surgery.
   b) **Obese girl**
   - Do TSH—t/r/o hypothyroidism.
   - Do USG—t/r/o PCOD (*polycystic ovarian disease*), adrenogenital tumour.

   If normal, treatment same as in '2(a)' and advise weight reduction. This may by itself establish menses.
   c) **Thin girl**
   - Do T_3, T_4, TSH t/r/o hyperthyroidism.
   - Do X-ray chest t/r/o tuberculosis.

   If normal, advise improvement in general health. Treat as in '2(a)'.

ABNORMAL AND EXCESSIVE UTERINE HAEMORRHAGE

Abnormality can be in the form of change in cycle or change in amount and duration.

GENERAL PRACTICE AS SPECIALITY

Accordingly, we can divide it into four types:

1. **Menorrhagia—cyclical but amount and duration increased—(5/28, 8/28)**
   Cause mostly lies in the uterus (fibroid, adenomyosis, etc.).
   Try haemostatic therapy first:
   - Tab. Ethamsylate (Sylate) 500 mg tds/qid (**or**)
     Tab. Gynac CVP tds (**or**)
     Tab. Stadren CKP 1–2 tds.
     Tab Tranexamic acid (Texid) 500 mg 1–2 tds (**or**)
     Inj. Stryptochrome 2 mL, if severe. Plus
   - Tab. Mefenamic acid (Meftal, Ponstan) 500 mg tds.

   If no relief, give hormonal treatment:
   - Tab. Norethisterone acetate (Regesterone) 5 mg
     i) 1 tds for 3 days, then
     ii) 1 bd for 3 days, then
     iii) 1 od for 15 days
   - OC pills

   If no response—investigate: Hb with platelet count and BT-CT (bleeding disorders), USG (fibroid), T_3, T_4, TSH (hypo or hyperthyroidism).
   If all investigations are normal: Advise curettage as a last resort which can be therapeutic.
2. **Polymenorrhoea—cyclical pattern changed but amount normal (5/21, 5/18)**:
   Cause lies in the ovaries (congestion, infection, endometriosis, etc.). Commonly seen for few cycles after pregnancy, following menarche and preceding menopause.
   - Reassurance for 3 cycles.
   - Hormonal treatment, as given above if no improvement.
3. **Polymenorrhagia—cyclical bleeding more frequent and excessive (9/20, 12/20)**:
   Disturbance in HPOA axis as well as in uterus, e.g., PID.
   - Do USG.
   - Treatment same as for menorrhagia plus give treatment for PID, i.e.,
   - Tab. Ciprofloxacin (Cifran) 500 mg bd plus
   - Tab. Metronidazole (Metrogyl) 400 mg tds × 14 days (**or**)
   - Tab. Doxycycline (Doxy 1)100 mg bd for 7–10 days plus inj. Ceftriaxone 250 mg IM (**or**)
   - Tab. Azithromycin 500 mg + Secnidazole 2 g + Cefixine 200 mg (ACT kit) stat in mild disease.
4. **Metrorrhagia—cyclicity lost and amount variable—irregular or continuous**:
   Mostly due to surface lesions of the genital tract, from vulva to endometrium.
   - Do p/s to r/o local lesions of vulva, vagina, cervix and uterus. Treat according to the cause found.
   - Do USG.
   - Refer if it shows conception products in uterus, ectopic gestation, cystic ovaries, etc.
   - Refer for diagnostic curettage, if no cause found.

- For satisfactory treatment, determine the cause and treat—no shooting in the dark.
- Younger the patient, more are the chances of menstrual disorder being functional and cure spontaneous.
- In the reproductive age group, always think of pregnancy related conditions like abortions, PID, etc.
- After the age of 40, functional disturbances are common but need complete evaluation to r/o malignancy.
- The more irregular the bleeding, the more need for investigations and curettage.
- Any postmenopausal bleeding episode warrants thorough investigations to r/o malignancy.
- Excessive and prolonged bleeding is never a feature of approaching menopause.

DYSMENORRHOEA

It is important to determine the type of dysmenorrhoea. The pain arising from the uterus is true or spasmodic dysmenorrhoea. The pain which is due to a pelvic organ or tissue other than uterus and is merely associated with menses in congestive dysmenorrhoea.

True Dysmenorrhoea

It is a 'first day pain' during menses though it may start a day or two prior. It occurs in 18–25 years age group and spontaneous cure after pregnancy is very commonly seen.

- Advise rest.
- *Give anti-inflammatory drugs first.*
- Tab. Mefenamic acid + Dicyclomine (Meftal spas).

If no Relief, Start Hormonal Treatment

- Tab. Oestrogen + Progesterone (Ovral L) od from 5–25 day of menses to suppress ovulation and hence pain.
- If spasmodic dysmenorrhoea is unilateral, advise USG to r/o uterine malformation.
- Dilatation of cervix or paracervical block, if no response to medical treatment.

Congestive Dysmenorrhoea

Pain starts 2–3 days before menses and reduces with the flow. It is a dull pelvic pain with backache.

- Advise USG to r/o PID, myomatas, etc.
- If there is evidence of PID clinically and/or on USG, treat for PID.
- If no relief, give Tab. Ovral L od from 5–25 days of menses for 3 cycles.

Pain with Endometriosis

Here, pain starts 2–3 days before the menses and reaches its climax at the end of menses.

- Do USG.
- Give Tab. Regesterone 5 mg from 5th to 25th day of menses for 3 cycles.
- If no response, refer.

PREPONEMENT AND POSTPONEMENT OF MENSES

Religious functions, sports activity, marriage, 'honeymoon', etc., are few of the reasons with which patients come to seek advice as how to prepone or postpone their menses. Postponement is more reliable than preponement.

To Prepone

- Tab. Oestrogen + Progesterone (Ovral L) od from 5th to 14th day of menstrual cycle **(or)**
- Tab. Ethinyl oestradiol (Lynoral) 0.05 mg tds from 5th to 14th day of menstrual cycle. This will prepone the menses by 1 week.
- Tab. Ranitidine (Zinetac) 300 mg od to prevent gastritis.

To Postpone

- Tab. Oestrogen + Progesterone (Ovral L) od **(or)**
- Tab. Norethisterone acetate (Regesterone) 5 mg bd at least 3 days before the expected date. Continue as long as postponement is desired, usually not exceeding more than 10–12 days.
- Tab. Ranitidine (Zinetac) 300 mg od.

VAGINAL DISCHARGE

It is one of the most common complaints in females worldwide. It gets the discredit of being the cause of many complaints like weakness, backache, etc. But, it is not always pathological.

"**Normal**" vaginal discharge is that which is enough to keep the introitus moist. It is white or cream in colour and may stain the underclothing brownish yellow. It is non-offensive and non-pruritic. It is more in ovulation, during pregnancy, before menses and during sexual excitement. Give firm reassurance. Advise to keep herself busy instead of concentrating on vaginal discharge.

Increased "normal" discharge (leucorrhoea)

- Do P/V examination to r/o local conditions like cervical erosion, polyp, tumours, etc. Treat the cause.
- If no local lesion found, reassure.
- Advise good genital hygiene.
- Improve general health.
- Try to reduce anxiety.

"**Abnormal**" vaginal discharge may be due to change in quality or quantity or both.

Abnormal discharge with pruritus—cause is usually trichomonal or candidial vaginitis. Treat as given in "*pruritus vulvae*".

Abnormal discharge with burning micturition—cause is mostly gonococcal infection—give Tab. Cifran 500 mg , single dose.

Abnormal discharge with pelvic pain is usually due to PID—give treatment as given in above section.

Any postmenopausal vaginal discharge, especially if bloodstained—do pap smear to r/o malignancy. If pap smear negative, treat as given in senile vaginits.

PRURITUS VULVAE

It is one of the most irritating and socially unaesthetic complaint. It is equally irritating for the treating physician as the list of causes of pruritus vulvae is a long one. We can make two broad categories:

1. **Pruritus vulvae with vaginal discharge** (80%)
   Most common causes are candidial (especially in diabetics, after antibiotics, during pregnancy, etc.) **or** trichomonal vaginitis (postmenstrually). Treat for both.
   - Tab. Metronidazole (Flagyl) 400 mg bd × 7 days.
   - Tab. Fluconazole (Forcan) 150 mg stat (or) Clotrimazole vaginal pessaries (Candid V_3) for 3 nights.
   - Clotrimazole + Beclomethasone dipropionate cream (Candid B)—apply 2 times a day.
   - Do BSL to rule out DM.
   - Treat the sexual partner also and advise aps finance till treatment continues.
2. **Pruritus vulvae without vaginal discharge** (20%)
   Skin diseases are ruled out by doing local examination. Itching can be due to scabies, pediculosis, threadworm, tinea cruris, contact dermatitis (deodorants, soaps, synthetic under-clothings, etc.).

- Treatment of each of these conditions is given in Chapter 7.
  - In atrophic vaginitis, give oestrogen cream (Evalon) bd.
  - If no local lesion seen, r/o diabetes. Glycosuria per se can cause pruritus.
- Treat symptomatically, if none of the above present:
  - Tab. Cetrizine (Cetzine) 10 mg od.
  - Clobetasone butarate + Miconazole cream (Eumosone M) bd.

CLIMACTERIC (MENOPAUSAL) SYMPTOMS

Though used synonymously, 'climacteric' is not the same as 'menopause'. Menopause means the time when menses ceases, which usually occurs between 45 and 50 years (average—47 years). Menopause before 40 years or after 55 years is considered abnormal and needs investigation. Climacteric is the phase of waning of the ovarian functions, which starts 2–3 years before menopause and continues for 2–5 years after menopause.

Symptoms

1. ***Hot flushes with sweating***: If severe to interfere with the daily activities, start with:
   - Tab. Ethinyl oestradiol (Lynoral) 0.01 mg od (**or**)
   - Tab. Ethinyl oestradiol + Desogesteral (Femilon) od (**or**)
   - Tab. Conjugated oestrogens (Premarin) 0.625 mg od.
   - Supplement with Tab. Regesterone 5 mg od
   - Tab. Menosan (Himalay) 1 bd for a month, then 1 od. Gradually increase the dose and maintain on a dose which is just enough to reduce flushes to 3–4 per day. The final dose is maintained for more than a month and then the drug should be tapered off slowly over a period of 3–4 months. Watch for a month. If symptoms reappear, restart (**or**)
   - Ethinyl oestradiol (Estraderm MX) patch (25 mg, 50 mg, 100 mg) can be used alternatively. It is applied on non-hairy areas of the skin below the waist. It is to be replaced every 3–4 days (2 patches/week) and each time the site has to be changed. Patches are to be discontinued when flushes reduce.
   - Avoid hot baths, tea, coffee, spicy food, and working near fireplace.
2. ***Senile/atrophic vaginitis***—causes itching, discharge, dyspareunia, etc.
   - Evalon cream once a day for 7 days then bi-weekly for 7 days, then once a week life-long.
3. ***Osteoporosis***:
   - Tab. Calcium carbonate (Ocal) 500 mg bd plus
   - Vit. D_3 (Calcirol granules) 60,000 IU 1 g sachet per week × 8 weeks.
   - Tab. Alendronate (Osteophos) 35 or 70 mg/week on empty stomach with glass of water. Advise not to eat or lie down for 1 hr after taking the medicine (**or**)
   - Tab. Ibandronate (Idrofos) 150 mg/month
   - Tab. Tibolone (Livial) 2.5 mg od.
   - Advise diet rich in soyabean, which contains natural oestrogens.
   - Advise exercise to prevent osteoporosis.
4. ***Psychological/neurotic symptoms***—irritability, depression, headaches, palpitations, precordial pain, paraesthesia in hands and feet, giddiness, etc.
   - Tab. Alprazolam (Restyl) 0.5 mg bd or hs.
   - Tab. Fluoxetine (Fludac) 20 mg od.
   - 'Active' listening , thorough examination to r/o organic cause & firm reassurance.

After the Age of 40, Advise

- Monthly self-breast examination.
- Yearly bi-manual pelvic examination. Yearly pap smear. Yearly mammography.
- No HRT as prophylaxis—its risks (Ca. uterus, Ca. breast, thromboembolism, CHD, etc.) outweigh the benefits (prevent osteoporosis).
- Thorough investigations to r/o malignancy of genital organs, if there is postmenopausal bleeding (any bleeding after a gap of 6 months) or blood-stained vaginal discharge.

ADVICE FOR CONTRACEPTION

Methods

Many methods of contraception are available and the choice depends on the circumstances in which it has to be applied and on its acceptance by the patient.

1. ***Oral contraceptive pills and depots***: This would be the best choice for young women below 35 years, especially newly married women, as here the contraceptive measure is independent of the sexual act.
   - Tab. Ovral L or Triquilar or Mala-D (oestrogen + progesterone) from 5th day of menses for 21 days (**or**)
   - Inj. Norethisterone enanthate (Noristerat) 200 mg 1 mL every 8 weeks, to be given on the 5th day of menses (**or**)
   - Inj. Medroxyprogesterone (Depo-provera) 150 mg 1 mL every 3 months, to be given on the 5th day of menses.

   The depot preparations have the advantage of not having to take the pills every day, but uncertain and acyclical breakthrough bleeding can occur and is many times unacceptable, especially in religious settings. OC pills should be taken after meals or with milk to avoid gastritis. The patient on OC pills should be warned to use some barrier contraceptive method during the first cycle as it may be ovular. Alternatively, OC pills can be started a month or two before marriage.
2. ***Intrauterine contraceptive device (IUCD)***: It is a method preferred for spacing between two children.
   - CuT 200, CuT 350, Multiload Cu-T 250 (copper based IUCDs)—effective for 2–3 years, or cu 375 for 5 years.
   - Progestasert (Progesterone based IUCD)—effective for 8–10 years.

   IUCDs can be inserted 6 weeks after delivery/abortion, 12 weeks after caesarean section or on 5th day of menses. Inserting IUCD is not a difficult procedure, which can be learnt and practised by a GP (see Chapter 34). Intermenstrual spotting, menorrhagia and dysmenorrhoea are common side-effects and the patient should be warned beforehand.
3. ***Barrier methods***: Condoms (Kamasutra) have the benefit of giving protection against STDs along with contraception. This method is advocated if other methods are not acceptable for medical or other reasons, but its failure rate is very high. Female condoms (Femidom) are freely available now.
4. ***Tubectomy or Vasectomy***: These methods of 'permanent' contraception are adopted when the family is complete. Vasectomy is much simpler and less hazardous procedure as compared to tubectomy. It can be done under local anaesthesia, without hospitalization (see Chapter 39).
5. ***Safe period***: It is advocated for couples not using any other contraceptive method and is far from being safe. It is applicable only if the woman has regular menstrual cycles. In a 28-day cycle, the safe period is 4 days of menstrual flow, 3 days postmenstrually and 9 days premenstrually. If the cycle is shorter than 28 days, time must be subtracted from the postmenstrual safe period; when it is longer than 28 days, time can be added to this phase.

LUMP IN BREAST

Confirm whether there is lump or not. Frequently there is no lump—the normal fat and glandular tissue between fibrous septa is perceived as lump. Confirm the presence or absence of the lump by the flat of your hand.

- In case of doubtful lump—call after 15 days, if patient is in premenstrual phase and re-examine to see if the lump persists.
- If lump confirmed, check if there is acute inflammation.
- If acute inflammation present—treat as given under '*breast abscess*'.
- If no acute inflammation and swelling is cystic —aspirate as given under "aspiration technique". Refer if:
  - Aspirate is blood stained.
  - Cyst refill.
  - There is lump after aspiration.
- If swelling is noncystic, firm to hard, smooth, mobile and lobulated, the clinical diagnosis is fibroadenoma. Confirm, if in doubt, by FNAC or incision biopsy. Excision biopsy is rarely required.
- If swelling does not fit in any of the above types—refer to experts for mammography, FNAC, etc.

> Any lump after menopause is considered malignant unless proved otherwise by mammography, FNAC or biopsy. Signs suggestive of malignancy are—lump that is hard, painless, irregular, attached to the skin or underlying muscle mass, nipple retracted, with or without axillary lymph nodes.

SCREENING FOR BREAST CANCER

The following screening procedure is to be followed for each woman but more stringently for those with high risk factors like multiparity, having family history of breast cancer, delayed age of first pregnancy, on HRT, etc.

1. ***Breast self-examination***: Every month on 7th day of menses for women above 40 years. Earlier, if with high risk factors. Pamphlets showing how to do this can be provided to the patient. Any new mass, change in size and shape of breast or nipple, nipple discharge, or skin changes should be reported.
2. ***Clinical examination of breast by a clinician***: Any mass felt by the 'flat of the hand' should be investigated. Axillary and supraclavicular nodes should be looked for.
3. ***Mammography***: Every 2 years for women between 40 and 50 years and every year for those above 50 years and those with high risk of breast cancer.

SCREENING FOR CARCINOMA CERVIX

Whom to Advise for Screening?

1. Every woman above 21 years—every year up to the age of 70 years, after which Ca. cervix is rare.
2. Postmenopausal bleeding, blood stained offensive discharge.
3. Postcoital bleeding.
4. Any cervical lesion bleeding on touch.
5. Fixed, friable, indurated cervix.
6. Every HIV +ve woman—every year.

The screening is done by doing cytodiagnosis either by cervical scrape technique using Ayre's method or vaginal cytology technique using Papanicolou's method. These methods are described in Chapter 34.

> One-half of all the patients of Ca. cervix present themselves when the growth has already reached incurable stage. Routine screening for Ca. cervix has been shown to drastically change this scenario.

ANTENATAL CARE

The ultimate goal of regular antenatal care is '*healthy mother with a healthy child.*'

The First Visit Check List

The first visit can be at 'just missed period' or at labour!!

- Record LMP (last menstrual period), confirm diagnosis (clinically or by urine pregnancy test) and calculate EDD (expected date of delivery). EDD is calculated by adding 9 months and 7 days to the 1st day of LMP.
- Record age, weight, height, BP.
- Record menstrual and obstetric history—H/o abortion, pre-eclampsia, preterm–post-term delivery, type of delivery, puerperium, APH, low birth weight baby, etc.
- Record if the woman has asthma, HT, DM, epilepsy, rheumatic heart disease, etc.
- Drug history especially OC pills, drugs taken for withdrawal bleeding, vaccines, etc.
- Investigations—Hb, blood group and Rh, ELISA for HIV, VDRL, Australia antigen, urine-routine, BSL.

Check List for Every Visit

One visit per month in first 7 months, thereafter every 15 days and weekly after 36 weeks. The visit should be more frequent, if there is a bad obstetric history.

- Record BP, pulse and weight.
- Check for oedema, pallor.
- Fundal height.
- FHS 24 weeks onwards (by stethoscope).
- Position, lie and presentation of foetus 36 weeks onwards.
- If possible, urine albumin at each visit. USG—ideally one per trimester, but at least one at 16–20 weeks.

Routine Treatment

- Tab. Folic acid (Folvite) 5 mg od in 1st trimester.
- Tab. Ferrous fumarate (Autrin) od after 2nd month.
- Tab. Calcium carbonate (Ocal) od
- Inj. Tetanus toxoid—2 in last trimester, 1 month apart. One will suffice, if taken in previous pregnancy.

Other than Drugs

- Dietary advice—Balanced and high protein diet, plenty of green vegetables and fruits.
- Adequate rest—Mental as well as physical.
- Regular isotonic exercises, yoga, physiotherapy.
- Breast and nipple care.
- Avoid long journeys in first and last trimester—if unavoidable, prefer train.
- Avoid sexual intercourse in first and last trimester or restrict to non-penetrative sex.
- Educate about importance of exclusive breast-feeding and immunisation of the baby to be born.
- Discuss future contraceptive measures.

High Risk Pregnancies

- Very young (<18 years) or old (>30 years)
- Multiparous
- Short statured (<140 cm)
- Obese
- Bad obstetric history
- Twin pregnancy
- Uterine height not corresponding to gestational age (IUGR).
- FHS not heard at 24–26th week.
- Breech or transverse lie at 36th week.
- Head not engaged at 36th week.
- Antepartum haemorrhage
- Abnormal FHS (<100/min or >160/min)

- Hypertension (rise in systolic BP by 30 and diastolic by 15 over and above the baseline value).
- Oedema, especially of face.
- Excess weight gain (>0.5 kg/week).
- Albuminuria
- Diabetic patient
- Cardiac disorders

> High-risk pregnancies require strict monitoring, preferably by an obstetrician.

Antenatal care schedule	
1st visit 5–7 wks	UPT + Consultation Sonography (TVS)
12–13 wks	Check up + NT scar (USG - Abd.) Investigations (Hmg, Bld. group, U-R & M, BSL-R, HIV, HBsAg, VDRL, Thalassaemia/Hb. electrophoresis)
16–17 wks	Check up + Triple marker test
20–22 wks	Check up + Anomaly scan
24 wks	Cardiac evaluation (USG) + Check up + Inj. TT – 1st dose
26 wks	Glucose challenge test with 50 g glucose
28 wks	Check up + Inj. TT – 2nd dose
32 wks	USG obst. Doppler + Check up
Check up every week	
36–37 wks	Check up, PV examination + NST
38 wks	USG

PROBLEMS IN PREGNANCY

Anaemia

No pregnant woman should land in labour in an anaemic state.

- If Hb is between 7 and 10 g%, start cap Autrin bd or tds.
- If not tolerated orally, start Inj. Imferon 2 mL deep IM alternate days AST.
- Blood transfusion is required, if there is no time for oral treatment.
- If Hb is below 6 g%, PCV is advised.
- Give Tab. Noworm 400 mg.

Morning Sickness

Very common and very unpleasant symptom.

- Bed tea with 1–2 biscuits or toasts.
- Frequent small feeds.
- Tab. Vitamin B_6 (B long) od.
- Tab. Meclizine (Pregnidoxin) 1–3 tabs/day (**or**) Tab. Doxylamine (Doxyla) 2 hs or 1 tds.

If not controlled with these measures and vomiting worsens leading to tachycardia with dehydration, admit the patient. She will require:

- IV fluids, especially DNS, dextrose 10%.
- IV 25% dextrose 4 amps daily.
- Inj. Multivitamin (Macraberin forte) 1 amp daily.

Preeclampsia

The diagnosis of preeclampsia is made if:

- Systolic BP >140 or diastolic BP > 90 mm Hg or 2 occasions 6 hrs apart beyond 20 weeks of pregnancy.
- Albuminuria present.

Advise

- Strict bed rest, especially in left lateral position.
- Tab. Labetalol (Lablol) Start with 50 mg bd and gradually increase up to100–200 tds.

- Tab. Methyl dopa 250–500 mg (Alphadopa) 3–4 tabs/day (or)
- Low salt or salt-free diet.
- Advise counting of foetal movements—should be more than 10 per 12 hr.
- Regular and stringent foetal monitoring—clinically and by weekly USG.
- Refer to obstetrician as soon as possible.

Refer immediately in the following conditions

- BP rises to above 160/100 mm Hg
- Headache
- Vomiting
- Visual disturbances
- Epigastric or right hypochondriac pain
- Reduced foetal movements (<10/12 hrs)
- Abnormal FHS (<100/min; >160/min)
- Oliguria
- Convulsions

P/V Bleeding in First Trimester

- Confirm it is pregnancy related bleeding and not 'delayed' menses.
- Bleeding sometimes occurs at menstruation time for first few months in some pregnant women.
- Advise bed rest.
- Tab. Natural progesterone (ETS, Naturogest) 200 mg bd × 5 days.

Do USG Pelvis to see if the Foetus is Alive

1. If yes, continue Tab. Naturogest and add:
   - Inj. Hydroxy progesterone (Fetugest) 250 mg IM 2/week up to 12 weeks (or) Inj. Progesterone (ETS) 100 mg 2 mL/2/week up to 12 weeks (**or**)
   - Inj. HCG (Profasi) 10,000 IU followed by 5000 IU 1/week up to 12 weeks.
2. If not, refer the patient to a hospital for D&E. It is important to explain the patient beforehand that only 50% of the threatened abortions conserve by the above measures; remaining 50% lead to abortion.

DRUGS FOR LACTATIONAL CONTROL

To Reduce or Stop Lactation

- Tab. Bromocriptine (Proctinal) 1.25 mg bd × 3 days, then 2.5 mg bd (**or**)
- Tab. Pyridoxine (B long) 2 tds (**or**)
- Tab. Stilbesterol 5 mg 2 tds for 4 days, then reduce to 1 tds (**or**)
- Inj. Oestradial + Testosterone (Mixogen) 1 mg IM—useful, if given early.
- Advise firm supporting brassiere or breast-binder.
- Regular breast evacuation, if congestion causes pain.
- Tab. Cabgoline 0.5 mg 2 stat.

To Increase Lactation

There is no better stimulation than regular suckling by the baby. Lactation is insufficient, if baby is failing to gain weight. If so, start:

- Tab. Metoclopramide (Reglan) 10 mg tds.
- Tab. Desamino oxytocin (Butocin) 1/2 hr before each feed.
- Shatavarex granules 2 tsf in milk twice daily.
- Plenty of water—Poor water intake is a common cause of poor milk quantity.

INFERTILITY AND STERILITY

Infertility is not an individual's problem, it is a couple's disease. So even though it is the woman who approaches for infertility treatment, the couple needs to be treated.

When should one Investigate for Infertility?

Medically speaking 12–18 months after consummate marriage (that is the period in which there were no contraceptive measures used by the couple). Till then, reassurance should be given, but may not help under family pressures or their own wishes.

Male Partner

- If h/s/o impotency, premature ejaculation—start Tab. Sildenafil citrate (Viagra) 50 mg half hour before sexual intercourse.
- If genital examination reveals phimosis, hypospadiasis, varicocoele, abnormalities of vas, epididymis or testes—refer to surgeon/urologist.
- If occupation involves exposure to high temperatures—advise change in occupation.
- Stop alcohol, smoking.
- Advise semen analysis.

Semen Analysis

The specimen is best collected by masturbation directly into a dry and clean glass container. Fresh sample (taken after 3 days of abstinence) should be processed within 2 hrs. Semen analysis should be carried out on two different occasions, if the first test suggests impaired fertility.

- If the number of sperms is <20 million/mL and/or motility is <50% and/or sperms of abnormal morphology are >20%—start with Tab. Clomiphene citrate (Clofert) 50 mg od × 3 months.
- If pus in semen examination—give Norflox 400 mg bd × 10 days or Ciplox 500 mg bd × 10 days plus Tab Doxy 100 bd plus Tab Metrogyl 400 bd.
- In azoospermia—refer for testicular biopsy and S. FSH.

Female Partner

- If infertility with amenorrhoea—treat as given in '*amenorrhoea*'.
- If h/s/o hyperprolactinaemia (discharge from nipples)—Tab. Bromocriptine 2.5 mg hs, increasing to 2.5 mg tds.
- If past h/s/o tuberculosis, PID, peritonitis, appendicitis—do USG and refer.
- If h/s/o endometriosis (severe menstrual pain with menorrhagia)—refer.
- HSG—postmenstrual (D 8,9,10) for tubal patency.
- S. FSH for ovarian reserve on day 3.
- If h/s/o ovulation failure, clinically or by USG, (PCOD, post-pill amenorrhoea), give Tab. Clomiphene citrate (Clofert) 50 mg od from 2nd day of menses for 5 days. If successful, ovulation occurs 7–12 days after the last day of treatment and coitus should be timed accordingly. If no response, increase the dose to 100 mg after 2 cycles. Refer if no success in 6 cycles. Watch for ovarian enlargement during this drug treatment by doing bimanual pelvic examination.

Both Partners

- The couple should be explained about ovulation cycle and *fertile period.* Conception is most likely between the 10th and 18th days of a 28-day cycle, at which time advise coitus at 48-hr interval.
- Avoid using lubricants—these are often spermicidal.
- Avoid alcohol 'in excess'.
- A long holiday is frequently an answer.

BREAST PAIN

The following clinical conditions can present as breast pain:

- Pregnancy

- Cyclical mastalgia
- Cracked nipple
- Mastitis, usually in a lactating woman
- Breast abscess
- Fibroadenoma
- Simple cyst
- Carcinoma of breast
- Drugs—OC pills

Management

In mastiti:

- Cap Amoxicillin + Cloxacillin 500 mg (Tab. Augmentin) 1 qid × 10 days (**or**)
  - Tab. Amoxicillin + Clavulunic acid 625 mg (Tab. Augmentin) 1 tds × 10 days.
- Tab. Diclofenac (Voveran) 50 mg 1 bd.
- If severe cellulitis—admit the patient for IV antibiotics.
- If breast abscess has developed—admit the patient for I and D under GA.
- Continue breast feeding.

In cyclical mastalgia:

- Tab. Ibuprofen+ Paracetamol (Combiflam) 1 tds
- Vitamin B1 (Thiamine)100 mg daily
- Vitamin B 6 (Pyridoxine) 100 mg daily
- Evening primrose oil 4–5 g daily.

DRUGS IN PREGNANCY

Drugs	Safe	Not safe
1. **Antibiotics**	Penicillins, Ampicillin, Amoxicillin Cephalosporins Erythromycin Azithromycin Lincomycin	Sulphonamides Tetracyclines Quinolones Chloramphenicol Cotrimoxazole
2. **Antifungals**	Fluconazole, except in 1st tri.	Ketoconazole Itraconazole
3. **Antivirals**	AZT, Acyclovir	
4. **Antitubercular**	INH, Rifampicin, Ethambutol	Streptomycin Ethionamide
5. **Anti-leprotic**	Dapsone, Rifampicin	Clofazimine
6. **Antimalarials**	Chloroquine	Primaquine Pyrimethamine
7. **Anti-infestives**	Gamma-benzene hexachloride Niclosamide	Mebendazole Albendazole
8. **Anti-protozoals**	Metronidazole	Tinidazole, 8-hydroxyquinolone Furazolidone

contd.

9. **Analgesics and antipyretics**	Paracetamol, Ibuprofen, Aspirin (only in 2nd tri)	Mefenamic acid Morphine Diclofenac sodium Nimesulide Piroxicam
10. **Antacids**	Cimetidine Famotidine Ranitidine	Omeprazole Misoprostol All antacids in 1st tri.
11. **Anti-emetics**	Promethazine Meclizine Doxylamine	Domperidone Cisapride Ondansetron
12. **Laxatives**	Bulkforming (Isabgol) Lactulose	Bisacodyl Castor oil
13. **Anticonvulsants**	All are teratogenic to some extent. Use mono-therapy with regular monitoring	Phenytoin Phenobarbitone Diazepam Carbamazepine Valproic acid
14. **Anti-anxiety Antidepressants**	Sertraline Fluoxetine Buspirone	Alprazolam Amitriptyline Imipramine
15. **Antitussives Anti-asthamatics Antihistaminics**	Salbutamol Terbutaline Theophylline Ipratropium bromide CPM Diphenhydramine Steroids (prefer prednisolone)	Cetrizine Loratidine Astemizole
16. **Antihypertensives**	Methyl dopa, Nifedipine, Amlodipine	ACE inhibitors
17. **Antidiuretics**	Hydrochlorthiazide Spironolactone Amiloride	Diltiazem Frusemide
18. **Antidiabetics**	'Human insulin'	All oral hypoglycaemic agents

If no response,

- Tab. Norethisterone (Primolut N) 5 mg from 14th to 25th day of menstrual cycle.

If still no response,

- Tab Danazol 200 mg 1 od.

If on OC pills, advise pills with low dose oestrogen.

If localized painful lump or cyst—advise FNAC, excision biopsy, mammography, USG, etc.

For cracked nipples:

- Masse cream for local application.
- Avoid feeding from cracked nipple for 4–5 days but empty breast by manual expression.
- Advise mother to feed baby with both areola and nipple, not only the nipple.

*This chapter has been reviewed by **Dr Harshad Gandhi**, MD, Gynaecologist, Pune.*

CHAPTER 13

Paediatric Conditions

- Febrile Convulsions
- Chronic Cough
- Epilepsy
- Wheezing Child
- Vomiting
- Constipation
- Nocturnal Enuresis
- Pica
- Weaning
- Tonics, Multivitamins, Iron & Calcium Preparations
- The Crying Baby
- Healthy Teething & Teething Complaints
- Poor Eater
- Recurrent Abdominal Pain
- Stridor
- Acute Diarrhoea

FEBRILE CONVULSIONS

A febrile child brought with a history of convulsions or is convulsing at the time of presentation is quite a common complaint. Proper history of the convulsive episodes is a must to diagnose the type of convulsion. Features of simple febrile convulsions (see below) differs from that of complex febrile convulsions or convulsions due to other causes. The latter two require investigations and should be referred to a paediatrician.

Features of simple febrile convulsions

- Age group of 6 months to 5 years.
- Generalized type convulsions.
- Occur within 24 hrs of onset of fever and at the peak of the fever.
- Only one convulsive episode during the fever.
- Lasts <10 min.
- No post-ictal stage, Todd's palsy, etc.
- Complete recovery within 6 hrs.
- Rarely develops into epilepsy.

Treatment

Most of the simple febrile convulsions require no treatment as convulsions usually stop before baby is brought to the clinic.

If the Child has Fever

- Remove baby's clothes and expose it to cool air.
- Tepid-water sponging.
- Tab. Paracetamol (Crocin) 10 mg/kg/dose 4–6 hourly **or** Suppol suppository 80 mg for fast effect.

If the Child is in Convulsions

- Give left lateral position to baby.
  - Midazolam(Nayzilam) nasal spray in child above 12 years of age.
- IV Diazepam (Calmpose) 0.2 mg/kg diluted in 20 mL of normal saline (**or**)
- Rectal Diazepam (Calmpose) 0.5 mg/kg diluted in 10 mL of normal saline.
- Search for cause of fever.

To Prevent Further Attacks of Convulsions

- Advise parents to continue sponging and add antipyretics as soon as fever begins to rise
- Give Lorazepam (Ativan) 0.1 mg/kg/dose bd till child is afebrile for 24 hrs.

CHRONIC COUGH

Cough should be called chronic if has lasted for more than 2 weeks.

> **Causes of chronic cough**
>
> *Chronic recurrent cough*
> - Variant asthma
> - Gastro-esophageal reflux disease (GERD)
>
> *Chronic continuous cough*
> - Post-nasal discharge due to sinusitis or adenoids
> - Pertussis
> - Tuberculosis
> - Tropical eosinophilia
> - Foreign body
> - Rarely, congenital anomaly such as tracheo-oesophageal fistula, etc.

Treatment

For chronic recurrent cough:

1. Treat as asthma (see Wheezing child).
2. If no response, and child is coughing only at night when it lies down, think of GERD and post-nasal drip. Give:
   - Tab. Famotidine (Famtac) 1 mg/kg/dose bd × 3 weeks.
   - Syr/Tab Domperidone (Domstal) 0.5 mg/kg/dose × 3 weeks.
   - To reduce cough due to postnasal drip, let the child sleep on abdomen.

For chronic continuous cough:

Advise

- X-ray chest PA view.
- Haemogram with ESR.
- X-ray skull—Water's view.
- Tuberculin test.
- AEC (absolute eosinophil count).

1. If cough has started abruptly, think and look for signs of foreign body. If history suggesting pressure of FB—Refer.
2. For sinusitis, give a course of antibiotics, steam, decongestants.
3. If adenoids enlargement (clinically and on X-ray of nasopharynx), refer for adenoidectomy.
4. If haemogram shows increased eosinophil count, give Tab. Hetrazan (1 mg/kg in 3 dd) × 3 weeks plus bronchodilator steam. Add steroids, if no response.
5. If tuberculin test shows induration > 10 mm, suspect tuberculosis and refer
   - Tab. Isoniazid 5 mg/kg/dose od × 6 months.
   - Tab. Rifampicin 10 mg/kg/dose od on empty stomach × 6 months.
   - Tab. Pyrazinamide 15–25 mg/kg/dose bd × 2 months.

EPILEPSY

Epilepsy is characterized by recurrent, episodic, seizures along with motor, sensory or psychomotor changes. Seizures can be generalized or partial. Epilepsy is "secondary," if there is a structural brain damage. These cases are to be referred. Epilepsy is "primary," if no cause can be identified. Primary epilepsy has early onset (6–7 years) and stereotyped pattern. There may be a positive family history and the child is normal in between the attacks.

Treatment is started, if there are two or more seizures in preceding 12 months. CT scan/MRI brain and EEG need to be done before starting treatment.

Principles of anti-epilepsy therapy

- Choose drug according to the type of seizure (see p. 440).
- Use mono-therapy as far as possible.
- Increase the dose gradually.
- Use two drugs if seizures recur in spite of optimum dose.
- Ensure strict compliance.
- Do LFTs at frequent intervals as all anti-epileptics are hepatotoxic.
- Continue the drugs after the child is free from seizure for at least 3 years. Then withdraw the drug(s) gradually over a period of 6 months after repeat EEG.

WHEEZING CHILD

Common Causes

1. *All that wheezes is not asthma, and all asthmatics do not wheeze.*
2. In infant < 6 months, wheezing is due to either bronchiolitis or pneumonitis.
3. If wheezing occurs with rhinitis and fever, never in-between, think of asthmatic bronchitis.
4. If unilateral wheezing, think of foreign body.
5. If wheezing is continuous (not episodic) and not responding to treatment, think of obstructive lesion like mediastinal mass, lymph nodes, etc.
6. Passive smoking is an important cause of wheezing in children.

Hospitalize Immediately, if

- Child is too dyspnoeic to feed.
- RR is > 50/min.
- Pulse is > 140/min.
- Chest is 'silent'.
- Child is drowsy.
- Severe respiratory distress with chest retraction.

For Moderate Cases

- Nebulise with Salbutamol (Asthalin) solution 0.02 mg/kg diluted in 2 mL of distilled water, 4 hourly, plus
- Inj. Hydrocortisone (Efcorlin) 4 mg/kg IV bolus and then every 4 hourly, plus
- Inj. Terbutaline (Bricanyl) 0.01 mg/kg SC.
- If no response, hospitalize.

In Mild Cases of Wheezing

- Syr/Tab. Salbutamol (Asthalin) 0.2 mg/kg/day in 3 dd.
- Syr/Tab. Theophylline (Theoped) 20 mg/kg/day in 3 dd.
- Tab. Prednisolone (Wysolone) 1–2 mg/kg/day in 3 dd.

Advise Parents to

- Give plenty of fluids.
- Give steam inhalation with tinc.Benzoin.
- Humidify baby's room with boiling water.
- If there is fever and on auscultation there are crepitations, add antibiotics & antipyretic.

VOMITING

Vomiting is a common symptom throughout childhood. It is important to recognize signs which indicate serious disease (see Box) and refer these cases immediately.

When to refer a child with vomiting

- Green vomiting (obstruction or severe infection).
- Persistent/projectile/profuse vomiting.
- Distended abdomen, abdominal mass, visible peristalsis.
- Drowsy.
- Bulging anterior fontanel.
- Fever with moderate to severe dehydration.
- Not responding to treatment.

Treatment

1. Liquid Ondensetron (Ondem): Less than 4 yrs —2 mg/day. 4–11 yrs—4 mg/day.
2. Liquid Domperidone (Domstal) 0.3 mg/kg/dose bd before feed.
3. ***If no response, give***
   - Inj. Metoclopramide (Reglan) 0.1 mg/kg/dose IM (**or**)
   - Inj. Trifluoperazine (Siquil) 0.25 mg/kg/dose IM.
   - Inj. Ondansetron (Emset) 0.15 mg/kg IV.
4. Advise parents to: **give clear liquids—ORS or *nimbu sharbat* continuously**. If baby vomits, stop for 10 min and restart. Give soft diet like apple, banana, khichdi, idly, orange juice after 6 hrs.
   If sign of dehydration, start IV DNS or refer.

CONSTIPATION

It is infrequent passage of small, hard and dry stools. Frequency of stools only should not be the criteria as it differs from child to child. One child may pass stools after every feed while another child may not pass even once in days. Both can be normal. Treatment is required if baby is uncomfortable (not parents). Most of the children have functional (non-organic) constipation caused by faulty or inadequate diet or because of faulty toilet training. Organic causes like hypothyroidism , aganglionic megacolon or anorectal stenosis are rare.

Auxiliary treatment

- In a breast-fed baby, constipation can be due to inadequate breast milk (as judged by inadequate weight gain). Start top feeds.
- In a bottle-fed baby, increase water intake and add sugar to the milk.
- Late weaning can cause constipation. Start weaning early, preferably at 4–5 months.
- Parents should not stress too early on toilet training. The bowel hardly requires training!
- In older children, advise high intake of tough residue foods like green leafy vegetables, salads, fruits, whole wheat, etc., plenty of water and regular exercise.

Medical Treatment

In acute constipation, without rectal pain:

- Stool softeners like docusates (Laxicon) 10–20 mg/day in infants.
- Osmotic laxative in lactulose (Duphalac) in older children.
  - 1–5 years 5 mL BD
  - 5–10 years 10 mL BD
  - >10 years 15 mL BD
- If no response, use Dulcolax suppositories or Neotomic enema.
- If nothing helps, manual removal of impacted stool with gloved lubricated finger has to be resorted to.

Acute constipation with rectal pain is usually due to fissure-in-ano. Give *Proctosedyl* rectal jelly with laxatives and painkillers.

In chronic constipation, if dietary measures fail, give Isabgol 1 tsf bd or tds in a glass of water for few days.

NOCTURNAL ENURESIS

About 15–25% of children above 6 years and 8% of 12-year-old children get wet in the bed. This suggests the high frequency of this embarrassing problem for children and parents. It is called *primary*, if the child was never dry in the past and *secondary*, if he/she had 6 months of night time dryness. Treatment for both remains the same. Before treating, organic causes like UTI, post-urethral valves in boys, ectopic ureter in girls, neurological cause like spina-bifida have to be ruled out. For this, do urine routine in each and every case. If result is s/o infection, go for USG and/or voiding cystourethrogram or refer.

Advice to the Parents

1. Do not start treatment till age of 6 years.
2. Do not blame or reprimand the child.
3. Motivate the child to take active part in the treatment plan like keeping a record in a diary for dry and wet nights.
4. *Bed-wetting alarms* have promising results, but the cost is prohibitive.
5. *Water therapy*: Restriction of fluids 2-hr prior to sleep. Going to toilet before going to bed.
6. *Desmopressin nasal spray* (D-Void) is useful for nocturnal polyuria, i.e., those with normal day-time voiding pattern. Start with 10 μg, half the dose in each nostril at bedtime. May increase to 20–40 μg. Treatment to be taken for 3–6 months and discontinued slowly. Relapse rate is high.
7. If no response, start Tab Imipramine (Depsonil) 2.5 mg/kg od HS. Reduce slowly over 2–3 months.

PICA

It is a very common problem in children, especially in emotionally deprived, undernourished children from low socio-economic class. Commonly consumed substances are clay, mud, paint, pencil, plaster, etc. Exact cause of pica is not established, though worm infestations and iron deficiency are commonly associated. Whether these are causes or effects are not known. Pica may present as a direct complaint from parents or as vomiting, abdominal pain, diarrhoea or with more severe complications like intestinal obstruction, lead poisoning, intestinal perforation, etc.

Treatment

- Tab/Syr Albendazole (Zentel) 400 mg if >2 years, 200 mg if <2 years.
- Tonoferon drops 6 mg/kg/day in 2–3 dd.
- Syr. Ostocalcium ½ to 1 tsf.
- High caloric diet if malnourished.
- Keep the substance for which the child is craving, out of reach.
- If emotional deprivation is the cause, the child needs to be given more parental attention and care.

WEANING

Weaning is a process by which food other than breast milk is introduced gradually into the baby's diet—first to compliment the breast milk and then to replace it with thicker feed. This is the most crucial period in child's growth as faulty weaning practice is one major contributing factor for infant malnutrition.

Weaning from Breast Milk to Top Milk

Child should be exclusively breastfed for first 4 months of life. Weaning is started at around 4 months (earlier if inadequate breast milk).

Cow's, buffalo's, goat's or infant formula can be used. If mother's milk is inadequate, give top milk in dilution as given below, give only pasteurized milk to prevent bovine tuberculosis.

- Dilution of milk
  - 1st month 1:1 (milk:water)

- 2nd month 2:1 (milk:water)
- 3rd month 3:1 (milk:water)
- 4th month 4:1 (milk:water)

- Cow's milk is to be given in undiluted form.
- Undiluted milk after 4 montha of age.
- Say emphatic 'No' to milk powder.
- No bottle-feeding. It is a cause of tons of problems. Only spoon and katori.

Weaning from Top-Milk to Thicker Feeds

It is done at around age of 6 months.

- Weaning food should be culturally acceptable, locally available, easy to prepare and inexpensive.
- Food should be started in small quantity and then very gradually increased.
- Any one food-type must be given for about a week and a new type added.
- Fruit and vegetable juices like tomato, orange, papaya or any other seasonal fruit should be given in diluted form (1:1). Slowly undilute it and increase its quantity.
- 'Kanji' prepared from wheat, rice, maize, jowar or bajra with milk or curds with sweet and/or salt added to taste. Mashed vegetables can be added to it.
- 'Khichdi' prepared from 3 parts of rice with one part of pulses with vegetables and 1 tsf oil. Beans, cabbage, soya-bean, groundnut, carrots or green leafy vegetables should be boiled, mashed and added to the khichdi to add vitamin and iron.
- Bread, biscuits, puddings, cakes, etc., can be given now and then just to break the monotony.
- Everyday one fruit—orange, papaya, apple, banana or any other seasonal fruit—should be given.
- By the 1st birthday, the child should be consuming full family diet—rice, dal, chapatti and vegetables from the family pot.
- Unlike adult, child's capacity of eating at one time is limited. So, it should be given food 6–8 times a day and not two.
- Malnourished children and children recovering from illness should be given frequent small meals with 1 tsf coconut oil 3–4 times a day. This is "*calorie-fortification technique*", which is a major remedy to break malnutrition–illness cycle.
- Mother should be advised to maintain adequate cleanliness while preparing food and serving the child.
- Child should be encouraged from the very beginning to feed himself with his own spoon, katori and glass.
- Add jaggery instead of sugar, whenever possible.

"*Weaning done properly is the key to healthy childhood.*"

TONICS, MULTIVITAMINS, IRON AND CALCIUM PREPARATIONS

Drug market is flooded with vitamins, iron, calcium and tonic preparations. But while choosing any brand, the doctor should look into the following points:

1. Concentration of iron, calcium or vitamins in the preparation.
2. Balance between various components.
3. Cost

We are supposed to supplement the child, not the drug company!

Multivitamins

- Breast milk lacks Vit. C and D. Therefore, multivitamin like Vi-syneral, ABDEC drop containing Vit. A and C should be given at a dose of 0.8 mL or 5 drops from 15 days of birth.

- Continue up to 9 months and then shift to syrup form.
- Stop when child starts taking complete balanced diet.

Vitamin A

- Deficiency presents as night blindness, xerosis or keratomalacia. Prophylactic treatment is Inj. Aquasol 4 mL or Inj. Arovit (2,00,000 IU) every 6 months.
- For treatment of mild deficiency, Cap Adexolin (5000) od-bd × 15 days.
- For severe deficiency, Arovit drops (1,50,000 IU/mL)—5000 IU/kg/day × 5 days followed by 25,000 IU/day till recovery occurs or Inj. Aquasol 4 mL IM on day 1, 2 and 30.

Vitamin D

- Deficiency presents as rickets after the age of 3 months.
- Prophylactic treatment is daily 400 IU after 4 months (from 10th day in premature infants), e.g., ABDEC drop.
- ***Treatment of deficiency***
  - Inj. Arachitol 6 lacs IM or Calcirol sachet in milk (60,000 units) to be repeated after 3 months, if no improvement. In severe def., Inj. Arachitol 6 lacs IM to be given on day 1, 15 and 30, if required **or**
  - Daily 1500–5000 IU of Vit. D for 4 weeks, e.g., D_3 granules – 6000 units.
  - Expose to sunlight.

Iron

- Prophylactic treatment to be started at the age of 2 months (earlier in premature). Tonoferon Ferbin or Feorsoft drops 5 drops bd < 1 year, 10 drops >1 year.
- Continue up to 1 year or till child starts taking complete balanced diet.
- For deficiency, 6 mg/kg/day should be given in 2 dd after breast-feed.
- Ferrous sulphate should be the 1st choice, then gluconate or fumarate.
- If oral iron not tolerated, which is rare, parental iron is given.
- Dose of parental iron = 0.3 × wt in pounds & % def. of Hb.

Tonics and Appetite Stimulants

1. Parents insisting for tonics are difficult patients to handle.
2. Don't straightaway refuse. Give multivitamins, iron, calcium as per the requirement.
3. Prescribe tonic with detailed dietary advice– 1 tsf of tonic to be taken with one laddu made of groundnut + jaggery + ghee tds. Stress that tonic will only work with this dietary product.
4. Start maintaining a growth chart to monitor the child's growth and development.
5. To increase appetite, give Cypon (Cyproheptadine) liquid 2 mg for 2–6 yr and 4 mg at bed time for 6–12 yr. This causes sedation. **Or**, Longiphene (Buclizine) 1 tsf before food. This does not cause sedation.

THE CRYING BABY

A shrilling baby rushed by a panicked mother in the clinic (breaking the queue) with 5–6 equally panicked relatives, is a common scenario. Sudden onset crying since few hours is the only complaint. What is expected is to keep our head 'cool' and go systematically to detect the cause of crying.

First Rule Out any Organic Cause

- Strip the child completely and look for marks of injury, insect bite or swelling anywhere on the body.
- Examine and palpate abdomen for tenderness, mass, and visible peristalsis to rule out GI infection, intestinal obstruction.

- Examine and palpate all extremities, head, chest and back for signs of trauma.
- Examine both ear-drums with otoscope to rule out acute otitis externa and media, especially if the baby is pulling its ear.
- Inspect genitalia for phimosis, torsion of testis or strangulated hernia.
- Palpate fontanels and check for neck stiffness.
- If a cause is found, treat it.

Common Causes of Crying without Disease

- Hunger—feed the baby.
- Discomfort—too hot, too cold, wet nappy, loud noises, pricking safety pin, etc. Look for and remove the cause.
- Evening colic—attack of sudden colic with flexion of thighs and flushing of face. It resolves spontaneously after 2–3 months. Drugs are rarely needed but to give symptomatic relief, prescribe:
  - Bonnisan (Carmicide) 1 tsf bd or tds.
  - Syp. Phenargan—0.2–2.0 mg/kg/day.
  - Colimex drops 0.5 ml sos.
- "Gases" —due to wrong feeding technique —gentle abdominal massage.
- Constipation—treat it as given in "Constipation".
- Loneliness—cuddle, carry the baby—it will stop crying. This won't spoil the baby, as is usually believed.
- Fatigue—rest the child in calm atmosphere.
- Teething—see "teething complaint".
- Drugs—Check the list of drugs the baby is taking and analyze if the drug is responsible, e.g., antihistaminic can cause drowsiness and irritability.

Don't be discouraged, if crying does not stop. The child may have a "*crying personality*".

"HEALTHY TEETHING" & "TEETHING COMPLAINTS"

Teething is a convenient condition to blame for every illness in a teething baby. Be it fever, cough, diarrhoea or convulsions, parents believe it to be due to teething.

Common Teething Complaints in Babies

- Irritability, fretfulness
- Sleeplessness
- Swollen, red gums
- Chewing on anything and everything
- Increased dribbling of saliva

Advice to Parents

- Gentle massaging of gums with a clean finger.
- Allow baby to chew on ice cubes wrapped in clean cloth.
- Do not keep anything on the floor as child tries to put everything in mouth leading to GI infections.
- Give Syr/Tab. Paracetamol (Crocin) 10 mg/kg/dose, if child is very uncomfortable.
- May require sedative at night for peaceful sleep.

'Healthy Teething'

1. Teething usually begins at the age of 6 months and primary set of teeth completes around 2–3 years.
2. It is a common tendency to neglect care of primary dentition as they are anyway going to fall off. This is a misconception. For healthy, properly aligned permanent set of teeth, you require healthy primary teeth.
3. Discourage bottle-feeding—it is a common cause of caries.
4. No lollipops, sweets, candies in between the meals or before bedtime.

5. Use of fluoridated toothpaste.
6. Rectify cause of mouth breathing, if present, like enlarged adenoids, DNS, etc.
7. Inculcate the habit of brushing teeth as soon as the 1st molar tooth appears around 1 year of age. Parents may require assisting him till he develops necessary motor skills of teeth brushing.
8. Tooth brushing and gargling after each meal.
9. Dental check-up every 6 months after the age of 3 years to detect and treat dental caries at an early age.

POOR EATER

Every mother complains that her child eats too less and she demands tonics. This is true for a child of 1–3 years of age. We cannot drive them away with a lecture on uselessness of tonics—– she will go to the doctor practising opposite you. At the same time, we should not write a tonic and succumb to their pressure. We have to strike a balance.

Evaluate child's appearance, activity and growth and record it on growth chart.

Only if he grades too low on the growth chart, examine and investigate for chronic infections like TB, UTI, CRF. Do haemogram, ESR, urine routine.

Investigations are unlikely to be productive, if history and examination do not suggest disease.

Look out for actual reason for mother's apprehension—illness or death of a sibling, relatives insisting that she is not taking proper care of her child, only child, marital or other stress.

Explain to the parents that the rate of growth is more in 1st year of life and then reduces in next 2–3 years along with physiological reduction in subcutaneous fat. Therefore, chubby child starts looking skinny. Explain that if the child is growing at a rate of 1½–2 kg/year, he is normal and to stop worrying.

Never try to force him to eat. Forcing food only leads to food refusal—and a vicious cycle starts. Increase physical activity of the child, appetite will automatically increase.

Monotonous food is another cause of food refusal. Child also requires variety to stimulate its appetite.

Respect his likes and dislikes to some extent. Be democratic not autocratic. Start maintaining growth chart and record it regularly.

Add last but not the least, a placebo tonic to keep family in doctor's treatment. It works wonderfully—the child keeps on growing naturally and the doctor takes credit!

RECURRENT ABDOMINAL PAIN (RAP)

It is defined as the presence of at least 3 episodes of abdominal pain in a child, severe enough to interfere with its activities for a period longer than 3 months. It is a very common complaint in children aged 2–6 years. As many of these cases are functional, it is essential to differentiate these from organic cases.

Features of NORAP (Non-organic RAP)

- Vague, ill-defined pain.
- Peri-umbilical or poorly localized.
- Non-progressive.
- Never wakes the child at night.
- No other symptoms like fever, jaundice, diarrhoea, urinary symptoms, abdominal distension, weight loss, vomiting, etc.
- Secondary gain present—like avoiding school, getting parental attention, etc.
- Accompanied or caused by stressful events, school phobia, sibling rivalry, parental conflicts, etc.
- Usually seen in children > 2 years.

Management of NORAP

1. Take thorough clinical history, and do proper clinical examination, even if features of pain suggest NORAP. This will help convince the parents that child's complaint has been taken seriously and nothing serious has been missed.
2. If convinced of pain being NORAP, ask the parents and child if old enough, to maintain a pain chart. This would identify the triggering factors and secondary gains the child is seeking.
3. Advise the parents not to 'fulfill' his secondary gain. Send him to school even if he has pain. Pay attention to the child, not his pain.
4. Advise parents to rectify the triggering factors—check out why child is fearing to go to school, find methods to reduce sibling rivalry, parental conflicts, etc. This will help reduce the pain.

Management of Organic RAP (ORAP)

When the features of NORAP are not present, think of ORAP. The most common causes of ORAP in India are giardiasis, worm infestation, recurrent UTI, constipation and gastritis.

Do haemogram, urine routine, stool routine.

- If UTI—Give Syr/Tab. Norfloxacin (Norilet) 6–8 mg/kg/dose in 2 days or Syr/Tab. Ofloxacin (Oflatoon) 4 mg/kg/dose bd for 7 days.
- If ova/worms—Tab/Syr Zentel 400 mg > 2 years and 200 mg < 2 years. Plus
- Tab. Metronidazole (Flagyl) 10 mg/kg/dose in 3 dd × 10 days.
- Tab. Famotidine (Famtac) 1–2 mg/kg/day in 2 dd × 2–3 weeks.
- If constipation—treat as given in "Constipation". If no response to above treatment, do USG to detect/r/o gallstones, abdominal tuberculosis, chronic appendicitis, etc., and treat accordingly.

Even after above treatment and investigations, some RAP remain undiagnosed. Refer these cases to paediatrician, as they may require invasive and expensive investigations like ERCP, CT scan abdomen, EEG, colonoscopy, etc.

STRIDOR

Causes of stridor

Acute

1. Viral croup
2. Bacterial—common, *H. influenzae*; rare, diphtheriae
3. Spasmodic croup
4. Allergic reaction—angioneurotic oedema
5. Foreign body
6. Bacterial tracheitis

Chronic

1. Laryngomalacia
2. Laryngeal webs

Acute stridor is a common and a frightening complaint (for parents).

The cause of the stridor in the baby should be accurately ascertained so as not to miss life threatening conditions like foreign body, angioneurotic oedema or acute epiglottitis.

All cases of chronic stridor, as they may require surgical intervention.

Acute stridor of abrupt onset with no fever—suspect inhaled foreign body—refer immediately. Acute stridor in a child > 3 years with high grade fever, toxicity, dysphagia, drooling—suspect acute epiglottitis. *Do not examine the throat*—refer immediately after giving Inj. Ceftriaxone (C-tri) 100 mg/kg stat.

Viral croup—In acute stridor with a h/o rhinitis, barking cough, hoarseness, give plenty of oral fluids.

Inj. Dexamethasone 0.2 mg/kg IV or 0.6 mg/kg IM stat.

For immediate relief, nebulise the child with salbutamol + budesonide. Antibiotics are not necessary.

Refer in viral croup, if:

- Stridor at rest with chest in-drawing.
- Toxic look.
- Poor oral intake.
- Age < 6 months.

ACUTE DIARRHOEA

Acute diarrhoea (<2 weeks) is one of the most common complaints for which baby is brought to a GP.

Management depends upon the cause of diarrhoea and status of hydration of the child.

Causes

- In an exclusively breastfed child, frequent passage of stools of whatever colour (green, yellow) or consistency is normal. No need to treat.
- Antibiotics-induced diarrhoea is an important cause of diarrhoea in children.
- Lookout for infections outside the GI tract—– tonsillitis, otitis media, pneumonia, UTI septicaemia, as a cause of diarrhoea. This is called 'parenteral diarrhoea'. Treat the cause.
- Most of the acute watery diarrhoeas are viral in origin and require no antibiotics—correction and maintenance of hydration is all that is needed.
- Unclean feeding utensils or bottles, lack of hand washing, are causes that have to be addressed to prevent further attacks of diarrhoea.
- Dentition per-se does not cause diarrhoea, it is the contaminated things that the baby keeps on chewing and biting that cause diarrhoea.

Having confirmed that the cause is GI infection, management of diarrhoea depends upon the status of hydration.

Management

For grade I dehydration (thirsty, irritable, alert, no changes in vital signs, normal skin turgor and adequate urine output), oral rehydration solution (WHO recommended) is the main stay of treatment.

Give ORS 1–2 tsp frequently and continuously. If child vomits, wait for 2 min and try giving ORS in smaller quantities at a time.

Age	ORS (no. of glasses/day)
<4 months	Exclusive breast feeding
4–12 months	2–3
12–24 months	3–4
24–44 months	4–6

Give 100 mL of ORS after every stool.

- In breast-fed child continue breastfeeding.
- In top-milk fed child, do not stop milk, may dilute it.
- In infant taking solid or semi-solid food, continue the food like rice-dal, rice-curd, ripe banana, apple, etc. Do not give fruit juices or oily food-stuff, soft drinks, etc.
- Once diarrhoea is corrected, give a teaspoon of coconut oil tds to make up for the lost weight. This 'caloric fortification' is very important to prevent the diarrhoea–malnutrition–diarrhoea cycle.
- Add antibiotics, if there is high-grade fever, toxicity, stools with blood or greenish foul smelling stools.
- **Do not give anti-motility drugs like Loperamide or opioids like Codeine.**
- If diarrhoea is severe, give racecodotril (Enuff) 1.5 mg/kg tds. It is an antisecretory drug.

- Give Vitamin A prophylaxis (200,000 IU) every 6 months to prevent diarrhoea.
- Prebiotics like *Sporolac* to be given.
- Stool examination should be done in almost every case of diarrhoea to avoid unnecessary use of antibiotics which will worsen the diarrhoea if it is viral.
- If fever or vomiting is present, amoebic infection is unlikely. So, Metronidazole or Ornidazole should be avoided.

Refer the baby, if

- Moderate to severe dehydration.
- Persistent vomiting.
- No response to treatment in 8–12 hrs.
- Develops complications like abdominal distension, oliguria, respiratory distress, drowsiness, etc.

| **Table 13.1** Antibiotics for diarrhoea |

Drug	Available as	Frequency of dose
Furazolidone + Metronidazole (5 mg/kg dose – 10 mg/kg/dose)	Susp. Metrogyl F Flagly F	tds
Nalidixic acid + Metronidazole (15 mg/kg/dose)	Susp Gramoneg or Susp Nilix M	tds
Norfloxacin + Metronidazole (10–15 mg/kg/day)	Normogyl susp Norspan susp	bd
Ciprofloxacin + Tinidazole (10–5 mg/kg/day)	Citi susp	bd
Ofloxacin + Ornidazole (10–15 mg/kg/day)	Zenflox susp	bd
Cefixime (8 mg/kg/day)	Zifi susp	bd

This chapter has been reviewed by ***Dr Rahul Khade*** *and* ***Dr Vaje****, MD Paediatrics, Pune.*

CHAPTER 14

HIV Related Conditions

- Diarrhoea
- Dysphagia
- Herpes Zoster
- Oral Ulcers
- Oral Candidiasis
- Itchy Folliculitis
- Other Skin Conditions
- Pulmonary TB
- Pneumonia
- Cervical Lymphadenopathy
- Course of HIV infection
- When to suspect HIV disease
- Paediatric HIV infection
- Prevention of common opportunistic infection

DIARRHOEA

1. During early and intermediate stage usually it is large bowel dirrhoea with colic, tenesmus, stools containing blood and mucus, and fever, etc. It is caused by the usual gastrointestinal pathogens like *E. coli*, *Shigella*, *E. histolytica*, etc.
   - ORS or IV fluids, if dehydration.
   - Tab. Norfloxacin (Norflox) 400 bd (**or**)
     Tab. Ciprofloxacin (Cifran) 500 bd (**or**)
     Tab. Ofloxacin 200 bd × 5 days.
   - Tab. Metronidazole (Metrogyl) 400 mg tds (**or**)
     Tab. Tinidazole (Tini) 600 mg bd × 5 days.
   - IV Ciprofloxacin, if dysentery is severe.
2. During intermediate or late stage usually it is small bowel diarrhoea, which is persistent or recurrent, profuse, watery without blood or mucus and without fever. It is caused by opportunistic organisms like *Isospora belli*, *Cryptosporidium*, microsporidia, etc.
   a) Tab. TMP/SMX (Ciplin DS) qid × 7 days.
   b) Tab. Metronidazole (Metrogyl) 400 tds × 7 days.
   c) Tab. Loperamide (Imodium) 2 mg tds × 7 days (**or**)
   Tab. Racecoditril (AD 100) 100 mg tds till diarrhoea stops.

If no response, advise stool examination. Inform the pathologist that the patient is HIV positive and to specifically stain and look for opportunistic organisms (mentioned above) and for *Mycobacterium tuberculosis*. If stool examination identifies:

a) *Isospora belli*: Repeat TMP/SMX qid × 14 days, then one tab daily, life long.
b) *Microsporidia*: Tab TMP/SMX as above plus Tab. Albendazole (Zentel) 400 mg bd × 2 weeks.
c) *Cryptosporidia*: No effective therapy. Try Tab. Azithromycin (Azithral) 500 mg od × 6 days.
d) *Mycobacterium tuberculosis*: Antitubercular treatment.

3. In advanced stage, if diarrhoea is severe or intractable, admit for further investigations and treatment.

DYSPHAGIA

Difficulty in swallowing (dysphagia) or painful swallowing (odynophagia) is a common complaint in intermediate or advanced stages.

Causes

1. Candidial oesophagitis
2. Herpetic ulcers
3. Drug-induced oesophagitis
4. Tuberculous ulcers
5. CMV ulcers
6. Idiopathic ulcers

The first three are the commonest causes and may or may not be associated with oral candidiasis or aphthous ulcers. Hence, give empirical treatment.

Treatment

- Tab. Fluconazole (Zocon) 150 mg od.
- Tab. Acyclovir (Ocuvir) 400 mg 5 times a day.
- Cap. Omeprazole (Omez) 20 mg × bd 2 weeks.

If no response, refer to gastroenterologist for endoscopy.

HERPES ZOSTER

Commonly encountered in early HIV disease.

- Tab Acyclovir (Acivir) 800 mg 5 times daily × 7 days or Tab. Valciclovir 500–1000 mg bd × 7–10 days. Most effective if started early, preferably within 48 hrs of onset of vesicles.
- Tab. Diclofenac (Voveran) 100 mg bd.
- Potassium permanganate soaks followed by application of Silver Sulphadiazine cream.
- Tab. Alprazolam (Restyl) 0.25 mg tds.
- Refer in case of ophthalmic zoster to ophthalmologist for treatment of possible involvement of eye.

ORAL ULCERS

In intermediate and advanced stages, two most common causes are herpes simplex ulcers and aphthous ulcers. It is many times difficult to differentiate between these two. Laboratory confirmation is also difficult.

Treatment

1. Initially treat as herpetic ulcers:
   - Tab. Acyclovir (Acivir) 400 mg 5 times a days × 7 days **or** Tab. Famciclovir (Famterx) 250 mg tds × 7 days.
   - Betadine mouthwash tds.
   - Acyclovir ointment—apply tds to ulcers.
2. If no response in 7 days, treat as for aphthous ulcers.
   - Tab. Prednisolone (Wysolone) 10 mg tds × 7 days.
   - Cap. Omeprazole (Omez) 20 mg bd × 7 days
   - Betadine mouthwash tds.
   - Kenacort oral paste, to be applied to ulcers.
3. If still no response, refer for biopsy to r/o lymphoma or CMV ulcers.

ORAL CANDIDIASIS

These are seen as creamy white patches in the oral cavity (thrush) or as erythematous patches on the tongue or palate (erythematous candidiasis) or as fissuring at the corner of the mouth (angular cheilitis).

- Clotrimazole trouches (Clenorush) 10 mg 5 times a day to be sucked. Avoid eating and

drinking for 20 min after use to increase contact time.
- Tab. Fluconazole (Fusys) 150 mg od × 10 days.
- Oral hygiene.

ITCHY FOLLICULITIS (Pruritic folliculitis)

Common eruption seen in the HIV infected individuals. Lesions are erythematous urticarial papules, seen mainly on the upper part of the body. There is moderate to severe pruritus. They wax and wane with time and usually resolve spontaneously over a period of months. The cause is not known but it could be scabies, insect bite allergy, drug sensitivity, etc. Treat empirically.
- Permethrin (Permite) cream 5%. Apply to the whole body on alternate days after bath × 4 weeks.
- Betnovate cream plus Moisturex cream. To be mixed in equal quantities. Apply on alternate days after bath and daily at bed time.
- Tab. Loratidine (Lorfast) 10 mg od in morning.
- Tab. Hydroxyzine hydrochloride (Atarax) 25 mg hs.

OTHER SKIN CONDITIONS

The following conditions are very commonly seen in HIV positive individuals. The treatment is as for HIV negative individual, although more vigorous and prolonged treatment is required. Please refer to Chapter 7 for details of treatment.
- Staphylococcal folliculitis—Antistaphylococcal antibiotics like cloxacillin.
- Scabies—Permethrin cream or Gamabenzene lotion
- Herpes simplex—Acyclovir
- Molluscum contagiosum—Electrocautery
- Insect bite reaction—Systemic and local steroids, antihistamincs.
- Seborrhoeic dermatitis—Topical steroids
- Psoriasis—Topical steroids and tar ointment
- Fungal infections of feet, nails and body—Fluconazole weekly and Clotrimazole cream
- Common warts—Local salicylic + lactic acid ointment or electrocautery.

PULMONARY TUBERCULOSIS

Incidence of pulmonary TB in HIV infected individuals is very high. Typical pulmonary TB involving the apical region is seen in early HIV disease, response to treatment is excellent and relapse rate is low. Atypical pulmonary TB involving the mid or lower zone is seen in late HIV disease. Give treatment as per Category I or Category II (see Chapter 2).

In Early HIV Disease

- Tab. Rifampicin + INH + Pyrazinamide + Ethambutol × 2 months (Forecox) 2 tabs in morning.
- Tab. Rifampicin + INH + Ethambutol (RHE -FD) 1 tab on empty stomach × 4 months.

In Late HIV Disease

- Treatment is initiated as above.
- Extend treatment by 3 months, if response is slow.
- Give treatment according to Category II, if it is a relapse case of pulmonary TB.
- Refer to specialist, if there is no response, as this could be Multi-Drug Resistance (MDR) tuberculosis.

PNEUMONIA

Two types of pneumonia are seen in HIV infected individuals—bacterial pneumonia and *Pneumocystis carinii* pneumonia (PCP).

Bacterial Pneumonia

Bacterial pneumonia is very commonly encountered in general practice. It presents with severe symptoms of acute onset (2–3 days), high grade fever, chest pain, cough with purulent sputum, toxicity, etc. Chest X-ray shows patches of consolidation. Clinical features, causative organisms and treatment are same as in a non-HIV infected patient.

- Tab Cefixime (Taxim O) 200 mg bd (**or**) Tab Cefuroxime (Ceftum) 500 mg bd × 14 days.
- Analgesic and antipyretic drugs.
- Cough expectorants like Zedex expectorant 2 tsf tds.
- IV fluids, if dehydration.

Pneumocystis Carinii Pneumonia (PCP)

PCP is seen in late stage and is not very commonly encountered in general practice. Typically the patient presents with low grade symptoms of insidious onset (1–2 months), cough (without expectoration), breathlessness (disproportionate to the minimal chest findings) and fever (which is low grade). Diagnostic confirmation is difficult in general practice as X-ray chest may be normal or non-specific and bronchoscopy may be required. Hence, give a trial of:

- Tab. Cotrimoxazole (Ciplin DS) 2 qid × 21 days.
- Analgesics and antipyretics.
- Cough suppressants like Cosome linctus

Admit if:

- No response to above treatment.
- Patient deteriorates clinically.
- Skin rash develops to Cotrimoxazole, which is common and could be life-threatening.

CERVICAL LYMPHADENOPATHY

If an HIV-infected individual presents with cervical lymphadenopathy, consider four causes:

1. ***Persistent generalized lymphadenopathy (PGL)*** seen in early stage. Persistent nonpainful, nontender, multiple, bilaterally symmetrical, freely mobile.
   - No specific treatment is required.
2. ***Tuberculous lymphadenopathy*** seen in intermediate stage, enlargement of 2–3 lymph nodes which are painful, tender, matted together and not bilaterally symmetrical. The lymph nodes soften and burst to form a discharging sinus. FNAC or biopsy confirms diagnosis.
   - Tab. Forecox 2 od on empty stomach × 2 months.
   - Then, Cap. Montonex forte 1 od × 4–6 months.
   - Repeated aspiration of pus from a nondependent area.
3. ***Secondary syphilis***: Bilaterally symmetrical, non-tender nodes with firm rubbery consistency. Advise VDRL test, which will confirm diagnosis.
   - Inj. Benzathine Penicillin 2.4 mega units once a week AST × 3 weeks.
4. ***Non-Hodgkin lymphoma***
   - Rare, seen in late stage. Firm nodules with uniform consistency.
   - Concomitant extra-nodal disease in brain, lungs, liver etc., may be present. Advise biopsy to confirm diagnosis. If confirmed, refer to oncologist for further investigations and chemotherapy.

COURSE OF HIV INFECTION

Window period	Initial 2–3 months	HIV antibody test is negative
Serocon-version	5–7 days after window period	Fever, rash, lymphadenopathy
Early HIV disease	5–8 years	Largely asymp-tomatic
Intermed-iate HIV disease	2–3 years	TB, recurrent diarrhoea, fever, herpes zoster, loss of weight, etc.
Late HIV disease (AIDS)	2–3 years	Opportunistic infections and malignancies

WHEN SHOULD YOU SUSPECT HIV DISEASE AND ORDER AN HIV ANTIBODY TEST?

1. Any person requesting the test, following unprotected sexual exposure.
2. All pregnant women.
3. Child born to an HIV positive mother (after 15 months of age).
4. All persons in high risk categories:
   - Commercial sex workers
   - Homosexuals
   - Intravenous drug users
   - Haemophiliacs, requiring repeated blood transfusions
5. Persons presenting with any of the following illnesses:
   - All persons with STD
   - Pulmonary or extrapulmonary TB
   - Generalized lymphadenopathy
   - Unexplained fever
   - Unexplained diarrhoea
   - Unexplained weight loss
   - Unexplained peripheral neuropathy
   - Skin lesion like herpes zoster, chronic herpes simplex, extensive psoriasis, extensive seborrhoeic dermatitis, extragenital molluscum contagiosum
   - Oral lesion like thrush, recurrent aphthous stomatitis
   - Recurrent pneumonia

WHAT A GP SHOULD KNOW ABOUT PAEDIATRIC HIV INFECTON?

1. Not all children born to HIV positive mother will be HIV infected. The risk of transmission of HIV from a pregnant mother to her baby is between 20% and 45%.
2. To make a diagnosis of HIV infection in a child, HIV antibody test should be done after 15–18 months of age, before which the maternal antibodies will give false positive results. Two negative results after 6 months rules out the infection.
3. About 20–30% of the infected babies are "rapid progressors", who develop advanced HIV disease in the 1st year of life and then progress rapidly. Around 70–80% are "slow or intermediate progressors", who remain asymptomatic for 1st few years of life.
4. Common clinical manifestations are generalized lymphadenitis, hepatosplenomegaly, parotitis, failure to thrive, delayed milestones, recurrent bacterial infections, recurrent upper and lower respiratory tract infections, TB, CSOM, recurrent diarrhoea, PCP, etc.
5. The baby should not be breastfed at all or exclusively breastfed (no water, no top feeds, etc.) for 4 months.
6. All babies born to HIV positive mothers should receive TMP-SMX (Septran) from 6 weeks onwards till proved HIV negative, or life long if the report is positive.

7. **PMTCT (prevention of mother to child transmission) of HIV**: Nevirepine 200 mg single dose to the mother after onset of labour and 2 mg/kg single dose to the newborn within 72 hrs of birth.
8. All babies born to HIV positive mothers should be vaccinated as per the National Immunization Schedule.

PREVENTION OF COMMON OPPORTUNISTIC INFECTIONS

- Do not give Rifampicin or Isonex to prevent TB, because of fear of development of resistance.
- Do not give Fluconazole to prevent oral candidiasis for the same reasons.
- Always start Tab. Fluconazole (Zocon) 150 mg od daily life-long, if the patient has suffered an attack of oesophageal candidiasis.
- Always start Tab. Cotrimoxazole (Ciplin DS) 1 od daily life-long, once the patient becomes symptomatic. This will prevent five diseases: toxoplasmosis, PCP, isospora diarrhoea, bacterial pneumonia and bacterial skin infections. This will cost just Rs. 1 per day to the patient and save thousands of rupees by preventing these diseases.
- If the patient is allergic to Cotrimoxazole, then give Tab. Dapsone 100 mg od life-long.

*This chapter has been reviewed by **Dr Prakash Mahajan**, HIV Specialist, Pune.*

CHAPTER 15

Miscellaneous Conditions

- Anaemia
- Loss of Weight
- Weight Gain
- Oedema
- Diabetes
- Simple Goitre
- Hypothyroidism
- Hyperthyroidism
- The Three-day Fever
- The One-week Fever
- The Three-weeks Fever
- Excessive Sweating
- Lymphadenopathy
- Cramps
- Intermittent Claudication

ANAEMIA

If a patient has vague symptoms like weakness, palpitations, dizziness, tingling numbness, etc., then look for pallor in the conjunctiva or palate. Also compare the patient's palms with your own palms to detect pallor. If pallor is present and especially if there are other evidences of anaemia like sore tongue, brittle nails, etc., order a full blood count. If Hb is low and the morphology of the RBC is "microcytic hypochromic" it is *iron deficiency anaemia*, which can be easily treated by a GP. If the Hb is very low (<5 g%) and the cell morphology is different (e.g., marked anisocytosis, marked poikilocytosis or spherocytosis), refer to a physician.

Treatment

- Treatment of the cause, e.g., DUB, bleeding piles, etc.
- Plenty of green leafy vegetables, fruits, meat, etc.
- Cap. Ferrous fumarate (Autrin) bd × 3–6 months (**or**)
  - Tab. Ferrous sulphate (Fersolate) 200 mg bd × 3–6 months (**or**)
  - Liq. Dexorange 2 tsf bd
  - Iron sucrose IV injection: (Orofer S 100 mg in 5 mL) 2 ampules are dissolved in 100 mL of normal saline and given over 20–30 min. Repeat on alternate days depending on severity of anaemia
- Tab. Zentel 400 single dose.

Who should be referred?

1. Active bleeding present, e.g., menorrhagia, bleeding piles, etc. (this has to be stopped.)
2. Any male patient with severe anaemia (usually the cause is not iron deficiency).
3. Huge splenomegaly with severe anaemia (could be haemolytic anaemia).
4. Jaundice with anaemia (could be haemolytic anaemia).
5. Melaena is present (could be cancer of the intestine).
6. Sudden severe anaemia (could be leukaemia or severe haemolysis).

LOSS OF WEIGHT

There are three types of patients seen in general practice as far as weight loss is concerned.

1. Mother complains that her school going child has lost weight, while in fact the child has increased in height and therefore looking thin. He is otherwise healthy and playful.
   - Santevini tonic 2 tsf bd.
   - Tab. Buclizine (Longiphen) 50 mg bd.
   - Nutriprot powder 2 tsf od with milk.
   - Increase food intake especially food rich in calories like sweet and fatty foods.
   - Reassurance to mother that the child is healthy.
2. An adolescent who because of sudden change in life-style (e.g., left home to live in a hostel or hectic work because of new job) or a newly married girl because of change in environment, has lost a few kilograms of weight.

Causes of weight loss
With good intake of food 1. Diabetes 2. Hyperthyroidism 3. Malabsorption syndrome
With reduced intake of food 1. Tuberculosis 2. HIV infection 3. Renal failure 4. Depression 5. Malignancy

3. An adult has over a period of a few weeks or months lost more than 10% of his original body weight. This is taken as pathological weight loss unless proved otherwise.

   Please refer to the box giving the common causes of weight loss. In general practice, it is not possible to order a "battery of investigations". So select the investigations to be carried out going by a thorough enquiry into the patient's symptoms.

If the Food Intake is Good

1. Does he have to pass urine at night? It could be diabetes—Do BSL and urine sugar.
2. Does he have tachycardia or tremors? It could be hyperthyroidism—Do T_3, T_4, TSH.
3. Does he have recurrent loose motions? It could be malabsorption—Do stool examination.

If the Food Intake is Reduced

1. Does he have prolonged cough, fever, cervical lymph nodes, etc? It could be tuberculosis—Do X-ray chest, ESR, FNAC, etc.
2. Does he give h/o unprotected exposure, herpes zoster or oral candidiasis? It could be HIV infection—Do HIV test.
3. Many times, weight loss is the only presenting symptom of chronic renal failure. So do S. creatinine and blood urea routinely.
4. Ask for symptoms like loss of interest, depressed mood, insomnia, etc. It could be severe depression.
5. Does he give h/o haemoptysis, PR bleeding, haematemesis, bleeding gums, etc. It could be malignancy. Refer to relevant specialist for investigations.

WEIGHT GAIN

Weight gain in an individual may be due to increase in body water or body fat. One has to rule out increase in weight due to water retention caused by renal, cardiac or hepatic causes before labelling that weight gain is due to obesity (i.e. excess of fat). This can be done by appropriate investigations like S. creatinine, blood urea, ECG, LFT, etc. Obesity can lead to various illnesses like hypertension, diabetes, dyslipidaemia, infertility, varicose veins, osteoarthritis, sleep apnoea, etc., leading to a shortened life expectancy.

Common Causes

- Simple obesity (most common)
- Hypothyroidism
- Drugs like corticosteroids, tricyclic antidepressants, OC pills, etc.
- Cushing's syndrome (mainly steroid induced)
- Polycystic ovarian disease
- Depression
- Premenstrual syndrome (Cyclical weight gain)
- Pregnancy

Management

- **Monitor BMI** (Body mass index) and W/H (Waist to hip) ratio periodically.
- **Diet**: Plenty of vegetables, salads. Chalk out a plan for the patient to lose weight gradually preferably under the guidance of a dietitian. 'Crash diets' usually fail. Junk foods, alcohol, soft drinks, bakery products, etc., should be avoided at all cost.
- **Exercise**: This should be a way of life not just a temporary method to lose weight. Dieting without exercise is useless. Brisk walk for 20–30 min each day or games like tennis, cycling, swimming goes a long way in reducing and maintaining weight.

Drug Treatment

- Tab. Orlistat (Orlistal, Xenical) 120 mg with each major meal. Take immediately after meal as it works by preventing absorption of fat.
- Sibutramin, Rimonabant and Fenfluramine have been banned in India.

OEDEMA

Unilateral Oedema

Localised to one lower limb. Treatment will depend on the cause.

Management

- ***Cellulitis***—diffuse swelling of one leg with severe tenderness.
  - Cap. Cefalexin (Phexin) 500 mg qid × 10–15 days (**or**)
  - Tab. Cefixime (Ceftas) 200 mg bd × 10–15 days (**or**)
  - Cap. Amoxiclav (Augmentin) 625 mg × 10–15 days (**or**)
- ***Gout***—tender swelling behind great toe.
  - Cap. Indomethacin (Indocap) 25 mg 2 qid (**or**)
  - Tab. Colchicine 0.5 mg, 2 tabs stat, then 1 tab. every 2 hr till attack subsides or diarrhoea starts (not freely available) (**or**)
  - Tab. Prednisolone (Wysolone) 10 mg tds.
  - Tab. Allupirunol (Zyloric) 100 mg tds in chronic gout.
- ***Deep vein thrombosis***—swelling of the legs with maximum tenderness on the calf. Admit for heparin treatment.
- ***Filariasis***—long-standing pitting oedema on one leg, which is non-tender. Patient gets intermittent fever with rigors.
  - Tab. Diethylcarbamazine (Hetrazan) 100 mg tds × 3 weeks.
  - Elastic stockings during day time.
  - Elevation of leg during night time.
  - Tab. Paracetamol 500 mg tds, if fever.

Generalised Oedema

Treatment will depend on the cause.

Management

- ***Anaemia with hypoproteinaemia***
  Seen in poor patients. Pallor, stomatitis, puffiness of face with oedema over feet.
  - Tab. Raricap bd × 6 months.
  - Tab. Multivit FM bd × 2 months.
  - Protinules powder 2 tsf bd.
- ***Drug-induced oedema***
  Sudden onset swelling of face and feet mainly following steroids, diclofenac, ibuprofen, nifedipine, oral contraceptives, etc. Withdraw the drug.
- ***Venous insufficiency oedema***
  Usually middle aged women, oedema over ankles after prolonged sitting or standing.
  - Elevation of legs at night.
  - Elastic stockings during day.
  - Tab. Hydrochlorothiazide (Esidrex) 50 mg od, intermittent courses off and on.
- ***Angioneurotic, i.e., allergic oedema***
  Sudden onset with intense itching, urticaria, hoarse voice, dyspnoea.
  - Tab. Prednisolone (Wysolone) 10 mg qid.
  - Tab. Cetrizine (Zyrtec) 10 mg bd.
  - Admit if hoarse voice or dyspnoea, as this could be life-threatening.
- ***Myxoedema or hypothyroidism***
  Non-pitting oedema, puffiness of face, weight gain, hoarse voice, lethargy, etc., of a few months duration. Do T_3, T_4, TSH. If TSH is raised and T_3, T_4 are reduced. Tab. Eltroxin life-long (see hypothyroidism).
- ***Premenstrual oedema***
  - Reduce salt intake.
  - Tab. Esidrex 1 od 1 week before menses.
- ***Cardiac***
  Oedema over legs in a known patient of heart disease. Admit.
- ***Renal***
  Generalised oedema more on face and in the morning. Advise urine examination. If albumin +++ present, admit.
- ***Hepatic oedema***
  Known alcoholic develops ascites and oedema over legs. Admit.
- ***Idiopathic oedema***
  Chronic mild oedema usually in middle aged females. Slight puffiness of face in mornings and mild oedema over feet in evenings, hardly any oedema present but marks of bangles and blouse seen. All investigations are normal. It is a diagnosis of exclusion.
  - Reassurance that oedema is harmless and will disappear spontaneously in a few years.
  - Low salt diet.
  - Tab. Esidrex od, intermittent courses, off and on.

CONTROLLING BLOOD SUGAR IN A DIABETIC PATIENT

How does the Diabetic Patient Present to a GP?

- Monilial balanitis in elderly males and itching of the genitalia (candidiasis) in elderly females.
- Peripheral neuritis. Tingling numbness and pain in both the legs.
- Non-healing wounds.
- Recurrent furunculosis.
- Tiredness, weakness and loss of weight in spite of good appetite.
- Frequency of urination, especially at night.

The classical of "3 polys", i.e., **polyuria** (excessive urination), **polydipsia** (excessive thirst) and **polyphagia** (excessive hunger) is not a common presenting feature. Under the above circumstances, order a fasting and a postprandial glucose blood test. A full glucose tolerance test is not required.

Criteria for Diagnosis

- Fasting plasma glucose > 126 mg/dL.
- Postprandial plasma glucose > 200 mg/dL.
- Random plasma glucose > 200 mg/dL, if symptoms of diabetes present.

Diet

Once diagnosed, give proper advice regarding diet and exercise.

- No food or drink containing sugar, e.g., chocolates, sweets, ice-creams, etc.
- Restrict fried foods, e.g., wafers, fast foods, papad, potato-wada, etc.
- Eat in moderation the following: Chapatis, bread, rice, meat, eggs, fish, chicken, cheese, butter, milk products, etc.
- Eat plenty of salads, green leafy vegetables, fruits (except bananas, mangoes and chickoo), beans, pulses, Marie biscuits, butter milk, clear soups, etc.
- Take small meals, four times a day.
- Take aerobic exercises or brisk walking for 3–4 km daily.

Plan the Initial Treatment

This will depend on the type of diabetes the patient has.

Type-I Diabetes

It was previously called insulin-dependent diabetes mellitus (IDDM) or juvenile diabetes. Occurs in young individuals in the second or third decade of life. There is no production of insulin by the pancreas.

Hence, insulin has to be given life-long. After discussing with the patient about his life-style and feasibility of taking multiple insulin injections daily, one of the following regimens is adopted:

- **4 injections per day**: Plain insulin before breakfast, lunch and evening snacks with intermediate acting Lente insulin before dinner.
- **3 injections per day**: Plain insulin before breakfast and lunch with long acting ultra Lente before dinner.
- **2 injections per day**: Mixtard twice daily before breakfast and dinner.

The first two regimens will have better control of blood sugar but with more frequent hypoglycaemic attacks. The two injections per day regimen is convenient and achieves a fairly good control of blood sugar. Premixed insulin of human origin (70/30, Mixtard or Actraphane) is preferred. Total dose of insulin to start with is 1/3rd the body weight, e.g., in a 60-kg diabetic, total daily dose is 20 units. Give 2/3rd of this dose (i.e., 13 units) in the morning before breakfast. Give 1/3rd of this dose (i.e., 7 units) in evening before dinner.

Type-II diabetes

It was previously called non-insulin dependent diabetes mellitus (NIDDM) or maturity onset diabetes. This is usually seen in the middle aged or elderly, obese and sedentary individuals.

- **Step 1**: First give proper trial with diet and exercise alone for at least 2 months. If BSL control is not achieved, give oral hypoglycaemic drugs.
- **Step 2**: *In obese* individuals, select metformin or aqcarbose. *In non-obese* individuals, select a sulphonylurea.

  A combination of one drug from each group is preferred (see Table 15.2). Start with a small dose initially, e.g., Glybenclamide (Semi-daonil) 2.5 mg before breakfast and Metformin (Glyciphage) 500 mg after lunch and dinner. Increase dose by ½–1 tablet of each after 2 weeks, if BSL is still high.
- **Step 3**: Measure BSL fasting and PP at weekly intervals to assess control.
- **Step 4**: If control is not achieved after 1 month, shift to mixtard insulin.

Achieving Long-term Blood Sugar Control

- Stress importance of good diet control. If during festivals, sugar intake has increased, compensate by either increase in exercise or more strict diet or increase in the dose of insulin.
- Stress importance of regular exercise. No holidays!
- Advise BSL every 3–4 months. Advice glycosylated haemoglobin test every year. This measures the average glucose level over a period of 3 months. It overcomes a pitfall in BSL estimation that the patient diets meticulously for the preceding 3–4 days before the BSL test in order to get a 'good' report!
- *When BSLs are not satisfactory in patients on oral drugs*: If both fasting and postprandial levels are high, change to (or increase the dose of) a long acting sulphonylurea, e.g., Tab. Glybenclamide (Daonil) 5–10 mg od. If only postprandial sugar remains high, change to a short acting sulphonylurea, e.g., Tab. Glipizide (Glynase) 5 mg od. Tolbutamide and chlorpropamide are outdated drugs. Repaglynide (Eurepa) 1 mg bd before meals or Pioglitazone 15 –30 mg od can be used if the above fails to achieve satisfactory control and the patient is reluctant to take insulin.
- *When BSLs are not satisfactory in patients on insulin*: Change to human insulin if on bovine insulin. While changing, reduce the dose by 30%. If PP sugar is persistently high, increase the dose of pre-breakfast insulin. If fasting sugar is high, increase the dose of pre-dinner long acting insulin.
- Dose adjustments can be made in rich patients by a home glucometer. In poor patients, this can be achieved by doing urine sugar by Benedict's test.
- Teach the patient to take injections at home. Educate patient about symptoms of hypoglycaemic attack. Tell him to make a habit of keeping sugar or biscuits in his pocket. Also ask him to keep an identity card mentioning his name, address and telephone number in the pocket. A mention should be also made on the ID-card that "*I am a diabetic on insulin. If found unconscious or behaving like a drunkard, take me to the nearest hospital for IV 25% dextrose administration.*"

SIMPLE GOITRE

A young girl at puberty complains of a swelling in the front of the neck, which has been pointed out by relatives and friends. But if large, it is quite obvious to the girl. This swelling can be either soft and diffuse or nodular. It is painless, not tender and moves up and down with deglutition. There are no symptoms of hypo- or hyperthyroidism.

Treatment

- Explain that it is a harmless swelling and may regress spontaneously.
- Check TSH and free T_4. If abnormal, Tab. Thyroxine (Eltroxin) 100 μg tds × 3–4 months. Then, 1 bd × 1 year.
- Diffuse soft goitre may regress. Nodular goitre usually does not. Refer for thyroidectomy for cosmetic reasons.

HYPOTHYROIDISM

It should be suspected in any patient who presents with the following complaints:

- Puffiness of face, which is mainly generalised, unlike renal oedema, which is mainly periorbital.

| **Table 15.1** Insulin preparations |

Type	Onset (hrs)	Peak (hrs)	Duration (hrs)
Short acting Soluble insulin Actrapid	½–1	3–4	6–8
Intermediate acting Lente, Monotard Lentard	1–2	8–10	14–16
Long acting Ultra Lente	3–6	12–18	18–20
Premixed Mixtard, Actraphane	½–1	8–10	12–16

| **Table 15.2** Oral hypoglycaemic agents (OHA) |

Drug	Trade name	No. of doses/day	Remarks
Sulphonylureas			
▪ Glybenclamide 5 mg	Daonil, Euglucon	1–2	Potent but slow acting
▪ Glipizide 5 mg	Glynase	1–2	Fast acting
▪ Gliclazide 80 mg	Diamicron	1–2	Has in addition antiplatelet action
▪ Glymeperide 1–2 mg	Glypride	1	Longer duration of action
Biguanides			
▪ Metphormin 500 mg	Glyciphage	1–3	Used in obese
α-Glycosidase inhibitor			
▪ Acarbose 50 mg	Glucobay	1–2	Blocks absorption of glucose Used to treat postprandial hyperglycaemia
New drugs			
▪ Repaglynide 1 mg/2 mg	Eurepa	2	Rapid action
▪ Pioglitazone 15 mg/30 mg			
DPP IV inhibitors			
▪ Sitaglyptin	Januvia	1	Prolongs action of incretins and causes endogenous insulin release after food
▪ Vildaglyptin	Galvus	1	

GENERAL PRACTICE AS SPECIALITY

- Slight oedema over the feet.
- Unexplained and rapid increase in weight.
- Physical and mental slowing, constipation, lethargy.
- Intolerance to cold. These patients put on a sweater even in warm weather. There is less sweating and dry skin.
- Hoarseness of voice has developed over a period of months.
- Thyroid gland usually is *not* enlarged.

All these symptoms require high index of suspicion; otherwise, diagnosis can be easily missed. When suspected:

1. **Elicit the ankle jerk**
   In this condition, after a quick contraction there will be slow relaxation. This can be learnt with practise.
2. **Order T_3, T_4, TSH**
   In hypothyroidism, T_3 and T_4 will be decreased and TSH will be increased. This is a costly investigation (approximately Rs. 600). In poor patients, order only TSH (approximately Rs. 150/-).

Treatment

Once diagnosed, the treatment is simple but has to be taken life-long.

- Tab. Thyroxine (Eltroxin) 100 µg od × 1 month.
- Repeat TSH after 1 month. If TSH is still not normal, increase the dose by ½ tab every month. Two or even three tablets may be required to achieve control.
- Tablets should be taken on empty stomach.
- In elderly patients and in patients with IHD, start with a smaller dose.

HYPERTHYROIDISM

The patient that will present to you will usually be a female with the following complaints:

- Rapid and excessive loss of weight in spite of *normal* appetite. (If there is loss of weight with decreased appetite, think of TB. If there is loss of weight with increased appetite, think of diabetes.)
- Cannot tolerate hot climate. Sweats excessively.
- Palpitations.

Examination

- Tachycardia even after resting in your OPD for ½–1 hr.
- Swelling of the thyroid gland.
- Big staring eyes (exophthalmos).
- Fine tremors of outstretched fingers.
  Under these circumstances, advise T_3, T_4, TSH. In hyperthyroidism, T_3 and T_4 are increased while TSH is decreased.

Treatment

- Refer to endocrinologist or a physician for either drug therapy **or** surgery **or** radioactive iodine therapy, a decision which is difficult to make.
- If the patient refuses to go to a specialist or in rural areas:
  - Tab. Carbimazole (Neomercazole) 5 mg 2 tds till TSH is normal or symptoms are under control. Then 1 tds.
  - Tab. Propranolol (Ciplar) 10 mg 1 tds to control tachycardia.

THE THREE-DAY FEVER

Viral fever

Most of the fevers of short duration seen in general practice are viral fevers. These are self-limiting and usually the patient becomes afebrile within 4–5 days spontaneously. Usually, there is no localizing symptom or sign to a particular system of the body. There is predominant mucous membrane involvement (rhinitis, watering of eyes, etc.) and muscle involvement (severe body ache). These fevers are highly contagious, so two or three members of the same family are down with fever. Treat symptomatically.

- Tab. Paracetamol 500 mg stat and repeat in case of a rise in fever.
- Inj. Diclofenac or Inj. Analgin 2 mL IM stat, if high fever and severe body ache.
- Add Ibuprofen or Analgin or Aspirin, if body ache is severe.
- Add anticold tablet like Actifed, Zyrtec D, if rhinitis.
- Rest in bed. No bath, but sponging may be done. Cold compresses over forehead. Bland diet.

Bacterial Fever

Not all fevers are viral though. Look for localizing symptoms and signs as evidence of bacterial infection. A thorough examination has to be done from head to toe.

1. **Is the headache severe?**
   If yes, r/o meningitis by testing for neck stiffness. Look for tenderness on the frontal or maxillary sinuses if there is h/o rhinitis.
2. **Is there pain in the throat?**
   Examine the throat properly with a tongue depressor and a powerful torch for exudates in the tonsils or congestion in the throat.
3. **Does the patient c/o pain in the ear?**
   Pressing the tragus will give rise to tenderness if there is a furuncle. Otherwise, it could be acute otitis media.
4. **Is there a toothache?**
   Examine for tenderness in the gums or an abscess in the palate or for caries tooth.
5. **Are there neck glands?**
   If these are of recent origin and are tender, they could be the cause of the fever.
6. **Is there chest pain?**
   Auscultate in detail for bronchitis, pneumonitis and effusion.
7. **Hepatomegaly?**
   Think of jaundice and examine the sclera. Keep typhoid fever and amoebic liver abscess in mind.
8. **Splenomegaly?**
   Malaria is the commonest cause, followed by typhoid.
9. **Is there a rash?**
   It could be chicken pox, drug rash or a viral exanthem.
10. **Is herpes labialis present?**
    If present, this favours the diagnosis of viral fever, malaria, pneumonia or meningitis.
11. **Is there burning micturition?**
    Could be urinary tract infection.
12. **Are inguinal glands tender?**
    Could be injury to the leg with secondary infection or STD.
13. **Are rigors severe?**
    If yes, the possibilities are malaria or UTI.
14. **Loose motions?**
    If present, it could be bacillary dysentery.

The treatment of each of these infections are given in the relevant chapters.

THE ONE-WEEK FEVER

If with the above treatment the fever does not respond, review your clinical diagnosis. If further clinical diagnosis is not possible, investigate keeping the following possibilities in mind:

- Prolonged viral fever
- Chloroquine resistant malaria
- Pulmonary TB
- Enteric fever
- Silent UTI
- Pneumonitis
- Pleural effusion
- Meningitis
- HIV infection

Treatment of malaria	
Tab. Chloroquine (Lariago DS)	→ 2 tablets stat, then 1 tablet after 6 hr, then 1 tablet daily × 2 days
followed by	
Tab. Primaquin 7.5 mg	→ 1 bd × 14 days (**or**)
Tab. Mefloquin (Larium) 250 mg	→ 3 tablets stat, then → 3 tablets after 6 hrs

Treatment of typhoid	
Tab. Ciprofloxacin	→ 500 mg bd × 10 days (**or**)
Inj. Ceftriaxone	→ 1 g bd IV X 7 days (**or**)
Cap. Chloram-phenicol	→ 500 mg qid × 14 days

Request for the following investigations:

- Haemogram
- ESR
- PBS for MP
- Urine—routine
- Widal test for typhoid
- X-ray chest
- HIV test

The WBC count is usually normal in viral fevers, malaria, UTI, enteric fever and pulmonary TB. In other bacterial infections, it is raised. If after these investigations, the diagnosis is clear, treat accordingly. If not, give empirical treatment for malaria as well as for typhoid (see Box).

THE THREE-WEEKS FEVER (PUO)

If in spite of the above treatment, the fever fails to subside, label the patient as having "**pyrexia of unknown origin**". This is defined as "*fever more than 3 weeks in duration, where routine investigations have not revealed the diagnosis and empirical treatment for malaria and typhoid has not brought down the fever.*"

Admit the patient in a hospital under a competent physician. The differential diagnosis now is either tuberculosis somewhere in the body or a rare bacterial infection or a hidden malignancy or a rare connective tissue disorder.

EXCESSIVE SWEATING

Sudden sweating may be caused by:

- Hypoglycaemia in a patient of diabetes on insulin
- Syncope
- Acute myocardial infarction
- Sudden, severe pain of any origin
- Fever like malaria
- Antipyretics
- Acute anxiety

Sweating of long duration may be due to:

- Congenital hyperhydrosis
- Hyperthyroidism
- Night sweats due to tuberculosis, lymphoma, etc.
- Rickets in children
- Alcohol abuse
- Anxious personality
- Recurrent sweating, hot flushes in menopausal syndrome

Management

Excessive sweating may be harmless like in congenital hyperhydrosis or in an anxious personality and only reassurance is required. In most of the cases, sweating is a manifestation of other diseases and treatment of the primary condition is required.

When symptomatic relief from sweating needs to be given, advise the following.

For hyperhydrosis of palms and soles:

- Avoid nylon socks and tight shoes.
- Ammonium chloride solution 20% or Gluteraldehyde solution. Immerse palms or soles once daily for 10 min (**or**)
- Tab. Dicyclomin (Cyclopam) 1 tds. This causes troublesome side effects like dry mouth, blurred vision, etc., which may not be acceptable to the patient.
- If no response, refer to dermatologist for iontophoresis (**or**) refer to surgeon for sympathectomy.

LOCALIZED ENLARGEMENT OF LYMPH NODES

Lymph nodes are normally palpable in children and even in adults. These are soft, mobile and <1 cm in diameter. They may enlarge to >2 cm during viral/bacterial respiratory infections.

The site of involvement, consistency etc. should give a clue to the probable diagnosis.

Site

- ***Cervical***: Tuberculosis, bacterial infections, nonspecific lymphadenitis, infectious mononucleosis.
- ***Axillary nodes***: BCG vaccine, breast infection, tuberculosis.
- ***Supraclavicular nodes***: Gastrointestinal malignancy.
- ***Occipital lymph nodes***: Folliculitis scalp, secondary syphilis.
- ***Inguinal nodes***: Injury or furuncle in the leg (vertical chain involved), venereal diseases like LGV, syphilis, granuloma inguinale (horizontal chain involved), tuberculosis.

Consistency

- Hard nodes—Carcinoma
- Rubbery nodes—Lymphoma
- Soft, multiple—Infections
- Soft, multiple, matted—Tuberculosis

A definitive diagnosis can be made by FNAC or by a lymph node biopsy. Treatment will depend on the cause.

Treatment

- In case of TB: Anti-TB treatment for 15 months.
- Bacterial infections: Antibiotics depending on the primary focus.
- Sexually transmitted diseases: See relevant section.
- Malignancy: Refer.

Practice Tips

Localized enlargement of Lymph nodes

- A swelling in area of lymph node may not be lymph node swelling. Rule out sebaceous cyst, dermoid cyst, brachial cyst, lipoma, thyroid nodule, parotid swelling, carotid body tumour, cervical rib, etc.
- Lymph nodes are normally palpable in children and are soft, mobile and <1 cm in diameter. They may enlarge to >2 cm during viral/bacterial respiratory infection.
- Knowledge of the areas drained by lymph nodes is must for diagnosis of cause of enlarged lymph node.
- For cervical lymphadenopathy, primary focus of infection can be in tonsil, teeth, scalp, throat or mouth.
- In children, benign lumps usually occur in anterior triangle while the rare malignant lumps usually occur in the posterior triangle.
- Suspicious node is that which is >2.5 cm in size, firm to hard and fixed to the surrounding tissues.
- In case of "localized" enlarged lymph node—look for enlarged nodes at other sites and for hepatosplenomegaly.

GENERALIZED ENLARGEMENT OF LYMPH GLANDS

The following possibilities should be considered:

- Tuberculosis
- Secondary syphilis
- Lymphoma, leukaemia, myeloma
- Infectious mononucleosis
- Persistent generalized lymphadenopathy (PGL) in HIV
- Rare—Toxoplasmosis, tularemia, CMV, serum sickness, juvenile chronic arthritis, Sarcoidosis.

All these patients require investigations depending on the clinical suspicion:

- Haemogram, ESR—in all patients
- Paul Bunnell test—Infectious mononucleosis
- Chest X-ray—TB, carcinoma lung, lymphoma
- HRCT, CT abdomen—Tuberculosis, malignancy
- VDRL—Syphilis
- HIV ELISA—PGL
- FNAC, lymph node biopsy—Malignancy, tuberculosis, PGL, etc.
- Treatment will depend on the cause.

CRAMPS

Cramps are '*involuntary contractions of a voluntary muscle accompanied with sharp pain.*' It can occur in any muscle in the body, but most commonly in the calves. When they occur in a normal healthy individual especially at night, usually no cause is found and idiopathic cramps form the largest group of patients. Cramps can also occur at rest in pregnancy, in hyponatraemia following excessive sweating and in hypocalcaemia in tetany. They occur during unaccustomed exertion like trekking or in persons whose occupation involves prolonged overuse of calf muscles like tailors.

Management

Treat the cause if possible. If cramps are occupation related, advise change of occupation. To relieve cramp, stretch the muscle. For example, to stretch the calf muscle, dorsiflex the ankle till the cramp is relieved.

Hypocalcaemia

- Injection calcium gluconate 10 cc slow IV stat followed by
- Injection Mecalvit 3 cc IM biweekly × 5 injections

Dehydration

- Plenty of oral fluids
- ORS powder
- IV fluids in case of severe vomiting

Neuropathy

- Tab. $B_1B_6B_{12}$ (Neurobion) od
- Cap. Vit E (Evion 400 mg) bd
- Tab. Pregabalin (Pregaba) 75–150 mg hs

If no cause found

- Tab. Quinine 300 mg hs × 2 weeks
- Tab. Voveron 50 mg sos

If cramps occur at night, advise alternate flexion and extension of ankle joint at bed time for 1–2 min.

INTERMITTENT CLAUDICATION

The term 'intermittent claudication' is used to describe calf pain that occurs during exercise and which is relieved by a short period of rest. It can either be caused by arterial or venous obstruction (vascular claudication) or by compression on a nerve (neurogenic claudication).

In *claudication due to arterial obstruction* caused by a thrombus, the most common complaint is intermittent claudication with pain of the calf, thigh or buttock. The patient often complains that after walking a certain distance, called the "**claudication distance**", the pain starts. There is decreased or absent peripheral pulses, decreased skin temperature, pallor on elevation of the extremity and redness when the limb is dependent, dystrophic nails and shiny hairless skin.

In *neurogenic claudication*, calf, buttock, or thigh pain and/or weakness with deranged reflexes are seen. It is mostly bilateral though can be unilateral. It is caused by lumbar canal stenosis or by radiculopathy. Pain is usually along a nerve.

Management

- Advise to stop smoking.
- Walking improves the symptoms of claudication.
- Tab. Asprin (Colosprin, Ecosprin) 75–100 mg od (or)
  Tab. Clopidogrel (Clopilet) 300 mg od.
- Surgery is only indicated in severe cases with limb-threatening ischemia or lifestyle-limiting claudication.

*This chapter has been reviewed by **Dr Parag Vaste**, MD, Consultant Physician, Pune.*

CHAPTER 16

Homoeopathy in General Practice

- Acid-Peptic Disease
- Acne Vulgaris
- Recurrent Aphthous Ulcers
- Burns
- Corns
- Hair-loss
- Warts
- Delayed Dentition
- Eczema
- Dysmenorrhoea
- Ganglion
- Herpes Zoster
- Keloid/Scars
- Morning Sickness
- Psoriasis
- Sciatica
- Chronic Otitis Media
- Migrainous Headache
- Toothache
- Urticaria
- Allergic Rhinitis
- Asthma
- Bell's Palsy
- Renal/Ureteric Stones
- Menopausal Complaints
- Anal Fissures
- Piles
- Musculoskeletal Problems
- Medicine Box

— **Madhu Oswal**

The basic principle of homoeopathy is '*Similia similibus curanter*', i.e., 'let like be cured by like'. Symptoms form the basis of drug selection and not the disease. A single remedy is used at a time. The beginners should use low (30C) or medium (200C) potencies. In acute conditions, the drug can be repeated frequently (2–4 hrly), while in chronic conditions, less frequent repetition (8–12 hrly) is required. The drug is usually dispensed in globules form, 3–4 globules (30 nos.) to be given at a time. The conditions described below are those where allopathic medicines have no or limited role to play and homoeopathic medicines have proved to be efficient.

(Symbols < denotes *aggravation*; > denotes *amelioration*)

ACID-PEPTIC DISEASE

- Complaints after eating sour things, ice-creams; severe burning pains > warm drinks; severe anxiety and weakness—**Ars. alb. 30C**
- Complaints from excess of alcohol, spicy food, drugs, etc., nausea and vomiting with severe retching > vomiting, epigastric pain, some time after eating—**Nux vom 30C**
- Gastritis with frontal headache; intensely sour eructations with sour vomiting—**Robinia 30C**.
- Pain in epigastric region radiating to all over the abdomen. Gastritis of drunkards with continuous loud belching; craving for sweets, < cold food—**Arg. nit 30C**.

ACNE VULGARIS

- Symmetrical in distribution—**Arnica 30C**
- Caused by cosmetics, < summer—**Bovista 30C**
- Predominantly on forehead—**Ledum pal 30C**
- On face, chest, shoulders; also scars after acne—**Kali brom 6x, 30C**
- With gastric derangements—**Nux vom 30C**

RECURRENT APHTHOUS ULCERS

- Ulcers with pricking pain, with clean moist tongue and central furrow—**Nitric acid 30C**
- Tongue pale, dry with great thirst, severe prostration—**Muriatic acid 30C**
- Thickly coated moist tongue with deep indentations of teeth; thirst excessive—**Merc. sol 30C**
- Ulcers with hot feeling in the mouth; no thirst; dry mouth—**Borax 30C**

BURNS

- Immediately after burns to prevent inflammation and reduce pain—**Arnica 200C**
- Burns with pain > cold application—**Cantharis 30C**
- Burning pain > hot application—**Arsenic album 30C**
- Non-healing wounds after burns with rawness and soreness—**Causticum 30C**
- Scars after burns with offensive sweat—**Silicea 6x, 30C**

CORNS

- Painful corns < pressure; tongue thickly coated; no thirst—**Antim. crud. 30**
- Corns with deep cracks of feet—**Graphites 30**
- Soft painful corn with sweaty feet—**Silicea 6x, 30**

HAIR-LOSS

- Handful, bunches in—**Phos 30C**
- Alopecia areata, with premature greying of hair—**Acid phos. 30**
- Hair fall after parturition—**Nat. mur. 30**

WARTS

- Pedunculated, large smooth—**Thuja 30C**
- Painful warts, large, bleeding—**Nitric acid 30C**
- Warts on face, hands—**Dulcamara 30C**
- Warts all over the body—**Nat. sulph 30C**

DELAYED DENTITION

- Child extremely irritable, snappy with dentitional diarrhoea—green coloured ; thirst increased—**Chamomilla 200C**
- Child emaciated with distended abdomen; irritable; less thirsty, wants to be carried all day; worm infestations—**Cina 200C**
- Child with recurrent profuse, offensive diarrhoea; always pressing gums together during dentition—**Podophyllum 30C, 200C**
- Slow and rapidly decaying teeth; peevish; craves salt; glandular enlargement; complaints of recurrent pain in abdomen and calves—**Calc. phos 200C**

ECZEMA

- Weeping eczema with watery sticky discharge in obese constipated individual < damp weather; skin dry, horny—**Graphites 30C**
- Profuse yellowish discharge; very sensitive to touch and cold wind; profuse perspiration—**Hepar sulph 30C**
- Eczema—dry or moist—disappearing in summer, appearing in winter; on hands, or behind ears, moist purulent discharge—**Petroleum 6x, 30C**
- Nummular eczema, worse in flexures of joints, on hands > warmth, < sea shore; heals with brownish pigmentation—**Sepia 30C, 200C**

- Eczema with intense itching in thin individual, which is worse at night and by warmth of bed, scratching relieves itching but is followed by burning; does not like to take bath—**Sulphur 200C**

DYSMENORRHOEA

- Severe labour like pain, pressing upwards with passage of large clots < heat—**Chamomilla 200C**
- Pain more on right side > warmth, > bending double, > pressure—**Mag. phos 200C**
- Pain in sacral area with constant urging to stool—**Nux. vom. 30C, 200C**
- Scanty painful menses with diarrhoea during menses—**Pulsatilla 200C**

GANGLION

- **Ruta 30**—if extremely painful
- **Benzoic acid 30—**with swelling of wrist
- **Calc. fluor 30**—if stony hard, painless.

HERPES ZOSTER/POST-HERPETIC NEURALGIA

- Severe burning pain with restlessness and anxiety, > hot application, thirst frequent for small quantities—**Ars. album 30C, 200C**
- Vesicular stage especially if with itching, great physical restlessness—**Rhus tox 200C**
- Severe burning pain; also post-herpetic neuralgia; < night—**Mezerium 30C, 200C**
- Bluish, blackish ulcers; severe intercostal or cranial postherpetic neuralgia < least touch, pressure—**Ranunculus 30C, 200C**

KELOID/SCARS

- Scars thick, with burning pain and general dryness of skin—**Graphites 30C**
- Scars with rawness, soreness—**Causticum 6x, 30C**
- Scars with itching—**Acid fluor 6x, 30C**
- Specific remedy—**Thiosinaminum 6X, 30C**

MORNING SICKNESS

- Vomiting < afternoon with weakness out of proportion, can tolerate hot drinks, thirst for small quantities—**Ars. alb 30**
- Severe nausea with vomiting, clean moist tongue—**Ipecac 30C**
- Vomiting with vertigo, clean tongue, retching severe > vomiting—**Nux vomica 30C**
- Vomiting with good appetite, tongue moist, coated white, > rapid walking—**Lobelia inflata 30C**
- Specific remedy—**Symphoricarpus 6x, 30C**

PSORIASIS

- Predominantly on hands with exacerbations in winter—**Petroleum 30C**
- Predominantly on scalp, sparing face, itching < night, >heat—**Merc. sol 30C**
- Predominantly on elbows, knees, < menopause, > scratching—**Sepia 30C**
- With heavy yellowish scales—**Kali sulph 6x, 30C**
- With white scales and severe itching—**Kali ars. 6x, 30C**
- With burning pain, < washing, < warmth—**Sulphur 200 single dose**

SCIATICA

- Lt sided sciatica, > hard pressure, hot application, cramping pain—**Colocynth 30C, 200C**

- Rt sided sciatica, < touch, > pressure, > warmth, very tender feet—**Mag. phos 200C, 30C**
- Sciatica with pain > continuous motion, < rest, < cold air, < night—**Rhus tox 200C**
- Specific remedy—**Gnaphalium 30C, 200C**

CHRONIC OTITIS MEDIA

- Thick yellow, offensive, acrid bloody discharge, < night, < warmth; increased thirst, offensive sweat—**Merc. sol. 30C, 200C**
- Bland, yellowish, offensive discharge < night, > open, < evening in a weepy and timid child —**Pulsatilla 200C**
- Discharge continuing even after merc. sol, in a rickety child with distended abdomen, chilly, obstinate; offensive foot sweat—**Silicea 200C**
- Fat, flabby, chilly child, profuse sour perspiration, does not like mental or physical exertion, very sensitive to cold air, hands and feet cold clammy—**Calc. carb 200C**

MIGRAINOUS HEADACHE

- Right sided headache, sudden onset, throbbing < every motion, > in dark in semi-erect position, flushed hot face—**Belladona 200C**
- Headache after exposure to sun, of welders, throbbing, head feels too large, < stooping, < lying down, < sunrise to sunset, left side > uncovering head—**Glonine 200C**
- Right sided migraine starts in the occiput, spreads upwards and settles over the eyes; every seventh day > lying down, > sleep, accompanied by bitter vomiting; unquenchable thirst—**Sanguinaria 30C, 200C**
- Headaches after fear, grief, exciting news; feels heavy as though a nail has been driven in the skull; temporarily relieved by change of position and bending head forward, < eating < morning—**Ignatia 200C**

TOOTHACHE

- Severe pain in decayed teeth, < cold drinks—**Coffea 200C**
- Agonising pain which is momentarily > cold fluids in mouth with great peevishness—**Chamomilla 200C**
- Pain in sound teeth with pain radiating to the ear—**Plantago 30C, 200C**
- Pain radiating to the head > warmth, > pressure—**Mag. phos 200C**

URTICARIA

- Severe stinging with swelling < heat—**Apis mel. 30C, 200C**
- Urticaria < excitement, < bathing, < warmth, < morning—**Bovista 30C**
- Violent itching < cold air, every year in winter—**Urtica urens 6x, 30C**
- In cold season, chronic urticaria—**Hepar sulph 30C**
- In wet damp weather—**Dulcamara 30C**

ALLERGIC RHINITIS

- Copious acrid nasal discharge with bland lacrimation, constant sneezing; polyps; < warm room, > open air—**Allium cepa 30C, 200C**
- Sneezing < open air, < winter season, discharge thin watery, excoriating with dull frontal headache; thirst for small quantities of water and frequent—**Ars. album 30C, 200C**
- Complaints after sitting in cold damp places; nose blocked up at night and in open air, fluent in warm room and during day; very chilly but > open air; tongue clean—**Nux. vomica 30C, 200C**

- Rhinitis with headache at root of the nose; atrophic rhinitis, continuous sneezing; < sudden change of weather—**Sticta 30C**
- Copious nasal discharge with sneezing with severe frontal headache, < cold air and cold drinks, > warm food and drinks; no thirst—**Sabadilla 30C**
- Coryza slow to progress after exposure to cold air; discharge excoriating with fullness of head, drowsy, prostrated, tongue coated yellow, < thunderstorm, < night, > open air—**Gelsemium 30C, 200C**

ASTHMA

- Attack starts after drinking cold things, most severe after midnight, cannot lie down, must sit bent forward, great anguish and restlessness, > warm food, severe prostration, thirsty —**Ars. alb 30C, 200C**
- Attacks mostly in warm moist weather, preceded by severe nausea and vomiting, violent dry cough, chest full of phlegm but cannot expectorate, tongue clean, no thirst, < lying down—**Ipecac 30C**
- Attack after digestive upset, most severe after midnight till morning, accompanied by bursting headache and fullness in epigastrium, < dry cold, belching, > damp weather, > rest —**Nux. vomica 30C, 200C**
- Attack accompanied by coarse rattles in chest but cannot expectorate with severe prostration, body covered with cold sweat, < 3 AM; no thirst; tongue coated thickly white; extremely drowsy; wants open air—**Antim tart 30C**
- Attack preceded by prickling sensation all over the body, cannot bear any exertion but > rapid walking, pain in epigastric region, < tobacco, < cold; profuse salivation with thickly coated tongue—**Lobelia inflata 30C**

BELL'S PALSY

- In the initial stage after exposure to cold wind, numbness and tingling of face, great restlessness and fear of death—**Aconite 30C, 200C**
- When no response to aconite with h/o exposure to cold air or after long lasting grief or sudden exertion; especially right sided, slowly progressive; accompanied by weakness, hopelessness, > heat—**Causticum 30C, 200C**
- Bad effects from fright, fear attack in cold damp weather; normal sensation, severe prostration and trembling; drowsy; > moving slowly—**Gelsemium 30C, 200C**

RENAL/URETERIC STONES

- Intolerable and constant urge to urinate, severe burning pain, stitching in lumbar region, < during cold weather—**Cantharis 30C, 200C**
- Left sided ureteric colic, burning pain, < standing < motion—**Berb. vulgaris 30C, 200C**
- Right sided colic with severe pain; bloody, flaky, sandy urine < sitting—**Sarsaparilla 30C, 200C**
- Right sided colic, pain before urination, > after flow, heavy red sediment, pain < 4–8 PM. > motion, > warm food, drink—**Lycopodium 30C, 200C**

MENOPAUSAL COMPLAINTS

- Sudden hot sensation in head and face followed by sweating, lot of anxiety, wants open air—**Amyl nitrosum 6x, 30C**
- Depressed, flushes < night after sleep < warm room < tight clothing—**Lachesis 30C, 200C**

- Flushes with left sided headaches, < day time, <sun, extremely irritable—**Glonine 200C**

ANAL FISSURES

- Severe pain after stools as if rectum is full of small sticks associated with backache up and down the spine < standing—**Aesculus 200C**
- Constipated but no desire for stools; fissure pain < warmth—**Graphites 30C, 200C**
- Pain in anal region as if full of glass splinters, pains hours after stools, > cold water—**Ratania 30C**
- Constricting, splincter like pains in rectal region; chilly, offensive sweat ; pain< night—**Nitric acid 30C**

PILES

- Constipated with constant ineffectual urge for stools; abuse of purgatives; blind piles—**Nux. vomica 30C, 200C**
- Bad effects from sedentary habits, piles large like bunch of grapes—sore, painful > cold application, standing < walking—**Aloes 30C, 200C**
- Large, purple piles covered with crusts with itching at anal region; burning hours after stools, with internal chilliness—**Paeonia 30C, 200C**
- Constant, ineffectual urge for stools with violent shooting pain in back; especially in overdrugged lean thin, shabby individual with unhealthy skin, hot, averse to bathing—**Sulphur 30C, 200C**

MUSCULOSKELETAL PROBLEMS

- Acute as well as chronic conditions; ailments from overexertion, exposure to wet weather when overheated; sprains; pain < sitting < beginning to move > continued motion—**Rhus. tox 200C**
- Acute as well as chronic joint pains; sharp stitching pain < least motion < warmth; > complete rest > pressure—**Bryonia 200C**
- Rheumatoid arthritis with soreness all over the body; tendons contracted; progressive loss of muscle power; severe weakness and trembling—**Causticum 30C, 200C**
- Joint pains on sudden change of weather, or in cold damp season; pain alternate with diarrhoea; > moving about—**Dulcamara 30C, 200C**
- Gouty joint pains, shifting from one joint to other, pain < evenly < least touch or movement; small joints affected; severe weakness—**Colchicum 30C**

MEDICINE BOX

Aconite 200C
Aloes 30C
Antimonium crudum 30C
Antimonium tartaricum 30C
Apis mellifica 30C
Arnica 200C
Arsenic album 30C, 200C
Belladona 200C
Bryonia 200C
Berberis vulgaris 30C
Borax 30C
Calcaria carbonica 200C
Calcaria phosphorica 200C
Calcaria fluor 6x
Cantharis 30C
Causticum 30C
Chamomilla 200C
Coffea cruda 200C
Colocynth 30C
Dulcamara 30C
Euphrasia 30C
Gelsemium 30C, 200C
Glonine 200
Graphites 30C, 200C
Hepar. sulph 30C
Hypericum 200C
Ignatia 200C
Ledum pal 30C
Lycopodium 30C, 200C
Mag phos 200C
Mercurius solubis 30C
Mezerium 30C
Nat mur 30
Nitric acid 30C
Muriatic acid 30C
Nux vomica 30C, 200C
Petroleum 30C
Podophyllum 30C
Pulsatilla 30C, 200C
Ranunculus bulbosus 30C
Ratania 30C
Rhus. tox 200C
Ruta 200C
Sepia 30C, 200C
Sabadilla 30C
Sulphur 30C, 200C
Silicea 30C, 200C
Thuja 30C, 200C
Urtica urens 30

*This chapter has been reviewed by **Dr Rita Shah**, MD, Practising Homoeopath, Pune.*

CHAPTER 17

Ayurveda in General Practice

- Viral Hepatitis
- Obstructive Jaundice
- Peripheral Neuritis
- Urticaria
- Obesity
- Excessive Belching
- Hemiplegia
- Allergic Rhinitis
- Hoarseness of Voice
- Chronic Colitis
- Constipation
- Hyperacidity
- Urinary Calculus
- Dysmenorrhoea
- Lipomas
- Anorexia
- Bleeding Piles
- Non-bleeding Piles
- Weight Gain
- Insomnia
- Viral Diarrhoea
- Viral Fever

– **Shyam Mhadekar**

Ayurveda is a science of life. The ancient vaidyas have discovered huge number of ayurvedic medicines after continuous study, observations, experiments and trials. These ayurvedic drugs are becoming more and more popular worldwide, because of their excellent results and minimal side effects.

In this section, the ayurvedic remedies are given where allopathic drugs have got certain limitations and ayurvedic drugs work more precisely.

VIRAL HEPATITIS

1. Tab. Arogyavardhini 250 mg tds (Liv 52 DS tds).
2. Tab. Sootashekhar sadha 250 mg tds.
3. Tab. Shankhabhasma vati 250 mg tds.

OBSTRUCTIVE JAUNDICE

1. Tab. Arogyavardhini 250 mg tds.
2. Tab. Sootashekhar sadha 250 mg tds.
3. Tab. Kaph-khuthar ras 100 mg tds.
4. Susp. Kumari asava no. 1–2 tsf with water.
5. Kalki choorna 1 gm hs with warm water.

PERIPHERAL NEURITIS

1. Tab. Chandrakala rasa 250 mg tds.
2. Tab. Praval pishthi vati 250 mg tds.
3. Susp. Chandanasava 2 tsf with water.
4. Tab. Navak guggula 250 mg 2 bd.
5. Local application of Chanadanadi taila.

URTICARIA

1. Hadridra khanda yoga 3 g tds.
2. Tab. Sootashekhar sadha 250 mg tds.
3. Trivang bhasma 250 mg tds.
4. Gandharva haritaki choorna 2 tsf hs with warm water.

OBESITY

1. Tab. Chandraprabha vati 250 mg 2 bd.

2. Tab. Medoher guggula 250 mg 2 bd.
3. Tab. Arogyavardhini 250 mg 2 bd.
4. Honey 2 tsf on empty stomach.

EXCESSIVE BELCHING

1. Tab. Vasant kusumakar 60 mg bd.
2. Ashwagandhawaleha paste 20 mg bd with warm milk.
3. Instruct patient to drink water, which is boiled with gold ornament.

HEMIPLEGIA

1. Narayan taila for massage.
2. Shatbindu taila 5 drops to be instilled in nose bd.
3. Tab. Mahayograj guggula 250 mg tds.
4. Tab. Ekangavir rasa 125 mg tds.

ALLERGIC RHINITIS

1. Tab. Nag guti 125 mg tds.
2. Susp. Bhallatakasava 2 tsf bd with water. (Ask the patient about the allergy to marking-nut before prescribing bhallatakasava.)
3. Anu taila 5 drops to be instilled in nose.

HOARSENESS OF VOICE

1. Tab. Khadiradi vati 4 tabs to be chewed qds.
2. Mixture of Jestmadh powder 500 mg and tankan 125 mg to be taken tds with honey.

CHRONIC COLITIS

1. Tab. Panchamrut parpati 250 mg tds.
2. Tab. Sanjivani vati 250 mg tds.
3. Susp. Kutajarista 4 tsf bd with water.
4. Advice to drink lot of buttermilk.

CONSTIPATION

1. Gandharva haritaki choorna 2 tsf hs with warm water. It is the best bulk forming laxative (**or**)
2. Tab. Sukhasarak 1 or 2 hs.

HYPERACIDITY

1. Tab. Praval panchamrut 250 mg tds.
2. Tab. Kamdudha 250 mg tds.
3. Susp. Efcid 2 tsf tds.
4. Tab. Shankabhasma 500 mg bd.
5. Avipattkar choorna 1 tsf hs.

URINARY CALCULUS

1. Tab. Chandraprabha 500 mg tds.
2. Tab. Gokshuradi guggla 500 mg tds.
3. Srup. Varunadi quatha 4 tsf bd with lot of water.

Prophylaxis—after passing of stone, continue only varuvadi quatha 2 tsf bd.

DYSMENORRHOEA

Srup. Dashanoolarishta 4 tsf bd × 3 months.

To increase intelligence in mentally retarded child

1. Tab. Smruti sagar rasa 250 mg bd.
2. Sup. Brahmiprash 2 tsf bd.
3. Sup. Saraswatarishta 2 tsf bd with water.

To increase sperm count in oligospermia

1. Tab. Makardhwaj vati 125 mg bd with honey.
2. Tab. Vasant kusumakar 60 mg bd with honey.
3. Say. Ashwagandharishta 2 tsf bd with water.

LIPOMAS

1. Tab. Kanchananar guggula 250 mg bd.
2. Local application of paste of Tab. Kanchananar guggula and water.

ANOREXIA

1. Hingashtak choorna 1 tsf powder with water before meals.
2. Tab. Aam pachak vati 250 mg bd.
3. Sup. Panchakolasava 2 tsf bd with water.
4. Shankhavati 250 mg bd.

BLEEDING PILES

1. Sama sharkar choorna 500 mg powder tds.
2. Sup. Abhayarishta 2 tsf bd with water.
3. Tab. Kutaj parpati 250 mg bd.

NON-BLEEDING PILES

1. Tab. Kankayan guti 250 mg bd.
2. Sup. Abhayarishta 2 tsf bd with water.
3. Local application of Pilex ointment bd.
4. Tab. Bhallatak parpati 250 mg bd.

(Ask the patient about the allergy to the marking nut before prescribing bhallatak parpati.)

FOR WEIGHT GAIN

1. Shatavari kalp 2 tsf with milk bd
2. Shatavari ghruta 1 tsf bd with milk.

INSOMNIA

1. Tab. Prasham 500 mg hs (or)
2. Tab. Jatmansi 500 mg hs.

VIRAL DIARRHOEA

1. Tab. Sanjivini 500 mg bd.
2. Tab. Kutaj paspati 500 mg bd.
3. Bilwa musta and Sunthi choorna, each 500 mg bd with warm water.

VIRAL FEVER

1. Tab. Sudarshan ghana 500 mg bd.
2. Liq. Dashamool arista 2 tsf bd with warm water.

The drugs mentioned in this section are mainly generic drugs of popular ayurvedic companies, usually freely available in any chemist shop.

Ayurved Rasashala, Charak, Himalaya, Zandu, Baidyanath are the few known ayurvedic pharmaceutical companies who prepare the above-mentioned drugs.

*This chapter has been reviewed by **Dr Shyam Mhadekar**, Pune and Dr Prajakte Bhosle, BMAS, MD, Pune.*

CHAPTER 18

Surgical Conditions

- Fissure-in-ano
- Fistula-in-ano
- Piles
- PR Bleeding in a Child
- Prolapsed Thrombosed Piles
- Anorectal Abscess
- Breast Lump

FISSURE-IN-ANO

Presents as *severely painful* PR bleeding during defaecation. Streaks of blood are seen at side of stools. O/e anal orifice tightly closed because of pain, does not allow PR examination. Longitudinal ulcer in posterior midline covered by sentinel tag of skin.

- Sitz bath. Ask patient to sit in a tub of lukewarm water containing potassium permanganate powder.
- Xylocaine 5% rectal jelly before defecation (**or**) 2% Glycerine trinitrate ointment in small amount only, to prevent headache.
- Tab. Ciprofloxacin (Cifran) 500 mg bd × 5 days.
- Tab. Metronidazole (Metrogyl) 400 tds × 5 days.
- Tab. Diclofenac (Voveran) 100 bd × 5 days.
- High fibre diet—to prevent constipation.
- Cremaffin liquid → 4 tsf hs.

  Refer to surgeon for anal dilatation or fissurectomy.

FISTULA-IN-ANO

Patient presents with pain and discharge at side of anus, which is recurrent for many months or years. O/e discharging sinus or an opening with granulation tissue or a scar is seen about 3–4 cm away from anal orifice; on PR examination, internal opening may be palpable to finger.

- Sitz bath—as above.
- Ciprofloxacin, diclofenac, metronidazole, Cremaffin as above.
- No local ointment.

Refer to surgeon for fistulectomy.

PILES

These are dilated varicose veins in rectum. They cause *painless* PR bleeding during defecation. Pain can occur in piles which are prolapsed and thrombosed. O/e in early cases, no abnormality seen at anal opening. In advanced cases, pile masses can be seen at 3, 7 or 11 o'clock position.

Grading of piles

- ***First degree***: PR bleeding only. Do not prolapse.
- ***Second degree***: Prolapse during defecation but reduce spontaneously.
- ***Third degree***: Have to be reduced by fingers.
- ***Fourth degree***: Cannot be reduced with finger and remain outside permanently.

Treatment

First and second degree piles

- High fibre diet.
- Cremaffin liquid 4 tsf hs.
- Proctosedyl ointment or Anovate ointment locally.
- Tab. R.B. Tone 1 hs, if anaemia.
- Tab. Venusmin (Diosmin) 300 mg (**or**) Tab. Daflon 500 mg bd till bleeding stops.

Third and fourth degree piles

Refer to surgeon for sclerosing injection, band ligation, excision of piles, stapler haemorrhoidectomy, etc.

PR BLEEDING IN A CHILD

Causes

1. ***Rectal polyp***, which is seen as a cherry like mass at the anal orifice or can be felt by PR examination.
   - No medical treatment.
   - Refer to surgeon.
2. ***Prolapse of rectum***, seen at anal opening or mother gives history that something comes out when child is defecating, which has to be reduced manually. This condition does not require surgery. It corrects spontaneously with time.
   - Reduce mass manually, if present during examination.
   - Give firm strapping to the buttocks with sticking plaster after reduction.
   - Control loose motions, if present.
   - Correct anaemia and malnutrition.

If no relief, refer to surgeon for '*Thiersh's stich*' operation.

DD of PR bleeding

1. *Painful PR bleeding*
   - Fissure
   - Thrombosed piles
2. *Painless PR bleeding*—Piles
3. *Bleeding independent of defaecation*
   - Amoebic dysentery
   - Prolapsed piles
   - Ca. colon
4. *PR bleeding in a child*
   - Rectal polyp
   - Prolapse of rectum

DD of anorectal pain

1. *Fissure-in-ano*: Painful PR bleeding during defecation.
2. *Fistula-in-ano*: Discharging sinus at side of anus.
3. *Prolapsed thrombosed piles*: Reddish tender mass at anal margin.
4. *Anorectal abscess*: Indurated swelling at side of anus.
5. *Perianal haematoma*: Cherry like mass at side of anus.

PROLAPSED THROMBOSED PILES

In a known case of piles, the pile mass suddenly prolapses and gets thombosed with severe pain and tenderness. To reduce the pain, the patient sits on edge of bed. O/e reddish or blackish mass is seen at 3, 7 or 11 o'clock position, which is tender to touch.

Management

1. Reduce mass by applying firm pressure with abundant Xylocaine jelly on gloved fingers.

2. If not possible to reduce, but pain is tolerable—treat conservatively.
   a) Bed rest with 2 pillows under the buttocks.
   b) Glycerine-magnesium sulphate compresses 3–4 times a day.
   c) Xylocaine rectal jelly—apply after compresses.
   d) Tab. Ciprofloxacin (Cifran) 500 mg bd.
   e) Tab. Diclofenac (Voveran) 100 mg bd × 5 days. Advise elective surgery for piles after one month.
   f) Tab. Chymoral forte 1 qid (or) Tab. Phlogam 1 tds.
3. If not possible to reduce, but pain not tolerable.
   a) Refer to surgeon for immediate reduction of piles and anal dilatation under GA.
   b) Elective surgery (excision of piles) after one month.

ANORECTAL ABSCESS

Severe pain in perianal and gluteal region usually on one side. Fever may be present. O/e diffuse erythematous, indurated swelling, which is tender to touch.

1. Inj. Diclofenac (Voveran) 3 mL IM stat.
2. Inj. Ceftriaxone (C-tri) 1 g IV stat.

> Refer the patient of anorectal abscess to a surgeon immediately for I & D under GA. Do not treat conservatively by giving antibiotics and waiting for abscess to 'point' like at other sites. If I & D is delayed, the abscess may burst inside the anal canal or rectum and fistula-in-ano might develop. This then requires major surgery and still recurrences are possible.

BREAST LUMP

Four conditions are commonly encountered in general practice.

Fibroadenoma

Seen in young women around 20 years of age. Usually solitary and it is called '**breast mouse.**'

a) Reassure patient that it is harmless.
b) Refer to surgeon for removal by simple excision and for biopsy.

Fibroadenosis

Seen in women close to menopause. Pain increases before menstruation. O/e indefinite but tender lump felt when breast is examined between finger and thumb. With the flat of hand, the lump can be felt only vaguely.

- Breast support with firm brassiere.
- Tab. Diclofenac (Voveran) 100 mg bd.
- Tab. Danazole (Danogin) 100 mg tds × 3–6 months. Costly but effective drug.
- Refer to surgeon for excision biopsy.

Breast Abscess

Seen commonly either in the first month of first lactation or in 6–7th month after teeth have erupted. Classical signs of inflammation are seen.

a) Breast support, hot fomentation.
b) Cap Ampicillin + Cloxacillin (Baxin) 500 tds × 7 days, only if inflammation is present and pus not formed.
c) Tab. Diclofenac (Voveran) 100 mg bd × 7 days.
d) Tab Metronidazole (Flagyl) 400 mg tds × 7 days.
e) Refer to surgeon for early drainage.

> i) Antibiotics should not be given if pus has already formed. A sterile abscess (antibioma) then forms which takes a long time to resolve.
> ii) **"To wean or not to wean"**: Feeding is continued from uninfected breast. From the infected breast, milk manually expressed, boiled for 5 min and then fed to baby is quite safe.

Carcinoma Breast

Any lump in breast seen in a woman after the age of 40 years should be suspected of malignancy and should be referred urgently.

Unfortunately, Indian women seek medical attention late "as there was no pain." O/E the lump is hard, irregular, fixed to skin and deep muscles, nipple is retracted and there are palpable lymphatic nodes in axillae. But these are late signs. Always refer at the earliest. Ca. breast is curable in early stages.

This chapter has been reviewed by ***Dr Arvind Kulkarni****, Pune.*

GP Tip

Grand old man. Hard of hearing?
No problem.
Just place the earpiece of your stethoscope in the patient's ears and speak into the diaphragm!

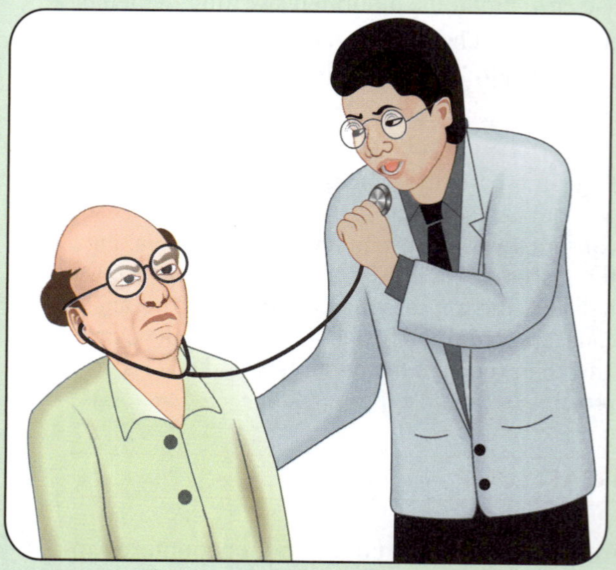

CHAPTER 19

Palliative Care in General Practice

- Fatigue
- Anorexia
- Constipation
- Nausea and Vomiting
- Dyspnoea
- Pain

Palliative care can be seen as part of continuum of supportive care, when the disease is no longer responsive to curative treatment. The aim is to give best possible quality of life to the patient. It includes management of symptoms that arise due to incurable diseases like cancer, HIV etc.

Patient suffering with cancer may not volunteer about the symptoms as they believe that suffering is inevitable. We need to proactively ask about the symptoms. As the patient may have multiple symptoms, we need to prioritize which needs urgent treatment with minimum drugs.

FATIGUE

Fatigue can be physical, emotional, or mental. Unlike fatigue in the general population, cancer-related fatigue does not improve with rest or sleep. It is important to distinguish physical weakness from dyspnoea on exertion, which is commonly reported as fatigue. Depression may also cause or exacerbate fatigue. Thoroughly assess the patient to identify any reversible causes of fatigue.

Causes

- Anaemia
- Poor appetite
- Insomnia, sleep disturbance
- Depression
- Medical co-morbidities: Renal, cardiac or pulmonary disease

In many cases, however, a reversible cause cannot be found.

Management

- Patients should be advised that fatigue has a fluctuating course and that they have a limited pool of energy, which they should conserve and use judiciously.
- Tab. Methylphenidate (Ritalin), a CNS stimulant, 5 mg bd. Adverse effects include anorexia, insomnia, anxiety, confusion, tremor and tachycardia.
- Treat the underlying depression and insomnia.
- Ensure sufficient caloric intake.

ANOREXIA

Most patients with advanced cancer experience anorexia, which is a marker of poor prognosis. In fact, anorexia frequently causes more distress to the family than to the patient. Decreased caloric intake leads to rapid, dramatic weight loss and cachexia. The first step in the management of anorexia is to identify any reversible causes, such as:

- Stomatitis
- Constipation
- Uncontrolled severe symptoms such as pain or dyspneoa
- Nausea, vomiting
- Depression
- Gastroparesis

Management

- Tab. Megestrol acetate (Megace) 80–160 mg daily.
- Tab. Olanzapine (Zyprexa) 5 mg bd.
- Tab. Dexamethasone (Dexona) 4–16 mg daily. Corticosteroids should be discontinued if the desired positive effects are not observed within 3–5 days. If prolonged survival is expected, wean to the lowest effective dose.
- High calorie foods and high-calorie, high-protein, high-fat drinks.
- Naso-gastric tube feeding in some patients with mechanical obstruction (e.g., oesophageal fistula, obstruction or proximal small bowel obstruction).

CONSTIPATION

Constipation is a very common symptom in a patient suffering from cancer. In fact, it is so common that it should be anticipated and prevented if possible.

Causes

- Drugs such as opioids, anticholinergics, antihypertensives, antacids, diuretics and iron supplements.
- Dietary factors such as a generally low intake of food, and specifically of fibre.
- Inactivity
- Dehydration
- Intestinal obstruction
- Comorbidities such as hypothyroidism, hypercalcaemia
- Uncomfortable toilet arrangements

Management

- Dietary modifications—Add a lot of fibre, green leafy vegetables, salads and sprouted beans to the diet.
- Plenty of liquids.
- Exercises, especially those which tone abdominal muscles—help in colonic movement.
- Advise not to suppress the call to defaecation.
- Always rule out organic cause before treating any case as functional constipation.
- Powder Isabgol (Naturolax, Isogel) 2 tsf in a glass of freshly prepared water (**or**) Sorbitol (Sorbilax) or Lactulose 10–20 mL (**or**) Tab Bisacodyl (Dulcolax) 10–20 mg (**or**)
- Dulcolax suppository. If still no relief,
- Neotonic enema (**or**) Soap water enema.

NAUSEA AND VOMITING

Nausea and vomiting may not always be due to chemotherapy as commonly believed. We should look for other potentially reversible causes of nausea and vomiting.

Causes

- Drugs
- Uraemia due to organ failure

- Infection
- Anxiety
- Constipation
- Gastric irritation
- Proximal gastrointestinal obstruction

Management

If no cause found, can try ***empirical approach*** with following drugs:

- Tab. Metoclopramide (Reglan) 10 mg by mouth before meals and at bedtime or as needed. Avoid if bowel obstruction is suspected **(or)**
- Tab. Haloperidol (Serenace) 12 hrly **(or)**
- Tab. Ondansetron (Emset) 4–8 mg by mouth or intravenously every 12 hrs **(or)**
- Tab. Olanzapine (Zyprexa) 2.5–5 mg sublingually is an alternative drug for patients who do not respond to Metoclopramide and Haloperidol.
- Tab. Dexamethasone (Decadron): Those with central nervous system metastasis can be treated with Dexamethasone as an adjuvant to the above therapies.

Some tips for choice of anti-emetic drug:

- Nausea due to chemical or metabolic factors: Haloperidol.
- Nausea due to gastric stasis: Metoclopramide, Domperidone.
- Nausea due to regurgitation: Metoclopramide, Cyclizine.
- Nausea due to cranial disease: Cyclizine.
- Cause unclear or multiple causes: Cyclizine, Haloperidol.

DYSPNOEA

At least half of patients with advanced cancer complain of dyspnoea. Most have primary pulmonary malignancies or metastatic lung disease, but almost 25% have no documented lung involvement or underlying cardiopulmonary diagnosis to attribute to.

Causes

- Anaemia
- Pleural effusion
- Pnuemonitis
- Collapse of lung
- Cardiac failure
- Primary lung malignancies or metastasis

Management

- Give a comfortable position to the patient—usually propped up position supported by pillow helps.
- Treat the cause like anaemia, pleural effusion, COPD, asthma, pneumonitis, etc.
- Tab. Morphine (5 mg) stat. if no treatable cause found. Can be repeated every 2 hrs as needed.

PAIN

Unrelieved pain in cancer is unacceptable. Pain relief is needed in all stages of cancer and is possible most of the time.

Causes

- Primary cancer or metastasis.
- Due to surgery, radiotherapy or chemotherapy.
- Increased perception of pain due to anxiety and depression.

Even if the cause of the pain is not apparent, the patient's complaint should not be disregarded.

- Simultaneous use of more than one NSAID or the concomitant use of an NSAID with a steroid is not recommended because the risk of toxicity is increased, and additional analgesia is not achieved.
- There is no "right dose". The right dose is that dose that relieves patient's pain.
- Analgesics should be given by clock at fixed intervals without waiting for the pain to come. This will give continuous pain relief.
- As far as possible, oral preparations are preferred.
- If oral route of administration is no longer possible (e.g., nausea and vomiting refractory to therapy, inability to swallow) then rectal, subcutaneous or IV route of drug delivery should be chosen.
- Transdermal fentanyl patches should be used in patients with stable pain who are noncompliant with oral medication or are unable to swallow or absorb.
- When increasing opioid dose, an increment of 25–50% is usually the minimum required to observe effect.
- Besides consideration of a change in opioid, an increase in pain intensity should prompt a re-evaluation of the cause of pain.
- Adjuvant drugs are those which are used along with analgesics to reduce the side-effects of analgesics or as co-analgesics for certain types of pain.
  - Laxatives and anti-emetics with opioids.
  - Antidepressants, anti-anxiety, anti-convulsant drugs for neuralgic type of pains.
  - Corticosteroids for pain due to increased intracranial pressure.

Management

The step ladder approach given by WHO is used for pain management in cancer.

Step 1: Non-opioid analgesics for mild to moderate pain.

- Tab. Acetaminophen (Crocin, Metacin) 650 mg 4 hrly (**or**)
- Tab. Keterolac 10 mg qid (**or**)
- Tab. Diclofenac (Voveran) 50–75 mg 8–12 hrly.

Step 2: If pain is not relieved or if moderate pain is present at presentation, give mild to moderate opioids.

- Tab. Codeine phosphate 10–15 mg 4 hrly,
- Tab. Tramadol (Tramazac) 50 mg 6hrly or
- Tab. Dextropropoxyphene with paracetamol (Proxyvon) 32.5–65 mg 6–12 hrly.

These are usually combined with a nonopioid analgesic.

Step 3: If no relief with Step 2, strong opioids are used along with NSAIDS.

- Tab. Morphine sulphate tablets 5–10 mg 4 hrly (**or**) 30–60 SR mg 12 hourly.
- Tab. Buprenorphine

*Section 1 has been reviewed by **Dr Bhagyashri D Rajopadhye**, MD (Pharmacology), Associate Professor of Pharmacology, Bharati Vidyapeeth Medical College, Pune.*

CHAPTER 20

Generic Drugs

UNDERSTANDING GENERIC DRUGS AND PRESCRIBING SENSIBLY

In Section 1 (Basic General Practice) of this book, I have given the **brand names** of the various drugs mentioned as treatment of the relevant conditions. *This policy has been used in this book keeping the convenience of the reader and the system of medicine prescribing in India.* Purists in the medical parlance will argue for the use of only the **generic drugs** (as against branded drugs), which is the method followed in all textbooks of medicine and surgery.

The Government of India has strongly advocated the use of generic drugs in clinical practice in India looking at the larger interests of the diverse Indian population. When a generic drug product is approved, it has met the rigorous standards with respect to identity, strength, quality, purity and potency.

Doctors need to know then the difference between the generic drugs and branded drugs and so many other names given below while classifying the drugs in a particular category. It is the intension of this chapter to clear the picture.

1. Brand Drugs
2. Generic Drugs
3. Authorized Generic Drugs
4. Branded Generic Drugs
5. Generic Generic Drugs

What are Brand Drugs?

A drug sold by a drug company under a specific name or trademark and that is protected by a patent. When a medicine is first developed, the pharmaceutical company that discovers it, receives a patent on its new drug. The patent usually lasts for 20 years, to give the originating company a chance to recover its research investment. This protects their investment in drug research by giving the drug company the sole right to manufacture and sell the **brand name drug** while the patent is in effect.

After the patent period expires, a "**generic**" **version** of the drug may become available. Multiple companies can then manufacture and sell generic versions of the brand name product.

What are Generic Drugs?

A generic drug is a medication that has exactly the same *active ingredient* as the brand name drug and yields the same therapeutic effect. It is the same in dosing, safety, strength, quality, the way it works, the way it is taken and the way it should be used. Generic drugs do not need to contain the same *inactive ingredients* as the brand name product.

For more clarity take the example of ***Sildenefil***. This drug was discovered by the pharmaceutical company **Pfizer** after spending billions of dollars in research. To recover the cost of the research, it was awarded a patent meaning it had the sole right to market its discovery under the brand name **Viagra** for the next 20 years. After the expiry of this period of patent this drug could be marketed by any authorized pharmaceutical company under the generic name **Sildenefil**.

Many questions are time and again come up in the patients and even the doctors' mind, which we will try to address:

- ***Why are generic drugs cheaper?*** Generic drugs are usually much less expensive than brand name drugs once they reach the market. This is because the drug manufacturer does not have to duplicate the original clinical trials for effectiveness and safety. Drug research is costly. Brand-name manufacturers also spend billions of dollars in marketing new drugs to doctors. They employ hundreds of medical representatives to visit doctors in their clinics to promote their products, they pay for physicians conferences to talk about their drugs with other doctors, etc.

  Generic manufacturers rarely spend money on advertising and marketing. Generics are not less expensive because they are lower in quality. Lower-cost generic drugs have been shown to increase the likelihood that patients take essential medications prescribed by their doctors and to improve patients' health outcomes.
- ***Are generic drugs as effective and safe as brand name drugs?*** Yes. The FDA must first approve all generic drugs before they are marketed. The FDA requires that generic drugs must be as high in quality, and as strong, pure and stable as brand name drugs. Generic drugs use the same active ingredients as brand name drugs and work the same way. They have the same risks and the same benefits as the brand name drugs.
- ***Why do generic and brand name drugs look different?*** Trademark laws do not allow generic drugs to look exactly like the brand name drug. However, the generic drug must have the same *active ingredients*. Colours, shapes and certain other *inactive ingredients* must be different. For example, **Viagra** was marked under patent as "*a little blue colour diamond shaped pill*" (for reasons best known to them!)
- ***Does every brand name drug is marketed as a generic drug after patency period is over?*** Not necessarily. Some drugs may never be marketed as a generic because manufacturers may decide these products to be unprofitable or too difficult to manufacture.
- ***Why do doctors not recommend generic drugs?*** The major reason why doctors may not prescribe unbranded generic medicine is the lack of confidence of physician and patients in their quality. Doctors are also influenced by aggressive promotion of branded generic medicines by the pharmaceutical companies.

What are Authorized Generics?

An "authorized generic" is an exact copy of the brand name version. It is a prescription drug that is produced by a pharmaceutical company and marketed as a generic. It is identical to the branded product in appearance (shape, colour, etc.) and unlike a generic, the authorized generic has exactly the same inactive ingredients.

What are "Branded Generics"?

Branded generics are generic drugs that have a brand name. These drugs are developed either by the original manufacturer after the patent expires for the original product or by a pharmaceutical company that is not the originator of the molecule but comes out with either new dosage forms or new manufacturing process.

In India, the generic drugs promoted by companies under their brand-names are referred to as branded generics and those sold by their chemical names are referred to as '**generic generics**' although both categories are off-patent drugs.

Many questions are time and again come up in the patients and even the doctors' mind, which we will try to address:

- ***What is the difference between generic and branded medicine in India?*** Drugs which are no longer subject to patent restrictions are to be sold only as pure generic, without using any brand name. It helps in making pure generics cheaper. But in India, most of the generic drugs are sold as their brand name which are called '**branded generics**'.

  Profits on sales of a brand name drug are much higher for everyone in the supply chain of branded generics. Since the company making branded generics can spend little on research and development, it is able to spend on marketing alone, thus earning higher profits and driving costs down. For example, the largest revenues of Ranbaxy, now owned by Sun Pharma, came from branded generics.
- ***Why do pharmaceutical companies prefer to give a brand name to the generic drug?*** The idea is to give the generic drug a distinctive name to market and in long-term users in chronic diseases like hypertension and diabetes to ensure that they continue to use the same product time after time.
- ***Any other important reason?*** Yes. Birth control pills are an example of a branded generic drug made by several manufacturers. **Ovral G** is an example. It can be hard for patients and relatives to pronounce and remember the generic name of the drug which is ethinyl estradiol and norgestrel.
- ***Are branded generics more expensive than the generic?*** Yes as a general rule. However, branded generics may be less expensive than the original brand.
- ***Are branded generics superior in quality than generic drugs?*** No, the branded generic is not of a higher quality product than a true generic, but this is the usual impression created by pharmaceutical companies for profit making.

Bottom Line

India is the biggest exporter of generic medicines in the world.

Several developed countries in the US and Europe are able to both develop and sell the generic medications at a much lower cost, not because the quality of the generic is inferior to the brand-name drug, but because the original manufacturer (patented) has already paid for the bulk of costs to discover and develop a prescription drug from scratch.

Generic drugs save money! Generic drugs improve adherence!!

It is the time when every stakeholder in the Healthcare game should work in the jointly towards Positive and Affordable Healthcare!

Did you know that...

- Generic drugs are NOT inferior in quality to branded drugs.
- Generic pills do NOT contain less active drug than branded pills.
- Inactive ingredients in generics do NOT affect absorption.
- Patients who are well-controlled on a branded medication CAN be switched to a generic medication.

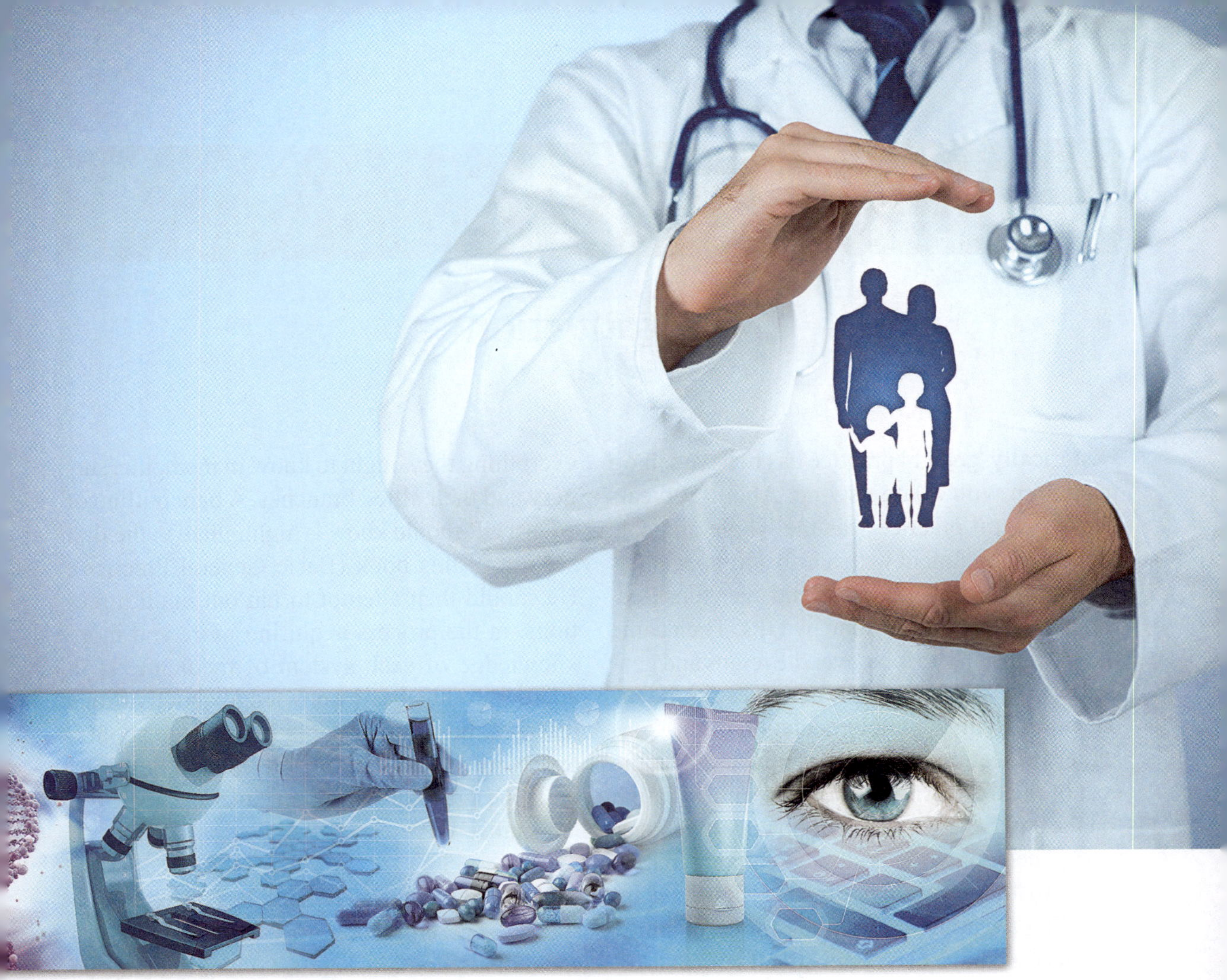

SECTION 2

SPECIALITY MEDICAL GENERAL PRACTICE

CHAPTER 21

Introduction

Historically, general practice has behaved like a pendulum with a large swing. About 50 years back, general practice was the whole and sole of medical treatment with hardly any specialists in the fray. Tooth extractions and even tonsillectomies were routinely done by GPs. Then came the specialists, who took over the reigns and general practice took a backseat, at least in the urban areas. With the implementation of the Consumer Protection Act, there is now a rise in the cost of the treatment, as specialists not wanting to take any risk, do not leave-out any investigations. The population is slowly realizing that by going to the specialists directly, they end up spending a whole lot of money for complaints, which could have been easily dealt with at a GP level, with much lesser cost. The pendulum is now swinging in the correct direction, and the family physician is receiving the dignity he deserves. In rural areas, where 80% of the Indian population resides, the specialists are a rare species, and virtually the whole population is catered to by the GPs.

In both the settings, a "specialist" general practitioner is always seen to have an upper hand and is by and large more successful than an "average" general practitioner. Who is this "specialist" general practitioner?

Concept of "Specialist" General Practitioner

General practice is a speciality in its own right. All GPs specialize in knowing something about everything they ought to know in medicine, surgery and their allied branches. A bare outline of what a GP should know is highlighted in the first section of this book (Basic General Practice). He should then attempt to fan out in all directions, in the process acquiring more and more knowledge of each system of medicine. If in addition to this basic knowledge about various diseases, he gains in-depth knowledge about a few more subjects of his interest and develops on it, he graduates from an 'average' GP to a 'specialist' GP.

In this endeavour, a GP snatches away from a specialist certain modalities, which belong to a specialist's domain e.g., a GP starts using an ECG machine belonging to a cardiologist's domain and gradually masters the electro- cardiogram. He buys a nebuliser, becomes a specialist in inhalation therapy and starts an 'asthma clinic'. He acquires knowledge about that upcoming science of acupuncture and gradually becomes a recognized acupuncturist. The list is endless.

And there is no reason for the specialists to crib. Even when the speciality general practitioner is transgressing the corridors of the specialists, the specialists in turn are reaching (or should be reaching) lofty levels. A cardiologist is no longer 'ECG dependent'. He has reached astronomical heights by getting equipped with 2D Echo, colour-dopplers and angiographies. A general surgeon has no hope if he remains 'general'. He should venture into specialities like endoscopic surgeries. So on and so forth.

What then can an ambitious GP snatch away from each individual specialist? A plausible list is given below.

To begin with, as an illustrative example, the use of an otoscope is described in the next chapter. It is very simple. The GP buys an otoscope, the price of which is almost the same as a standard BP instrument. In a few weeks or months he will realize that many diseases of the external ear or the tympanic membrane (which he used to treat with "all in one" ear drops) has now fallen in his domain. What is required is only a little additional effort in knowing about otoscopic examination coupled with a burning desire to learn! His therapeutic range will increase. And I am sure by the time he has finished reading this chapter and practised on a few patients, he has become an external ear specialist or a qualified "otoscopist".

Speciality	"Snatch away"
ENT	Otoscope, foreign bodies in ENT, minor surgeries in pinna and nasal cavities, etc.
Ophthalmology	Use of ophthalmoscope, surgery of eyelid lesions, e.g., chalazion, refractory errors, removal of foreign bodies, etc.
General Physician	ECG, inhalation therapy, pleural fluid tapping, ascitic fluid tapping, diabetic clinic, asthma clinic, etc.
Dermatology	Intralesional steroids, skin biopsies, establishing a PUVA therapy unit, chemical and electrocautery, etc.
Urology	Catheterization, minor surgeries on the penis e.g., circumcision, dorsal slit, etc.
Paediatrics	Immunization, well-baby clinics, administration of IV fluids.
Dentistry	Extraction of tooth, reduction of dislocated TM joint, professional cleaning of teeth, etc.
Gynaecology & Obstetrics	Minor surgery of external genitalia, ANC, use of Doppler, minor procedures like Cu T insertion, Pap smear, HRT, D&C, MTP, etc.
Orthopaedics	Intra-articular injections, plastering techniques for minor fractures, etc.
Radiology	Use of ultrasound machine or X-ray unit.
Surgery	Minor surgeries like draining of abscess, taking biopsy, removing ganglion, etc.
Pathology	Collection centre, use of glucometer for BSL, rapid ELISA for HIV testing, pregnancy detection kits. Benedict's test for urine sugar, Hb by Sahli's method, buying an auto-analyser for other lab tests, etc.
Physiotherapy	SWD, ultrasound machine, wax bath, cervical and lumbar tractions, etc.

CHAPTER 22

The Otoscope

- Instruments Used
- How to Use an Otoscope
- Normal EAC
- Abnormalities in the EAC
- Normal TM
- Abnormalities in TM

INSTRUMENTS USED TO EXAMINE EXTERNAL AUDITORY CANAL AND EAR DRUM

Otoscopic examination requires good illumination and some degree of magnification, which can be obtained by the following equipments:

1. **Bull's lamp and head mirror**: Here, the source of light is a 100 watts lamp called the Bull's lamp. This is placed behind the left shoulder of the sitting patient. The light is projected on to the concave mirror worn on the forehead by the examiner. The mirror converges the light into a sharp focal point to fall inside the auditory canal and on to the tympanic membrane through a speculum which contains a magnifying lens.
2. **Electric head light**: These are worn on the forehead of the operator and works on dry cells, which are incorporated in the unit itself, just like in miner's lamp. Magnification can be obtained by means of a speculum.
3. **Fibre-optic headlight**: These are similar to the electric headlights described above, but they work on electricity. They give a very powerful beam of light but are very expensive.
4. **Operating microscope**: This is the best method for examining the ear but very very expensive to be used in a GP's clinic. For an ENT specialist, it is indispensable for correct diagnosis and treatment.
5. **Electric otoscope (or auroscope)**: Here the source of light is in the handle itself. The handle is attached to the speculum (Fig. 22.1) which contains the magnifying lens. The advantage of the electrical otoscope is that, it is a portable instrument and is simple to use without any training. The only disadvantage is that it is dependent on batteries and bulbs, which are notoriously unreliable. The examiner suddenly finds himself without the means of examining the ear for weeks, before the instrument is repaired. Otherwise, it is a very convenient instrument for use in general practice and is strongly recommended. The Indian made costs around Rs.

700 (almost the same as a good BP instrument) and the imported version about Rs. 2500. These are readily available in any surgical shop.

HOW TO USE AN OTOSCOPE?

The otoscope should be held like a pen between the thumb and index finger of the right hand with the ulnar border resting lightly on the head of the patient so that any sudden movement by the patient is largely neutralized, thus preventing damage to the ear. The left hand pulls the pinna backwards and upwards, which makes the external auditory meatus and the tympanic membrane clearly visible to the examiner.

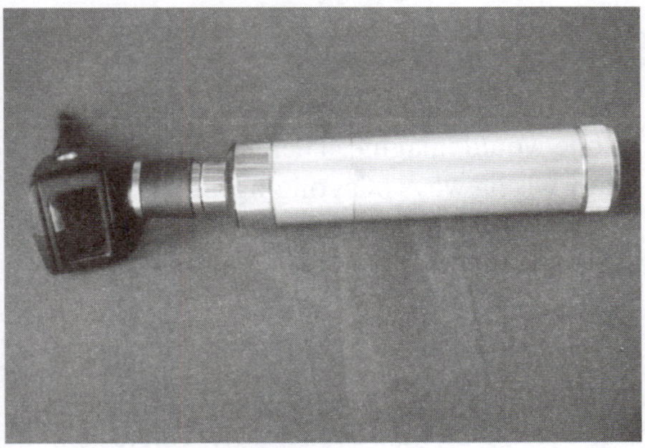

| **Fig. 22.1** Electric otoscope |

HOW DOES THE NORMAL EXTERNAL AUDITORY CANAL (EAC) LOOK?

The canal that you now see extending from the otoscope to the tympanic membrane (identified by its pearly grey shiny appearance) is the external auditory canal (EAC). It is about 2.5 cm in length and is composed of two parts—the *outer cartilaginous part* and the *inner bony part*. The skin of the cartilage of the pinna will be seen to continue on to the outer cartilaginous part of the EAC. As it is firmly adherent to the underlying cartilage, furuncles in this part are very painful. Even contact of the furuncle with the otoscope will cause severe pain, making the patient resist the otoscopic examination. This part also contains ceruminous glands which secrete wax. If wax (or other debris) is seen through the otoscope, withdraw the instrument, clean the canal as described below and reintroduce the otoscope. The canal will be seen to narrow down at about 1 cm from the pinna. This is called the *isthmus*, which connects the outer and inner portions. It is in this portion that foreign bodies usually get stuck. Beyond the isthmus the canal will curve making the whole EAC 'S' shaped. The skin on the inner bony layer is loosely attached to the underlying bone and does not contain any hair follicles or ceruminous glands. Hence, furuncles are not found in this area.

WHAT ABNORMALITIES DO YOU EXPECT TO FIND IN THE EAC?

Otomycosis (Aural Aspergillosis, Aural Candidiasis)

This is a fungal infection of the EAC caused by *Aspergillus niger* or *Candida albicans*. It can be a primary disease, the fungus getting established in the canal during swimming, but usually it complicates chronic otitis externa or chronic suppurative otitis media. Also, prolonged use of antibiotic ear drops kill the local bacteria and facilitates the fungal growth. The patient presents with either intense itching, a scanty black discharge or with marked pain in the ear (due to secondary bacterial infection or invasion of the fungus into the skin). On examination with otoscope (Fig. 22.6), the EAC will either show:

- *A cotton like growth*, which resembles the fungal growth seen on a slice of bread kept in the open, overnight in the rainy season.

Interspersed in this white background, black fungal spores of *Aspergillus niger* may also be seen.

- *Wet blotting paper like deposits*, which are white, brown or black. This picture is usually caused by *Candida albicans.*

The condition readily responds to clotrimazole or tolnaftate ear drops for 2–3 weeks. Treat the secondary bacterial infection if present, with systemic antibiotics.

Furuncles (Boils)

The patient presents with severe pain in one ear, severe enough to cause insomnia. This is because there is no room for expansion for the furuncle as the skin is firmly bound down to the cartilage. Pain is increased by any movement of the meatal cartilage, e.g., during mastication or pressure on the tragus. In addition, because the presence of the furuncle causes the walls of the meatus to come in opposition, otoscopic examination is still more difficult. Nevertheless, if gently and carefully pursued, the erythematous boil with the pus pointing may be visualised. A deep seated furuncle may not be visible but even then a definite spot of tenderness may be found, if careful palpation is done all over the cartilaginous portion with a vectis (or even with the tip of the otoscope).

Hot fomentations are useful. Systemic antibiotics effective against Staphylococci (e.g., cloxacillin) will be needed along with analgesics. Large furuncles need incision and drainage but incision of small unripe furuncles is highly mischievous, as it is more likely to spread the infection than cure it.

Foreign Bodies (FB) in the EAC

The otoscope is invaluable in identifying FB in the ear, which are commonly encountered in children. The method of removal of FB in the ear is described in Chapter 40. Suffice it to mention here at the cost of repetition that FBs in the ear for the purpose of removal are divided into two categories—those which are vegetable, and those which are not. Vegetable FBs (e.g., a pea) should never be syringed as they swell and have to be removed piecemeal. The 'non' vegetable FBs (e.g., beads, stones, buttons) can be syringed out.

Wax in Ear

This again can be identified by the otoscope as a brownish black mass in the EAC. The patient presents with either pain or deafness or both. The method of removal of wax is dealt with in Chapter 9. The easier option for removing the wax is by hooking it out with a wax hook or a vectis. The hook is passed beyond the wax and wax hooked out by gentle but firm traction along the canal. Syringing out the wax is not as simple as one would imagine. There is a right way and many wrong ways of syringing an ear. The right way is to syringe it out after it has been softened with lukewarm oil. A jet of lukewarm water should then be directed upwards and backwards on the posterior wall of the meatus. If the wax is impacted, a chink is made along the posterior wall behind the wax, so that water enters behind the wax and pushes it out. The many wrong ways will not be described here as they are best forgotten!

Exostosis

Occasionally on otoscopic examination, a hard bony outgrowth is encountered in the EAC. Usually, it is asymptomatic. If symptomatic however, refer the patient to an ENT surgeon as the treatment is operative removal with an electric drill, a procedure which can damage important structures like the facial nerve.

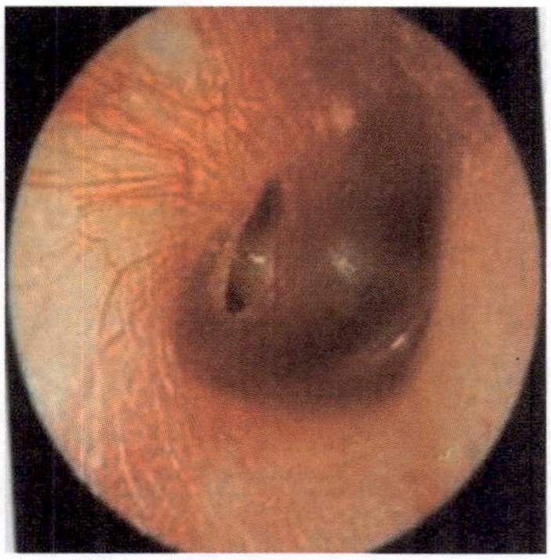

| Fig. 22.2 Perforation of ear drum |

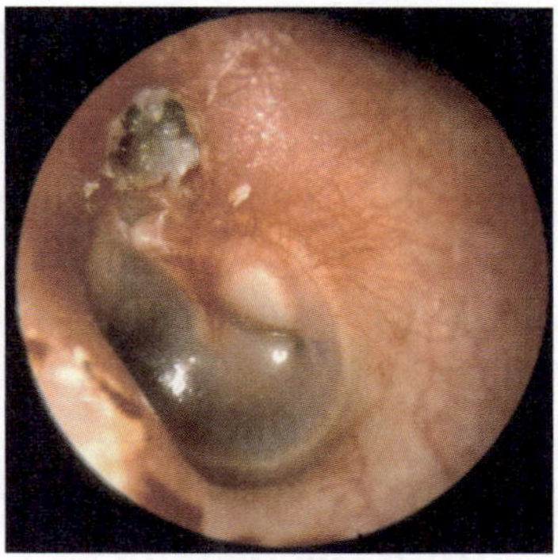

| Fig. 22.3 Cholesteatoma |

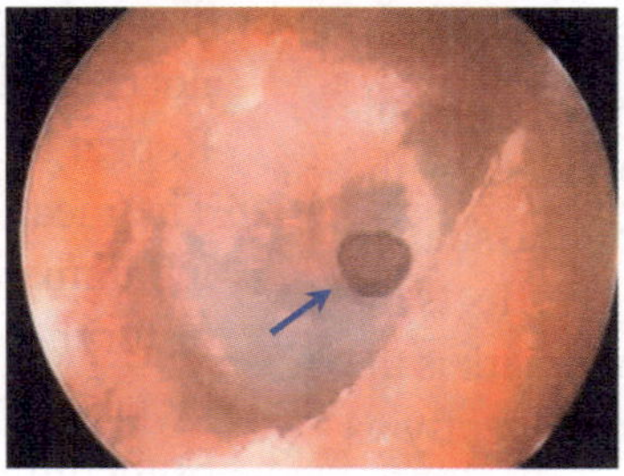

| Fig. 22.4 Perforation of ear drum |

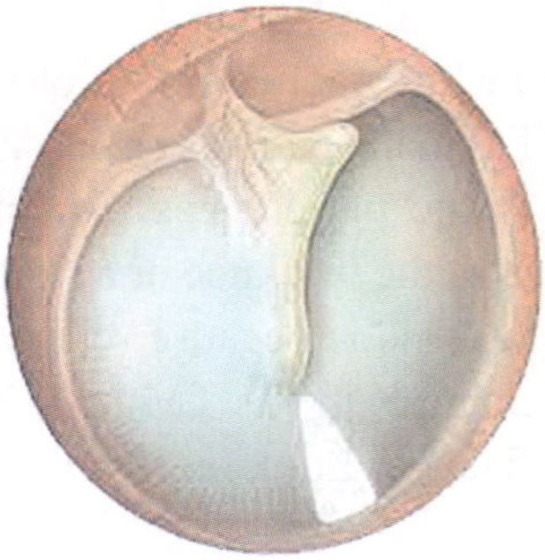

| Fig. 22.5 Otoscopic view of ear drum |

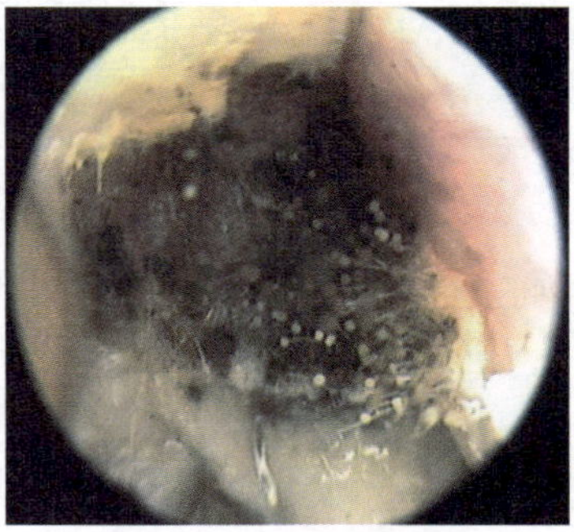

| Fig. 22.6 Otomycosis |

Keratosis Obturans

The patient presents with very severe pain in one ear. On examination, a blackish brown mass of wax mixed with desquamated epithelium of skin of the EAC is seen totally occluding the meatus. By continued enlargement, it may cause pressure on other important structures, e.g., the facial nerve. Refer to an ENT specialist as removal under general anaesthesia may be required.

HOW DOES THE NORMAL TYMPANIC MEMBRANE (TM; EAR DRUM) LOOK?

Fig. 22.7 showing parts of the ear drum should be self-explanatory. But for the novice, the problem is to identify the TM and its parts through the otoscope. Having retracted the pinna upwards and backwards in adults and backwards in children, the examiner should be able to identify the TM through the otoscope as an egg-shaped pearly grey membrane. It shines and reflects the light. The most easily identifiable landmark is the *short process*, which stands out prominently as a white knob. The *handle* of the *malleus* then can be seen as a white streak extending downwards and backwards from the short process.

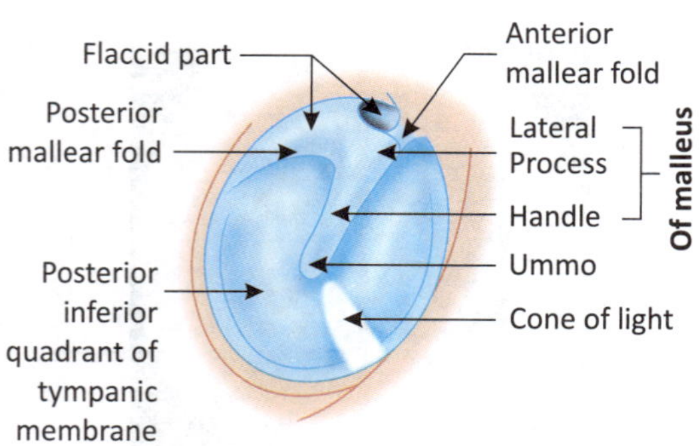

| **Fig. 22.7** Parts of tympanic membrane |

The lower end of the handle of the malleus is the *umbo*, from which a triangular cone of reflected light is seen extending downwards and anteriorly. This is due to the sectional shape of the TM. Because of the curvature of the EAC, the anterior inferior portion may be hidden from the view by the anterior wall of the EAC.

The examiner should again concentrate on the short process of the malleus and try to identify the folds running anteriorly and posteriorly, called the anterior and posterior *malleolar folds*. The part of the TM below these folds is the *pars tensa* (tense part) and part above these folds is the *pars flaccida* (flaccid part or the attic).

If the Drum Cannot be seen, the Following could be the Reasons

1. The light is not properly focused or the meatus not properly straightened by pulling the pinna. Repeat the otoscopic examination properly.
2. The meatus has become narrow because of inflammation of the walls like in otitis externa or furuncles. Call back the patient after antibiotics.
3. Something is obstructing the meatus e.g., wax, discharge, etc. Clean the canal properly and repeat the examination.

In order to get thoroughly conversant with the normal TM, the GP who has bought a new otoscope, should for practice do an otoscopic examination of as many patients as possible; it does not matter if the patient has pain in the ear, osteoarthritis of the left knee or a right sided inguinal hernia. This is because relatively minor and subtle changes in the TM may have diagnostic significance. Look out for the following abnormalities.

COMMON ABNORMALITIES ENCOUNTERED IN THE TYMPANIC MEMBRANE

1. The normal TM is pearly grey in colour and the surface is smooth and shiny. If this normal glistening appearance is lost then the TM is probably thickened because of fibrosis caused by *chronc otitis* media or externa.
2. Scarring of the membrane because of *healed perforation* is either seen as a thin, transluscent *scar* or as chalky white patches (tympanosclerosis). They are not indicative of disease.
3. If the TM looks fiery red, bulging and with loss of normal features described above, it could be *acute otitis media* associated with fluid in the middle ear cavity.
4. If the TM has retracted into the middle ear cavity as diagnosed by the undue prominence of the short process of the handle of malleus, it could be due to obstruction of the eustachian tube. Because of the *eustachian block*, the trapped air in the middle ear cavity gets gradually absorbed and cannot be replaced. Hence, a vacuum develops resulting in the retraction of the ear drum. Gradually, serous exudation takes place in the middle ear, which may be seen as a fluid level or as bubbles if the obstruction is partial.
5. Perforation of the TM can be appreciated well with the otoscope (Figs. 22.2 & 22.4). Perforations in the pars flaccida are called *attic perforations*. Perforations in the pars tensa are either *marginal* or *central*, depending on whether a rim of normal TM is surrounding the perforation or not. *Marginal and attic perforations are 'dangerous or unsafe perforations'* because they are associated with life-threatening complications, which may be so silent initially that they can be overlooked. It is in order that an ENT opinion should be sought.

   If there is an ear discharge and there are no signs of otitis externa or furunculosis, the discharge must come from the middle ear. If the perforation is not seen through the otoscope, try either Valsalva manoeuvre (forced expiration with mouth and nose closed) or Toynbee manoeuvre (swallowing with nose closed by thumb and forefinger). Secretion then, will be seen coming out through the TM and the perforation visualized.
6. Finally, a few words about the entity called "**cholesteatoma**" (Fig. 22.3), which a GP should know and have a high index of suspicion in its diagnosis. Cholesteatoma is not a tumour as the suffix "oma" might suggest, but is designated so, because of its property to destroy surrounding tissue and bone. A highly simplified explanation about its pathogenesis is given below.

The skin overlying the TM and EAC is unique in the body for two reasons:

- Firstly, it has the property of migration (an ink dot placed on the TM is seen at the opening of the EAC in a few weeks). This property is provided by nature for 'autocleaning' of the canal, which being a blind duct cannot be cleaned easily by external friction, as is the case in the skin of the other parts of the body.
- Secondly, this skin is also very thin as it lacks a corium, so that the epithelium lies directly on the perichondrium and can be easily destroyed. Now, in case of perforation of the TM, this skin can migrate into the middle ear cavity. As this is a "skin in the wrong place", it can provoke a reaction and a cholesteatoma is formed. Because of its destructive property, it can erode the surrounding structures and also get secondarily infected, giving rise to a discharge with a foul smell.

If the cholesteatoma lies in the attic, it can destroy important structures lying in this area such as the facial nerve or the ossicles. On the other hand, it may remain quiescent throughout life without giving rise to any complications whatsoever. Hence it has been described as a 'live bomb, which may or may not explode'. Nevertheless, it is always better to take an ENT opinion under the slightest suspicion of its presence.

Conclusion: A knowledge about few common diseases of the external ear and the tympanic membrane is all that is required to become an external ear specialist and push the ENT specialist into the middle and inner ear cavities!!

This chapter has been reviewed by ***Dr Naina Karodpati****, MD, ENT Specialist, Pune.*

CHAPTER 23

The ECG Machine

The ECG machine is such an important tool for a general practitioner that it should rank 4th amongst his armamentarium, the 2nd and 3rd important tools being the examination table and the stethoscope! The first and foremost is of course the patient himself! It is an extremely useful or indispensable instrument in a rural setting, where the GP when confronted with a patient of chest pain, has to decide on the spot whether referral of the patient to the nearest city with an ICU facility, is necessary or not.

The ECG machine should be used judiciously by a GP. As one of my cardiologist friend once said in a lighter vein "*The only contraindication for using an ECG machine is that the patient does not have money (unethical)*". There are hundreds of indications for taking an ECG like "chest pain in the body". I'll go further and say that an ECG is indicated sometimes even if there is no chest pain. We all know that myocardial infarction can present without chest pain in diabetics and in the guise of vomiting, syncope and even mental confusion. It is like vaccination. A few ECGs will be wasted, but unexpectedly an ECG tracing will show an infarct and save a life. Used in this manner, approximately 95% of ECG tracings in a GP setting are likely to be normal, in contrast to an ICCU setting where 95% ECG tracings are likely to be abnormal. Hence, I will describe the normal ECG with its normal variations in detail. This will be followed by a brief description of the abnormal ECG tracings where the GP's job is to recognize these abnormalities, identify those patients who can be managed in his own clinic and those cases which should be referred to an ICCU.

TAKING AN ECG RECORDING

Don't leave this procedure entirely to your compounder or nurse. A faulty recording can lead to a faulty diagnosis and in a cardiac patient this could be potentially dangerous.

- Use owner's manual and get well versed with your machine.

- Make the patient lie down and relax to prevent muscle tremor.
- Connect the limb electrodes. Confirm that the proper electrode has been connected to the proper limb. The limb electrodes are usually labelled or marked by a specific colour for identification. The electrodes should be applied just above the ankles or wrists.
- Calibrate with the 1 mV signal shown on the machine.
- Check that the paper speed is correct (25 mm/sec).
- Adjust the temperature of the stylus.
- First record the six extremity leads.
- Then record the six chest leads by means of 'suction cup electrodes' holding it in place on the chest. The positions of the chest leads are given in Fig. 23.1.

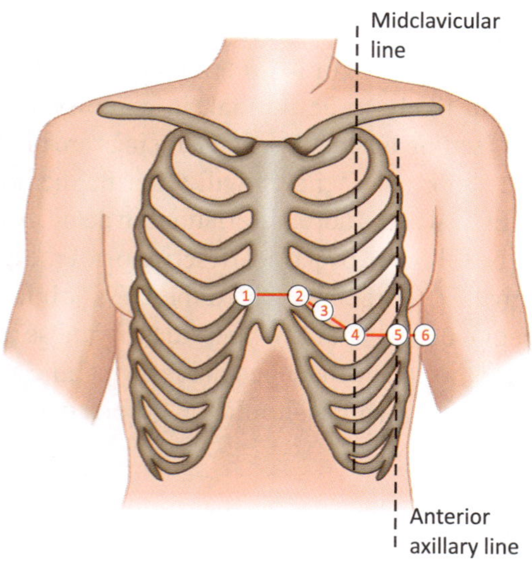

V_1 : Fourth intercostal space at right sternal border.
V_2 : Fourth intercostal space at left sternal border.
V_3 : Midway between V_2 and V_4
V_4 : Midclavicular line in the 5th intercostal space.
V_5 : Anterior axillary line at same level as V_4.
V_6 : Midaxillary line at same level as V_4 and V_5.

| **Fig. 23.1** The positions of chest electrodes |

Shaving may be required in males. In females, the electrodes should be placed under the breast and not on the breast. The fourth intercostal space is just below and lateral to the angles of Louis on the sternum. This can be located just 2 cm below the top of the sternum as a horizontal ridge. Most modern machines have six chest electrodes, which are labelled or coloured. Older machines may have only one chest electrode which requires to be positioned one by one from V_1 to V_6.

ECG Paper

All ECG machines run at a standardized rate and use standardized paper strip (roll). The paper strip is divided into 1 mm² squares with heavier lines between every five squares. The ECG paper strip usually moves at the speed of 25 mm/sec. Hence one small square measured horizontally corresponds to 0.04 sec and five small squares (i.e., one large square) correspond to 0.2 sec. Five large squares are covered in 1 sec and 300 large squares in 1 min. The voltage or amplitude of a given deflection is measured vertically (Fig. 23.2).

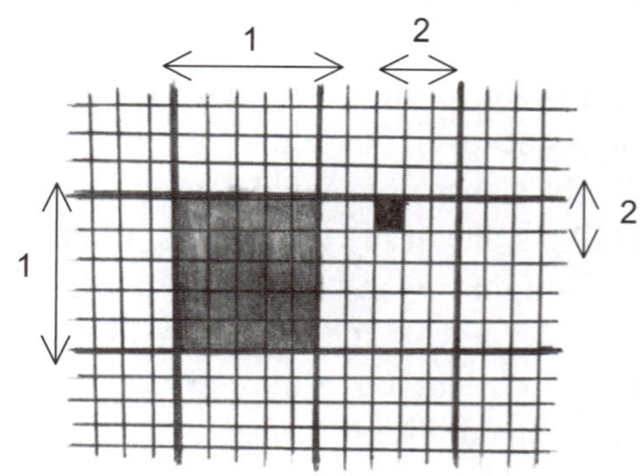

With the paper speed adjusted to 25 mm/sec
1. One large square represents 0.2 sec on horizontal axis and 5 mm voltage on vertical axis
2. One small square represents 0.04 sec on horizontal axis and 1 mm voltage on vertical axis

| **Fig. 23.2** Measurements on ECG graph paper |

Standardization or Calibration

Your ECG machine may have a special standardization button, which when pressed gives a deflection of 1 mV (10 mm). Before the ECG is taken you must check that the machine is properly calibrated, which means a square wave 10 mm tall (2 large squares) (Fig. 23.3) is produced on pressing the button. If not properly calibrated, a small complex may lead to a mistaken diagnosis of pericardial effusion or a tall R wave can be thought of due to left ventricular hypertrophy. On electronic machines, standardization is displayed on the bottom of the paper.

Artifacts

Especially for beginners, it is important to identify a particular wave as an artifact, as otherwise this could lead to wrong interpretations (Fig. 23.3).

- *Misplacement of electrodes*: The limb electrodes are commonly swapped by oversight. If you see an unexpected wave inversion or aVR is seen to be predominantly positive, it is a good practice to recheck the electrode placement.
- *Patient movement* or poor electrode contact can produce deflections in the ECG recording giving an impression of an abnormal beat. Ask the patient to relax and lie still.
- *Wandering baseline*: The baseline does not remain steady but moves up and down making recording very difficult.
- *External electrical interference*: Other electrical appliances in the room (AC, refrigerator, etc.) produce 'fine tooth comb' artifacts. This can make reading of the ECG tracing impossible. This can be eliminated by turning off the appliances in the room or connecting the ECG machine to a different plug.
- *Incorrect calibration* can give false high or low voltage pattern (normal 1mV pulse = 10 mm). Faster paper speed will document waves which are wider than normal (normal—25 mm/sec).

BASIC CARDIAC ELETROPHYSIOLOGY

Under resting conditions, the myocardial cells are *polarized*, i.e., they carry an electrical charge on the surface. The outside of the resting cell is positive and the inside is negative. When these cells are stimulated they rapidly *depolarize,* i.e., they reverse their membrane polarity. The outside of the cell becomes negative while the inside becomes positive. This depolarization process spreads in a wave like manner through the atria and the ventricles. After a time the cells begin to return to their original resting state. This is called *repolarization*, where the outside of the cell becomes positive and the inside of the cell becomes negative again. When the atria are stimulated, i.e., depolarized, it produces the P wave on the ECG. Stimulation and depolarization of the ventricles produces the QRS complex.

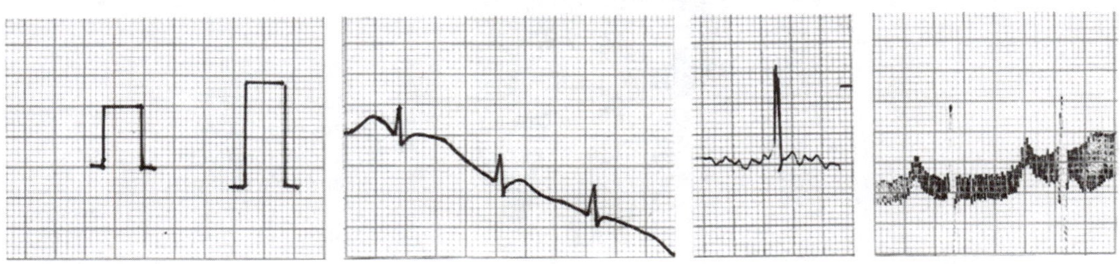

Correct and incorrect calibration — Wandering base line — Patient movement — External electrical interference

| **Fig. 23.3** Artifacts |

Ventricular repolarization produces the ST segment, T wave and U wave on the ECG tracing.

The depolarization stimulus originates in the normal heart in the *sino-atrial node* (Fig. 23.4). This is a collection of specialized cells located near the opening of the superior vena cava in the right atrium. This functions as the pacemaker of the heart. It has the capacity of spontaneously generating electrical impulses (automaticity). Initially, the impulses stimulate the right and the left atria causing it to contract and pump blood into both the ventricles simultaneously.

Next, the impulse stimulates the AV junction, which is a collection of specialized cells connecting the atria to the ventricles. There is a delay of this impulse at the AV junction during which time ventricular filling takes place. The AV junction is formed by the AV node and the bundle of His. The His bundle bifurcates into two main branches.

The right bundle branch stimulates the right ventricle and the left bundle branch stimulates the left ventricle. The main left bundle bifurcates into two subdivisions, the anterior fascicle and the posterior fascicle. The depolarization wave then spreads by way of these fascicles, through the Purkinje fibres located in the ventricular walls, from the endocardium to the epicardium. The ventricles contract, pumping blood into the lungs and into the general circulation.

Understanding this basic electrophysiology helps us to explain many ECG abnormalities, e.g., depression of the SA node as seen in the sick sinus syndrome produces bradycardia and many rhythm disturbances on ECG. Blockage of the impulse at the AV junction and bundle branch produce heart blocks and bundle branch blocks, respectively. Damage to the muscles of the ventricles in MI produces specific ECG abnormalities diagnostic of the condition.

BASIC ECG WAVES, COMPLEXES AND INTERVALS

By convention, the ECG waves are labelled alphabetically P, Q, R, S, T and U. These letters were selected arbitrarily soon after the discovery of the ECG machine. The upwards and downwards deflections P, Q, R, S and T are called *waves*. The Q, R and S deflection together constitute a *complex*. The time between two waves is called an *interval*. The interval between S wave and the beginning of T wave is called the ST *segment*. The J point is the junction between the end of QRS complex and the beginning of the ST segment (Fig. 23.5).

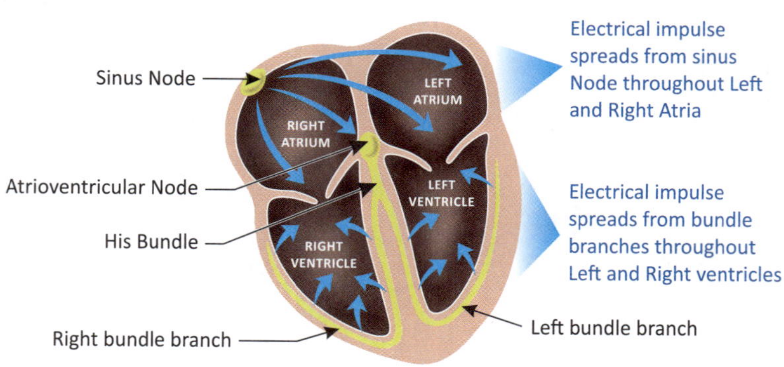

| **Fig. 23.4** The conduction system of the heart |

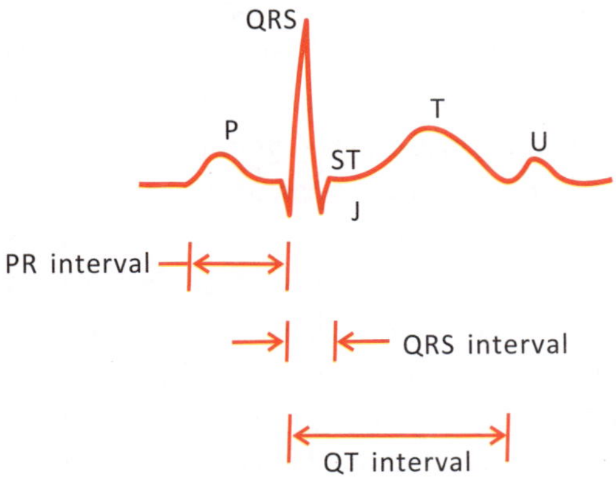

| **Fig. 23.5** Basic ECG waves and intervals |

Each phase of cardiac activity produces a specific wave or complex. The *P wave* represents atrial depolarization, the *QRS complex* represents ventricular depolarization and the *ST segment* and *T wave* represent ventricular repolarization. Then what represents atrial repolarization? The '*atrial T wave*' (*Ta*). It is so small that it is usually not observed on the normal ECG. U wave is a small deflection seen occasionally after the T wave. Its genesis is uncertain, but could be the final phase of ventricular repolarization.

There are four major intervals. The *R–R interval* denotes the ventricular rate and is used to measure the heart rate. The *P–R interval* measures the time taken by the impulse to spread from its origin in the SA node, across the atria and through the AV junction. During this interval, the ventricles get time to fill with blood. The *QRS interval* measures the duration of ventricular depolarization, while the *QT interval* measures the time taken for ventricular depolarization and repolarization. These are described in some detail below (vide infra—Genesis of the normal ECG).

ECG LEADS

Simply stated, a lead is an electrical picture of the heart depicted graphically. It does not mean the wires that are connected to the limbs as is the common misconception.

The heart is a three-dimensional structure producing an electric current just like any dry cell battery. This electric current fans out all over the body, which is recorded by the ECG machine. This machine records the electric events taking place in the heart from different positions by means of metal plates (electrodes) placed on the surface of the body. An ECG lead (graph) shows the differences in voltage detected by these electrodes. Conventionally these voltages from the heart are recorded by 12 'standard' leads, which can be subdivided into two subgroups: the six *extremity* (*limb*) leads and the six *chest* (*precordial*) leads. The extremity leads are further divided into *bipolar* leads (I, II and III) and the *unipolar* leads (aVR, aVL and aVF).

The chest leads are designated as V_1, V_2, V_3, V_4, V_5 and V_6. The extremity leads re-cord the electrical events in the frontal plane while the chest leads do this in a horizontal plane.

The frontal plane cuts your body into an anterior and a posterior half, the cut going through both the ears, both the shoulders, etc. The horizontal plane cuts the body into an upper and lower half. All these 12 leads therefore give a three-dimensional picture of the electrical activity going on in the heart.

To understand this concept more clearly, compare a 12-lead ECG recording to a cricket match being recorded by 12 TV cameras placed in different positions in the stadium. With these cameras, we get a different view of the same cricketing event from different angles. The situation is analogous. The only difference is that, in a cricket match a camera cannot be placed underground (i.e., inferior surface of the heart) and in an ECG recording, there can be no posterior leads.

Bipolar Leads I, II and III

These leads are called bipolar because they record the difference between the electrical voltage between two limb leads.

- Lead I = Left arm–right arm
- Lead II = Left leg–right arm
- Lead III = Left leg–left arm

A schematic diagram of these leads is drawn (Fig. 23.6), which is called **Einthoven's triangle**.

An important rule concerning the bipolar leads is that the sum of the voltages in the Lead I and Lead III is equal to the voltage in Lead II (i.e., Lead I + Lead III = Lead II). Thus, when a cardiologist and an electronic engineer come together the equation is, one plus three equals to two! This is a fundamental rule and if in your ECG tracing this is not so, probably the electrodes have been put wrongly. As shown in Fig. 23.6b, the Einthoven's triangle can be modified by just shifting all the three leads inwards, giving rise to the *triaxial diagram*.

Unipolar Leads aVL, aVR, aVF

These leads are called unipolar as they record the voltage at one site relative to zero potential. Augmentation is done by your machine to make the ECG graph more apparent. The unipolar leads can be represented schematically as a triaxial lead diagram as shown in Fig. 23.6c. As you can see the positive pole of aVR points towards the right shoulder, of aVL towards the left shoulder and of aVF towards the left foot. The rule applicable to unipolar leads is that the sum of voltages of all the leads equals zero (i.e., aVR + aVL + aVF = 0). Check in your ECG tracing if this is so. If not, again the electrodes have been put wrongly.

If now the triaxial diagram of bipolar and unipolar limb leads are superimposed on each other, what we get is a **hexaxial lead diagram** (Fig. 23.6d). This is a very useful reference diagram needed for explaining the complexes in your ECG as well as calculating the mean QRS axis. This diagram should be committed to

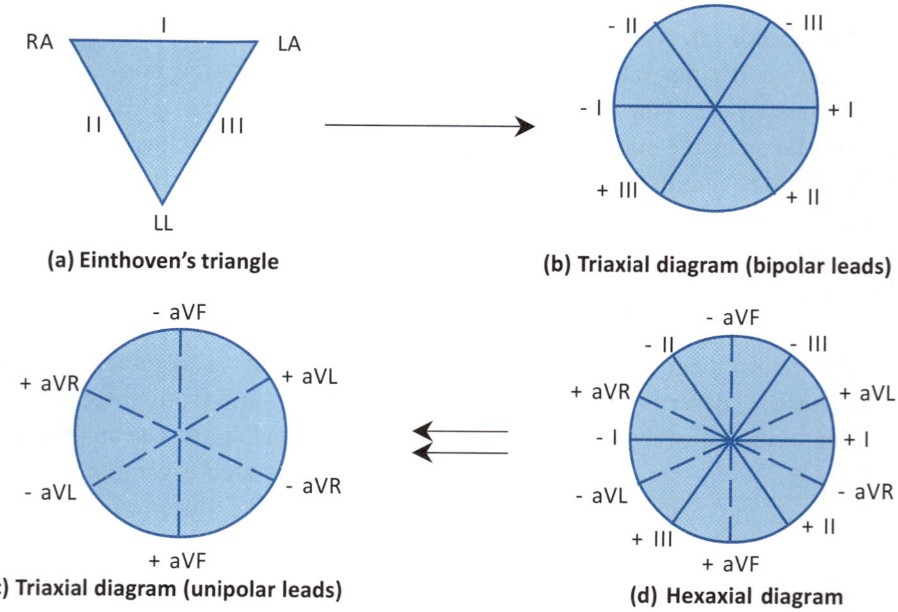

Fig. 23.6 How the hexaxial diagram is formed

memory or stored in your clinic for instant reference. Time and again we will be referring to this diagram in this chapter.

Chest Leads V_1–V_6

These leads record voltages in the horizontal plane of the body. The positive pole of each lead is directed towards the anterior chest wall while the negative pole is directed towards the posterior chest wall. So now, we have a 12-lead system which takes pictures of the same cardiac event at a given moment from 12 different angles:

- LI, aVL—left lateral surface of the heart.
- LII, LIII, aVF—inferior surface.
- aVR—right atrium.
- V_1–V_2—right ventricle.
- V_3–V_4—interventricular septum and anterior wall of left ventricle.
- V_5–V_6—lateral wall of left ventricle.

GENESIS OF THE NORMAL ECG

In a normal ECG, the P wave is positive (upwards) in some leads while it is negative (downwards) in other leads. Similarly about the QRS complex, T wave, etc. Why is it so? What is the reason for the variety of ECG complexes in different leads? An explanation of the above questions is given below without going into too much details. Fundamentally we have to understand that an impulse (mean wave of depolarization) flowing towards the positive pole of a lead produces an upwards deflection on the ECG, whereas an impulse flowing away from the positive pole (towards the negative pole) causes a downward deflection. If an impulse is flowing at right angles to any lead, a biphasic deflection is produced which consists of an upward and a downward deflection of equal size. So once you know the direction of the impulse through the heart, it is easily possible to understand the pattern of waves in the lead in question.

P Wave

The atrial depolarization wave originates in the SA node and spreads downwards to the patient's left, towards the AV node. Since this wave points towards the positive pole of Lead II and away from the positive pole of aVR, the normal P wave is positive in Lead II and negative in aVR (refer to hexaxial lead diagram). Normal P wave is <2.5 mm (2½ small squares) in amplitude and <0.12 sec (3 small squares) in width. P-wave exceeding these limits is abnormal.

PR Interval

PR interval measured from the beginning of P-wave to the beginning of R-wave, represents the time taken by an impulse to spread through the atria and AV junction. The normal PR interval should not be <0.12 sec (3 small squares) and should not be >0.2 sec (5 small squares).

Q Waves

They result from septal depolarization, which occurs from left to right in a normal individual. Hence, a small Q wave ('Septal Q') is normal in left sided leads LI, LII, aVL, V_5 and V_6. A small Q wave may also be seen normally in Lead III. This usually disappears on holding breath in deep inspiration while taking the ECG. A normal septal Q wave is <2 small squares deep and 1 small square wide.

QRS Complex

QRS complex represents ventricular depolarization. The ventricles are depolarized in two phases one after another. In the *first phase*, the stimulus spreads from the left side of the interventricular septum, across the septum and to the right. In the *second phase*, both the ventricles are stimulated simultaneously, but as the left ventricle has a great muscle mass than the right, the direction of the depolarization wave is towards the left ventricle and inclined downwards, from the 11 o'clock to the 5 o'clock position (Fig. 23.9).

Chest Leads

In lead V_1, which is placed in the 4th intercostal space at right border of the sternum, what we see is a rS complex. The initial small positive deflection is due to the impulse going from left to right through the septum towards the positive pole of V_1 (septal 'r'). The large negative S wave that follows is due to the second phase of ventricular depolarization going from right to left away from the positive pole of V_1. In contrast, lead V_6 will show a qR complex. As an exercise try and explain the genesis of this complex ('septal Q' with a tall R). As you move from V_1 towards V_6, the R wave gradually increases in height becoming maximum in V_5 or V_6 and the S wave gradually decreases in height. At V_3 or V_4 both R wave and S wave become almost equal in size. This is called the *zone of transition*.

Limb Leads

The limb leads will show a lot of variations in the normal ECG except in aVR which always registers a negative QRS complex (Qr, Qs and rS) as the wave of depolarization is going away from its positive pole. The complex registered in the remaining five leads will depend on the direction of the impulse, i.e., the mean QRS axis. If this points vertically downwards, the ECG will show predominantly positive QRS complex (qR) in L-II, L-III, aVF. If it points horizontally, the ECG will show predominantly positive QRS complex (qR) in L-I and aVL. Normally, the QRS width is not more than 0.1 sec (2½ small squares).

Confused by the QRS nomenclature and configurations? You need not be if you remember the following points:

- The first negative deflection of the QRS complex is called a **Q wave**.
- The first positive deflection is called **R-wave,** whether or not it is preceded by a Q wave.
- A negative deflection after a R wave is called a **S wave**.
- Large waves are denoted by capital letters (Q, R, S) and small waves are denoted by small letters (q, r, s).
- If the whole complex is positive, it is called a R wave. But, if the whole complex is negative, it is called a QS complex (and not a Q wave or S wave).
- If an additional R wave is present, it is called R′ (R prime).

ST Segment

The ST segment represents the beginning of ventricular repolarization. It lies between the end of S wave and beginning of T wave. Normally it is isoelectric, although slight deviations of <1 mm are common in normal individuals. Notice the marked elevation of ST segment in Fig. 23.7. This is called *early repolarization pattern*. This is seen in normal individuals and is quite benign. It can be mistakenly interpreted as an 'infarct' but notice that reciprocal ST depression is not associated.

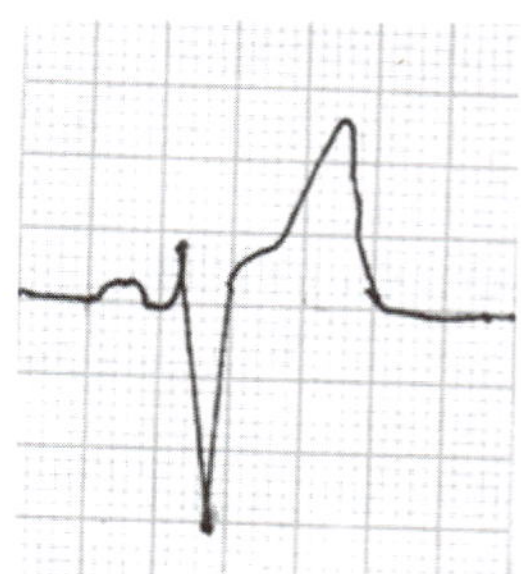

| **Fig. 23.7** Normal variant of ST segment. Early repolarization |

T Waves

T waves correspond to ventricular repolarization. As a general rule, T wave is in the same direction of the mean QRS complex. An inverted T wave is considered normal in leads aVR, V_1, V_2 and in L III. In other leads, an inverted T wave is generally considered pathological.

QT Interval

It represents total duration of ventricular activity (depolarization and repolarization) and is measured from the start of Q wave and end of T wave. The normal values depend on the heart rate. A decrease in heart rate increases the QT interval and predisposes the patient to ventricular arrhythmias. Normal QT interval is from 0.32 to 0.4 sec.

CALCULATION OF HEART RATE (HR)

By this, we mean calculating the **ventricular rate,** which is the same as the patient's pulse. The method of calculating the HR will depend on whether the rhythm is regular or not.

If the rhythm is **regular**, count the number of large squares between two successive R waves and divide the number 300 by this number. In Fig. 23.8b, there are five large squares in between two R waves. Therefore, the HR = 300/5 = 60 per min. If very accurate HR is required, divide the number 1500 by the number of small squares in between two successive R waves. If the rhythm is **irregular**, count the number of R waves in 30 large squares and multiply by 10. In Fig. 23.8c, the HR is 11 × 10 = 110 per min.

REPORTING OF AN ECG

All the 14 points mentioned below should be interpreted and reported. In practice, reporting a series of normal findings is tedious, time consuming and many times dispensed with. This often leads to mistakes in reporting. Interpretation should be done by correlating with clinical findings; otherwise, this could lead to a mistaken diagnosis. For example: T wave inversions in V_1, V_2 and V_3 are abnormal finding in an elderly

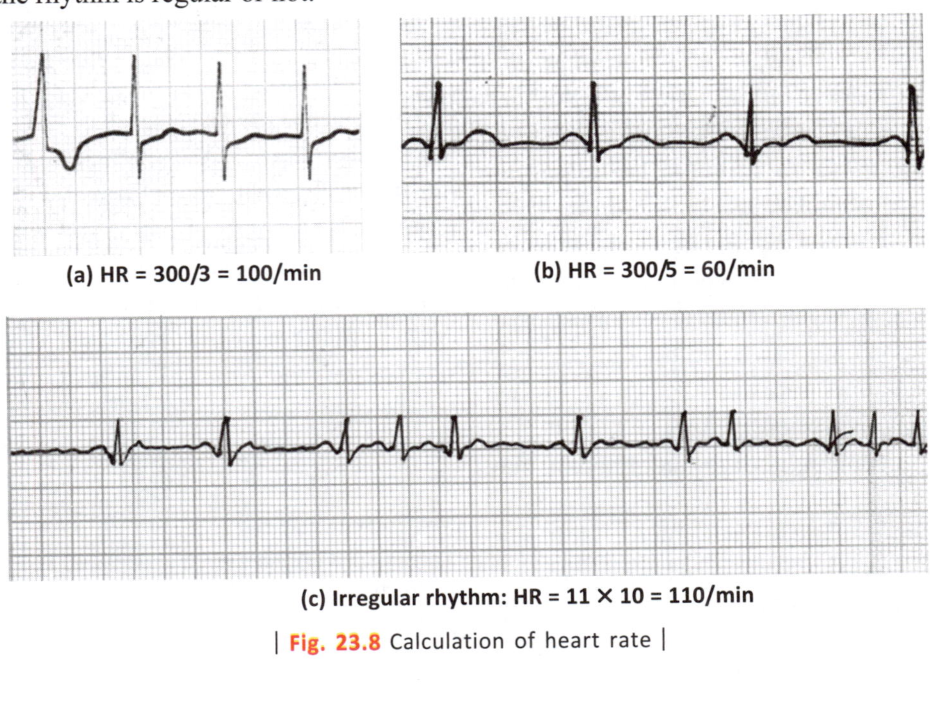

(a) HR = 300/3 = 100/min

(b) HR = 300/5 = 60/min

(c) Irregular rhythm: HR = 11 × 10 = 110/min

| Fig. 23.8 Calculation of heart rate |

patient complaining of acute chest pain suggestive of myocardial infarction. However, it is a normal variation in a young boy who has come for a routine ECG for insurance purposes.

a) Calibration
b) Heart rate
c) Rhythm
d) Mean QRS axis
e) P wave
f) Q wave
g) PR interval
h) QRS interval
i) QRS voltage
j) ST segment
k) T waves
l) QT interval
m) R wave progression in chest leads
n) U waves

MAJOR ECG ABNORMALITIES

1. Electrical Axis and Axis Deviation

The mean direction of spread of the depolarization wave through the ventricles is called the *cardiac axis* or *mean QRS axis*. Normally, this depolarization wave starts at the top right hand corner and flows towards the bottom left hand corner towards L-I, L-II and L-III, i.e., from 11 o'clock to 5 o'clock (Fig. 23.9). Hence, there is a prominent upward deflection in these leads.

If the right ventricle is hypertrophied, the axis will swing towards the right. The deflection in L-I will become negative and the deflection in L-III will become more positive. This is known as **right axis deviation** (**RAD**). When the left ventricles become hypertrophied, the axis may shift to the left so that there is a negative deflection in L-III. This is known as **left axis deviation** (**LAD**).

The '**hexaxial lead diagram**' is very useful in determining whether the axis is normal or there is LAD or RAD. It is also useful for calculating the mean QRS axis. By convention, the positive pole of lead I is said to be 0° and the negative pole is 180°. All leads above this level are negative leads and those below this level are positive leads. If the depolarization wave is directed below this level, then the axis is said to be positive and above this level the axis is said to be negative. The normal axis lies between -30° and +90°. RAD exists if the axis is found to be +90° or more positive. LAD exists if the axis is found to be -30° or more negative.

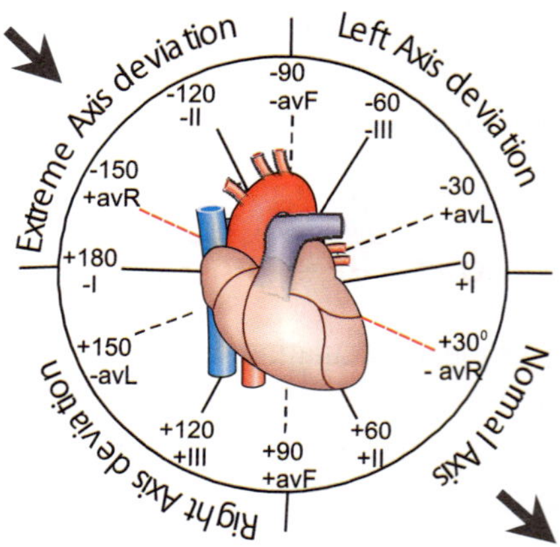

| **Fig. 23.9** Hexaxial lead diagram |

Why Determine the Axis?

Determining the axis need not necessarily diagnose a particular condition but it definitely gives supportive evidence for a suspected condition. Hence, axis should be determined routinely as a part of interpretation of all ECGs. Mild LAD (0° to -30°) may be seen in ECGs of normal persons, especially obese persons or in patients with ascites. Significant LAD (-30° to -90°) always indicates organic heart disease especially left ventricular hypertrophy and left bundle branch block. RAD is usually seen in right ventricular hypertrophy, which in turn is due to pulmonary conditions that put a strain on right side of the heart like chronic obstructive pulmonary disease or congenital heart disease.

Determining the axis causes unnecessary confusion amongst general practitioners. It need not be so, if the following simple rules are followed (Fig. 23.10):

- **Normal**—positive QRS deflection in both L-I and L-III.
- **LAD**—positive QRS deflection in L-I and negative in L-III.
- **RAD**—negative QRS deflection in L-I and positive in L-III.

For a quick estimate, imagine the ECG tracing in L-III below L-I. If the QRS deflection in these leads point away from each other, then it is LAD (Left = *Leave* each other). If they point towards each other, then it is RAD (Right = *Reach* each other).

Calculation of Axis

For a general practitioner, I feel it is sufficient to know whether the axis is normal or there is LAD or RAD.

Nevertheless, if so required the axis calculation can be done by referring to the hexaxial lead diagram and by following the three simple rules given below:

a) Look for the *tallest R wave* in the limb leads (Fig. 23.11). If the R wave is tallest in L-II, the axis is either +60° or -120°. Now, if the axis is normal, it cannot be -120°. Hence, the axis is +60°.
b) If there is no single tall R wave but there are *two tall R waves of equal height* then the general rule is that the axis points midway between these two leads, e.g., in Fig. 23.12, the R waves are of equal height in L-I and L-II. Hence, referring to the hexaxial diagram the axis is either +30° or -150°. As there is no axis deviation, the axis in this ECG is +30°.
c) If there is no single tall R wave or there are no two tall R waves of equal height, look for a *biphasic complex*, which is seen in the L-III in the same figure. Now, the rule is that the mean QRS complex is oriented at right

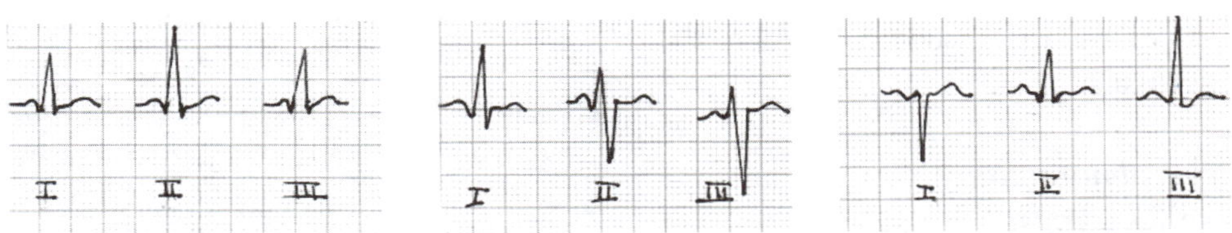

Normal axis   Left axis deviation   Right axis deviation

| **Fig. 23.10** Determining the axis |

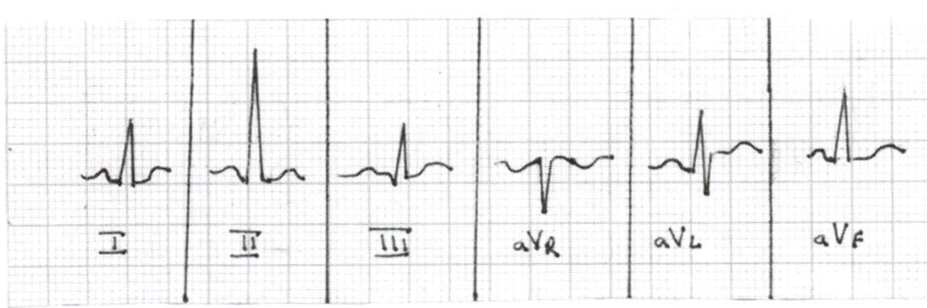

Tallest R-wave' in lead II. Axis = +60°.

| **Fig. 23.11** Calculation of axis |

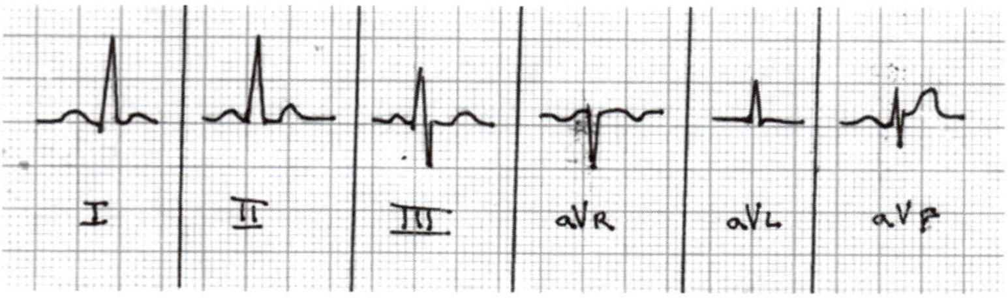

Tall R-wave' of equal height in L-I and L-II Axis = +30°.

| **Fig. 23.12** Calculation of axis |

angles to the lead showing a biphasic complex. Hence, referring to the hexaxial diagram, the axis is either +30° or -150°. As there is no left axis deviation, the axis cannot be -150°. Hence, the axis is +30°.

2. Atrial Abnormalities and Ventricular Hypertrophy

Atrial Abnormalities

As the SA node is situated in the right atrium, the right atrium is activated first followed by the left atrium. The impulses which are directed downwards and towards the left, merge together to form the P wave. P wave is best seen in L-II and V_1. Normal P wave is <2.5 mm (2½ small squares) in height and <0.12 sec (3 small squares) in width. Any P wave of greater dimensions than this is abnormal.

Right atrial abnormalities

This is manifested by *tall peaked P waves* (more than 2.5 mm in height) best seen in inferior leads II, III and aVF and sometimes in V_1. The term *P pulmonale* is used to designate these tall peaked P waves as right atrial enlargement often occurs with severe pulmonary disease like chronic cor pulmonale and sometimes in congenital heart disease **(Fig. 23.13)**.

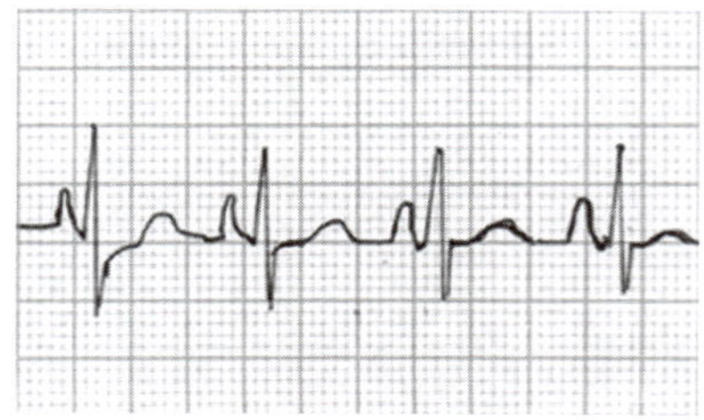

| **Fig. 23.13** Right atrial hypertrophy. Tall peaked P waves "P pulmonale" |

Left atrial abnormalities

In left atrial enlargement, it takes longer time than normal to depolarize. Consequently, a wide P wave with a duration of 0.12 sec or more, i.e., 3 small squares or more is produced **(Figs. 23.14 & 23.15)**.

Normally, the left atrium depolarizes after the right atrial and hence the later part of the normal P wave corresponds to left atrial depolarization. Consequently, in isolated left atrium enlargement, a broad *notched P wave* is often seen in extremity leads. This is called *P mitrale* as it was first described in patients of mitral valve disease. The chest lead V_1 however, shows a *bi-phasic P wave* **(Fig. 23.15)** with a small initial positive deflection because of right atrial de

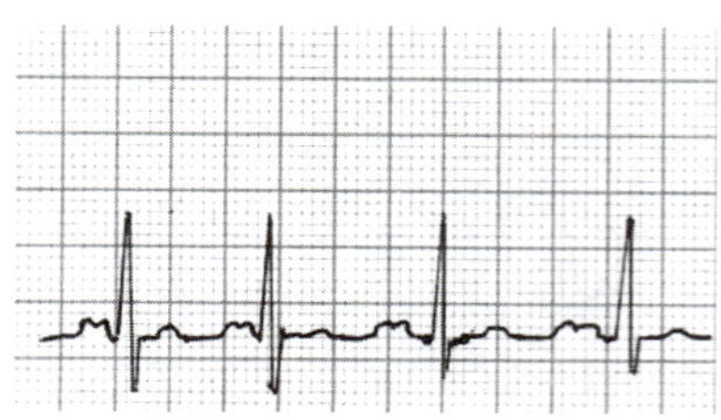

| **Fig. 23.14** Left atrial hypertrophy: broad and bifid P-waves. "P-mitrale" |

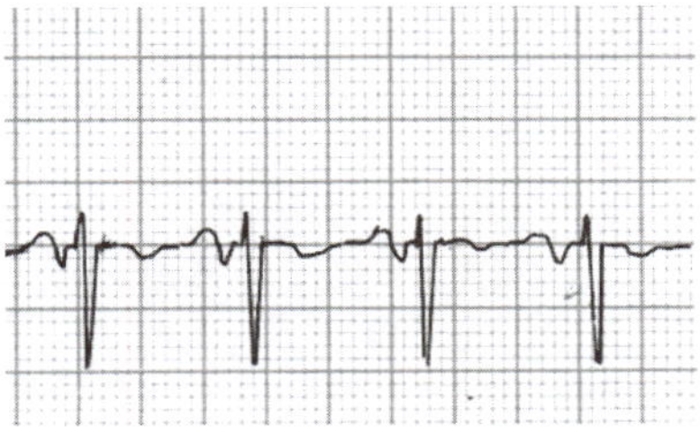

| **Fig. 23.15** Left atrial hypertrophy. Biphasic P wave in V1 |

polarization and a subsequent wide negative deflection because of left atrial enlargement.

Ventricular Hypertrophy

Just as P wave changes are produced by atrial enlargement, QRS changes are produced by ventricular hypertrophy. Left ventricular hypertrophy exaggerates the normal pattern of QRS complexes in the chest leads, while in right ventricular hypertrophy the normal pattern of QRS complexes are reversed.

Left ventricular hypertrophy (LVH)

The leads oriented to the left ventricle, i.e., L-I, aVL and V_5, V_6 record tall R waves while V_1 and V_2 record deep S waves (mirror images). This is because stronger than normal impulses are conducted by the hypertrophied left ventricle towards the patients left and downwards. The following criteria and guidelines have been established for diagnosis of LVH (Fig. 23.16):

- The R wave in V_5 or V_6 exceeds 25 mm.
- The S wave in V_1 or V_2 exceeds 25 mm.
- The sum of height of R wave in V_5 or V_6 and the depth of S wave in V_1 or V_2 exceeds 35 mm.
- Associated left ventricular strain pattern in LVH with ST segment depression and T wave inversion, mainly in the left chest leads.
- Associated left axis deviation and LBBB pattern.

These criteria are not necessarily diagnostic of LVH as healthy young individuals and athletes with thin chest wall often have tall R waves and deep S waves. Please correlate clinically. LVH occurs when there is either obstruction to the flow of blood from left ventricle (systolic overload) as in hypertension or when there is overflow of blood into the left ventricle (diastolic overload) as in mitral regurgitation.

Right ventricular hypertrophy (RVH)

The leads oriented to the right ventricle namely V_1 record a dominant R wave, i.e., bigger than the S wave (normally in V_1, R wave is smaller than the S wave). This is due to the spread of the depolarization wave towards the right because of the hypertrophied right ventricle. RVH is also associated with (Fig. 23.17):

- Deep S wave in lead V_5 and V_6.
- Right axis deviation.
- Right bundle branch block.
- Right ventricular strain pattern with ST segment depression and T wave inversion in right and middle chest leads.

Right ventricular hypertrophy occurs when there is obstruction to the flow of blood from the right ventricle. This occurs in pulmonary hypertension and in pulmonary stenosis.

3. Bundle Branch Blocks

This refers to conduction block in the right or left main branches of the bundle of His. The QRS complex is caused by depolarization of the ventricles, which in normal individuals does not take more than 0.12 sec (3 small squares). A block of the left bundle branch delays the depolarization of the left ventricle as it must now be indirectly activated via the right branch. This then widens the QRS complex to more than 3 small squares. Also the shape of the QRS complex is

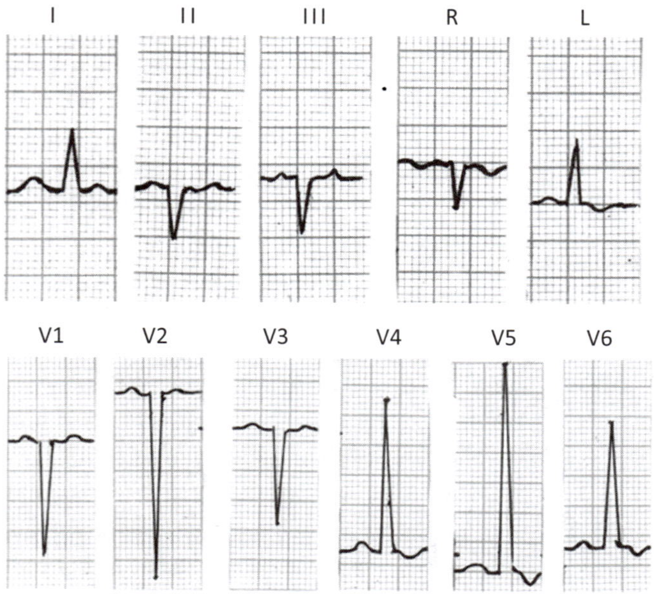

1. Height of R-wave in V_5 is 35 mm
2. Deep S-waves in V_1 and V_2
3. Inverted T-waves in V_4, V_5, V_6 (strain pattern)

| **Fig. 23.16** Left ventricular hypertrophy |

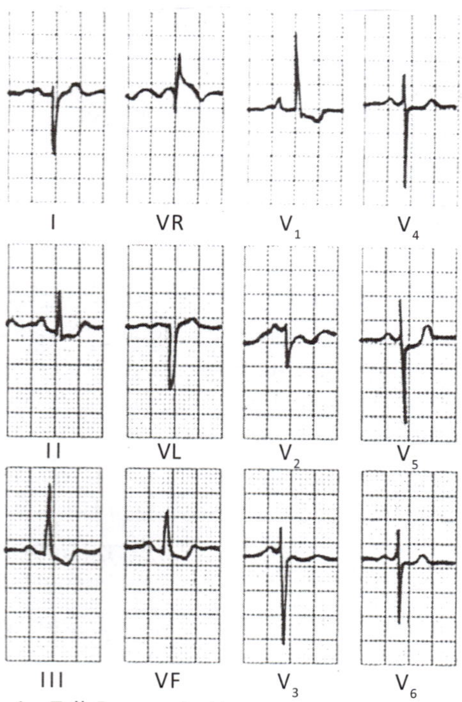

1. Tall R wave in V_1
2. Deep S wave in V_6
3. Inverted T waves in V_1 and V_2
4. Right axis deviation

| **Fig. 23.17** Right ventricular hypertrophy |

distorted because in the presence of LBBB, the septum depolarizes from right to left instead of from left to right. Hence, there is no septal r wave in V_1 and no septal q-wave in V_6. This gives rise to QS complex in V_1 (instead of the normal rS pattern) and a tall R wave without a q wave in V_6 (instead of normal qR pattern). Sometimes a small notch is present at its peak.

In RBBB, as the left bundle branch is intact the septal depolarization and the left ventricular depolarization is normal giving rise to the normal rS complex in V_1 and the normal qR complex in V_6. Because of the block in the right bundle branch, the right ventricle is then depolarized by the intact left bundle branch, the impulse going from left to right. This gives rise to an additional positive deflection (R′ [prime]) in V_1 and a deep slurred S wave in V_6.

Occasionally the QRS complex has the classic appearance of a bundle branch block described below but is only 0.1–0.12 sec wide. This is called an *incomplete block*, where the conduction in the bundle branch is delayed but not completely blocked.

Left Bundle Branch Block (LBBB)

- In leads oriented to the left ventricle mainly V_6, a wide tall R wave with slight notching at its peak ("M" pattern) is seen. LBBB is best appreciated in left chest lead V_6.
- Lead V_1 will show a wide negative QS complex, sometimes with a small notching at its peak.
- Another characteristic ECG finding in LBBB is the secondary T wave inversion in leads with tall R waves, i.e., the left sided chest leads **(Figs. 23.18–23.20)**.

Right Bundle Branch Block (RBBB)

- In leads oriented to the right ventricle mainly V_1, rSR pattern or ('M' pattern) is seen. RBBB is best appreciated in right chest lead V_1.
- Lead V_6 will show a qRS pattern with a deep slurred S wave.
- Secondary T wave inversions occur in RBBB just like in LBBB, but in right sided chest leads along with rSR pattern **(Fig. 23.19)**.

Clinical Significance

LBBB is almost invariably a sign of organic heart disease unlike RBBB, which may be seen without apparent cardiac disease. Most patients with LBBB have underlying LVH following long standing hypertension, valvular heart disease or cardiomyopathy. Virtually any condition that affects the right side of the heart (ASD, COPD, pulmonary stenosis, etc.) can give rise to RBBB.

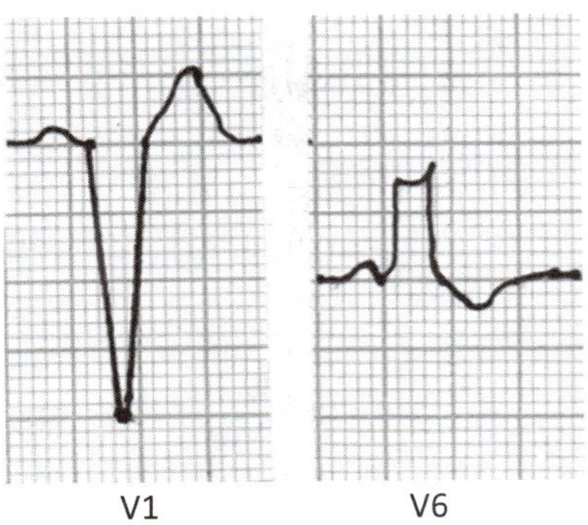

| **Fig. 23.18** Left bundle branch block. V1: Wide QS complex; V6: Wide R wave with a notch |

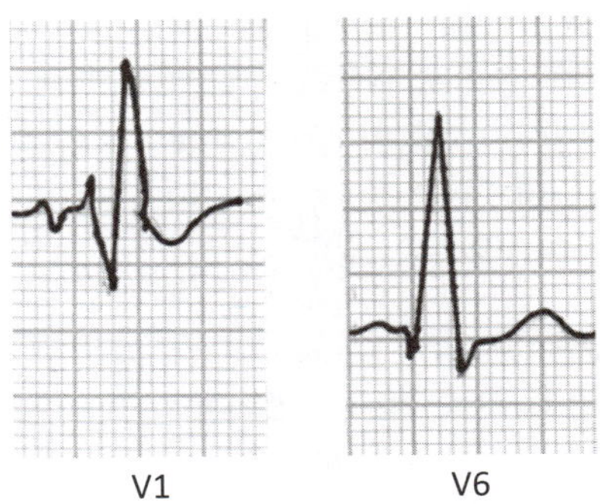

| **Fig. 23.19** Right bundle branch block. V1: Wide rSR complex; V6: Wide qRS complex |

	Typical QRST pattern	RBBB	LBBB
V_1	rS	rSR	Notched QS = "W"
V_6	qR	qRS	Notched S = "M"

| **Fig. 23.20** V1 and V6 in RBBB and LBBB |

In the elderly, degenerative changes in the conducting system may lead to both LBBB and RBBB.

Fascicular Blocks or Hemiblocks

The left bundle branch subdivides into an *anterior fascicle* and a *posterior fascicle* unlike the right bundle branch, which remains single. A block in either fascicle of the left bundle branch is called a *hemiblock* or a fascicular block. A hemiblock does not widen the QRS complex markedly but causes either a *left axis* or a *right axis deviation*.

Left anterior hemiblock leads to left axis deviation (-30° or more). Left posterior hemi-block leads to right axis deviation (+120° or more).

4. Myocardial Ischaemia and Infarction

The ECG is a cornerstone in the diagnosis of ischaemic heart disease (IHD). It is also one of the most important topics for a GP as far as electrocardiography is concerned. Recognition of this life-threatening emergency on an ECG tracing and prompt referral to an ICCU after primary treatment is vital.

Basic Facts

The term IHD refers to a group of heart diseases where there is deficient blood supply to the myocardium. This could be transient, as in angina pectoris and produce transient changes in ECG. If the ischaemia is more severe, necrosis of a part of myocardium results, which is called myocardial infarction (heart attack) and produces persistent changes in the ECG.

Either of the three main coronary arteries supplying to the heart can get occluded resulting in ischaemia (Fig. 23.21). The **right coronary artery (RCA)** supplies the right ventricle and the inferior part of the heart. The **left circumflex coronary artery (LCX)** supplies the lateral wall of the left ventricle. The **left anterior descending coronary artery (LAD)** supplies the major portion of the ventricular mass and the ventricular septum. With this knowledge, a rough assessment of the likely artery thrombosed can be made from the ECG tracing.

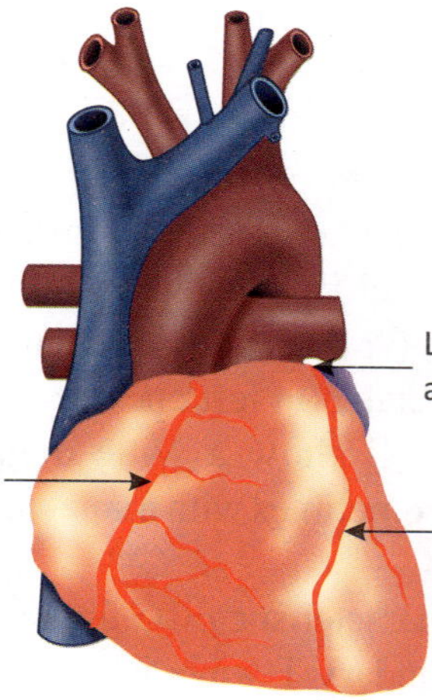

| **Fig. 23.21** The blood supply of the heart |

The left ventricle mass consists of two layers. From within outwards, these are the subendocardium and the epicardium. Traditionally when the whole thickness of the ventricle wall is affected usually due to complete occlusion of a coronary vessel, it is called **transmural ischaemia**. When only the inner half is affected, it is called **subendocardial ischaemia**. Transmural infarcts are many times associated with Q waves on ECG, which is usually associated with a bad prognosis.

But, this is not always the case. Hence, the current tendency to use the terms **Q wave** infarcts and **non Q wave** infarcts, while describing infarctions, instead of transmural infarcts or subendocardial infarcts.

ECG Changes

These are easy to understand, if the following three facts are remembered:

a) Transmural infarction usually produces changes in both myocardial depolarization (represented by QRS complex) and repolarization (ST–T complex) giving rise to ST segment and T wave abnormalities as well as pathological Q waves.

Subendocardial infarction, on the other hand, usually affects only the ventricular repolarization (ST–T complex) and hence Q waves do not appear.

b) Acute transmural ischaemia and infarct produces ST elevation while acute subendocardial ischaemia and infarct on the other hand produces ST depression. Involvement of the epicardium also produces ST elevation.

c) In the classical and the prinzmetal anginas, the ischaemia is transient and produces only transient ST depression and elevation, respectively, and that too only during the attack of pain.

The ECG patterns seen in IHDs can be conveniently divided into the following four categories Table 22.1:

| **Table 23.1** Myocardial ischaemia and infarction produces a variety of ECG changes |

1. Transmural infarction (Q wave infarcts)	→	Persistent ST elevation with hyperacute T waves followed by T wave inversion and Q waves
2. Subendocardial infarction (Non-Q wave infarcts)	→	Persistent ST depression with T wave inversion without pathological Q waves
3. Transmural ischaemia	→	Transient ST elevations (Prinzmetal's angina)
4. Subendocardial ischaemia (Classical angina)	→	Transient ST depressions

a) ***Transmural infarction (Q wave infarct)* (Fig. 23.22)**: The ECG changes occurring here can be divided into three sequential phases. The *hyperacute* phase occurs in the first few hours of the event. ST segment elevations are recorded with tall widened T waves, which may exceed the height of R wave. The *evolving* phase occurs hours or days later and here we get T wave inversions and appearance of Q waves in the leads that previously showed T wave elevations. In the resolution phase, which occurs a few weeks after the infarct, the ST segment starts returning to the baseline and T waves gradually return to their normal configuration. The pathological Q waves may persist for months or even years, and may remain as the only evidence of a previous infarct.

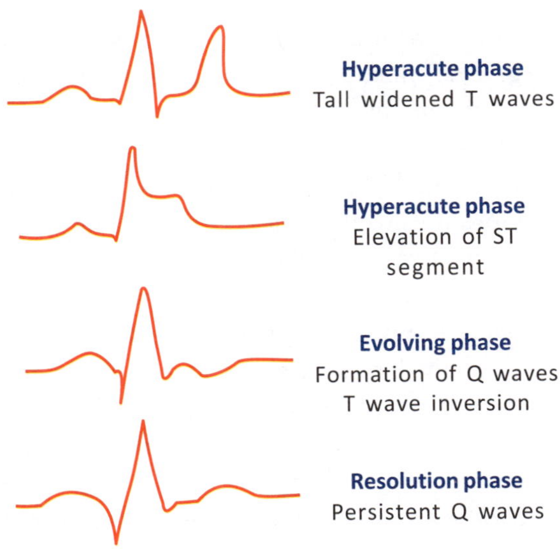

| **Fig. 23.22** Evaluation of myocardial infarction on ECG |

b) ***Subendocardial infarction (Non-Q wave infarct)***: As stated previously, this usually affects the ventricular repolarization (ST–T complex) and not depolarization (QRS complex). Hence, Q waves are usually not seen. Another important point to be noted is that the ECG shows *persistent ST segment depression*, as against ST elevation seen in transmural infarcts. T wave inversions are sometimes seen.

| **Table 23.2** Localization of myocardial infarcts |

Changes seen in leads	Location	Likely artery thrombosed
V_3–V_4	Strictly anterior	Left anterior descending
V_1–V_3	Anterioseptal	Left anterior descending
I, aVL, V_1–V_6	Anteriolateral	Left circumflex
I, aVL, V_5–V_6	Lateral	Left circumflex
II, III, aVF	Inferior	Right coronary

c) ***Transmural ischaemia: (Prinzmetal's angina)***: Prinzmetal's variant angina (or vasospastic angina or atypical angina) is characterized by transmural ischaemia. In acute transmural MI, the ECG shows persistent ST elevations while in classical angina the ECG shows transient ST depression (see below). Prinzmetal's angina is called atypical for two reasons. Firstly, we get transient *ST elevation* only during the attack of pain. Secondly, the attack of pain comes at rest unlike classical angina where it is precipitated by exercise.

d) ***Subendocardial ischaemia (Classical or typical angina)***: Here, the inner portion of the ventricle becomes ischaemic while the epicardium remains normal. This is reflected in the ECG as *ST segment depression*. In angina pectoris where there is chest pain precipitated by exertion and relieved by rest, ST depression appears only during the attack of pain, i.e., the changes are *transient*. They revert back to normal with relief of angina. Its presence may be demonstrated by recording the ECG during exercise (stress test) where ST depression of 1 mm or more is diagnostic.

Localization of Infarcts

In *anterior* wall infarcts (Fig. 23.23) (which means involvement of the interventricular septum and anterior/lateral walls of the left ventricles) these changes are seen in chest leads V1 to V6 and extremity leads I and aVL. With *inferior* wall infarcts (Fig. 23.24), these changes are seen in leads II, III and aVF. These changes are seen in the leads that face the site of infarction while the leads that are opposite the site of infarction show *reciprocal ST depression*, which is a characteristic feature of myocardial infarction. Thus, in anterior wall infarction (with ST segment elevations in leads V1 to V6, lead I and aVL) ST segment depression is many times seen in inferior leads II, III and aVF and vice versa. Another characteristic feature of anterior wall infarct is the loss of normal R wave progression in the chest leads. A more specific localization of the area of the infarction and not merely 'anterior' or 'inferior' can be done by using Table 23.2.

Posterior infarction may be difficult to diagnose because none of the 12 conventional leads face the true posterior wall of the heart. The diagnosis is made by mirror image changes seen in lead V1 and V2. Thus, the pathological Q wave is seen as a tall R wave, ST segment elevation is seen as ST segment depression and inverted T wave will appear as tall upright T waves in lead V1 and V2.

Q wave infarction and non-Q wave infarction: The traditional difference between transmural and subendocardial infarcts is a subject of debate. Many transmural infarctions do not have

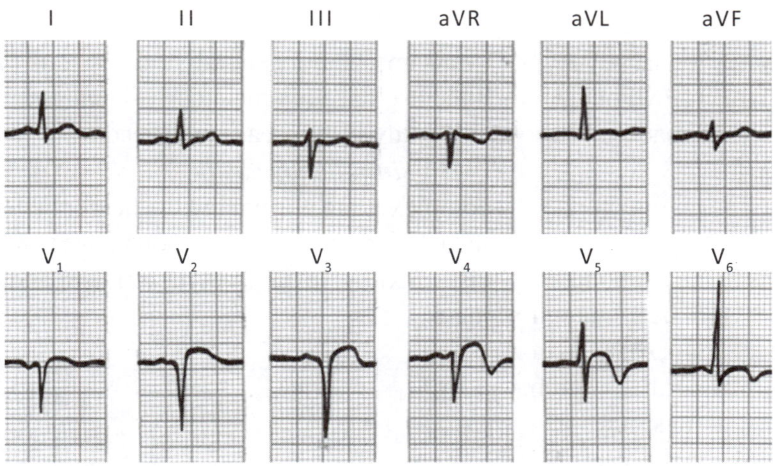

1. Pathological Q waves in V_2 and V_3
2. Inverted T waves in V_4, V_5, V_6

| **Fig. 23.23** Anterior wall infarction |

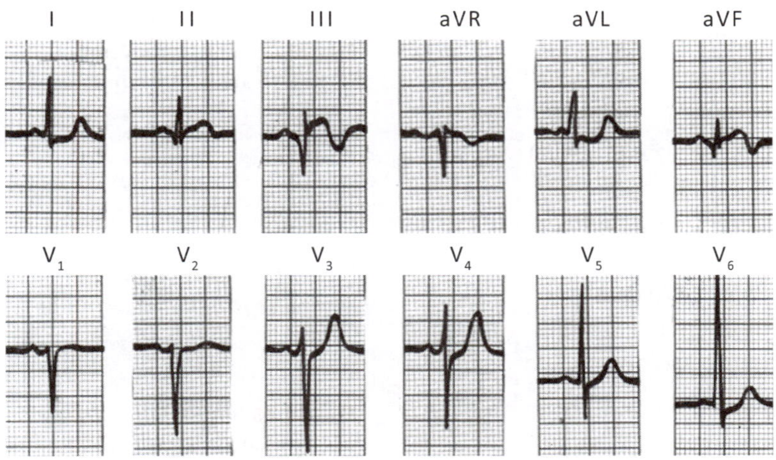

1. Pathological Q waves and ST segment elevation in III, aVF
2. ST segment depression in aVL and V_6

| **Fig. 23.24** Inferior wall infarction |

a Q wave. Many so-called mild partial thickness subendocardial infarction have high mortality and morbidity and are reported to have a higher risk of reinfarction. Hence instead, the terms Q wave infarcts and non-Q wave infarcts and non-Q wave infarcts (non-transmural) were proposed.

Q wave infarct implicated a through- and-through endocardial to epicardial necrosis, while the non Q wave myocardial infarct (absence of Q wave) implicates less extensive myocardial damage. Non Q wave myocardial infarct has been defined as acute MI without a new onset deep Q wave on ECG after days of evolution. However, for various reasons these terms were not recommended for use. Instead Acute coronary syndrome are is now classified as unstable angina (UA), non-ST elevation MI (non-STEMI) and ST elevation MI (STEMI).

Non STEMI is caused by partial occlusion of the coronary arteries and typically presents with ST segment depression and T wave inversion. Many of these patients will develop MI. STEMI is caused by complete coronary artery occlusion and virtually all these patients will develop MI. The rationale to classify ACS patients as having NSTEMI or STEMI or UA is that the clinical management for each of these differs.

5. Arrhythmias

When depolarization begins in the SA node, the heart is said to be in sinus rhythm beating regularly between 60 and 100 beats/min. An arrhythmia is a disturbance of normal cardiac rhythm when depolarization begins at sites other than SA nodes like atria, AV node or the ventricle. Then the arrhythmia is named after the site of origin, e.g., atrial tachycardia, atrioventricular block, ventricular fibrillation, etc.

The topic of arrhythmia is quite complex and can tax the brains of the most experienced cardiologist. Also these arrhythmias are mainly encountered and treated at a setting of an ICCU and very infrequently at a general practitioner's clinic. Hence the following brief discussion, by no means complete, is intended to provide only a brief outline of the most common arrhythmias. Interested general practitioners are advised to consult larger essays on this subject.

Sinus Arrhythmias

Sinus bradycardia, sinus tachycardia and sinus arrhythmias originate in the SA node and the path of their electrical impulse is exactly the same as normal sinus rhythm. Hence P wave, PR interval and QRS complexes are of normal configuration. The difference lies in the regularity and rate of impulse.

In ***sinus bradycardia*** (Fig. 23.25), all the complexes are normal but the heart rate is <60 beats/min. It can be seen as a normal variant in healthy individuals or in athletes or in hypothyroidism. But, the most common cause seen in practice is the sinus bradycardia in patients on beta-blockers or digitalis. The popular sick sinus syndrome is a degenerative disease of the SA node itself seen in the elderly. It causes significant bradycardia occasionally leading to syncope.

In ***sinus tachycardia*** (Fig. 23.26), all the complexes are normal but the heart rate is more than 100 beats/min. Common causes are exercise, anxiety, fever, hyperthyroidism and anaemia.

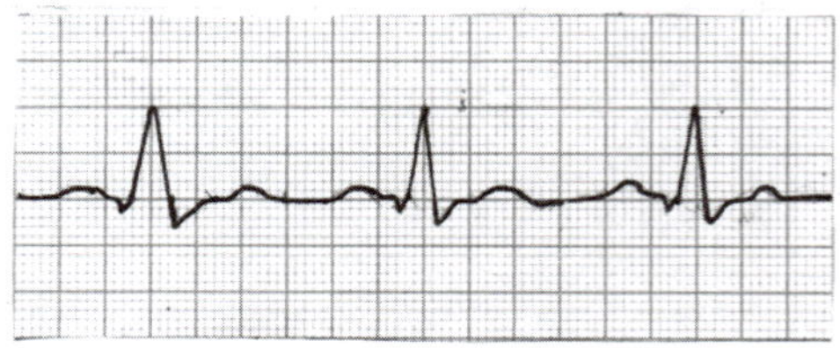

| **Fig. 23.25** Sinus bradycardia
Heart rate = 50/min |

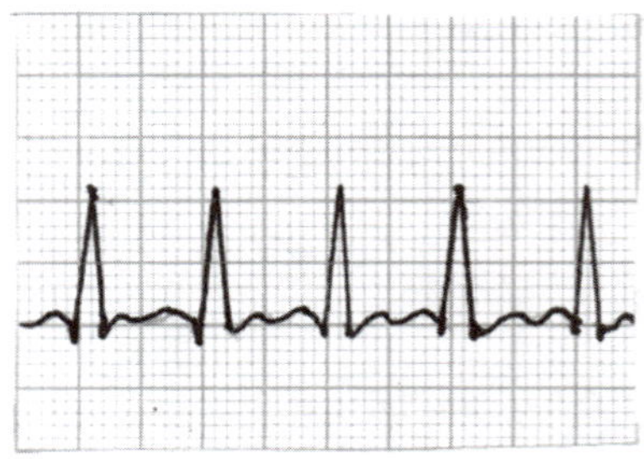

| **Fig. 23.26** Sinus tachycardia
Heart rate = 150/min |

In ***sinus arrhythmia*** (Fig. 23.27), again all the complexes are normal but the heart rate increases with inspiration and decreases with expiration. The ECG shows variation in RR interval. It is commonly seen in children and is benign. Even in adults, it does not decrease cardiac output and does not lead to serious arrhythmias.

Extrasystoles or Ectopic Beats or Premature Beats

Ectopic beats arise from foci in the heart other than the SA node. They are often premature, i.e., they occur before the next beat is due and are followed by a compensatory pause. If the ectopic beat comes after a pause then it is called

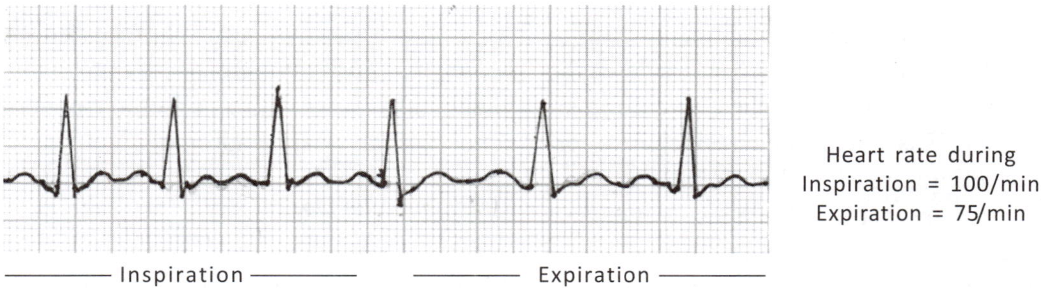

| **Fig. 23.27** Sinus arrhythmia |

an *escape beat*. Depending on the origin, ectopic beats are either atrial premature beats (APBs), atrioventricular junctional premature beats (JPBs) or ventricular premature beats (VPBs).

In APBs, the P wave is slightly different in shape but the QRS complex, which is depolarized in a normal way, is of normal width. In JPBs, the atria are stimulated in a retrograde manner, the wave of depolarization points upwards. This produces a positive P wave in lead aVR and a negative P wave in lead II. Ventricles are depolarized normally, producing a QRS complex of normal width. In VPBs, however, the focus is either in the left or right ventricle stimulating them sequentially. This produces a wide QRS complex (more than 0.12 sec) with T wave pointing in the opposite direction of the QRS complex (Fig. 23.28). A VPB comes before the next normal beat is due and this is followed by a compensatory pause. It does not affect the SA node, so the next P wave arrives at the expected time after the pause. A sudden run of three or more APBs constitutes a *supraventricular tachycardia* while run of three or more VPBs constitutes a *ventricular tachycardia* (Fig. 23.29).

Ectopic beats can be recognized by feeling the pulse and by auscultation. They can occur in healthy persons when they are quite benign. In patients with organic heart disease, however, they could be associated with increased risk of cardiac arrest or ventricular fibrillation.

Paroxysmal Supraventricular Tachycardia (PSVT)

PSVT is a series 3 or more premature supraventricular beats, the last beat of the series being followed by a compensatory pause. The P wave is abnormally shaped or not seen because it is buried in the preceding wave. QRS complexes are normal.

Clinically, the patient complains of sudden pounding in the chest. The heart rate is usually between 140 and 250 beats/min. The heart is beating so rapidly that the ventricles do not have time to fill completely resulting in diminished

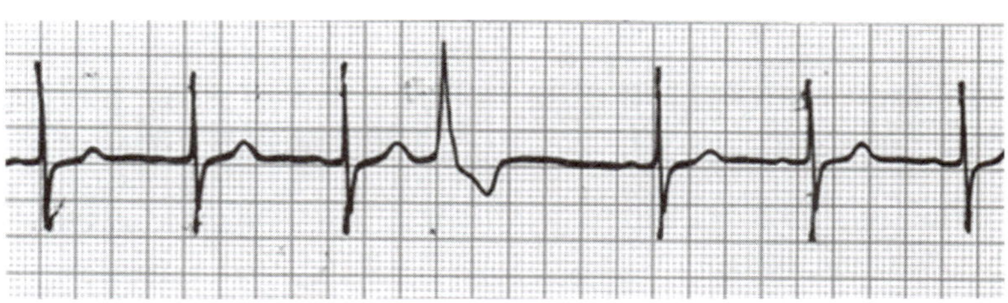

| **Fig. 23.28** Ventricular premature beat |

cardiac output. This causes extreme weakness or breathlessness. The usual treatment is stimulation of the vagus nerve, which slows down the heart. This can be accomplished by carotid sinus massage, Valsalva manoeuvre, including forcible vomiting, pressing the eyeballs or even putting a thermometer in the anus. If the heart continues to beat rapidly in spite of the above measures, Verapamil can be given in slow IV drip. Failing this, cardioversion can be achieved by DC shock.

Atrial Flutter and Fibrillation

These are due to rapid discharge from an ectopic focus in the atria. With PSVT the atrial rate is more than 250 beats/min. In atrial flutter, it is generally 250–350 beats/min. In atrial fibrillation it is more than 400 beats/min. At this fast rate, the AV junction cannot transmit all the impulses. Often alternate beats are transmitted when 2:1 AV block is said to be present.

Occasionally, 3:1 or 4:1 block is present. The ECG in atrial flutter shows multiple P waves on the baseline having a "*saw tooth*" appearance called *flutter (F) waves* (Fig. 23.31). In atrial fibrillation, the ECG shows irregular "tremulous" waves on the baseline called *fibrillatory (f) waves* (Fig. 23.30), which may be difficult to locate when the rate is very rapid. Atrial flutter always occurs in diseased hearts while atrial fibrillation can occur even in normal young individuals with an excessive bout of alcohol (holiday heart syndrome).

Atrioventricular Block

Heart block occurs when transmission through the AV junction is impaired. The mildest form is *first* degree heart block when all the impulses reach the ventricles but are delayed resulting in prolonged PR interval (more than 0.2 sec). When some impulses reach the ventricles but others do not, it is called *second* degree heart block. In the *third* degree heart block, no impulses are transmitted to the ventricles. Atria and ventricles beat independently, i.e., they are 'dissociated'.

Ventricular Fibrillation

This is an arrhythmia which is fatal within 3–5 minutes if not treated properly. There are no distinct QRS complexes but bizarre indulations of irregular height and rate (Fig. 23.32). There is no effective cardiac output and the patient becomes unconscious immediately. Ventricular fibrillation requires immediate defibrillation with DC shock.

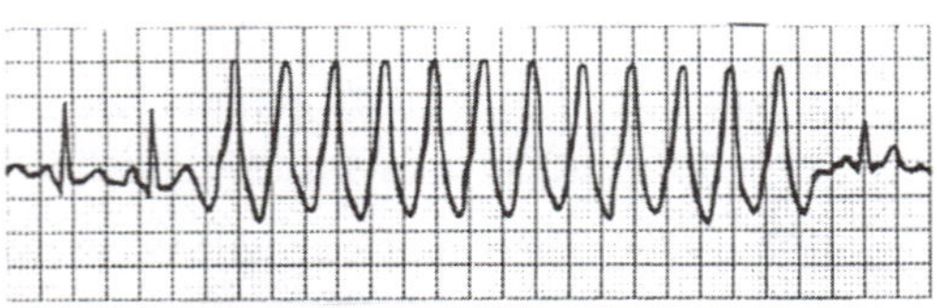

| Fig. 23.29 Ventricular tachycardia |

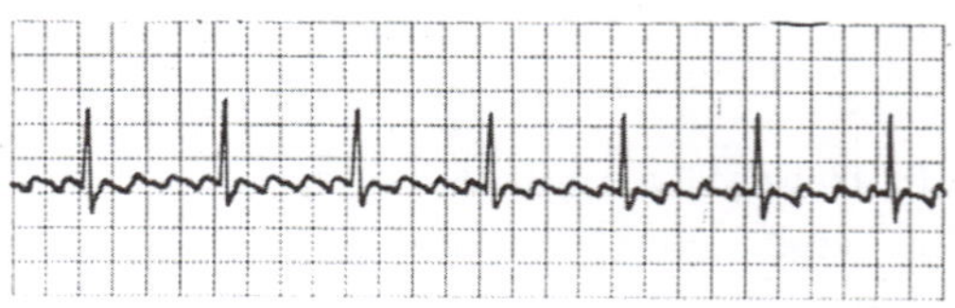

| Fig. 23.31 Atrial flutter |

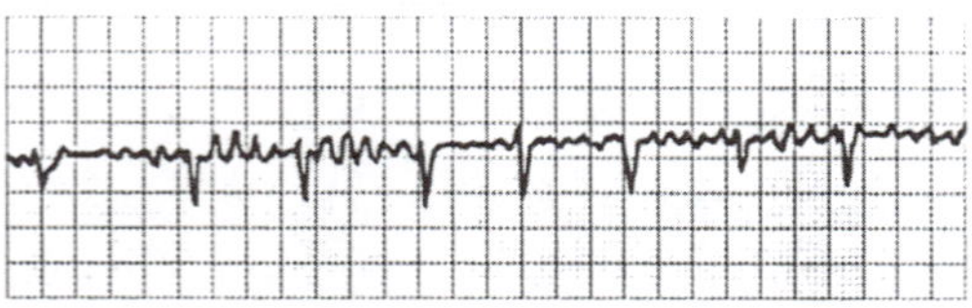

| Fig. 23.30 Atrial fibrillation |

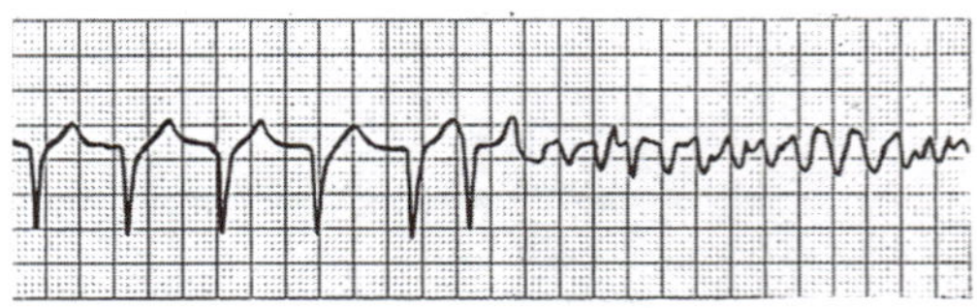

| Fig. 23.32 Ventricular fibrillation |

| **Table 23.3** Bradyarrhythmias |

Type	Main ECG findings		Causes
Respiratory sinus arrhythmia	▪ Minor changes in the R–R interval during respiration: reduction during inspiration and increase during expiration		▪ Physiological, particularly in athletes
Sinus bradycardia	▪ Rate < 60 beats/min		▪ Physiological, particularly in athletes ▪ Sinus node syndrome
	▪ Normal p wave before every QRS complex		▪ Drugs: beta blockers, calcium channel blockers
Tachycardia-bradycardia syndrome	Intermittent tachyarrhythmias and bradyarrhythmias		▪ Abnormal supraventricular impulse generation and conduction ▪ Sick Sinus syndrome
Atrial fibrillation with bradycardia	Absent P waves with bradycardia		
Atrio ventricular block	First degree block	PR interval > 200 ms	▪ Physiological response ▪ Increased vagal tone ▪ Drugs: beta blockers or calcium channel blockers
	Second-degree block	**Mobitz type I/Wenckebach**: progressive lengthening of the PR interval until a beat is dropped **Mobitz type II**: irregular dropped beats	▪ Drugs: Digoxin, beta blocker, calcium channel blocker ▪ Increased vagal tone ▪ Sinoatrial conduction disease
	Third-degree block	AV dissociation: no relationship between P waves and QRS complexes	▪ Right coronary infarction ▪ Complete block: no communication between the atria and ventricles

contd.

		▪ Abnormal supraventricular impulse generation and conduction
Intraventricular block	As in left bundle branch block and Right bundle branch block	▪ Conduction of the electrical impulse is blocked on the ventricular level ▪ Myocarditis

| **Table 23.4** Ventricular Arrhythmias |

Type	Main ECG findings	Causes
Premature ventricular beats	▪ Premature, wide QRS complex that is not preceded by a P wave ▪ Compensatory pause after the premature beat	▪ Ectopic beat that originates from a ventricular focus ▪ Due to hypoxia, hyperthyroidism, electrolyte abnormalities
Ventricular tachycardia	▪ Regular, rapid rhythm ▪ Wide QRS complexes ($\geq$3 consecutive premature ventricular beats)	▪ Coronary artery disease ▪ Myocardial infarction ▪ Structural heart diseases
Ventricular fibrillation	▪ Fibrillatory baseline without rhythm usually >300 bpm ▪ Erratic, unrecognizable wavy QRS complexes	▪ Myocardial infarction ▪ Structural heart disease

| Table 23.5 Supraventricular Arrhythmias |

Type	Main ECG findings	Causes
Supraventricular premature beats	P wave abnormalities or absent P waves	▪ Physiological ▪ Electrolyte imbalances ▪ Underlying cardiovascular disease
Sinus tachycardia	▪ Gradual onset ▪ Regular rhythm ▪ Rate: Max 180 bpm ▪ P wave: Normal morphology ▪ Narrow QRS complex	▪ Sympathetic activation or vagal withdrawal on the SA node
Atrial flutter	▪ Very abrupt onset ▪ Regular rhythm ▪ Rate: Atrial 250–350; Ventricular < 200 ▪ P waves - Occur before every QRS complex - Sawtooth appearance of regular P waves (flutter waves), especially in leads II, III and aVF ▪ Narrow QRS complex	▪ Macro reentrant rhythms within the atria
Atrial fibrillation	▪ Very abrupt onset with rate variation ▪ Rhythm: Irregularly irregular ▪ Rate: 350–450 bpm; <200 ▪ P-waves are not recognizable	▪ Multiple mechanisms which are not completely understood

Differential Diagnosis of Q wave, ST ↑↓ and T wave ↓

Not all ST–T changes and the presence of Q waves reflect ischaemia or infarction. A list of other important causes is given below:

1. **Pathological Q waves:** Small Q waves are normally present in leads which look at the heart from the left: I, II, aVL, V_5 and V_6 (septal Q waves). A small Q wave may be present in L-III due to high diaphragm, which disappears on deep inspiration. Q waves in other leads are abnormal (pathological), especially if they are more than two small squares deep or more than one small square wide. They are seen in:
   - Myocardial infarction
   - Left ventricular hypertrophy
   - Bundle branch blocks
2. **ST elevations:** ST segment elevation is sometimes seen as a normal variant in young healthy individuals called the *early repolarization pattern* and is quite benign. ST elevations are also seen along with LVH and LBBB, which are chronic diseases. Rest of all the ST elevations should be taken seriously as all the following remaining causes are life threatening:
   - Acute MI: Persistent ST elevation
   - Left ventricular aneurysm: ST elevations persisting for weeks after MI.
   - Prinzmetal's angina: Transient ST elevations.
   - Acute pericarditis: ST elevations in almost all leads.
3. **ST depressions**
   - Subendocardial infarction
   - Subendocardial ischaemia (Classical angina)
   - Reciprocal ST depression in transmural infarct
   - Acute posterior myocardial infarct
   - LVH with 'strain'
   - Digitalis effect/Hypokalaemia
4. **T wave inversions**
   - Normal variant in aVR, V_1, V_2 and L-III.
   - Myocardial ischaemia and infarction
   - Ventricular hypertrophy with 'strain'
   - LBBB and RBBB
   - After a bout of tachycardia
   - Mitral valve prolapse syndrome, etc.
5. **Tall upright T waves**
   - Hyperacute phase of MI
   - Prinzmetal's angina
   - Hyperkalaemia
   - LVH
   - LBBB

CHAPTER 24

Medical Urgencies

- Emergency Drugs
- Cardiopulmonary Resuscitation
- Respiratory Urgencies
- Psychiatric Urgencies
- Dermatological Urgencies
- Miscellaneous Urgencies

A few years back I met one of my colleagues who was practising in the same locality where I practised. "You didn't come to our monthly meeting yesterday?" I asked him. He said he could not attend because "one of my depressed patient committed suicide yesterday and I had to attend his funeral". A thought crossed my mind, 'who is responsible for the death, the depressed patient or the physician (mis)treating him?'

That reminded me of an incident that occurred during internship at Sassoon General Hospital, Pune. The police brought a patient who was rowdy and ataxic to the casualty. The police said that they picked him up for creating disturbance in the community under the influence of alcohol. I rushed for the ampoule of injection haloperidol, for my priority was to calm down the patient. The senior resident doctor stopped me, ordered the nurse to fill an ampoule of 25% dextrose and give it to the patient IV bolus. The patient soothed down in minutes. A case of mistaken diagnosis on my part. It was not a case of alcohol intoxication, it was hypoglycaemia. When I asked my senior, how he had made the diagnosis without even examining the patient or asking the history, he said 'hypoglycaemia was written all over his face.' That was experience backed by sound knowledge of emergency medicine. So after 25 years in this field, I look back and reflect about a few of the mistakes committed by my colleagues and myself in treating emergencies and what experience has taught me.

- An elderly person coming to me with isolated vomiting (i.e., vomiting without any leading symptoms such as epigastric pain, fever, headache, etc.), the first consideration that comes to my mind is acute myocardial infarction presenting atypically and not gastritis.
- If I am called for a home visit to see a middle-aged woman and my diagnosis is hysterical convulsions, I cannot go back and sleep because probably this could be epilepsy or a space-occupying lesion in the brain.
- Similarly, an acute onset swelling on the face with hoarseness of voice is for me "angioneurotic oedema," even if non-pruritic. I take the

BP, give Inj. Adrenaline SC and a shot of IV Efcorlin plus Phenargan, and await the result.

- If I confront a patient who has acute dyspnoea and on auscultation I do not find rhonchi, I resign to my fate of having to consider a large number of differential diagnosis, right from the apparently innocuous hysterical hyperventilation to life-threatening pulmonary embolism.
- A number of times I have referred patients of psychosis to a psychiatrist not because they cannot be managed at a GP level but because I find it difficult to rule out 'organic' psychosis. I have always hoped that there is blood test for the diagnosis of psychiatric conditions.

So on and so forth. Such mistakes can kill a good practice. I repeat, mismanaging manageable emergencies can kill a good practice. On the other hand, successfully managing an emergency, which a neighbouring GP has refused to handle, can boost a practice. Need I impress on you more the importance of correctly handling emergencies at a GP level? So read on. And best of luck to my doctor colleagues for a perfect diagnosis and perfect treatment, and for their patients for a quick recovery.

But, before you read on let me explain this term 'medical urgencies'. This term has been purposely used by me. If a GP encounters a dire emergency like a patient in shock or a case of organophosphorous poisoning, his only passive role is to actively refer him to an ICU. There are many books in the market written by foreign and Indian authors on how to manage these dire emergencies in the set-up of a hospital or an ICU.

But even after a diligent search, I could not find a book on emergency medicine keeping the requirement of a GP in mind. What the GP requires is the treatment of emergencies which are not life-threatening, and treatable at his own clinic. That is what I mean by 'medical urgencies'.

Ten golden rules for diagnosis in emergencies

1. In an unconscious patient, always consider the possibility of hypoglycaemia and opium over dosage.
2. Always consider the possibility of myocardial infarction in an adult presenting with acute chest pain.
3. Always consider the possibility of ectopic pregnancy in any women of child bearing age presenting with acute abdominal pain.
4. Always consider upper airway obstruction first, if a patient is found cyanosed.
5. An asthmatic patient is always serious, if he is severely dyspnoeic and on auscultation the chest is 'silent'.
6. In a young adult who presents with severe headache, always consider the possibility of subarachnoid haemorrhage.
7. If a child with sudden onset of dyspnoea is found to be pale, consider epiglottitis as the first diagnosis.
8. Consider the possibility of depression in a post partum women presenting with vague symptoms and with problems with coping with the baby.
9. Consider ventricular fibrillation or other arrhythmias in a patient who collapses suddenly.
10. In a patient who complains of pain in abdomen and suddenly collapses, always consider intra abdominal bleeding.

EMERGENCY DRUGS (IDEAL KIT)

Injections

Inj. Atropine 0.6 mg/mL—2 amps.
Inj. Aminopylline 4 mg/mL—2 amps.
Inj. Adrenaline 1 mg/mL—2 amps.
Inj. Chlorpromazine (Largactil) 25 mg/mL—4 amps.
Inj. Haloperidol (Serenace) 5 mg/mL—4 amps.

Inj. Lorazepam (Calmese) 2 mg/mL—2 amps.
Inj. Diazepam (Calmpose) 10 mg/2 mL—2 amps.
Inj. Phenytoin (Dilantin) 100 mg/mL—4 amps.
Inj. Promethazine (Phenargan)—2 amps.
Inj. Prochlorperazine (Stemetil) 12.5 mg/mL—2 amps.
Inj. Metoclopramide (Reglan) 10 mg/2 mL—2 amps.
Inj. Pentazocine (Fortwin) 30 mg/mL—2 amps.
Inj. Frusemide (Lasix) 20 mg/2 mL—4 amps.
Inj. Hydrocortisone acetate (Wycort) 25 mg/mL—3 amps.
Inj. Terbutaline (Bricanyl) 0.5 mg/mL—2 amps.
IV Glucose 25% 50 mL—5 amps.
IV DNS 450 ml—5 bottles.
Inj. Dexamethasone (Dexona) 4 mg/mL—4 amps.

Aerosols

Salbutamol aerosol
Glyceryl trinitrate spray
Ipratromium bromide solution

Tablets

Tab. Aspirin (Loprin) 75 mg—5
Tab. Nifedipine (Depin) 10 mg—5
Tab. Glyceryl trinitrate (Angised) 0.5 mg—4

CARDIOPULMONARY RESUSCITATION (CPR)

Cardiopulmonary resuscitation (CPR) is an emergency procedure which is performed in an effort to preserve brain function until further measures are taken to restore blood circulation and breathing in a person who is pulseless and is not breathing following a cardiopulmonary arrest. It should be noted that CPR alone is unlikely to restart the heart. The main purpose is to restore flow of blood to the brain and heart temporarily to prevent permanent damage to these structures.

Administration of an electric shock to the subject's heart, termed defibrillation, is usually needed in order to restore heart rhythm. CPR is generally continued until the patient's circulation is established or the patient is dead.

Procedure

1. **Attempt to wake victim**: If the victim cannot be awakened and is not breathing (or is gasping for breath), call an ambulance.
2. **Begin chest compressions (C)**: Place the heel of your hand in the middle of his chest. Put your other hand on top of the first. Keep elbows straight. Push down using upper body weight (compress). Push hard and fast. Compress the chest at least 2 inches (4–5 cm). Allow the chest to completely recoil before the next compression. Compress the chest at a rate of at least 100 pushes per minute. Perform 30 compressions at this rate. If you are not trained in CPR, do not do rescue breathing but continue to do chest compressions until help arrives or the patient wakes up.
3. **Begin rescue breathing**: If you have been trained in CPR, after 30 compressions, open the patient's airway (A) by lifting up the head and chin. Pinch the patient's nose and fix your lips over the patient's lips. Use a CPR mask if available.

   Give the patient a breath (B) big enough to make the chest rise. Let the chest fall, and then repeat the rescue breath once more. If the chest doesn't rise on the first breath, adjust the head position and try again. Whether it works on the second try or not, go to step 4.

   (Please note: If you don't feel comfortable with this step, just continue to do chest compressions at a rate of at least 100/min. Chest compressions are extremely important.

If you are not comfortable giving rescue breaths, still perform chest compressions! It's called "Hands Only CPR". Current recommendations place emphasis on chest compressions performed well over rescue breathing).

4. **Repeat chest compressions**. Do 30 more chest compressions just like you did the first time.
5. **Repeat rescue breaths**. Give 2 more breaths just like in step 3 (unless you are skipping the rescue breaths).
6. **Keep going**: Repeat steps 4 and 5 for about 2 min (about 5 cycles of 30 compressions and 2 rescue breaths).
7. Repeat the process, checking for breathing every 2 min (5 cycles or so), until help arrives. If the victim wakes up, you can stop CPR.

American Heart Association (AHA) CPR guidelines

In 2010, AHA released the Association's newest set of guidelines for CPR. Changes for 2010 include the following:

- The initial sequence of steps is changed from ABC (airway, breathing, chest compressions) to CAB (chest compressions, airway, breathing), except for newborns.
- The compression depth for adults should be *at least* 2 inches (instead of *up to* 2 inches).
- The compression rate should be at least 100/min.

Importance of CPR

Heart disease is the number one killer all over the world. Half of these cases will die suddenly, outside the hospital, because their heart stops beating. The most common cause of death from a heart attack in adults is a disturbance in the electrical rhythm of the heart called ventricular fibrillation. This can be treated, but it requires applying an electrical shock to the chest called defibrillation. If a defibrillator is not readily available, brain death will occur in <10 min.

One way of buying time until a defibrillator becomes available is to provide artificial breathing and circulation by performing cardiopulmonary resuscitation, i.e. CPR. The earlier you give CPR to a person in cardiopulmonary arrest (i.e., no breathing, no heartbeat), the greater the chance of a successful resuscitation. By performing CPR, you keep oxygenated blood flowing to the heart and brain until a defibrillator becomes available.

CPR in three simple steps: "CALL-PUMP-BLOW"

1. Call

Call the patient's name loudly. If the person is not responsive and not breathing or not breathing normally, call for an ambulance.

2. Pump

If the victim is still not breathing normally, coughing or moving, begin chest compressions. Push down in the centre of the chest 2 inches 30 times. Pump hard and fast at the rate of at least 100/minute.

3. Blow

After 30 compressions, tilt the head back and lift the chin. Pinch nose and cover the mouth with yours and blow until you see the chest rise. Give 2 breaths. Each breath should take 1 sec.

Continue with 30 pumps and 2 breaths until help arrives.

Note: *This ratio is the same for one-person & two-person CPR. In two-person CPR, the person pumping the chest stops while the other gives mouth-to-mouth breathing.*

Please note: *This is not a substitute for actual CPR training. It is always better to get proper hands on training from an instructor in emergency medicine.*

RESPIRATORY URGENCIES

- Acute Breathlessness
- Tension Pneumothorax
- Pulmonary Embolism
- Acute Pulmonary Oedema
- Massive Pleural Effusion
- Acute Severe Asthma
- Community Acquired Pneumonia

Acute Breathlessness

This is a relatively common emergency presenting to a family physician. In some cases, the diagnosis can be made very easily. For example, a known asthmatic coming with an attack of bronchospasm. At times, the diagnosis can be difficult, e.g., when in a patient having nocturnal attacks of bronchial asthma, paroxysmal nocturnal dyspnoea due to pulmonary oedema of cardiac origin is to be ruled out.

Acute breathlessness occurs as a symptom in many diseases as listed in Table 24.1. On encountering a patient with acute breathlessness, the family physician should immediately pose the following questions to himself:

1. Is it due to involvement of the respiratory system?
2. Is it due to involvement of the cardiac system?
3. Is it due to one of the uncommon causes listed under "other causes"? (Table 24.1)
4. Is it a functional complaint?

Dyspnoea due to involvement of the respiratory system are by far the commonest emergencies encountered by a family physician in his day to-day practice. Out of the causes shown in Table 24.1, asthma, COPD, pneumonia and pleural effusion can be managed by the physician in his clinic, the treatment of which is detailed separately. The rest are dire emergencies and if the physician fails to recognise them and does not hospitalize the patient immediately the patient might die. How do these patients then present to a GP? A short resume of each is given below.

| **Table 24.1** Causes of acute dyspnoea at rest |

Respiratory
1. Acute asthma
2. Acute exacerbation of COPD
3. Pneumothorax
4. Pulmonary embolism
5. Pulmonary oedema
6. Pneumonia
7. Massive pleural effusion
Cardiovascular
1. Acute LVF
2. Valvular heart disease, e.g., MS
3. Cardiac tamponade
Others
1. Acute renal failure leading to volume overload
2. Metabolic acidosis, e.g., diabetic ketoacidosis
Psychogenic
1. Panic attack
2. Hysterical hyperventilation

Tension Pneumothorax

Admit immediately! In this condition, air leaks into the pleural cavity from the lungs. Due to valve like mechanism air enters but cannot leave the cavity. This causes marked rise in intrapleural pressure, which completely collapses the lung, shifting the mediastinum to the opposite side. This prevents cardiac filling, which results in fall in cardiac output and shock. Clinically, the patient presents with *a classical triad of chest pain, severe dyspnoea and shock*. Chest pain is very severe, of sudden onset and always unilateral. Physical signs would be absent breath sounds, decreased vocal resonance, a hyperresonant note and a shift of the mediastinum to the opposite side as demonstrated by the shifting of the trachea and the apex beat. Admit immediately.

If the patient is acutely ill and the physician is experienced and confident, insert a wide bore needle into the 2nd intercostal space in the midclavicular line on the right side and in the 5th intercostal space in the midaxillary line (to avoid puncturing the heart, allowing the air under tension to escape, pending an insertion of an intercostal drain in the hospital setting.

Pulmonary Embolism

Admit immediately! It is obstruction of the pulmonary arterial vessels by an embolus, which has in 95% of cases originated from deep vein thrombosis (DVT) of the legs and pelvis. This means that pulmonary embolism is not a primary disease, but a life-threatening complication, which may occur during the course of another disease which predisposes to the formation of DVT, e.g., prolonged immobility following a major surgery, fractures or even pregnancy. The patient has been discharged and is under the care of family physician,when he suddenly dies (because of a massive embolus) or gets symptoms mimicking an acute myocardial infarction (because of a medium size embolus). Admit immediately. Do not waste time in looking for evidence of thrombosis in the deep veins of the calf. Absence of DVT does not rule out a pulmonary embolism, because by the time you have seen the patient, all the clots may have travelled to the lungs.

Acute Pulmonary Oedema

Admit immediately! It is a grave medical emergency complicating a variety of clinical conditions, cardiac (e.g., MI, hypertension, cardiomyopathy, etc.) or non-cardiac (e.g., pulmonary embolism, rapid IV infusions, eclampsia, etc.). Most of the attacks come during sleep unless there is a particular precipitating factor like rapid large IV infusions in an elderly patient with cardiac disease. The patient has to suddenly wake up from sleep because of severe cough and a feeling of breathlessness and has to sit up. The blood-tinged secretions of the respiratory tract mix with air to form a pink frothy sputum. There may be reflex bronchoconstriction leading to noisy respiration (cardiac asthma).

On examination, you find a patient who is extremely anxious and pouring with sweat. The extremities are cold and clammy and there is marked tachycardia. BP may be high with a narrow pulse pressure. Auscultation of the lungs reveals widespread loud crackles and rhonchi all over the lungs. Auscultation of the heart is difficult because of the loud respiratory noises. The immediate job at hand is to distinguish this from acute severe asthma because in both the conditions the patient is severely dyspnoeic, sitting up and has tachycardia. *In asthma*, the wheeze is more high pitched. There is a quick inspiratory snatch followed by an extended expiration.

In very severe bronchospasm, there will be a silent chest. The sputum will be white and sticky. In *pulmonary oedema* where the sputum is pink and frothy, the chest is full of respiratory noises and the patient is in extremis. Having ruled out asthma, summon the ambulance immediately. If the ambulance is getting delayed, give IV Frusemide 40–80 mg slowly. Above all, do not look anxious. This will needlessly increase the patient's anxiety and diminish his respiratory drive!

Massive Pleural Effusion

It can be managed in day care clinic. A pleural effusion can present as an emergency only if it is massive, virtually occupying the whole lung up to the clavicle. Small effusions do not cause any symptoms. The only symptom that can be attributed to an effusion is breathlessness and the severity depends on both the size and rate of accumulation of fluid. There may be history of pleuritic pain. On examination, movements of chest wall are reduced or absent, the mediastinum is displaced towards the opposite side, the percussion note is dull, air entry is decreased or absent on that side and finally, above the effusion a pleural rub may be audible. An X-ray chest confirms the diagnosis.

Management

The only way breathlessness can be relieved is by aspirating the pleural fluid. In smaller effusions, the optimal site for aspiration can be marked with the help of an ultrasound but in large effusions this is unnecessary. The 8th intercostal space posteriorly just below the tip of the scapula is a convenient site for aspiration. However, aspiration can also be done from the 6th ICS in the midaxillary line or the 7th ICS in the posterior axillary line. Insertion of the needle in the 10th or 11th space is likely to penetrate the diaphragm and enter the peritoneal cavity. The GP should make himself familiar with the working of a 3-way stop cork. The patient is made to sit up and lean forward with his arms on the top of a small bed table. The predetermined area for aspiration is anaesthetized and the needle introduced at right angles to the skin in the 8th intercostal space and advanced into the pleural space. Please note that the neurovascular bundle lies just below each rib. Hence, the needle should be inserted just at the upper border of the lower rib to avoid injury to the neuro vascular bundle. The correct position of the needle into the pleural space is confirmed by aspiration when a straw coloured fluid comes into the syringe. The needle is now attached to the 3-way stop cork and about 1–1.5 L of fluid is aspirated at one time by applying suction to the syringe. It is adventurous to remove more fluid than this, as this may induce reflex pulmonary oedema.

Discontinue, if

1. The patient has central chest pain, which could mean that there is a mediastinal shift. This could lead to a cardiovascular collapse.
2. The patient has haemoptysis, which means that the lung is punctured. This is usually harmless but is frightening for the patient and his relatives.

Acute Severe Asthma

It can be managed in day care clinic. This term has replaced the old term 'status asthamaticus,' which was in the past used to describe a severe attack of asthma lasting for more than 24 hrs in spite of adequate bronchodilators. It was realised that it is the severity of attack that matters and not the duration, as asthmatics were seen to die within 2–3 hrs of an attack of acute severe asthma. Hence, it is a prudent policy for all GPs to assess the severity of attack of bronchospasm even before the management is started and hospitalize the patient, if necessary.

| Table 24.2 |

A word of caution: Even before undertaking the management, the GP should remember the old adage *"all that wheezes is not asthma"*. It still holds good. Be sure of your diagnosis by considering the following possibilities:

1. A first attack of asthma in a person in his 4th or 5th decade of life is rare (consider the possibility of *acute left ventricular failure*).
2. Even in a known case of asthma, *acute myocardial infarction* with left ventricular failure is a possibility. Diffuse expiratory rhonchi (which is the sine qua non of bronchial asthma) are also seen in acute LVF. Look for cardiac signs and do an ECG.
3. A case of *COPD with acute exacerbation* because of secondary infection can present with wheezing. It is essential to be sure of the diagnosis because here the mainstay of the treatment is antibiotics.
4. A *tumour pressing on the bronchus* can cause wheezing and dyspnoea similar to asthma. Of course, here the rhonchi are unilateral.

Who should be Hospitalized?

Those patients with the following life-threatening features:

1. Respiratory rate >30/min
2. Pulse rate >120/min
3. The patient who is too breathless to speak complete sentences.
4. Pulsus paradoxus—in a severe attack, the fall in systolic arterial pressure between expiration and inspiration may be more than 18 mm Hg. (The normal difference is not more than 5 mm Hg.)
5. A silent chest—bronchospasm is so severe that hardly any air moves inside the bronchus to cause a wheeze.
6. Cyanosis, bradycardia, hypotension, exhaustion, etc.

Admit urgently! If the above features are not present, the patient can be treated in a GP's OPD, especially so if provisions for a day care management is available in his set up.

Management

So once you have decided that it is indeed a case of severe attack of asthma and definitely manageable in your clinic, immediately put an IV drip and reverse back the bronchospasm in a stepwise manner:

1. ***Corticosteroids*** are life-saving under the circumstances. They are not bronchodilators but act by way of reducing the airway inflammation, which is implicated more and more in recent years in the pathogenesis of asthma. The effect may not be evident for at least 6 hrs. Hence, they should be given at the first opportunity. Hydrocortisone hemisuccinate 200 mg stat IV followed by 100 mg in IV drip is to be given for 4–6 hrs. Oral prednisolone 10 mg tds should be started at the same time.
2. Simultaneously ***nebulize with salbutamol***. This can be repeated after 2–4 hrs depending on the response. If a nebulizer is not available, salbutamol can be given as a metered dose inhaler (MDI) with a spacer device. A good alternative is Inj. Terbutaline subcutaneously.
3. ***Ipratropium bromide*** causes bronchodilatation by blocking the vagus. It can be usefully combined with nebulized salbutamol or used alternatingly 2 hrs apart. In almost all the carefully selected patients, these measures should suffice.
4. If the above measures fail to reverse the bronchospasm, give Inj. Aminophylline. If the patient is not taking oral theophylline, give loading dose of 250 mg IV slowly over 20 min diluted in 25 mL of normal saline. This is

followed by a slow IV infusion at the rate of 0.5 mg/kg/hr. If in spite of all these measures there is no response, admit the patient.

5. As a last desperate attempt before admitting the patient, Inj. Adrenaline is worth a trial, as it can give dramatic results. 0.5 mL of an 1:1000 solution is given subcutaneously, which can be repeated after 15 min. Avoid in patients over 40 years and those who are suffering from any heart disease, hypertension or diabetes.

Other Measures

Dehydration is common in a panting patient and should be corrected. Physicians feel comfortable after giving antibiotics, though their role is debatable. Do not give sedatives to allay anxiety, as these may suppress the respiratory drive. Instead, give a massive dose of reassurance! Finally, keeping the patient in your day care clinic will automatically remove the patient from an allergen present at home.

Community Acquired Pneumonia

Is it an emergency? It is occasionally difficult to answer this question. Pneumonia is often a terminal illness at extremes of age. It can come very suddenly in a normal healthy individual and by the time any aggressive treatment can be initiated, the patient is dead. Such cases are thought to be due to superadded *Staphylococcal* infection on a lung which has been already damaged by a viral pneumonia. Luckily for everybody this is a rare event. About 80% of the pneumonias are pneumococcal pneumonias, which are less severe. Mycoplasma, Chlamydia and Legionella are responsible for the so-called atypical pneumonias, which are again common and have a less severe presentation. These can be managed by a GP.

Who should be Hospitalized?

1. Extremes of age.
2. Respiratory rate > 30 breaths/min, tachycardia (>140/min), hypotension (<90/60 mm Hg).
3. Underlying illness (diabetes, cardiac disease, immunocompromised state, etc.).
4. Concomitant pleural effusion on X-ray chest (could be empyema).
5. The mentally confused patient with pneumonia.
6. Very low or very high WBC (less than 4000 or more than 20,000 WBC per microlitre).
7. Suspected *Staphylococcal* or Gram -ve pneumonia.
8. S. urea > 45 mg/dL
9. Failure of out-patient management.

Mnemonic: "CURB"

C – **C**onfusion
U – **U**rea
R – **R**espiratory rate
B – **B**lood pressure

If none of the above are present, the decision to manage as an outpatient should be appropriate. Ideally, antibiotics should be instituted after the aetiological agent has been identified by suitable means. But in a setting of a general practice, you will probably have to give antibiotics even before you know which organism you are dealing with. Nevertheless, a rough assessment can be made from the following:

1. ***Clinically***: Two different presentations are seen. Traditionally, these are called typical and atypical pneumonias. The *typical pneumonia* caused by *Streptococcus pneumoniae* or *H influenzae*, presents with high grade fever, severe pleuritic pain, cough with rusty purulent sputum and signs of consolidation (decreased resonance, coarse crackles, bronchial breathing). The *atypical pneumonias* have a more gradual onset, dry

cough, predominant extrapulmonary symptoms (such as headache, myalgias, fatigue, vomiting, diarrhoea, etc.) and abnormalities on chest X-ray, although there are hardly any auscultatory findings. They are most commonly produced by *M. pneumoniae* and *Legionella* species. Antibiotic selection in GP will depend on whether the pneumonia is typical or atypical and usually not on the culture sensitivity report.

2. ***X-ray chest***: It can confirm the presence of pneumonia, show the extent of the disease and give a rough idea as to the aetiological agent.
3. ***Sputum examination***: If done before instituting antibiotics, it can give an indication of the possible pathogen and thus aid in the choice of antibiotics.

Antibiotic Treatment as an Outpatient

Having then decided to treat the patient as an outpatient and having got a rough idea about the aetiological agent, the patient is treated as follows:

1. Young adult with typical pneumonia:
   a) Inj. Procaine penicillin 12 lac IM daily for 2 weeks **(or)**
   b) Cap. Amoxicillin 500 mg tds × 2 weeks **(or)**
   c) 2nd generation Cephalosporins (e.g., Tab. Cefuroxime axetil 500 mg bd × 2 weeks) **(or)**
   d) Tab. Amoxicillin 500 mg + Clavulanic acid 125 mg 1–2 tds.
2. Young adult with atypical pneumonia :
   a) Tab. Erythromycin 500 mg qid × 10 days **(or)**
   b) Tab. Azithromycin 500 mg od × 6 days **(or)**
   c) Tab. Doxycycline 100 mg bd × 14 days.
3. Young or old patients with preexisting respiratory disease like chronic bronchitis.
   a) Tab. Amoxicillin + Clavulanate **(or)**
   b) Tab. Cefuroxime axetil **(or)**
   c) Tab. Azithromycin (as above)

Some authorities believe that all patients of community acquired pneumonia should receive a combination of antibiotics likely to cover all pathogens, e.g., cefuroxime + azithromycin. This I feel is a reasonable and practical approach and not necessarily unscientific. The newer quinolones like Gatifloxacin and Levofloxacin cover most of the pathogens causing typical or atypical pneumonias, are effective orally and have to be given only once a day. These make them the drug of choice in the treatment of community acquired pneumonia on OPD basis. However, they should be used only after TB has been ruled out as they are anti-TB agents. They can cause partial recovery from TB, and given as monotherapy can cause drug resistance.

PSYCHIATRIC URGENCIES

- Acute schizophrenia
- Acute mania
- Acute severe depression
- Panic attacks
- Hysterical fits
- Epileptic convulsions
- Acute psychosis

Acute Schizophrenia

A schizophrenic patient may present to a family physician as an emergency in a psychotically agitated state with poor behavioural control. These patients must be immediately dispatched to a hospital and put under psychiatrist care. Alternatively, he may present more subtly with strange bizarre complaints. For example, a healthy 25-year-old male student has been noticed by friends as behaving in an odd manner. Sometimes there is burst of anger and sometimes he laughs to himself for no apparent reason. Sometimes he is preoccupied with his own thoughts for hours together. When asked he confesses to hearing voices talking to him. He also feels that the police are conspiring against him along with his teachers to poison him. He adds further that people close to him can read his thoughts, so on and so forth.

Every first episode even with a subtle presentation should be ideally referred to psychiatrist. Subsequently, episodes can be dealt with by the family physician. Chlorpromazine 25 mg orally or IM should be initiated, the dose being adjusted according to response, the usual maintenance dose required is 75–100 mg daily. Acute dystonia (extrapyramidal reaction) if it occurs should be dealt with by giving IM Phenargan.

The sedation action is immediate but the antipsychotic effect requires 2–3 weeks. When rapid response is required, haloperidol is preferred in a dose of 10 mg IM stat.

Acute Mania

Patients with manic episodes may become angry, agitated or even violent, if thwarted and may then present to the family physician as an urgency. Mania is characterized by elevation of mood, increased physical overactivity and self-important ideas. In a typical patient, the sleep is reduced and the patient wakes up early feeling lively and energetic. He does not believe in wasting time in sleeping and busies himself noisily. Throughout the day, he is euphoric and hyperactive. He will wear bright coloured clothes to match the mood. The speech is rapid but disoriented moving from one topic to another in rapid succession. Appetite is increased and he will gulp down food greedily. Expansive ideas are common and he will make many grandiose plans and leave them unfinished. Many patients are extravagant and will spend their money recklessly. Sexual desires are increased. Finally, this physical overactivity leads to exhaustion.

Antipsychotic drugs such as chlorpromazine and haloperidol usually bring the symptoms of acute mania under control rapidly. However, large doses may be needed and are hence preferably managed by a psychiatrist.

Acute Severe Depression (Major Depression)

The patient presents to a general practitioner with the following features of a few days duration. More often he is brought forcibly by relatives.

1. Low mood, a black cloud pervading all his thoughts.
2. Lack of interest in things that he usually used to enjoy.
3. Relatives have observed apathy in the patient, i.e., psychomotor retardation (not just that the patient is complaining of a feeling of weakness or fatigue).
4. Significant weight loss or weight gain.
5. Sleep disturbance, usually insomnia with early morning wakefulness but many times hypersomnia.
6. Feeling of worthlessness.
7. Diminished ability to think.
8. Reccurent thoughts of death (i.e., suicidal ideation) with or without a specific plan.

At least 5 of the above symptoms should present for the diagnosis of a major depressive episode. Refer immediately to a psychiatrist, if: (1) There is a high suicidal risk; (2) The patient has profound psychomotor retardation; (3) There is superimposed psychosis. If these three symptoms are absent, the patient is less severely depressed and can be managed by a general practitioner.

Management

With a new antidepressant being introduced in the market every alternate month (mainly for commercial reasons), it becomes difficult for nonpsychiatric physicians and general practitioners to keep track of all the antidepressants. Despite tall claims made by manufacturers, there is no hard evidence that these new drugs act more quickly and are more effective than the time tested conventional tricyclic antidepressants (TCA) like amitryptyline, imipramine, trimipramine, etc. The main advantage of the newer antidepressants is their safer side effect profile. They are less cardiotoxic, have less serious anticholinergic side effects and are relatively non-sedating. The general practitioner should become thoroughly familiar with 2–3 antidepressants and start the treatment as follows:

Tab. Amitryptyline (Tryptanol) 25 mg daily (**or**)
Tab. Imipramine (Depsonil) 25 mg daily (**or**)
Tab. Trazodone (Trazonil) 25 mg daily (**or**)
Cap. Fluoxetine (Fludac) 20–40 mg daily (**or**)
Tab. Sertraline (Serta) 100 mg daily
Tab. Escetalopram (Nexito) 10 mg orally od (**or**)
Tab Venlafaxine (Venlor) 25 mg BD or tds (**or**)
Tab. Venlafaxine extended release (Venlor XR) 37.5 mg bd

The doses can be increased after a week depending on the response or the extent of the side effects. The full dose should be given for at least 6 weeks, after which reduced doses should be given for at least 6 months.

Panic Attacks

Which general practitioner has not faced this situation in his clinic? During his most busy hour, a young boy or a girl in his late teens or early twenties comes to the clinic with an attack of tremors, apprehension, choking sensation, dyspnoea, palpitations, chest pain and faintness. The patient believes that he is having a heart attack and is dying and wants to see the doctor urgently. This is a typical "panic attack", which in older textbooks is referred to as neurocirculatory asthenia, Da Costa's syndrome, effort syndrome, etc. This typical attack often begins abruptly without warning when the patient is doing his day-to-day activity like driving a car or taking his lunch. Like a bolt from the blue the patient gets the above symptoms, which peak within 10 min and resolve within 30 min. Many times when the patient manages to reach his family physician the attack has subsided only to come back again after a few days or months.

By definition, a panic attack is "*a sudden episode of free flowing extreme anxiety with marked physical symptoms*." A patient is said to be suffering from a *panic disorder* when more than 4 attacks have occurred in 4 weeks or one attack has been followed by 4 weeks of persistent fear of another attack. When the patient gives a history of multiple visits to multiple physicians who have time and again taken multiple ECGs, the diagnosis is obvious. However, during the first few attacks medical conditions like hypoglycaemia, angina pectoris, hyperthyroidism, cardiac arrhythmia or pheochromocytoma have to be ruled out.

Treatment

If the patient comes in severe panic, a short acting benzodiazepine like Inj. Lorazepam (Calmese 2–4 mg IM or IV) or Inj. Diazepam (Calmpose 5–10 mg IV slowly) will control the panic immediately.

If the patient is seen after the attack has subsided, a tricyclic drug like imipramine in low doses initially is the drug of choice. The initial effect of these drugs is sleeplessness, anxiety and palpitation. For this reason small doses, i.e., 10–25 mg are used at first and the dose is gradually increased. Lorazepam (Ativan) can be used to cover panic episodes till such time imipramine takes effect. Or newer antidepressants like fluoxetine or sertraline can be used instead of imipramine, which do not have these side effects.

Beta-blockers like propranolol can be used to block the peripheral manifestations of panic attacks like palpitations, tremors, etc.

And finally a sane advice to the general practitioner in charge: Give a strong verbal dose of reassurance to the patient and please do not panic!

Table 24.3 Symptoms of a panic attack (from DSM IIIR)
1. Shortness of breath
2. Choking
3. Palpitations
4. Chest pain
5. Sweating
6. Dizziness
7. Nausea or abdominal distress
8. Depersonalization or derealization
9. Tingling numbness
10. Flushes or chills
11. Trembling or shaking
12. Fear of dying
13. Fear of going crazy

Hysterical Fits (Acute Conversion Reaction)

It is another common situation faced by a general practitioner. The nearest physician is called for an urgent home visit because a young lady has suddenly got a 'fit'. The physician on reaching the place finds the young lady lying 'unconscious' on the bed with clenched teeth, froth coming out of the angle of the mouth, arms and legs in a bizarre position or movements. Some well meaning friend is trying to put a spoon in the mouth, another neighbour is making the patient smell a chappal, while yet another family member is trying to push a key into the clenched palm. Two immediate differential diagnosis will come to our mind. "*Is it hysteria or is it epilepsy*"? The main differentiating points between the two are summarized in Table 24.4.

What is Hysteria ?

It is an old fashioned word literally meaning "wandering of the womb", because ancient Greek physicians thought it to result from the movement of the uterus from its normal position. It is better called **'acute conversion reaction' (ACR)** as a severe mental stress is converted into a physical symptom like a fit or another mental symptom like amnesia. Psychogenic convulsion or psychogenic paralysis is commonly seen by general practitioners because of its dramatic onset and the availability of the general practitioner during the attack. Other conversion reactions like psychogenic blindness (ophthalmologists), deafness (ENT specialist), tremors (neurologist) or hiccups (gastroenterologists) are usually seen by the respective consultants.

A few additional points are to be noted so as to have a clear idea about ACR and to minimize diagnostic errors:

1. First, age is important. It is rare after 40 years, as most predisposed persons would have already experienced the stress that would have produced the disorder.
2. Secondly, in the absence of stress the diagnosis is doubtful.
3. Thirdly, an attack of ACR carries some sort of advantage to the patient, e.g., a woman suffers an attack of "hemiplegia" so that she does not have to care for her ailing mother-in-law. This is called "secondary gain".
4. A notable feature is the disproportionate indifference shown by the patient to his or her 'serious' disease. This is called "belle indifference".

| **Table 24.4** Difference between Hysteria & Epilepsy |

	Hysteria	Epilepsy
Onset	Precipitated by emotional stress	No such stress
Situation	Attack occurs in presence of known people and surroundings. Never during sleep.	Anywhere Any time
The attack	Unconvincing, exaggerated, bizarre, thrashing movements. Patient in a safe position—never falls or incurs any trauma. No tongue bite or voiding of urine. Attack is prolonged for several minutes to impress the spectators. A repeat attack may occur when the physician arrives. Recovery is sudden.	Tonic or clonic movements. Patient may fall, passes urine or bites tongue during the attack. Convulsions hardly last for a minute or so. Recovery is gradual.
Examination	Patient screws up the eyelids when the physician tries to open them (easily elicited and an important sign). Plantar reflexes are normal (difficult to elicit under the circumstances). Corneal reflex present.	Eyelids open easily without resistance. Plantar reflexes are extensors. Absent

5. Finally, two of the most common misconceptions about ACR are that the patient is always a young woman and that the symptoms are being faked. In ACR, the symptoms are never faked and always occur at a subconscious level. When the symptoms are faked, condition is called *malingering*.

Management

If the patient is throwing bizarre convulsions, she can be calmed down by Inj. Lorazepam (Calmese 2–4 mg IM or IV) **or** Inj. Diazepam (Calmpose 5–10 mg IV slowly) **or** Inj. Haloperidol (Serenace 5–10 mg IM). Otherwise, drugs have hardly any role to play. At the same time, some face saving measures for the patient is called for, e.g., putting a swab of smelling salt (aromatic spirit of ammonia) on the nostrils in case of psychogenic unconsciousness or starting 'rapid' IV fluids in case of psychogenic vomiting.

Once the acute phase is over (and sanity prevails!), it is necessary to identify the stress and deal it with psychotherapy, anxiolytics and antidepressants.

Epileptic Convulsions

Epilepsy, though not a psychiatric condition is discussed here for immediate comparison with acute conversion reaction. In an epileptic patient, the convulsions start without warning, although there may be a momentary vague nonspecific sensation before the event. There is a sudden loss of consciousness and the patient falls to the floor often injuring himself. This is followed by tonic contraction of all muscles and the patient lies in an opisthotonic position on the ground.

Even the respiratory muscles contract, the forced expiration giving rise to a cry and the decreased respiration giving rise to cyanosis. This is followed by a clonic phase where there are rhythmic contractions of all limbs. The violent contractions suddenly stop within a minute or so, the muscles relax and the patient lapses into unconsciousness for a few more minutes. There is a gradual return to consciousness but the headache and drowsiness may remain for days. During the attack, there may be voiding of urine or biting of tongue. This is *grand mal epilepsy* (or generalised tonic-clonic seizure).

There are other types of seizures like partial seizures (simple or complex), absence seizures, myoclonic seizures etc. Apart from grand mal seizures, only *partial complex seizures* will present as an acute emergency. Here there is recurrent contraction of muscles of only one part of body (e.g., hand) followed by unconsciousness.

Management

1. ***If seen during the acute attack***, the following measures should be taken:
   - Place the patient on his side to prevent aspiration. Loosen the clothes.
   - Ensure that the airway is patent by removing food, vomit or dentures from the mouth.
   - Place the patient in a safe place to avoid injury.
   - It is harmless to put a key in the fist or make the patient smell a chappal, but forcing the mouth open with a hard spoon could be dangerous. A loose tooth could get dislodged and aspirated by the patient. A rolled up cloth is a better alternative.
   - Try to find out from the relatives (if available) if the patient is a known epileptic. If yes, there is no advantage in calling an ambulance for hospitalisation. Reassessment and adjustment of doses of anticonvulsant drugs should be advised. If it is the first attack, advise hospitalisation.
2. ***If seen during the post ictal state***: The diagnosis is easy, if the physician actually witnesses the attack. But more often than not, the convulsions are over before he arrives and the patient is either fast asleep or in a confused state. He may have hurt himself, passed urine or bitten his tongue. No drug treatment is necessary as the patient will regain consciousness spontaneously.
3. ***If the convulsions persist or recur***: Advise immediate hospitalisation because it could be a life-threatening case of *status epilepticus.* Till the time the ambulance arrives, 10 mg of Inj. Diazepam should be given IV slowly. Please note that intramuscular diazepam has no anticonvulsant effect and if given rapidly by intravenous route may cause respiratory depression. If the ambulance has still not arrived, Inj. Phenytoin IV should be given as the action of diazepam is very short lived. 200–300 mg should be given as an IV drip in normal saline (and not in dextrose where it can precipitate) and again slowly as it can cause severe hypotension though not respiratory depression. Needless to add this is best done in a hospital setting.

| Table 24.5 |

1. IV Phenobarbitone should never be given as outpatient treatment after IV diazepam. This can cause severe respiratory depression and even arrest.
2. If you encounter an epileptic fit on the road, declare your identity as a doctor, place the patient in a safe position and place a call for the ambulance (no IV diazepam on the road please!)

Acute Psychosis

The young agitated hostile patient! A general practitioner may be called in to treat a very young agitated, excited or hostile patient in his clinic or at the residence of the patient. This is a psychiatric emergency. The first step under this circumstance is for the general practitioner to try his best to calm him down (not an easy thing to do), elicit the history from the relatives and observe the patient's behaviour and mental state. Now is the time for the general practitioner to remain calm and tackle the situation in a stepwise manner.

Step I: Rule Out Organic Psychosis

Hypoglycaemia, postepileptic state, recent h/o head injury, fever or alcohol abuse can cause acute psychosis. Treat them accordingly. Incontinence of urine during the attack is an important sign of organic psychosis.

Step II: Try to Come to a Diagnosis

Acute psychosis could be acute mania, acute schizophrenia, acute depression or acute hysterical state. But in the highly charged atmosphere and in the very early stage of the disease, it is not an easy task to make a precise diagnosis.

Step III: Control the Violent Patient

Whatever the diagnosis, the violent patient has to be calmed down. Listen to the patient, talk to him but do not argue. If the patient does not cooperate and refuses treatment the only option left is to physically restrain the patient using relatives and friends to hold him down firmly to administer him the antipsychotic drug. Do not place yourself in a vulnerable position.

Step IV: Immediate Drug Treatment

For the patient who is frightened, Inj. Diazepam (10 mg slowly IV) or Lorazepam (2–4 mg IM or IV) is useful. For the severely agitated or violent patient Inj. Haloperidol is advocated 10 mg stat IM or IV, which can be repeated every hour if necessary to maximum of 60–80 mg/day. If sedation is desired, Inj. Phenargan can be usefully added to Inj. Haloperidol. This also prevents the acute dystonic reaction so commonly seen to haloperidol.

When the patient has calmed down, shift the patient directly to a hospital for further psychiatric management.

DERMATOLOGICAL URGENCIES

- Acute urticaria and angioedema
- Herpes zoster
- Lepra reaction
- Cutaneous drug eruptions
- Henoch-Schonlein purpura
- Erythema multiforme (EM)

Dermatology is basically a benign speciality but the cool life of a dermatologist is occasionally punctuated by life-threatening emergencies, the so called "*acute skin failure*". The following dermatological emergencies are best managed by the dermatologist–physician combination in a hospital, as they can be life-threatening. The GP should however, have a high index of suspicion in recognising these emergencies. If they are missed, it could lead to disastrous consequences. How to recognise these conditions?

Pemphigus Vulgaris

There is an extensive vesiculobullous eruption on the skin and the mucous membrane. The bullae are quickly denuded by friction or pressure. The normal skin may display Nikolsky's sign—if lateral pressure is put on the skin surface with the finger, the epidermis appears to slide over the underlying dermis. Untreated, pemphigus is fatal (Fig. 24.1).

Stevens-Johnson Syndrome

This is extensive erythema multiforme (described later) with additional involvement of the mucous membranes of the mouth, eyes and genitalia. Also there is severe constitutional disturbance.

Toxic Epidermal Necrolysis (TEN)

This is also a severe variant of erythema multiforme with extensive shedding of the skin but less mucosal involvement. The epidermis peels off in large sheets, leaving a dark red oozing dermis like in a case of burns. However, TEN carries a worse prognosis than burns of the same extent because of systemic involvement. Mortality is high (Fig. 24.2).

Staphylococcal Scalded Skin Syndrome (SSSS)

Staphylococcal scalded skin syndrome is a blistering disorder caused by *Staphylococcus aureus* toxins. The condition is common in children than in adults. There is sudden onset of high grade fever with formation of large flaccid bullae, which rupture immediately. Large sheets of epidermis then separate, leaving painful raw areas. Mortality in adults is almost 50% (Fig. 24.3).

Exfoliative Dermatitis (Exfoliative Erythroderma)

There is involvement of almost the whole skin by extensive erythematous and extensive scaly rash. Persistent generalised peripheral vasodilatation and heavy shedding of scales gives rise to loss of fluids, electrolytes, proteins, vitamins, etc., which have in turn a profound effect on the renal and cardiovascular systems. Also, exfoliative dermatitis is always secondary to skin disease or malignancy. All in all, this needs hospitalization.

Disseminated Herpes Zoster

Disseminated herpes zoster refers to the presence of more than 5 vesicles outside the primary dermatome. This is usually seen in immunocompromised patients where the number of vesicles are so many that the differential diagnosis becomes chicken pox.

Under the circumstances, dissemination to vital organs like brain is a distinct possibility. As you can see, all the above life-threatening skin conditions are vesiculobullous disorders with extensive bullous rash with or without systemic manifestations. Under such circumstances, hospitalize the patient under the care of a dermatologist. But, the following dermatological conditions which are serious but not life-threatening can be safely managed by general practitioners as outpatients, and will be described in some detail now:

a) Acute urticaria
b) Herpes zoster
c) Lepra reaction
d) Drug eruptions
e) Henoch-Schonlein purpura
f) Erythema multiforme

Acute Urticaria and Angioedema

Urticaria (hives) are transient lesions that have a central wheal surrounded by an erythematous halo. Individual lesions are round, oval or bizarre. They appear with alarming speed and disappear spontaneously within a few hours. Urticaria involves only the dermis, whereas in angioedema, the subcutaneous tissue as well as the mucous membrane of the eyelids, lips, tongue, larynx and bronchus may be involved. Severe extensive urticaria may lead to potentially life-threatening anaphylaxis. Angioedema involving the larynx and bronchus (causing hoarseness and wheezing) may lead to respiratory obstruction, cyanosis and death. As such, these are dermatological emergencies (Fig. 24.4).

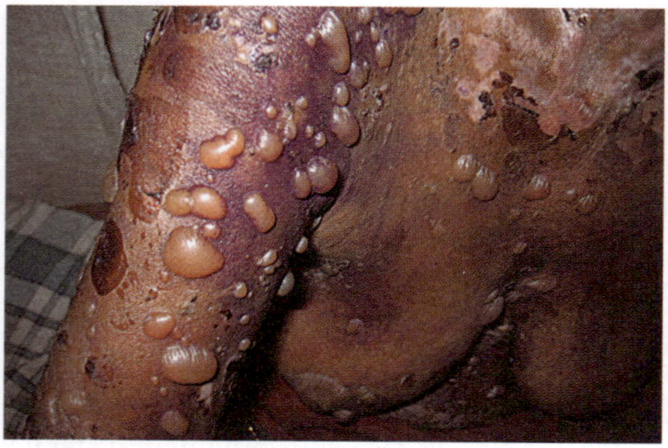

| **Fig. 24.1** Pemphigus vulgaris |

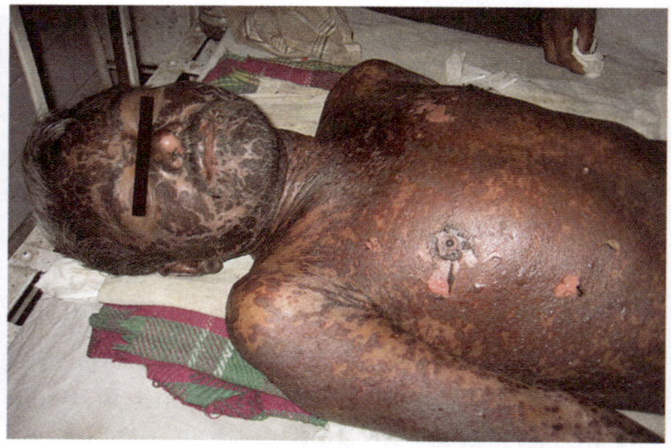

| **Fig. 24.2** Toxic epidermal necrolysis |

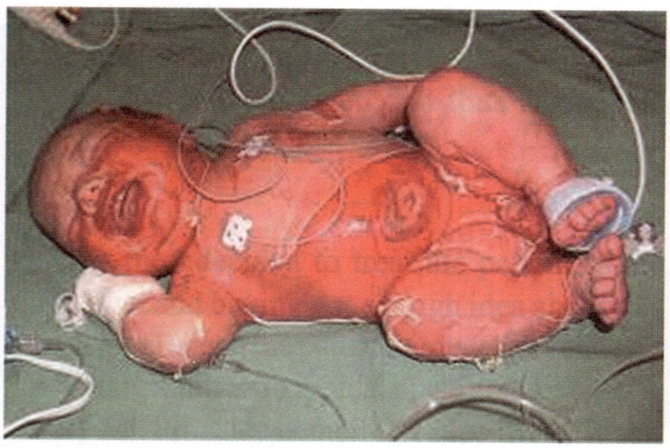

| **Fig. 24.3** Staphylococcal scalded skin syndrome |

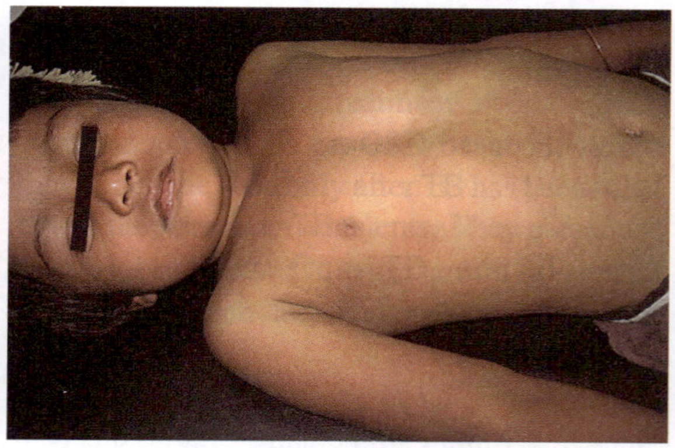

| **Fig. 24.4** Urticaria |

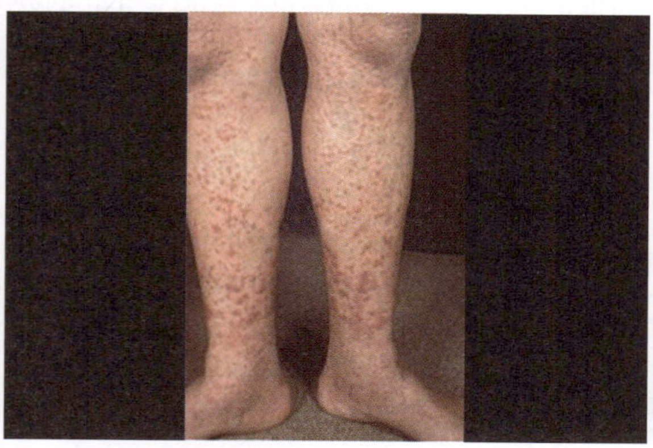

| **Fig. 24.5** Purpura |

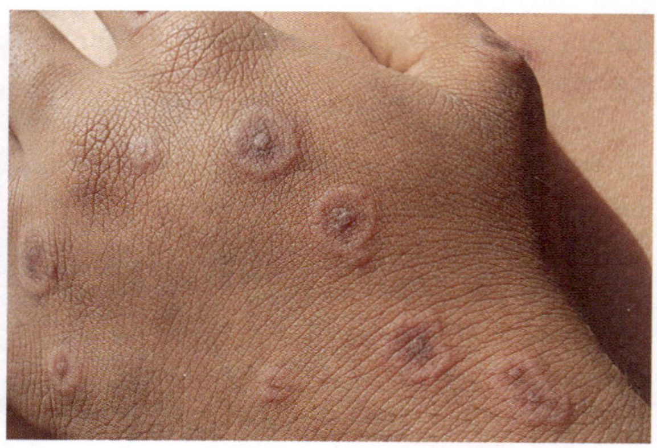

| **Fig. 24.6** Erythema multiforme. Note: 'Target' lesions |

Treatment

1. *Inj. Adrenaline* 0.3–0.5 mL SC, if there is angioedema or extensive urticaria.
2. *Antihistaminics* are the mainstay of treatment and should be given in adequate doses. It is better to err on the higher side, as except sedation there are no side effects. Newer antihistaminics like cetrizine, levocetrizine, loratidine, desloratidine or fexofenadine are less sedating and can be usefully combined with conventional antihistaminics like Pheniramine (Avil 20–50 mg oral, IM or IV) or Promethazine (Phenargan 25–50 mg oral, IM or IV).
3. *Corticosteroids* like Inj. Efcorlin 100 mg IV stat or oral Prednisolone 5 mg tds.
4. *Topically*, Calamine lotion or Crotomiton (Crotorax).

Herpes Zoster

Otherwise a self-limiting condition without any sequelae (except postherpetic neuralgia), herpes zoster can become a medical urgency in the following circumstances:

1. All cases of involvement of ophthalmic division of trigeminal nerve (*ophthalmic zoster*). Presence of vesicles at the tip of the nose indicates infection of the nasociliary branch and hence an important sign that keratitis might follow. Conjunctivitis, ocular muscle palsy, ptosis and mydriasis are other complications.
2. *Ramsay-Hunt syndrome* is due to the involvement of the geniculate ganglion. It comprises severe facial palsy associated with loss of taste in the anterior tongue and vesicles in the external auditory canal and pharynx. Often the 8th nerve is involved as well, giving rise to tinnitus, hearing loss and vertigo.
3. Involvement of the 1st and 2nd *sacral ganglia* may cause severe ulcerations in the genital region giving rise to urinary retention.
4. *Immune deficiency states* secondary to HIV infection, diabetes, leukaemias, Hodgkin's disease and non-Hodgkin's lymphoma.

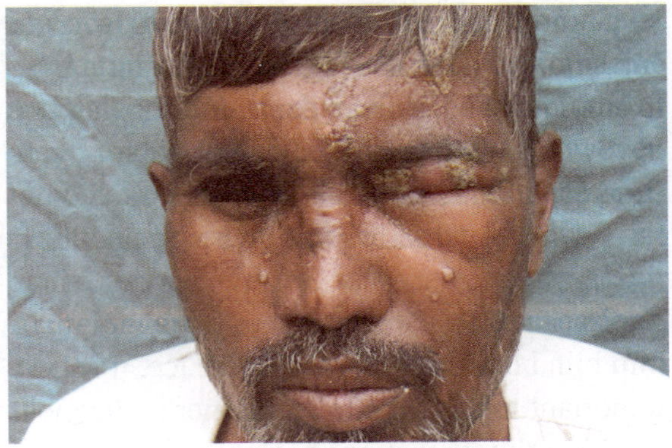

| Fig. 24.7 Herpes zoster ophthalmicus |

Management

1. *Acyclovir* 600–800 mg 5 times a day for 7 days is indicated in all the clinical varieties of zosters mentioned above. To be effective the drug should be started within 48 hrs of the onset of vesicles. Famciclovir 250 mg, needs to be given 3 times a day only, and therefore has better compliance. Valacyclovir 1000 mg tds is also a superior alternative because of convenience of dosage.
2. *Analgesics* in adequate doses.
3. *Local* treatment with potassium permanganate soaks and some antibiotic cream. Local acyclovir ointment has no value. Wet compresses are preferred to drying lotions like calamine.
4. *Steroids* 40–60 mg of prednisolone daily may prevent postherpetic neuralgia.
5. Take opinion of ophthalmologist in case of ophthalmic zoster and an ENT specialist in case of Ramsay-Hunt syndrome.

Lepra Reaction

Many general practitioners manage leprosy patients and I strongly recommend that they do, because the course of the disease is quite indolent and treatment of leprosy requires a thorough knowledge of a very few drugs. These general practitioners are suddenly faced with a situation where the patient has suddenly become worse when everything was going on fine. He is probably facing a 'lepra reaction'. This term is used when there is erythema, swelling and tenderness of the original patches and new patches have suddenly developed. Other complications like acute neuritis, iritis or orchitis can occur, which can cripple the patient overnight or make him blind or sterile in a week. Hence, it is very important for a general practitioner to diagnose and treat these reactions promptly.

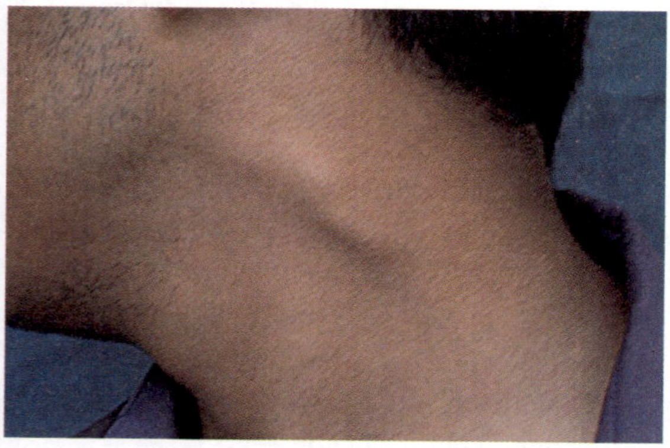

| **Fig. 24.8** Hansen's disease. Note: Thickened greater auricular nerve |

Treatment

Treat the patient according to whether he has a mild reaction or a severe reaction. Dapsone should be continued in all cases unless the reaction is very severe.

1. Patients with *mild reactions*. Reactions in which:
   a) Skin is not so severely inflamed.
   b) Nerves are not tender.
   c) ENL reactions with minor skin lesion and mild systemic manifestations.

   Aspirin—600 mg qid is still the cheapest and the best anti-inflammatory drug.

   Chloroquine—is added for its anti-inflammatory action in the dose of 300 mg tds.
2. *Severe reactions* are those in which:
   a) Skin ulcerations are present.
   b) There is severe neuritis.
   c) Iritis or orchitis develops.

   All cases of iritis or orchitis should be hospitalized. Severe neuritis can be successfully managed by the general practitioner.

   Steroids—prednisolone 40–60 mg daily and gradually tapered off.

   Clofazimine (Lamprene) is unique in the treatment of leprosy as it has both antileprotic and anti-inflammatory action. Dapsone can be withdrawn and steroids can be gradually tapered off when this drug is given 300 mg tds.

   Thalidomide if available, is a wonderful drug for ENL reactions.

   Antibiotics, if intercurrent infections are present.

Cutaneous Drug Eruptions

Clarification of a few well established but not widely known facts about cutaneous drug eruptions are highlighted:

1. A rash may be only one part of a generalised drug reaction, which simultaneously affects other organs of the body as well.
2. A common misconception is that the rash develops only after the first exposure to the drug. This is never the case. In fact, the rash develops only after the patient has developed sensitivity to the drug which could be days or weeks or months after repeated exposures. Once sensitivity occurs, the patient remains sensitive for life.

The following drug eruptions require emergency treatment:

1. *Severe urticaria, angioedema, anaphylaxis*.
2. *Severe phototoxic and photoallergic eruptions*—these are more marked in the sun exposed areas but may extend to sun protected areas.
3. *Morbilliform eruptions* (toxic erythema)—here a widespread erythematous eruption mainly affects the trunk with moderate pruritus and fever. It usually starts 1 week after initiation of therapy and lasts for about 2 weeks after the drug has been withdrawn.
4. *Exfoliative dermatitis*: This usually follows untreated toxic erythema or develops independently. Severe metabolic disturbance may require hospitalization.
5. *Acute vasculitis and purpura*: Urticaria, haemorrhagic blisters, palpable purpuric lesions are common.
6. *Bullous eruptions*: These may vary from a few bullae to extensive bullae indistinguishable from bullous pemphigus or pemphigoid.
7. *Erythema multiforme major* (*EM*): This is characterized by vesicles, bullae and the distinctive iris or target lesions, with fever and mucous membrane involvement.
8. *Toxic epidermal necrolysis* (*TEN*): This is a toxic erythema of the skin where the skin peels off in sheets like in burns. Mortality is very high.

The last three conditions (which are bullous disorders) require hospitalization and vigorous treatment. The rest can be managed on OPD basis.

Management

1. Immediately stop all drugs that the patient is taking.
2. In case of anaphylaxis, give Inj. Adrenaline and shift the patient to a hospital.
3. Steroids—in severe cases, IV Efcorlin should be given. In mild cases, oral prednisolone 10 mg tds should suffice.
4. Fever should be preferably treated with ice water sponging. Only if fever does not subside paracetamol should be given and that too starting with a low dose.
5. Antihistaminics
6. For photosensitive reactions, bed rest in a dark room is recommended.
7. Locally, potassium permanganate soaks followed by steroid creams.

And finally, never give a trial of a drug in a known sensitive patient. It could spell disaster.

Henoch-Schonlein Purpura

Typically, a young adolescent is brought to a general practitioner with an erythematous rash mainly confined to the buttocks and lower extremities. On examination, the rash is a palpable purpura (i.e., the lesions are erythematous papules, raised above the skin and do not blanch on pressure). There is moderate pruritus and a history of sore throat 2–3 weeks back. In addition to the skin involvement which is seen in all patients, there may be involvement of three other systems of the body (Fig. 24.5):

1. Gastrointestinal—involvement is seen in almost 70% of patients and is characterized by colicky pain in abdomen, vomiting, diarrhoea and occasionally haematemesis.
2. Joints—arthralgia is seen in almost all patients with typical arthritis in knees, ankles and elbows seen in a few.
3. Renal involvement is usually characterised by mild glomerulonephritis leading to haematuria with RBC casts.

This is *Henoch-Schonlein* purpura also called *anaphylactoid purpura*. The disease, though frightening to the parents usually ends in spontaneous resolution in a few weeks or months without any complications, although there is a remarkable tendency to recur several times. Urine and stool exam might reveal RBCs, haemogram is normal and platelet count is also normal. (This is in contrast to thrombocytopenic purpura where the platelet count is decreased.) A rare but serious complication is nephrotic syndrome.

Management

1. Bed rest.
2. Antibiotics are usually given if there is a h/o sore throat. Penicillin or macrolides are preferred.
3. NSAIDs—usually aspirin.
4. Steroids are usually prescribed for severe multisystem involvement though their role is debatable. Prednisolone should be given 40–50 mg/day.
5. Urine analysis should be done every week during the attack and every month thereafter for 3 months. If abnormalities persist, refer to a nephrologist.

Erythema Multiforme (EM)

It is not that all cases of erythema multiforme are medical urgencies. In EM, the clinical spectrum varies from a localized eruption on the skin (erythema multiforme minor) to a severe fulminating multisystem disorder (erythema multiforme major). It is the major variety that we are concerned with here, both because of its multisystem involvement and its potentiality to shade into SJS and TEN, which have been previously described. Apart from the papular, maculourticarial and vesiculobullous eruptions (hence 'multiforme'), it is the classical 'iris (*target*) lesions' that gives away the diagnosis. These are round *erythematous* lesions which expand centrifugally slowly in concentric circles. The centre is dark in colour where a vesicle may eventually form (Fig. 24.6).

EM can be produced by viral infections (mainly herpes simplex virus), bacterial infections and drugs. In many cases, however, the precipitating factor cannot be identified.

Treatment

1. Withdraw offending drugs if any.
2. Antibiotics, if bacterial infection is suspected.
3. Topical steroids.
4. Prednisolone 10 mg tds × 10–14 days.

MISCELLANEOUS URGENCIES

- Vertigo
- Haemoptysis and haematemesis
- Acute red eye
- Acute vomiting
- Ischaemic heart disease (IHD)
- Stable angina pectoris (Classical angina)
- Unstable angina (Preinfarction syndrome)
- Acute myocardial infarction (AMI)
- The unconscious diabetic
- Syncope
- Anaphylactic shock
- Tetany

Vertigo

When we are dealing with vertigo as an emergency we do not mean those patients who come to your clinic on their own and have lightheadedness, giddiness, blurred vision, etc., and say "Doctor, I am feeling dizzy. I have an attack of hypertension". We also do not have in mind those patients who have cerebellar ataxia, hypoglycaemia or the hyperventilation syndrome.

By vertigo as an emergency we mean "true vertigo", which is defined as a "*hallucination of motion*" where the person feels that either his surroundings are going around him or he himself is rotating. We are dealing with vertigo which has an abrupt onset, is severe enough to make the patient lie down and is associated with either nausea, vomiting, tinnitus, nystagmus or hearing loss.

Clinical Features

Broadly speaking there are two types of vertigo—peripheral and central:

- ***Peripheral vertigo*** results from diseases of the inner ear. The vertigo is acute in onset, severe and is characterised by a recurrent course, each attack lasting for minutes or days. Tinnitus, deafness, nystagmus, nausea and vomiting are usually present.
- ***Central vertigo*** results from neoplasm or inflammatory disease of the cerebellum or medulla. Here, vertigo is at best an accessory symptom with symptoms such as palsy or other neurological deficit predominating. The vertigo is slow in onset, usually mild and is characterised by a chronic course. Tinnitus and deafness are usually absent though nausea and vomiting may be present.

An "***emergency vertigo***" brought to your clinic will probably be a peripheral vertigo. Under the circumstances, consider four well known definite clinical entities, viz., Meniere's disease, vestibular neuronitis, BPPV and acoustic neuroma.

1. ***Meniere's disease***: It is characterised by a triad of vertigo, tinnitus and deafness. There is an attack of severe vertigo associated with nausea, vomiting and tinnitus. This attack subsides within minutes or may last for days. After a variable period, these attacks recur. With each attack there is progressive deafness. The tinnitus may be continuous or present only during the attack.
2. ***Vestibular neuronitis***: The main symptom here is severe vertigo, which strikes like a bolt from the blue and subsides within a few days. This usually follows an URTI and hence is presumed to be a viral infection of the vestibular nerve. There are no cochlear symptoms like deafness or tinnitus. This is a self-limiting disease and the attack usually does not recur. In a minority of the cases where it recurs, each attack is milder than the previous one.
3. ***Benign paroxysmal positional vertigo*** (***BPPV***): There is a momentary vertigo which arises only when the head is placed in certain critical positions. After attaining the offending head position the vertigo does not start immediately but after a few seconds (latency). If in spite of the discomfort the offending position is maintained, the vertigo disappears (fatiguability). Also, after repeatedly placing the head in the offending position, the intensity of the vertigo decreases (habituation). Latency, fatiguability and habituation are characteristics of BPPV. There are no cochlear symptoms like deafness and tinnitus.
4. ***Acoustic neuroma***: This is a neurofibroma arising from the 8th cranial nerve and may or may not be associated with generalised neurofibromatosis (Von Recklinghausen's disease). When within the confines of the inner ear, the symptoms are gradually progressive unilateral deafness and tinnitus in addition to vertigo. At a later stage, features of a space occupying lesion are also seen. Early diagnosis is important, which can be achieved by a CT scan or MRI.

Management

1. ***Symptomatic relief***: During the acute attack, bed rest is essential and the patient usually finds a position in which vertigo is minimal. Immediate relief can be obtained by giving Inj. Promethazine 25–50 mg IM (Phenargan) or Inj. Prochlorperazine 12.5 mg IM

(Stemetil). This is followed by oral labrynthine sedatives such as Cyclizine (Marzine), Dimenhydrinate (Gravol, Dramamine) or Cinnarazine (Stugeron) all 25–50 mg tds. The vasodilator Beta-histine 8 mg tds (Vertin) is another useful drug which can be given along with the above drugs.

2. ***Further management***: After the acute phase is over, the opinion of the ENT specialist should be sought in every case for a more specific diagnosis and treatment like vestibular exercises in case of BPPV or surgical destruction of the labyrinth in case of Meniere's disease.

Haemoptysis and Haematemesis

Haemoptysis is an alarming symptom for most of the patients and even for a few general practitioners.

1. The immediate problem faced by a GP is to find out whether the patient has haemoptytis or haematemesis, because invariably the patient will describe the episode as "*There was a bout of cough followed by vomiting of blood.*"

   Eliciting an accurate description of the present episode is all too important for the diagnosis.

   In haemoptyss, the blood coughed up is bright red, frothy and mixed with sputum. In haematemesis, the blood vomited out is dark red in colour and mixed with food particles. In case of doubt, ask the patient to demonstrate haemoptysis by spitting in your basin—you will be able to see blood-streaked-sputum. In haemoptysis there is past h/o cough, while in haematemesis there is past h/o abdominal pain and vomiting. The following day even if the hemoptysis has stpped, the patient continues to have rusty sputum. In haematemesis, the next day there is melena.

2. Having established the exact nature of the problem, the next problem is which patients are to be referred for the hospital management and which patients are to be managed on OPD basis:
   a) Ideally, *all cases of haematemesis* should be hospitalised. There are three main causes of acute haematemesis: i) Bleeding peptic ulcer; ii) Liver cirrhosis with oesophageal varices; iii) Ca. stomach. All these lesions produce massive bleeding. Recurrences are common and unpredictable. A case of varices can land up in acute liver failure following heavy bleeding. Treatment includes multiple blood transfusions and at times surgery. This is all beyond the scope of a general practitioner's setting.
   b) Any *case of massive haemoptysis* should be immediately referred because the patient can die suddenly due to shock or aspiration of large amounts of blood into the respiratory passages. Multiple blood transfusions or even emergency lobectomy may be required.
   c) *Mild to moderate haemoptysis* can be managed on OPD basis. The patient should be made to lie down in the lateral decubitus position with the diseased side in the dependent position. This prevents the aspiration of blood to the unaffected bronchi. A mild sedative like diazepam to allay the anxiety is of value. In case of moderate haemoptysis, IV fluids to maintain hydration and to prevent shock should be started. Many so-called haemostatic agents like calcium gluconate, stadren, vitamin-K, ethamsylate, etc., are of dubious value in stopping the bleeding. In any case, the haemoptysis which is scant will stop spontaneously without any pharmacotherapy.

As soon as the patient is settled, the patient should be sent for an X-ray chest in order to ascertain the cause of the bleeding. The most common cause in India is of course pulmonary tuberculosis. The important causes of haemoptysis are listed in Table 24.6.

| Table 24.6 Causes of haemoptysis |

Respiratory:	Tuberculosis
	Bronchiectasis
	Lung abscess
	Pneumonia
	Bronchial carcinoma
Cardiac:	Mitral stenosis
	Aneurysm of aorta
	Pulmonary hypertension

A plain X-ray chest usually will reveal the cause of the bleeding. If not, the patient should be referred for a CT scan or a bronchoscopy.

The further management will depend on the final diagnosis.

Acute Red Eye

When this condition is encountered by a general practitioner, the immediate objective is to make sure that the condition he is going to deal with is definitely conjunctivitis, which can be easily treated by a general practitioner. Other conditions which can present as an acute red eye are iritis, acute glaucoma and corneal ulcer, for which immediate referral to an ophthalmologist is necessary. Iritis should not be misdiagnosed as conjunctivitis, because improper treatment of iritis can lead to glaucoma or cataract. Again, the diagnosis of acute glaucoma and corneal ulcers should not be missed, as they require urgent treatment under expert guidance in order to prevent disastrous complications.

First, ask if there is pain in the affected eye. Conjunctivitis results in "the non-painful red eye", and there is a gritty sensation only. Keratitis, iritis, glaucoma however result in "the painful red eye" and here the vision is also reduced.

Next, identify whether the inflammation is in the conjunctiva or is of the deeper structures. The type of congestion seen in conjunctivitis (conjunctival congestion) is quite distinct from the type of congestion seen in the acute inflammation of the cornea, iris, ciliary body or in acute glaucoma (ciliary congestion). This is shown in Table 24.7.

A more specific diagnosis can then be made with the help of features shown in Table 24.8.

So in summary, in bacterial conjunctivitis, pain is absent, congestion is more marked in the fornices, is bright red in colour, there is mucoid or mucopurulent discharge, eyelids stick on waking in mornings.

Treatment

1. Local antibiotic drops like chloramphenicol, gentamicin or norfloxacin to be instilled 4–5 times a day.
2. Local antibiotic ointment, like chloramphenicol eye ointment or applicaps at bed time.
3. Dark glasses, if there is photophobia.
4. Avoid touching the unaffected eye with the same handkerchief used for the affected eye.

Finally, never pad the affected eye. It favours bacterial growth.

Acute Vomiting

Many times a GP is faced with a situation where there is persistent severe vomiting in a patient lasting for a day or two, with only minimal additional symptoms and signs. A patient who gets just 1 or 2 vomits which have stopped spontaneously does not approach a GP. A patient who has unexplained vomiting for a few weeks or months (chronic vomiting) is a hospital case.

Symptomatic treatment can be given by correcting the dehydration by IV fluids and by controlling the vomiting with antiemetic drugs. Inj. Stemetil (12.5 mg IM) and Inj. Metoclopramide (10 mg IM) are good antiemetics but both these drugs can cause sedation, acute muscle dystonia and other extrapyramidal side effects. Oral Domperidone (10 mg tds) and oral Cisapride (10 mg tds) are devoid of these side effects but the antiemetic efficacy is low. Ondansetron (2–4 mg in slow IV infusion) is also devoid of these side effects and has a potent antiemetic activity.

But, the curative treatment will rest on a firm diagnosis which many times cannot be made so early in the evolution of the disease. However, the patient will have a few additional symptoms and signs albeit minor, the so called 'associated symptoms' or 'pointers'.

1. The associated symptom could be a *loose motion or two* in which case the patient might land up with acute gastroenteritis the following day.
2. The patient may have *fever*, in which case the management will be like any other fevers.
3. Severe *headache and high grade fever* could be a pointer towards meningitis or encephalitis. Watch for meningeal signs.
4. The patient may have *heart burn*, in which case the diagnosis of acute gastritis is usually made. But, it is important to remember that spontaneous gastritis is very uncommon and the gastritis is seen usually when there is an insult to the gastric mucosa, e.g., acute alcohol abuse, drug abuse (NSAIDs, steriod), eating very spicy foods, etc. Under such circumstances, especially in the elderly individuals, consider the possibility of acute myocardial infarction.
5. If there is a h/o *amenorrhoea* in a female, it could be a case of hyperemesis gravidarum.
6. If the vomiting is associated with *pain in abdomen* the diagnosis will depend on the site of pain, e.g., pain in the right hypochondriac region could be due to hepatitis or acute cholecystitis. Pain in the right iliac fossa could be due to acute appendicitis. Pain in the loin could be due to acute pyelonephritis and so on and so forth.
7. If there is vomiting with severe *peripheral vertigo*, the cause could be in the inner ear, e.g., vestibular neuronitis or Meniere's disease.
8. If the patient is an uncontrolled *diabetic*, ketoacidosis could be the cause of the vomiting.

And lastly, the ill-defined entity of periodic syndrome or cyclical vomiting should be kept in mind. Recurrent attacks of unexplained vomiting is usually seen in the young. It is a diagnosis of exclusion.

Ischaemic Heart Disease (IHD)

These are a group of heart diseases where the myocardium is inadequately perfused with oxygen. There is imbalance betwen oxygen supply and demand. The most common cause of this myocardial ischaemia is atherosclerosis of the coronary arteries, which decreases the coronary blood flow. Coronary thrombosis and vasospasm further limit the blood supply to the myocardium. Similarly, diseases which increase the demand of oxygen to the myocardium like ventricular hypertrophy can cause myocardial ischaemia. Depending on the degree and duration of ischaemia, a *spectrum of IHD* is encountered:

Stable Angina Pectoris

The ischaemia is transient. Hence, there is decreased blood supply to the myocardium but

| Table 24.7 |

	Conjunctival congestion	Ciliary congestion
Colour	Bright red	Dark purple
Site	Mostly marked in the fornix	Mostly marked around the cornea (circum-corneal)
Discharge	Pus	Watery or none
Vessels	Network of tortuous vessels (arborization) Individual vessels can be made out Inflamed vessels move with the movement of the conjunctiva On releasing pressure the vessels fill up rapidly	Vessels arranged radially around cornea Individual vessels cannot be made out (diffuse red blush) Inflamed vessels are stationary
Indicates	Conjunctivitis	Iritis, glaucoma

| Table 24.8 |

	Conjunctivitis	Iritis	Acute glaucoma
Congestion	Conjunctival	Corneal	Corneal
Discharge	Mucoid or purulent	Watery or none	Watery or none
Onset	Acute or gradual	Gradual	Acute
Pain	Gritty sensation	Moderate	Severe
Vision	Normal	Reduced	Greatly reduced
Pupil	Normal	Constricted & reacting sluggishly to light	Dilated and fixed
Cornea	Normal	Normal	Hazy
Intraocular pressure	Normal	Normal	Raised
Refer?	No	Yes, urgently	Yes, urgently

necrosis does not occur. Ischaemia is due to coronary artery spasm on a pre-existing atherosclerotic coronary artery.

Unstable Angina Pectoris

This occurs when there is sudden fissuring and disruption of a previously stable atheromatous plaque. This invites platelet aggregation and thrombus formation. The blood supply to the myocardium is thus partially cut off. The thrombus may undergo spontaneous lysis and the crisis is over. However, the thrombus may increase and completely occlude the artery leading to acute myocardial infarction.

Acute Myocardial Infarction (AMI)

This occurs if the ischaemia is prolonged leading to myocardial necrosis and scarring.

Stable Angina Pectoris (Classical Angina)

The typical patient of angina is a 50–60-year-old man who comes to you complaining of acute onset chest pain, which is radiating to the left shoulder and to the ulnar surface of the arm and hand following some such precipitating factor such as a heavy meal, walking hurriedly up the stairs, anxiety and stress, straining at stools, etc. This pain can also radiate to the back, neck, jaw or the epigastrium. It is relieved by rest and by sublingual nitroglycerine or nifedipine.

However, classical angina pectoris can also present in an atypical fashion. It can occur at night when the patient is recumbent. This is called *angina decubitus*. In *Prinzmetal's or variant angina*, the chest pain occurs at rest and is accompanied by palpitations and dyspnoea, which is severe and frightening. In *Wenckebach's second wind angina* or breakthrough angina, there is initial chest pain while walking, but on continued walking the pain stops spontaneously without coronary vasodilators.

Physical examination is usually normal. ECG reveals typical ST segment and T wave changes, which are present only during the episode but disappear subsequently.

Management

1. ***Treatment during the attack***: A short acting nitrate like glyceryl trinitrate (Angised) 0.5 mg or isosorbide dinitrate (Sorbitrate or Isordil) 5 mg are the drugs of choice, administered sublingually or as a Nitroglycerine spray. Usually, the pain subsides in 2–5 min. If not, a second dose may be given after 5 min. Once the pain stops, the remaining tablet may be spit or swallowed. A throbbing headache is the most common side effect.
2. ***Prevention of attacks***: Modification of life style, reduction of risk factors, advising adequate rest and allowing exercises which do not precipitate angina, form an integral part of treatment programme. The following drugs are used to prevent attacks:
   a) *Nitrates*: They act by causing dilatation of the coronary arteries. All nitrates have the same action—they differ only in their duration of action. They are either short acting like glyceryl trinitrate or long acting like isosorbide dinitrate or mononitrate.

      Long acting nitrates are preferred for prophylaxis. Tolerance with loss of efficacy develops with 12–24 hrs of continuous use. Hence, only a minimum effective dose must be used and a minimum of 8-hr drug-free interval each day is recommended. Isosorbide dinitrate (Isordil or Sorbitrate) 5 mg 8 hourly or Isosorbide 5 mononitrate (Ismo-20 or Monotrate) 20 mg tds is used. Glyceryl trinitrate is readily absorbed via the skin and therefore is also available as ointment or as transdermal patches.

   b) *Beta-blockers*: These reduce the oxygen requirement of the heart by reducing the heart rate, blood pressure and myocardial contractility. Atenolol (Aten, Tenormin) 25–100 mg/day, which requires to be given once a day is preferred to propranolol. It should be started along with nitrates in all cases. This combination not only reduces the frequency of anginal attacks but also the occurrence of myocardial infarction.

c) *Calcium antagonists*: A calcium antagonist like nifedipine is added to the above combination, if the frequency of the attacks is not reduced. Given alone, it is not of much value.

Calcium antagonists are powerful coronary and peripheral vasodilators. Hence, they increase the oxygen supply to the heart as well as reduce the oxygen demand. Also by blocking the entry of calcium into the myocardial cells they decrease the myocardial contractility. Nifedipine (Depin, Calcigard, Nicardia) 10–40 mg tds, amlodipine (Amlogard) 5–10 mg od, verapamil (Isoptin) 80–120 mg tds and diltiazem (Dilzem) 30–90 mg tds are the common preparations used.

d) *Antiplatelet therapy*: Aspirin should be started for its antiplatelet effect as early as possible. The inhibitory effect of aspirin on platelet aggregation starts immediately after a single dose and remains effective for 5–6 days. The dose is controversial but 100–150 mg daily is adequate. It is cheap, of proven efficacy and with a well understood side effect profile. Only if aspirin is contraindicated (because of hypersensitivity or peptic ulcer), Ticlopidine (Tyklid) 250 mg bd should be used. The maximum effect of ticlopidine is delayed till 3–5 days and it also has a dreaded side effect—neutropenia. In comparison, Clopidogrel (Clopiget) 300 mg stat followed by 75 mg od, has quicker onset of action, is more potent and has minor side effects as compared to ticlopidine. It can be effectively combined with aspirin (the magic bullet).

Amongst the newer antiplatelets, *Pasugrel* is used along with aspirin to prevent thrombosis of coronary arteries. Loading dose is 60 mg followed by 10 mg maintenance dose. It is contraindicated in patients with active bleeding or H/O stroke. It is also not recommended in over 75 years of age because of increased risk of intracranial bleeding. *Tecogrelol*, a newer antiplatelet drug, can be used in the entire spectrum of acute coronary syndrome.

Unstable Angina (Preinfarction Syndrome)

This refers to the IHD spectrum which, is midway between classical stable angina and acute myocardial infarction (AMI). Clinically, in a known patient of classical angina, *preinfarction syndrome is suspected when*:

1. The pain becomes more severe, lasts longer and occurs with increasing frequency.
2. The pain now occurs at rest.
3. The pain is associated with vomiting, dyspnoea or perspiration.
4. It is not completely relieved by sublingual nitrates.

The diagnosis is established by these clinical features along with transient ECG changes like ST depression or elevation and/or inversion of T wave. These ECG changes revert back to normal within 24 hrs, because in unstable angina there is no necrosis of the myocardium.

Acute myocardial infarction is suspected when:

1. ECG changes do not revert back to normal within 24 hrs.
2. There is increase in levels of cardiac enzymes.

Frequently, it is difficult to ascertain at which particular point the patient lies. The safest bet under the circumstances is to make a presumptive diagnosis of myocardial infarction and admit the patient in an ICCU for heparinization/ thrombolytic therapy, etc.

Acute Myocardial Infarction (AMI)

The typical patient of myocardial infarction presents with a severe constricting pain in the retrosternal area, which may radiate to the left or both the shoulders or arms. Occasionally, the pain radiates to the neck, infrascapular region, epigastrium or the jaw. This may be accompanied by features of sympathetic hyperactivity like restlessness, tachycardia, palpitation or profuse sweating. Occasionally, however, signs of parasympathetic hyperactivity are seen such as bradycardia and hypotension.

| Table 24.9 Atypical presentations of AMI |

These are chiefly responsible for mistaken diagnosis:

1. Silent infarct—there may be no pain, especially in long standing diabetes, hypertension, elderly or middle aged post-operative patients.
2. Sudden onset sweating and vomiting, with or without chest pain.
3. Sudden onset breathlessness, with or without chest pain.
4. Acute confusion, severe unexplained profound weakness, arrhythmia, syncope or sudden death are other common presentations.

Physical Examination

Most patients are restless, anxious and sweating profusely. There is a striking pallor and the extremities are cold. There may be bradycardia, tachycardia or a normal pulse. The blood pressure may be normal, high or low. On auscultation of the lungs, there may be basal crepitations.

Diagnosis and Investigation

This is a clinical diagnosis. An ECG may be normal at first and changes may evolve slowly over a period of next 72 hrs. Hence, if the initial ECG is normal and the suspicion of AMI is strong, always advise a repeat ECG after a few hours.

The earliest change is ST elevation, which starts reversing within 24 hrs. T wave then begins to get inverted. Q wave appears when transmural infarction occurs. Cardiac enzymes (Myoglobin, CPK MB, SGOT, LDH, cardiac troponins) are released into the blood from the damaged heart muscles. Myoglobulin rises in the first 30 min and is thus an important marker for early detection and/or exclusion of cardiac damage. Troponin levels typically start to elevate in the blood within 2–3 hrs from the onset of chest pain and is used in practice for early detection of cardiac damage. CPK MB, SGOT and LDH rise only after 6–8 hrs.

Do not waste time in investigating. About 25% of the patients of AMI die before reaching the hospital. Give an urgent call for a cardiac ambulance. Till the ambulance arrives, the following treatment is given:

Immediate Prehospital Treatment

1. Give an aspirin tablet 300 mg orally to be chewed as buccal absorption of the drug is faster than gastric absorption.
2. Give in addition one tablet of glyceryl trinitrate (Angised) 0.5 mg or isosorbide dinitrate (Sorbitrate) 5 mg sublingually. This will be followed by a nitroglycerine drip in the hospital.
3. In case of bradycardia, give Inj. Atropine 0.3–0.6 mg IV.

4. Tachycardia, if <120/min, does not require treatment.
5. If the patient has left ventricular failure, give Inj. Frusemide 40–80 mg IV.

When the ambulance arrives, rush the patient to the hospital. Immediate treatment in the hospital can be life-saving.

The Unconscious Diabetic

The immediate differential diagnosis to be considered in such a situation is (1) Hypoglycaemic coma caused by excess insulin or sulphonylureas or (2) Hyperglycaemic coma (diabetic ketoacidosis) or (3) Alcohol-induced hypoglycaemic coma and (4) Unconsciousness unrelated to diabetes, like encephalitis, cerebral malaria, head injury, etc.

The immediate concern is to differentiate between hypoglycaemic coma and hyperglycaemic coma because both are life-threatening. The former can be easily treated at the patient's residence while the latter requires hospital management, preferably in an ICU. How do you differentiate between these two? Plainly speaking there is hardly anything common between these except both are diabetics and both are in coma!

1. Glucometer if available, will settle the issue immediately. In hyperglycaemia, BSL is >400 mg/dL & in hypoglycaemia, it is <40 mg/dL.
2. Take the history. In hyperglycaemic coma, the onset of symptoms is gradual (days), the coma being preceded by polyuria, polydipsia, abdominal pain and vomiting. There is h/o default in insulin and usually there is some precipitating factor like intercurrent infection or surgery. In hypoglycaemic coma, the onset is abrupt and there is h/o having skipped a meal following insulin or there is h/o unaccustomed exercise.
3. Examine the patient. In hyperglycaemic coma, the patient is febrile and looking toxic. The skin is dry, the pulse is feeble, BP is low and the breathing is rapid with a sweet odour to the breath (mainly due to dehydration and electrolyte disturbance). In hypoglycaemic coma, the skin is moist, the extremities are cold, clammy, the pulse is bounding, the BP and RR are normal (attributable to discharge of adrenalin in response to low glucose in blood).

Treatment

If the issue of hypo or hyper is still not settled, 50 mL of 50% glucose solution should be given IV as bolus. The patient with hyperglycaemia will not regain consciousness but no harm is done.

He should be shifted to a hospital for further management. The patient with hypoglycaemia will regain at least partial consciousness immediately. If not, one or two more bolus injections may be required. If hypoglycaemia is because of long acting insulin or sulphonylureas, the patient should be put on an IV drip of 10% glucose to prevent further hypoglycaemic episodes.

Note: In order to prevent the patient slipping into coma, a knowledge about the early warning symptoms is necessary.

Hypoglycaemic Precoma

The patient must be educated about these symptoms. They are so common that they are a part and parcel of a life of a type I DM patient. The patient gets symptoms depending on the rapid or gradual fall of blood sugar.

1. *Adrenergic symptoms*: These symptoms mimic symptoms caused after an injection of adrenaline, viz., tachycardia, palpitations and a sinking sensation. These symptoms are experienced when the blood sugar falls rapidly, as after short acting insulins.
2. *Parasympathetic symptoms* mimic symptoms experienced in a vasovagal syncope, viz., dizziness, pallor, sweating, etc.

3. *Neuroglycopaenic symptoms*: These symptoms are seen because of inadequate glucose supply to the brain. Patients are mentally confused, ataxic and behave abnormally (as in acute alcohol abuse). In severe cases there may be convulsions. Usually neuroglucopaenic symptoms are seen when the BSL falls gradually, as after long acting insulins or sulphonylureas.

Hyperglycaemic Precoma

Usually the presentation is subacute, spanning over a day or two. The early warning symptoms are severe polyuria, drowsiness and vomiting.

Abdominal pain because of distension of stomach is an important symptom which can cause confusion in diagnosis. Polyuria gives rise to dehydration and sodium and water depletion manifested clinically as dry skin, sunken eyeballs, bradycardia, hypotension and hypothermia. Acidosis gives rise to deep sighing respiration and ketosis to fruity breath odour.

Syncope

Syncope means a *transient loss of consciousness* that results from a sudden reduction of cerebral blood flow leading to cerebral ischaemia. If there is no loss of consciousness, it would mean that the patient had a simple faint. Vasovagal syncopes are most commonly encountered in general practice.

Description of Typical Vasovagal Syncope

1. The patient is almost always in an upright position to begin with.
2. He is forced to encounter an emotionally painful or stressful stimuli (e.g., tooth extraction, sight of blood or dead body, etc.)
3. He experiences warning symptoms like dizziness, blurring of vision, sinking sensation, nausea and may even vomit.
4. This is followed by a striking pallor of the face, tongue and lips along with profuse cold sweat.
5. O/e, the pulse is feeble and there is marked bradycardia. The BP is low or unrecordable, the patient is hardly breathing and lies motionless. Incontinence of urine is rare.
6. If the patient is forced to lie down, further progress is arrested. If not, this is followed by a loss of consciousness and the patient falls. The recumbent position restores the blood flow to the brain. The pallor reduces; the pulse, BP and breathing come back to normal. Finally, consciousness is regained.
7. The whole episode usually lasts for 2–3 min although it might sometimes last for 30 minutes or so. Convulsions may even occur if well meaning friends and bystanders prevent the patient from falling down.
8. A complete recovery is the rule although some degree of weakness may remain for a few minutes more.

Types

1. ***Vasovagal syncope***: These occur in adolescents who are otherwise healthy. They are extremely common and benign and as described above always occur in an upright position.
2. ***Cardiac syncope***: The syncope is due to fall in cardiac output because of a primary cardiac lesion. They differ from vasovagal syncope in that the patient may not be in an upright position at the onset of the attack.

   They are diagnosed by history, physical examination, by an ECG, cardiac imaging or by Holter monitoring.
3. ***Carotid sinus syncope***: In many individuals massage of the carotid sinus can cause hypotension and bradycardia. In elderly individuals with a hypersensitive carotid sinus even a small stimulus like shaving or turning

the head to one side can provoke a syncopal attack.

4. ***Others*** like micturition syncope, cough syncope, breath holding spasm in children or postural syncope in the elderly.

Differential Diagnosis

A proper history will usually differentiate syncope from the following conditions where there may be transient loss of consciousness:

1. Epilepsy
2. Severe hypertension
3. Hyperventilation syndrome leading to tetany
4. Hypoglycaemia
5. Hysterical fainting
6. Peripheral vertigo

Treatment

Patient should be immediately placed in a supine position with the legs raised. All tight clothing should be loosened. In case of the benign vasovagal syncope, this is all that is required. In case of life threatening syncopes of cardiac origin, a referral to the relevant physician is required for a thorough evaluation.

Anaphylactic Shock

This is a severe life threatening emergency which the GP has to manage in his own OPD till the condition of the patient stabilizes and he can be shifted to a hospital. In a GP's set up, two kinds of patients are encountered:

1. Following an injection or a tablet given by the practitioner, the patient suddenly develops a hypersensitive reaction.
2. A patient is brought in a shocked state, having exposed himself to an allergen like fish, eggs, pollens, etc.

Clinical Features

The hallmark of an anaphylactic reaction is the development of the following manifestations within seconds to minutes after the introduction of the antigen into the body.

Early symptoms include severe itching all over, change in voice and tightness in the chest. If these are ignored, the patient develops severe manifestations of a typical hypersensitivity reaction, viz:

- Hoarseness or stridor, due to laryngeal oedema.
- Wheeze, because of bronchospasm.
- Severe urticaria.
- Angioneurotic oedema.
- Itching of the eyes, chemosis of the conjunctiva and lid oedema.
- Abdominal cramps, vomiting and diarrhoea.

Very severe cases may collapse with a thready pulse, severe hypotension, acute respiratory failure and even death.

Differential Diagnosis

Confusion may arise in the following situations:

1. Severe bronchospasm in an asthamatic after NSAIDs. Here there is absence of hypotension and urticaria.
2. Hypoglycaemic coma after insulin. Here there is a bounding pulse and a normal BP.
3. Syncope after a painful injection like Imferon. Here there is bradycardia and hypotension.
4. Severe urticaria and angioedema induced by a drug. Here the patient is haemodynamically stable.

Treatment

Patient should be immediately placed in a supine position with the legs raised. All tight clothing should be loosened.

1. Do not panic—be in firm control of the situation.
2. Make the patient lie down, apply a tourniquet above the injection site and immediately start a fast IV drip before the veins collapse.

3. Injection *adrenaline*: Mild reactions can be controlled by giving 0.5 mL of 1:1000 adrenaline subcutaneously. Severe collapsed patients will require intramuscular injection of adrenaline to be repeated every 10–15 min till the patient is stable. This will correct both the hypotension and the bronchospasm.
4. *Antihistaminics* like diphenhydramine IV.
5. *Steroids*: IV 200 mg of hydrocortisone hemisuccinate (Efcorlin) should be given even though the action is delayed for many hours. It is useful for persistent bronchospasm and hypotension.
6. Shift the patient to a *hospital* for observation for 24 hrs even if the patient recovers. If the patient does not show signs of recovery in spite of the above treatment, shift the patient to an ICU for cardiac monitoring, dopamine drip, O_2 administration, tracheostomy, etc.

Tetany

Usually, a young female is brought to the general practitioner in a frightened state because of an attack of carpopedal spasm. This is 'tetany', which is a state of muscular hyperexcitability when a minor stimulus may produce cramps and spasms. In a frank case because of the characteristic carpal spasm the diagnosis is quite obvious. If the diagnosis is in doubt because the patient gives a history suggestive of tetany but you have not witnessed the cramp, you can reproduce the carpal spasm by a BP cuff inflated above the systolic BP for 2–3 min (*Trousseau's sign*). Another way of confirming the diagnosis is by tapping lightly with a patellar hammer about 3 cm below and in front of the ear, i.e., at the exit of the facial nerve from the skull. The facial muscle will twitch briefly with each tap (Chvostek's sign).

Management

A very common cause of tetany seen in general practice is the *hyperventilation syndrome.* This is a functional disorder usually an acute conversion disorder (i.e., hysteria). The history is always classical.

Usually, a young woman presents with an episode of severe anxiety followed by breathlessness → circumoral paresthesia → tingling numbness of the arms and legs → and finally carpopedal spasm, all because of the lowered CO_2 in blood.

The mainstay of treatment here is to ask the patient to breathe in and out of a paper bag. The CO_2 that is thrown out is again inhaled thus correcting the CO_2 levels in the blood. The relief of tetany itself has a soothing effect on the anxious patient (and the relatives). This can be followed by an anti-anxiety drug like diazepam. I have found that a straight talk with the patient and relatives immediately after the episode is most fruitful in establishing the cause of anxiety and for further management.

Other common causes of tetany in general practice are:

1. *Hypocalcaemia* caused by prolonged diuretic therapy, in which case IV 10% calcium gluconate slowly over a period of 5–6 min gives immediate relief, and
2. Marked *alkalosis* caused by prolonged vomiting, when IV infusion of normal saline should be given.

Other causes mentioned in the textbooks like tetany following thyroid surgery are rarely seen in the set up of a GP.

*This chapter has been reviewed by **Dr Parag Vaste**, MD Medicine, Consultant Physician, Deenanath Mangelkar Hospital, Pune.*

GP Tip

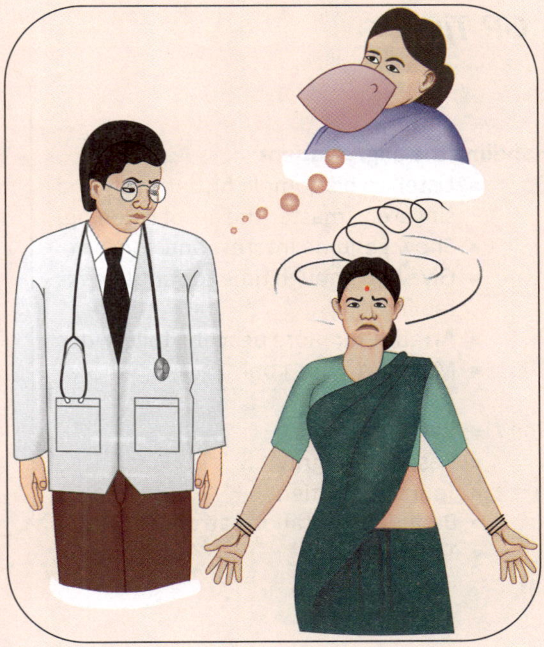

A neurotic patient is in panic and is hyperventilating. She might faint because of the consequent low levels of CO_2 in the blood.

Prevent this by asking the patient to breathe in and breathe out of a plastic bag.

GP Tip

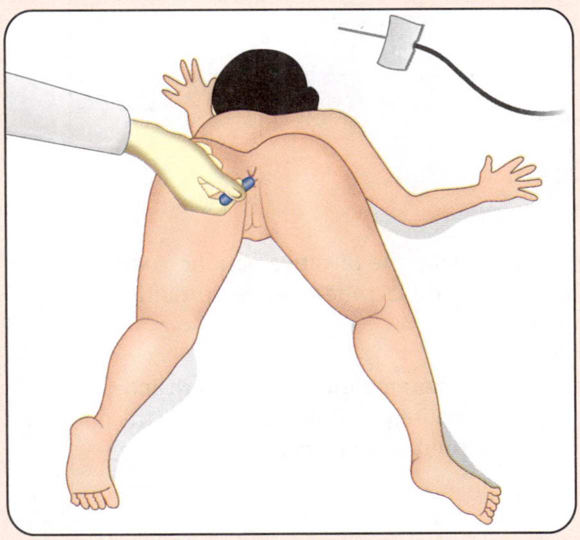

Stopping convulsions in a baby, the easier option to intravenous diazepam

Cut off the butterfly of the scalp vein and push the rubber tube in the rectum. Administer injection diazepam via this tube per rectally.

GP Tip

Handling the angry patient:

Do
- Listen to his complaint, seriously and sincerely (master the art of listening)
- Show genuine interest and concern
- Give him enough time to ventilate his feelings
- Arrange for more peaceful follow-ups
- Maintain your cool

Don't
- Raise your voice
- Respond angrily
- Touch the patient
- Be judgemental or patronising
- Talk too much

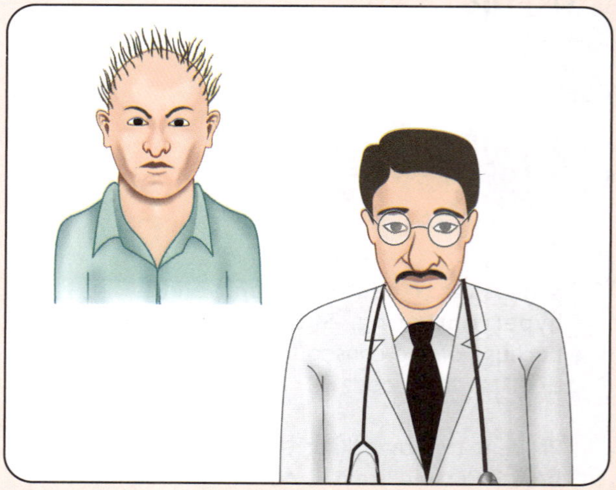

GP Tip

How to stop the talkative patient from her verbal diarrhoea, while ausculta-ting?

Thrust a thermometer in her mouth and ask her politely to shut (up) her mouth, even if there is no fever!

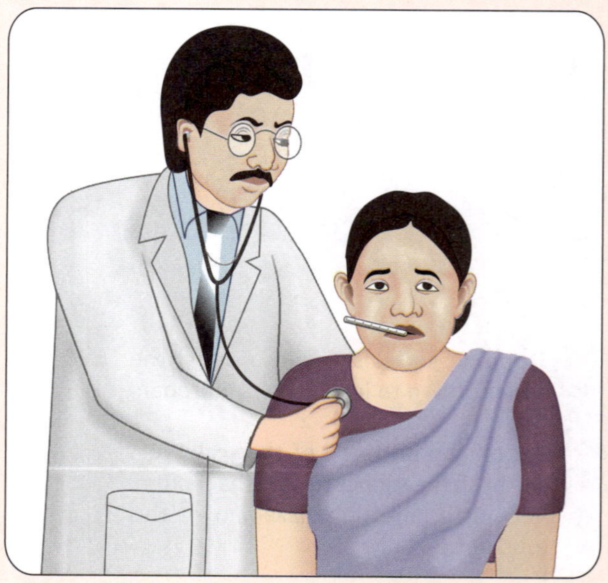

CHAPTER 25

The Asthma Clinic

- Introduction
- Equipments
- Inhalation Devices and Techniques
- Making a Diagnosis
- Drugs Used in Asthma
- Managing an Attack of Acute Severe Asthma
- Management of Chronic Asthma

INTRODUCTION

Twenty years back the management of an asthmatic patient was very different from what it is today. The patient was given a prescription of bronchodilator tablets to be taken daily life-long. In an exacerbation, the patient was prescribed a corticosteroid preparation, which was to be taken for 8–10 days. (In India, where self-medication and over-the-counter sale is rampant, even steroids were taken daily, life-long!) In spite of this, if the patient got an attack of dyspnoea, he was rushed to the family physician. The family physician usually gave him Inj. Deriphylline + Inj. Decadron intramuscularly or Inj. Adrenaline subcutaneously or Inj. Aminophylline intravenously, depending on the severity of the bronchospasm and the readiness of the GP to take a calculated risk in administering the above injections.

This practice has taken a 'U' turn for the better. No more adrenaline or aminophylline injections because better and less risky treatment modalities have been developed by which the patient treats himself most of the time at home. Rushing to the family physician is not required. The result? General practitioners started seeing less and less number of asthmatic patients in their day-to-day practice, affecting their income. Some doctors resigned to their fate. Other more innovative general practitioners came out with the concept of "asthma clinic" and quite successfully too. This is not surprising as a cure of the condition called asthma, described more than 2000 years ago, is still not in sight. The prevalence of asthma is on the rise as with the new definition of asthma many ill defined conditions like 'wheezy bronchitis', 'asthmatic bronchitis' and 'allergic bronchitis' have been brought under the asthma category, so that now a population of 2500 people will have at least 125 asthmatics on the average. The asthmatics are benefitted largely because of these clinics in terms of safer and more convenient treatment resulting in near normal life-style for the asthmatic.

What does a General Practitioner do in an 'Asthma Clinic'?

1. Identifies an asthmatic by making an initial diagnosis. Diagnosis of asthma can be difficult at times.
2. Refers to a chest physician in case of doubt about diagnosis.
3. Educates the patient about his disease.
4. Educates the patient about the various inhalation devices available and the proper technique to be used. Also assists him in making the correct personal choice of the inhalation device suitable to him for the treatment of his chronic disease.
5. Treats a severe attack preferably by drugs delivered through a nebulizer.
6. Refers to a hospital in case of life-threatening asthma or status asthmaticus.

Difficult in a GP setup? Not at all. All it requires is purchasing a few equipments as an initial not too large investment and training your compounder in the above mentioned aspects of an 'asthma clinic'.

EQUIPMENTS

1. **Nebuliser** (Fig. 25.1)
A nebuliser is an instrument, which converts liquid into fine mist. Various nebulisers are available in the Indian market and is an essential component of an asthma clinic. Based on the method of aerosol generation, nebulisers are either jet nebulisers or ultrasound nebulisers. Jet nebulisers are commonly used in India and cost about Rs. 2500.

A nebuliser is to be used in a severe attack of bronchospasm, when airway narrowing limits the inspiratory airflow to such an extent that metered dose inhalers are not effective. Your compounder should be trained about the method of delivery of the drugs and the method of cleaning the instrument as cross infections may occur. A constant stock of a salbutamol respiratory solution and ipratropium bromide respiratory solution need to be kept with him. Discourage the use of nebuliser by the patient at home. While it adds to the convenience of the patient, the worry is that a patient will stay at home using the nebuliser during a severe

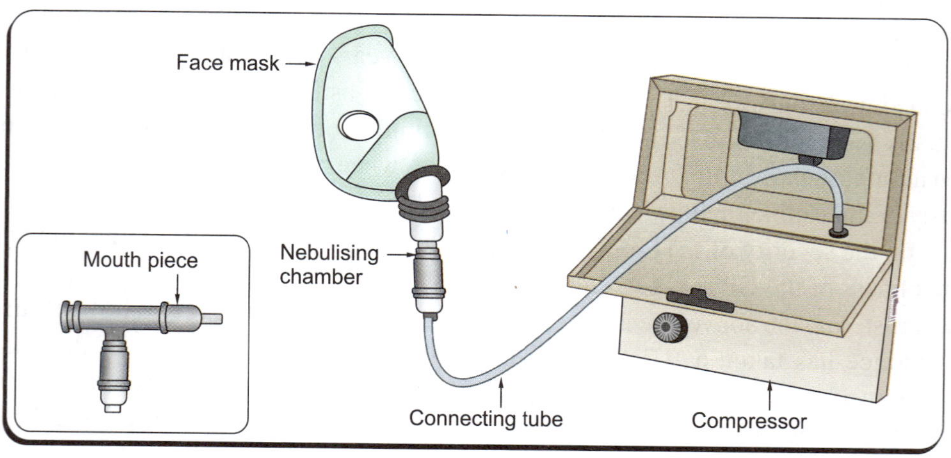

| **Fig. 25.1** Nebuliser |

attack while in fact other treatment like IV corticosteroids are necessary, which could be life-saving.

2. **Peak flow meters** (Fig. 25.2)
   Peak flow meters are inexpensive (costing about Rs. 600/-) and portable instruments used for diagnosis as well as monitoring treatment. It can be looked upon as an equivalent to blood sugar estimation in the management of diabetics or a sphygmomanometer in the management of hypertension. Every asthma clinic should have a peak flow meter and a few should be stocked to be sold to asthmatics for home monitoring of his condition.

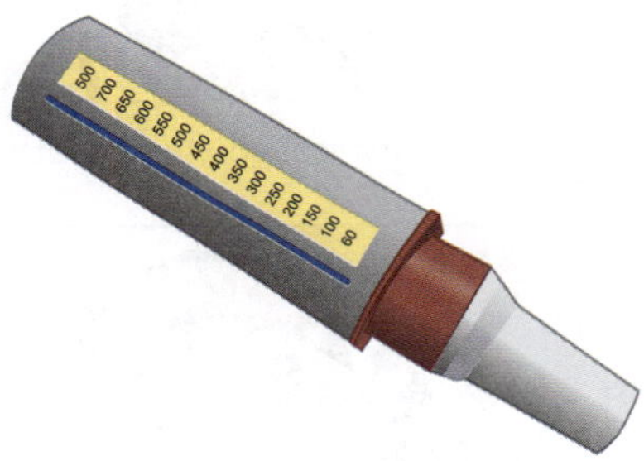

| **Fig. 25.2** Peak flow meter |

3. **Placebo inhalers**
   The trained compounder will need a variety of placebo inhalers, a spacer device and placebo rotacaps for demonstration. The asthmatic is shown the way these are used, so that he can select the most suitable device for himself. These can be obtained from pharmaceutical companies who will readily oblige. They may also provide literature for patient education, which should be kept in the clinic.
4. **Oxygen**
   A small cylinder of oxygen (if possible), to deal with hypoxia in an attack of acute severe asthma, before being shifted to a hospital.
5. **Drugs to be stocked**
   Injections: Adrenaline, aminophylline, salbutamol (Asthalin), terbutaline (Bricanyl), hydrocortisone (Efcorlin).
   Nebuliser solutions:
   a) Salbutamol respiratory solution (Asthalin).
   b) Ipratropium bromide respiratory solution (Ipravent).
   c) Salbutamol + ipravent respiratory solution (Duolin).

INHALATION DEVICES AND TECHNIQUES

Delivering drugs by the inhaled route is usually regarded as a modern invention. The fact is it is not, though the last 4–5 decades have seen rapid advances in this field. Mention is found in the most ancient cultures like India, China, Rome, etc. The Indian "Hookah" which is used in the northern parts of India for tobacco smoking as well as for giving indigenous medicine is probably the most time tested inhalation device in the world. The recent advances in the inhalation route started about 60 years back when adrenaline was first given by aerosol through a crude nebuliser. Twenty years later, steroids were delivered by this route. In 1956, the break came when the first metered dose inhaler (MDI) was developed. From then onwards, there is no looking back and modification in these techniques to give maximum benefits to the asthmatic is the order of the day.

But why the inhaled route of delivery? This route obviously is the most logical way of treating respiratory diseases just as it is logical to treat skin diseases with skin ointments and eye diseases with eye drops. The only problem that needs to be overcome is to find out the best way to deliver a drug inside the body deep into the respiratory tract, unlike the skin or the eye, which are easily accessible to local therapy. Otherwise advantages galore:

- Much smaller doses are required to achieve the therapeutic effect by inhalation route as compared to the systemic route. For example, the inhaler of salbutamol provides 100 μg (microgram) per puff, which is approximately equal to the therapeutic effect provided by 4 mg (milligram) of a salbutamol tablet, i.e., 40 times the inhaled dose.
- Obviously, the adverse effects of the drug are significantly minimized.
- Again obviously, as the drug is delivered directly at the desired site, the onset of action is more rapid.

Inhalation Devices

A wide variety of inhalers are available in India, with a wide variety of drugs to go along with:

1. Metered dose inhalers
2. Spacer devices
3. Single dose dry powder inhalers
4. Multi dose dry powder inhalers
5. Nebulisers

Metered Dose Inhalers (MDIs)

The MDIs have become the most widely used inhalation devices in the treatment and prophylaxis of asthma. It has now been in use for the last 30 years. It is a device containing the drug in a suspension form in a canister. It delivers a fixed amount of drug in aerosol form, which remains the same actuation after actuation.

The original MDIs contained the non-selective β-agonists isoprenalin and adrenaline, but these were soon superseded by selective β_2 adrenergic agents salbutamol, terbutaline and formoterol. Finally, delivery of topical steroids by MDIs made treatment of asthma revolutionary (Fig. 25.3).

Particles inhaled through the mouth have to turn a corner to enter the respiratory tract through the larynx. This requires a propellant, the commonly used being chloroflurocarbon (CFC

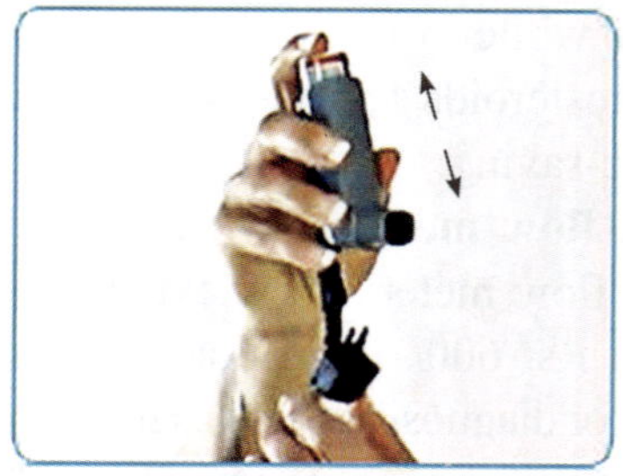

(a) Take off the cap. Shake the inhaler well.

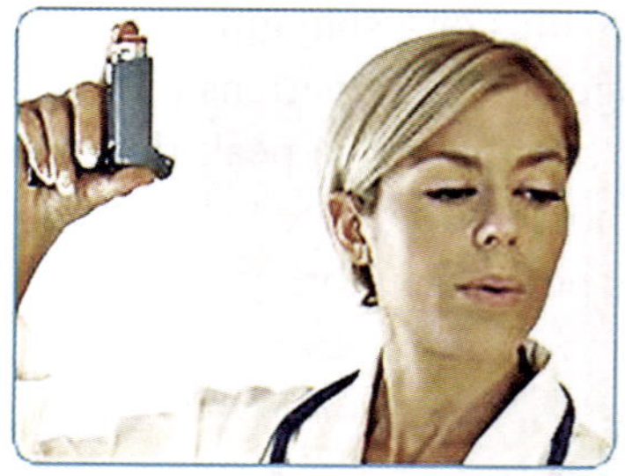

(b) Breathe out through your mouth.

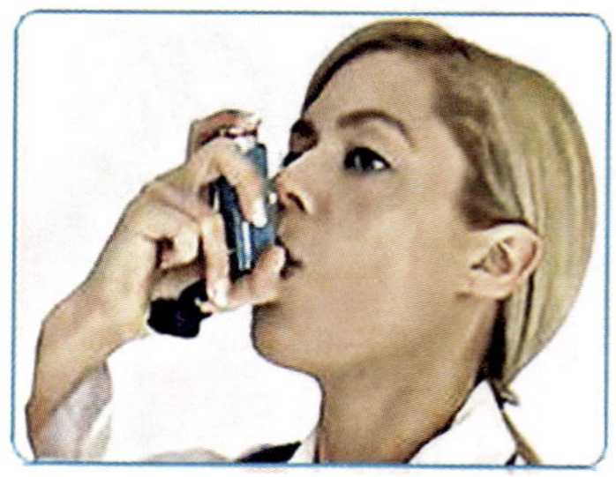

(c) Place the inhaler between your lips. As you start to breathe in, press the top end of the inhaler & keep breathing in steadily and deeply.

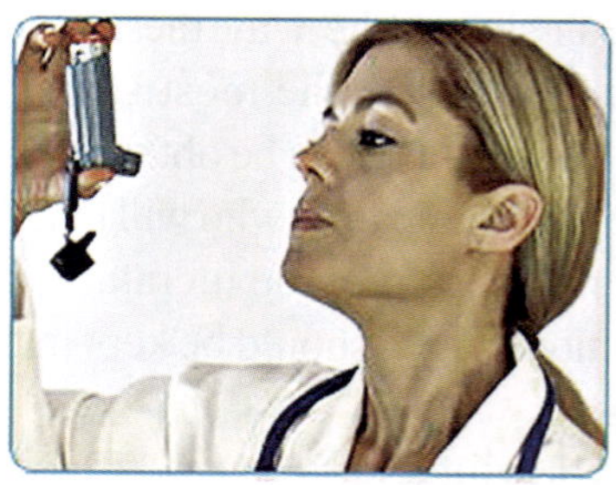

(d) Remove the inhaler from your mouth. Hold your breath for 10 sec/as long as you find comfortable. Breathe out.

| **Fig. 25.3** Correct inhalation technique for using MDIs |

or Freon). These particles then strike the back of the throat with considerable velocity. The larger heavier particles simply impact in the oropharynx and are subsequently swallowed and wasted. The lighter smaller particles, which form only about 10% of the dose delivered through the MDI reach the lungs.

However, this tiny dose is sufficient to give a clinical response. CFCs are not environment friendly as they damage the ozone layer and has been banned in many countries. They however, do not have any adverse effects on the patient. Many companies are now using hydroxy fluorene instead of CFC.

Correct inhalation technique

The key to successful MDI therapy is to deposit aerosol in any part of the lungs and this requires some skill and experience on the part of the patient. Time spent on teaching the correct technique for using MDIs to the patient is time well spent.

| **Table 25.1** Correct technique for using MDIs (Figs. 25.3a–d) |

1. Remove the cap.
2. Shake the canister.
3. Hold the canister upright.
4. Breathe out gently.
5. Place the inhaler mouth piece between the teeth and seal lips around it.
6. Fire the inhaler while taking deep breath.
7. Continue to inhale deeply till lungs are full.
8. Remove the inhaler from the mouth.
9. Hold the breath for 10 sec.
10. Breathe out.

Used correctly, MDIs are a boon to the asthmatics. They are economical, easy to carry and contain at least 200 accurately metered doses of the drug that are immediately ready for use. However, in spite of the best instructions it is a sad fact that some asthmatics will just fail to use DIs correctly. Secondly, poor 'actuation-inhalation' coordination or 'press-breath' coordination, especially in children and older individuals, reduce the clinical response. Finally, the so-called '*cold freon effect*', where the patient stops inhaling completely when the cold blast of CFC strikes the pharynx makes the dose ineffective. All in all this meant that MDIs were not totally perfect and there was a need for modifications of the MDIs. These were then made commercially available in the form of *spacer devices*.

Extension Tubes and Spacer Devices

In order to overcome the problem of actuation-inhalation coordination and the 'cold freon effect', many patients started using a number of commonly used day-to-day hollow objects such as empty bottles, plastic bags, etc., to store the aerosol before inhalation. Falling in line with this usage finally a large number of spacer devices became commercially available. It is important to note that these are all additions to the standard MDIs and not separate type of inhalers by themselves in the strict sense. The spacer, usually a 280-mL plastic chamber is attached to the MDI. The aerosol released from the MDI stays in suspension inside the spacer chamber (or holding chamber). The patient can inhale from this chamber shortly afterwards without having to coordinate actuation and inhalation. For infants and young children who cannot inhale through the mouthpiece, a face-mask is attached to the mouthpiece of the spacer or to the newly introduced 'baby haler'. This has virtually eliminated the use of nebuliser in this age group **(Fig. 25.4)**.

Spacers do not benefit asthmatics whose inhalation technique is already adequate. In those with poor technique, they increase the lung deposition to 20–30% with a parallel reduction in the oropharyngeal deposition. This is important for

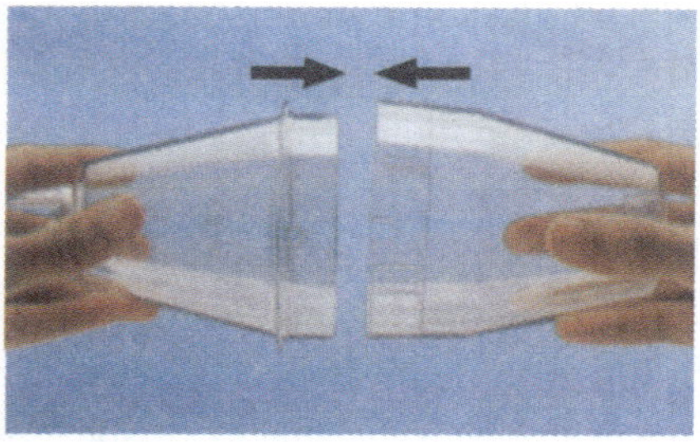

(a) Assemble the spacer by pushing the notch of one half into the slot of the other half

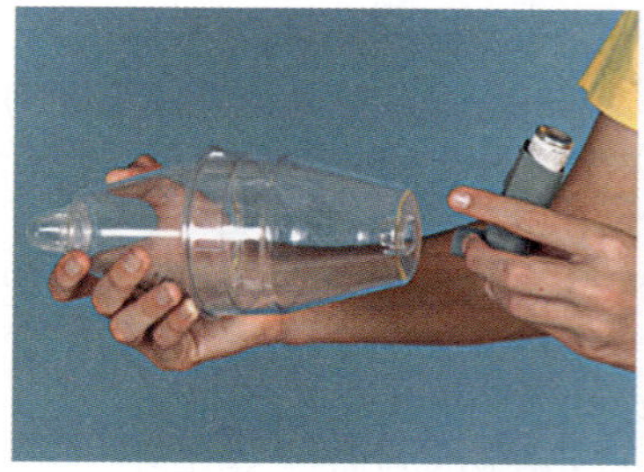

(b) After shaking the inhaler well, fit it into the spacer

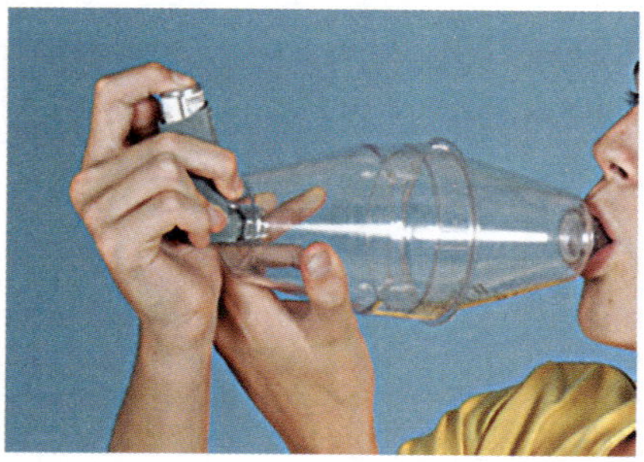

(c) Breathe out through your mouth. Then close your lips around the spacer, as shown

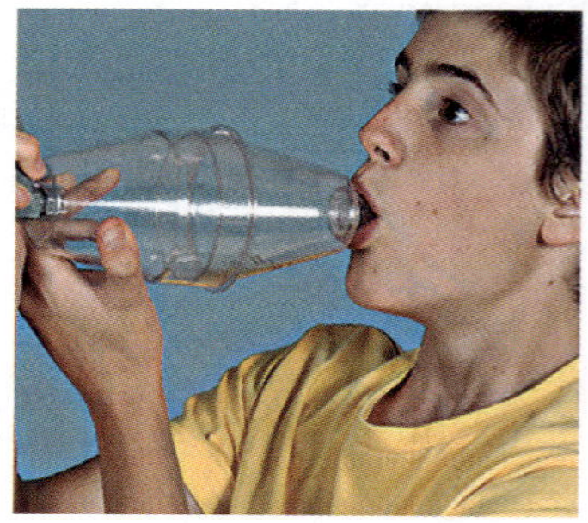

(d) Press the top end of the inhaler. Then, breathe in deeply through your mouth

| **Fig. 25.4** How to use spacer |

pressurized corticosteroid aerosols, which cause oral thrush and dysphonia as side effects but is of no consequence for inhaled bronchodilators, which do not cause any local side effects.

Drug particles are deposited gradually inside the wall of the spacer chamber, which attracts freshly released drug particles by electrostatic energy resulting in reduced drug delivery. This problem can be reduced by cleaning the spacer once a week and by changing the spacer every year or so. Alternatively, a small volume spacer device made of polyamide material (Zerostat spacer) has been introduced, which is static free and hence increases the amount of inhaled aerosol. Spacers are suitable for home use but are too bulky to be carried around easily.

Obviously, a compact device was needed, which could be kept in pocket or purse and at the same time did not require coordination between actuation and inhalation. The breakthrough came in the form of *breath-actuated pressurized inhalers.*

Single Dose

Dry powder inhalers (DPIs): Since the major problem with MDIs was poor coordination between firing the MDI and inhalation, it was logical to think in terms of a device, which was triggered by the patient's own inhalation. Such a device was introduced as the dry powder inhalers (DPIs).

A very popular single dose DPI available in India is the transparent *rotahaler*. It has an efficiency equal to that attained by the pressurized MDI, does not require coordination, easy to teach, portable and has a low initial cost as compared to MDIs. Further, it does not contain CFCs and hence problems of 'cold freons' are overcome. Being transparent, it also has the added advantage of allowing the patient to see whether he has fully inhaled the dose.

In the rotahaler (Fig. 25.5), a capsule (called the rotacap) is inserted into the raised square hole of the rotahaler, transparent end first. Holding the mouth piece with the hand, the patient rotates the base. A sharp fin inside the rotacap separates the two halves of the capsule and the powder inside the capsule falls into the body of the rotahaler. The patient then inhales the powder deeply into his lungs, the action comparable to the inhalation of a cigarette. During the act of inhalation the rotar and capsule rotate making a rattling sound. In case of lack of clarity and understanding, take the help of the medical representatives who will be only too eager to demonstrate the use of the rotahaler in addition to the correct use of the MDIs and spacers.

Although single dose DPIs circumvented problems with MDIs, a separate group of problems were found to be associated with its use. Only children above the age of 6 years

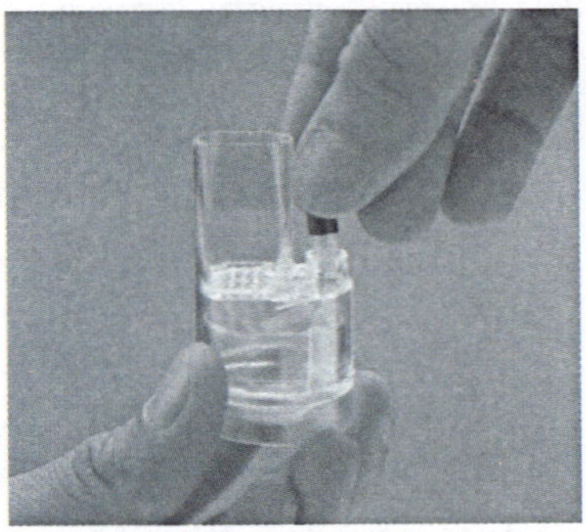

(a) Insert the transparent end of the rotacap into the raised square hole of the rotahaler

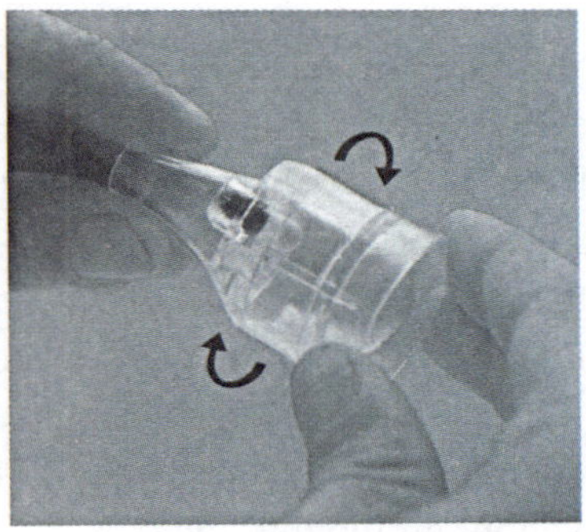

(b) Hold the top of the rotahaler firmly with one hand and rotate the base until the capsule breaks

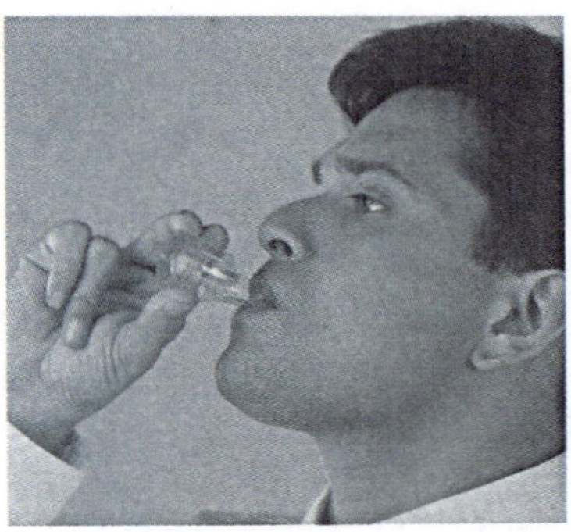

(c) Breathe out through your mouth. Then, placing the rotahaler between your lips (as shown), breathe in through your mouth as deeply as possible

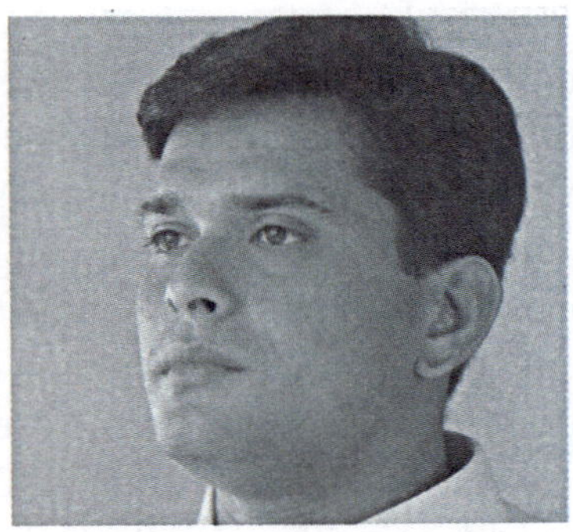

(d) Remove the rotahaler from your mouth. Hold your breath for 10 sec or as long as you find comfortable. Breathe out.

| **Fig. 25.5** How to use rotahaler |

could generate the inspiratory flow rates required for complete inhalation of the dry powder. Capsules soften in humid weather and do not then break correctly. But, the most important limitation of the single dose DPI was the requirement of loading the capsule every time before use, in contrast to pressurized MDI where at least 200 metered doses were immediately ready for use. This was especially important in an acute attack. Hence, the concept of ready to use multi-dose powder inhalers was mooted, which combined the ease of use of the DPIs with the convenience of the MDIs. The result: *multidose MDIs*.

Nebuliser

Narrowing of the airways in an acute attack of asthma may be so severe and the patient so distressed that MDIs, MDIs with spacer or DPIs cannot be used effectively (Fig. 25.1). In these circumstances, treatment with nebulisers will still be effective as nebulization requires only relaxed tidal breathing. In acute severe asthma, nebulised therapy with salbutamol produces as good a response as intravenous aminophylline.

A nebuliser is an instrument that converts a liquid solution into a fine mist, which can then be inhaled easily using a face mask. This only requires relaxed tidal breathing, eliminating the need for coordination as required with MDIs. Also large doses of bronchodilators can be nebulised, which makes a nebuliser an ideal instrument of delivering the drug in an attack of acute severe asthma at all ages and may be the only type of inhaler suitable for infants and small children in a similar situation. Nebulisers can also be used for maintenance therapy in infants although MDI with a spacer and a face mask is an alternative. Thus, the nebuliser, which is the oldest genuine aerosol inhaler used since 1872, still retains its popularity although not as the original crude hand-held nebuliser but as the modern jet nebuliser or the ultrasound nebuliser.

However, there are a few disadvantages. Treatment with a nebuliser is time consuming, taking 10–15 min to deliver the dose, the instrument is bulky and expensive. In addition, the solution can get contaminated if cleaning of the instrument is not adequate.

Selecting the right device

The choice at the time of writing is mainly between pressurized MDIs, MDIs with spacer, DPIs (single or multidose) and nebulisers. Selecting the appropriate device for your patient will depend on the following factors:

1. **Age**
   - Infancy to 3 yrs : MDI with spacer + baby mask or nebuliser
   - 3–6 yrs : MDI with spacer
   - 6–12 yrs : MDI with spacer or DPI (rotahaler)
   - Adult : MDI or DPI
2. **Acute severe asthma**
   Nebulisers are preferred as large doses of a bronchodilator can be given. Also during the attack, patients may have reduced tidal volume making it difficult for the drug to reach the lungs by any other inhalation device.
3. **Initial cost**
   Nebulisers are the costliest while rotahalers are the most economical. MDIs are also comparatively economical, though the cost increases with the addition of the spacer and the face mask.
4. **Intelligence of the patient**
   The rotahaler is very easy to use even by illiterate patients. MDIs without spacer require good training and a lot of practice.
5. **Home versus hospital use**
   At home, for mild exacerbations, MDIs,

MDIs with spacer or DPIs are all good choices. In hospitals when the attack is severe, the nebuliser is preferred.

MAKING A DIAGNOSIS

In my opinion, asthma is grossly underdiagnosed and undertreated by general practitioners. Firstly, mild cases of asthma are often misdiagnosed as 'asthmatic bronchitis', 'allergic bronchitis' or 'wheezy bronchitis'. Even severe attacks of bronchospasm presenting for the first or second time to the physician are not diagnosed as asthma either because of the lack of confidence on the part of the general practitioner or because he fears that if the patient is told that he is suffering from asthma (which is a frightening label), the patient will change the doctor to seek a second opinion. Failing to diagnose and label the patient as asthmatic has led to gross underdiagnosing this condition, resulting in gross under-treatment.

Pitfalls in Diagnosis

Typical young asthmatics, who present with breathlessness and wheezing which is recurrent in nature, are easy to diagnose. However, all patients do not present typically. Particularly in children, an intractable cough, which is most troublesome at night may be the only symptom. In infants, attacks of wheezing are very common under one year of age.

The wheeze may be caused by mucosal thickening of the already contracted airways. But it should be noted that over one-third of such infants go on to have asthma later in childhood. Even in older children, there is a tendency on the part of general practitioners to diagnose repeated attacks of wheezing as 'wheezy bronchitis' because he feels that 'declaring' the diagnosis to the parents will cause undue anxiety. In adults, asthma is misdiagnosed as 'chronic bronchitis' even in non-smokers and wrongly treated with 'higher' and 'higher' antibiotics. In elderly individuals, paroxysmal nocturnal dyspnoea and chronic cor pulmonale are often misdiagnosed as asthma with disastrous results.

In case of doubt about the diagnosis, it is better to approach the patient systematically—first take a proper history, then conduct a thorough examination and finally confirm your diagnosis by a peak flow meter and pulmonary function tests.

History

If the patient presents to his physician when he is asymptomatic and not during the attack, inquire about the following points in history:

- Are there recurrent attacks of dyspnoea?
- Does he have troublesome cough, especially during night time?
- Is the dyspnoea seasonal?
- Does he get breathless during his day-to-day activities or after minimum exercise?
- Does he have associated allergic rhinitis or eczema?
- Does his common cold 'go to the chest'?
- Does he get breathless after taking certain medications, e.g., aspirin or propranolol?

If the answer to the above questions is affirmative, in all likelihood, it is asthma.

Physical Examination

The following signs are likely to be present if the patient presents to the physician during the time he is experiencing symptoms:

- Wheezing, considered as the *sine qua non* of asthma, is a high pitched whistling sound while breathing. This is what the patient experiences and is heard by the physician without the stethoscope.
- Rhonchi, mainly expiratory, are heard with the stethoscope. Absence of rhonchi may be

misleading however, in very mild or very severe bronchospasm.

- Flaring of the nostrils while breathing in.
- Patient prefers to sit hunching forward making maximum use of accessory muscles.
- Talks in short sentences.
- Tachycardia, tachypnoea, hyperinflation of the chest.

Pulmonary Function Tests (PFT)

They are useful to confirm the diagnosis of asthma, establish the severity of the disease and monitor the response to therapy. The most common test is the peak expiratory flow rate (PEFR) measurements as detected by a peak flow meter (Fig. 25.2). This can be easily measured at the GP's clinic or by the patient himself at home. PEFR is the fastest rate at which air can move through the airways during a forced expiration starting with fully inflated lungs.

How to use a Peak Flow Meter

1. Adjust the pointer to zero.
2. Tell the patient to breathe in fully and encircle the lips tightly around the mouth piece.
3. Now tell him to blow as hard and as fast as possible into the peak flow meter.
4. Note down the reading as shown on the scale by pointer.
5. Take three such readings and note down the highest of these readings. This is the patient's 'personal best' reading if the patient is tested when he is asymptomatic.

A diagnosis of asthma can be made if after giving inhaled salbutamol, there is at least 15% increase in the PEFR.

DRUGS USED IN ASTHMA

Drugs used in the treatment of asthma can be classified in a number of ways depending on the mode of action, chemical structure, etc. Traditionally, the most common classification was to group them into two classes, i.e., bronchodilator drugs and anti-inflammatory agents. However, in practice a more useful way is to group them in the following two categories:

1. **Relievers**: These are the drugs, which give immediate relief from dyspnoea by causing bronchodilatation.
2. **Preventers**: These are the drugs, which do not give immediate relief but suppress inflammation of the airways, thereby preventing an attack of bronchospasm.

A brief description of the drugs commonly used in asthma follows:

Injection Adrenaline

It causes immediate and dramatic bronchodilatation, but the action lasts for a very short time. However, blood pressure may rise and heart may be stimulated leading to palpitations, tremors and a throbbing headache. It is rarely used now because of the availability of safer drugs.

Theophyllines

The short acting theophyllines are used as 'reliever' drugs (Theobid) while their sustain release preparations (Theobid SR) are used as 'preventers'.

Theophylline has proved to be an effective bronchodilator for many years. However, it is no longer considered the drug of choice because of its narrow margin of safety. The adverse effects are primarily referrable to GIT, CNS and CVS. The side effects increase as the dose is increased. Rapid IV injection of aminophylline can cause syncope and even sudden death due to marked fall in BP, ventricular arrhythmias or asystole.

Today, inhaled therapy is being advocated more and more. Hence, the use of theophylline has declined. But over the last few years it has made a significant comeback as it has found a place in the management of asthma in the following situations:

- In *acute episodic mild asthma*, where attacks are mild and very occasional.
- When an inhaled steroid used as a preventer does not adequately control symptoms.
- In *acute severe asthma*, when salbutamol given through a nebuliser does not control symptoms, IV aminophylline is many times effective.

Short Acting Bronchodilators (β_2 Agonists)

Salbutamol and Terbutaline

The only significant side effects of these drugs are tremors and muscle cramps, which are transient and mild. The bronchodilator action of inhaled salbutamol and terbutaline is very rapid, the action starting within minutes and lasting about 6–8 hrs. This has made these two drugs the most widely used bronchodilator drugs for the past 2–3 decades. In the past, both salbutamol and terbutaline were used on a regular basis three to four times a day for the prevention of asthmatic attacks. Large multicentric trials have proved that their regular administration may be responsible for the diminished response seen after long-term use of these drugs. All international guidelines have recommended them only as reliever drugs to be used under the following circumstances:

- In *mild episodic asthma* as and when required.
- In *children* below 5 years who cannot take inhaled therapy, these drugs can be given orally on short-term basis.
  - *Salbutamol* (Asthalin) is available as 2 and 4 mg tab, 2 mL/5 mL syrup, and 100 μg metered dose inhaler containing 200 metered doses and as 200 μg rotacaps.
  - *Terbutaline* (Bricanyl) is available as 2.5 mg and 5 mg tab, 3 mg/5 mg syrup, 0.5 mg/mL injection and as bricanyl misthaler 250 mg/metered dose.

Long Acting Bronchodilators (β_2 Agonists)

Two agents from this class are available in the Indian market for inhalation therapy. *Salmeterol* (Serobid) was introduced in 1994 while *formoterol* (Foratec) has been recently introduced. Both have the advantage over salbutamol and terbutaline in that the duration of action is at least 12 hrs. Hence, given twice a day as prophylactic therapy they can achieve better control of asthmatic symptoms than salbutamol given four times a day. This is especially true in those patients having nocturnal attacks. However, the onset of action of salmeterol is slow (2½ hrs to peak its action) and is therefore not useful in relieving acute attack.

Long acting β_2-agonist should always be used along with inhaled steroids. Used alone, the inflammatory element in asthma remains untreated which can worsen the long time prognosis. Exercise induced asthma especially in children is probably the only situation where they can be used alone. A single inhalation taken in the morning can provide symptom free period for the child throughout the day.

Bambuterol is a newly introduced oral drug having an action lasting for 24 hrs. 10 mg of the drug can be conveniently given orally once daily in the evening, which prevents bronchospasm for 24 hrs.

| Table 25.2 Bronchodilator drugs for inhalation |

Preparation	Form	Dose per actuation	Presentation
Salbutamol (Asthalin)	MDI Rotacaps	100 µg 200 µg	200 metered doses 400 metered doses
Ipratropium bromide (Ipravent)	MDI Rotacaps	20 µg 40 µg 40 µg	200 metered doses 120 metered doses
Salmeterol (Serobid)	MDI Rotacaps	25 µg 50 µg	200 metered doses
Formoterol fumarate (Foratec)	MDI Rotacaps	12 µg 12 µg	120 metered doses

Anticholinergic Drugs

The only agent used from this group today is *ipratropium bromide* (Ipravent) given by the inhaled route. It is an atropine substitute. *Datura* smoke (which is also an anticholinergic compound) has been used for centuries in India in the inhaled form for the treatment of respiratory disorders.

Ipratropium bromide or tiotropium bromide, as compared to salbutamol are weak bronchodilators and cannot be recommended as a monotherapy in asthma. It is indicated in those patients whose asthma is not adequately controlled by salbutamol alone. Concurrent administration of ipratropium bromide and salbutamol gives greater relief of bronchospasm than either agent alone. A combination of salbutamol with ipratropium bromide (Duolin) is available for use by the inhaled route.

GENERAL PRACTICE AS SPECIALITY

Mast Cell Stabilizers

Sodium Cromoglycate

It is an anti-inflammatory agent that acts by stabilizing mast cells thus preventing the release of histamines, interleukins, etc., which cause bronchospasm. Hence, it is used in the prophylactic treatment of asthma. It is not a bronchodilator and therefore it is ineffective if given during an attack of bronchospasm. Sodium cromoglycate is not absorbed orally and is administered as an aerosol in a metered dose inhaler (Chromal inhaler 5 mg/dose) or as rotacaps (Chromal rotacaps 20 mg/dose) for the prophylactic treatment of mild asthma. The drug has to be inhaled at least four times a day for adequate prophylaxis. Hence, compliance is often poor. It may be preferred in children, as a substitute to inhaled steroids, if adverse effects on growth because of inhaled steroids is feared (which are unfounded at the dose routinely given). It is a very safe drug without any side effects except for throat irritation and cough in some patients.

Systemic Corticosteroids

With the development of inhaled corticosteroids, which have a high safety profile along with a rapid outset of action, systemic corticosteroids are now indicated in only a few situations:

Acute Severe Asthma

Exacerbation in an asthmatic must be treated with oral prednisolone 30–40 mg/day along with nebulised salbutamol. In very severe exacerbations hhydrocortisone hemisuccinate 200 mg IV should be given every 6–8 hrs. This could be life-saving.

Severe Chronic Asthma

In a small proportion of cases not adequately controlled by high dose inhaled corticosteroids and inhaled bronchodilator, long-term oral corticosteroids will be necessary. Initiate with oral prednisolone 30–40 mg/day. Keep dose to the minimum for the shortest period of time aiming at partial relief of symptoms only, thus avoiding the side effects (Table 25.4). Short acting prednisolone is preferred and there is no advantage of using long acting betame-thasone, dexamethasone or a depot preparation like triamcinolone acetonide. The whole daily dose is best given single dose in the morning or on every alternate mornings in order to minimize hypothalamus-pituitary-adrenal (HDA) axis suppression and other side effects (Table 25.3).

Table 25.3 Side effects of steroid therapy

During short-term treatment	: Acute gastritis : Fluid retention, puffiness of face : Precipitation of diabetes : Mild euphoria or frank psychosis
During long-term treatment	: Adrenal suppression : Fluid retention : Susceptibility to infection : Delayed wound healing : Peptic ulceration : Fat redistribution : Psychiatric disturbances : Muscle atrophy : Skin atrophy, purpura, telangiectasia, etc. : Hyperglycaemia, precipitation of diabetes : Osteoporosis : Premature cataract : Growth retardation in children

Status Asthmaticus

Initiate with high dose of Inj. Hydrocortisone hemisuccinate 200 mg IV repeated 6–8 hourly. Shift to oral prednisone once the crisis is over and then withdraw gradually.

Inhaled Corticosteroids

Asthma is now proved to be due to inflammation of the bronchial mucosa by inflammatory cells, which are present even in the asymptomatic patients. Hence, it is logical to think in terms of suppressing this process by inhaled steroids. Systemic corticosteroids given for a prolonged period are associated with many adverse side effects. Inhaled steroids on the other hand effectively suppress inflammation without significant adverse side effects, e.g., 2000 μg of inhaled beclomethasone diproprionate or budesonide are as effective as 30–40 mg of prednisolone, whereas their side effect profile is equivalent to 5 mg of oral prednisolone. Hence steroid inhalation is now considered the *first line therapy* for chronic asthma.

Beclomethasone Dipropionate (Beclate Inhaler)

The introduction of inhaled beclomethasone dipropionate (BDP) in 1972 has radically changed the treatment of chronic asthma. Hoarseness of voice and oropharyngeal candidiasis are the only side effects reported. These can be minimised by gargling after every puff to wash off the drug deposited in the oropharynx. Treatment of these conditions consists of local clotrimazole paint along with a single dose of fluconazole 150 mg. Even in the high doses (800–1600 μg/day) that have been recommended for severe asthma, beclomethasone dipropionate has a good safety profile. In cases requiring higher doses than this, it is usefully combined with an inhaled long acting β_2-agonist (e.g., salmeterol) twice daily and using short acting inhaled β_2-agonist (salbutamol) for breakthrough symptoms.

| **Table 25.4** Corticosteroids available for inhalation |

Preparation	Form	Presentation
1. **Beclomethasone dipropionate** (Beclate)	MDI Rotacaps Nebuliser solution	200 metered doses
2. **Budesonide** (Budecort)	MDI Nebuliser solution	200 metered doses
3. **Fluticasone proprionate** (Flohale)	MDI Rotacaps Nebuliser solution	120 metered doses

Doses:

Mild asthma: 100–200 μg twice daily
Moderate asthma: 200–400 μg twice daily
Severe asthma: 400–800 μg twice daily

Budesonide (Pulmicort, Budecort) and **Fluticasone proprionate** (Flohale) are more potent inhaled corticosteroids available as metered dose inhalers, rotacaps and nebuliser solutions. Being more potent, once daily dosing may achieve a sustained clinical effect throughout the day.

Leukotriene Receptor Antagonists (LR-As)

It is now proved that asthma is a chronic inflammatory disease regulated by a variety of mediators like histamines, prostaglandins, leukotrienes, etc., which cause bronchoconstriction. Leukotrienes are more potent than even histamines as bronchoconstrictors. LRAs block this bronchoconstrictor response to leukotrienes. They are the available *Zufirlukast* and *Montelukast* (Montair 4 mg, 5 mg, 10 mg tablet).

The effects of these drugs are much weaker than those of inhaled steroids although the onset of action is relatively rapid. Advantage of these drugs is that they are orally administered once daily only which gives better compliance. As such they have been recommended as an add-on therapy to inhaled steroids and do not have any role as monotherapy.

MANAGING AN ATTACK OF ACUTE SEVERE ASTHMA

An attack of severe asthma in a known asthmatic hardly ever causes alarm to the relatives (because it is "the usual story") and to the physician (because of the availability of potent drugs).

| **Table 25.5** Who should be hospitalized? |

If the answer to any of the following questions is 'yes' hospitalize immediately:

1. In the case of adults, is the patient too dyspnoeic to talk or complete a sentence in one breath?
2. In the case of children, is the baby too dyspnoeic to eat?
3. Is he cyanosed?
4. Is the patient exhausted?
5. Is the respiratory rate more than 30 breaths/min in adult or more than 50 breaths in a child?
6. Is the heart rate more than 120 beats/min in adult or more than 140 beats/min in a child?
7. Is the peak flow meter reading below 50% of the predicted patient's personal best value?
8. Has the patient not responded after adequate treatment?

Occasionally, even the patient himself fails to assess correctly the severity of the attack. This has led to less than optimum and vigorous treatment of the attack leading to a sudden unexpected death. It is therefore crucial to assess the severity of the attack immediately when the patient is seen and hospitalize the patient if necessary as per the guidelines given in Table 25.5.

| Table 25.6 Summary of drug management in asthma |

Relievers (Quick relief medications)
▪ *Short acting β_2 agonists*: First line therapy for acute attack. ▪ *Anticholinergics*: Add-on therapy to above. ▪ *Systemic corticosteroids*: For moderate to severe exacerbations. ▪ *Adrenaline and aminophylline*: In case of severe exacerbations not responding to above.
Preventers (Long-term preventive drugs)
▪ *Inhaled steroids*: Most potent anti-inflammatory agents. ▪ *Long acting β_2 agonists*: Add-on therapy to above and to prevent nocturnal attacks. ▪ *Sustained release oral theophylline*: Add-on therapy to above. ▪ *Sodium cromoglycate inhalation*: For mild disease especially in children. ▪ *Leukotriene receptor antagonists*: Further trials needed to establish exact role in asthma.

Having satisfied yourself that the patient does not require hospitalization, the 'attack' may be managed in your own 'asthma clinic' as follows:

Drug Therapy During the Attack

The conventional treatment in the recent past used to be IV aminophylline, SC adrenaline or IM or IV steroids. This approach has undergone a radical change in the past two decades.

High Dose Nebulised β_2 Agonist Treatment

Most asthmatics brought with a severe attack will be already on inhaled or oral bronchodilators. The first step should be to give a high dose of a bronchodilator usually the same agent taken at home but through a nebuliser. If the response is suboptimal, nebulised ipratropium can be added.

Subcutaneous Terbutaline

If there is no response after nebulised salbutamol plus ipratropium, terbutaline can be given subcutaneously in a dose of 0.25–0.50 mg.

Corticosteroids

Corticosteroids are life-saving in such a situation and it cannot be emphasized enough that steroids are quite safe as a short-term therapy and definitely safer than a poorly controlled attack of asthma. The usual mistake is to postpone initiating steroids or to give too small a dose for too short a time. Failure to initiate systemic steroids early and in high doses has been shown to be a factor responsible for deaths during a severe attack. The maximum benefit obtained from steroids is seen after 6–8 hrs after the initial dose and hence they must be initiated as early as possible. Hydrocortisone hemisuccinate (Efcorlin) 200 mg stat IV should be given followed by oral prednisolone 40–60 mg/day.

Adrenaline

If in spite of the above measures the bronchospasm fails to get relieved, injectable adrenaline is worth a trial. It is administered subcutaneously in a dose of 0.2–0.5 mL of a 1 in 1000 aqueous solution. The relief is usually dramatic. If not, the same dose can be repeated after 15 min. The injection may be accompanied by palpitations, headache or tremors. It is absolutely necessary to check that the needle is not in a vein before injecting as intravenous adrenaline could be disastrous. Adrenaline can be dangerous in patients with any cardiac disease, hypertensives and in elderly asthmatics. With the availability of more safer drugs, the use of adrenaline has declined.

Aminophylline

If adrenaline fails to relieve the bronchospasm in about half an hour, intravenous aminophylline is given. It is a drug with low safety profile and may cause death if given too quickly or if a large dose is given, particularly in the presence of cardiac damage or to a patient who is already on theophylline therapy. Aminophylline is given as an initial loading dose of 250 mg (or 5 mg/kg body weight) diluted in 20 mL of 5% dextrose given intravenously slowly over a period of 20–30 min. The loading dose should be omitted, if the patient is already on oral theophylline. If necessary, the loading dose can be followed by slow intravenous infusion at a rate of 0.5 mg/kg/hr.

Antibiotics

Unfortunately, in practice, antibiotics are given routinely in every severe attack of bronchospasm. Severity of the attack is no indication for antibiotic therapy. Even when the attack is preceded by an infection, the causative organism is usually a virus not susceptible to antibiotic therapy. Only when the patient has purulent sputum during the attack, antibiotics are indicated and then amoxicillin is most appropriate.

An attack of moderate severity is usually terminated within 2 hrs by these measures, which can be easily carried out in the clinic itself and little else is necessary. The patient can be sent home with a prescription of prednisolone 30–40 mg/day (to be gradually tapered off) and an increased dose of inhaled bronchodilator and inhaled corticosteroid. However, if the patient does not respond by this time, it should be treated as a case of status asthmaticus and shifted to a hospital.

MANAGEMENT OF CHRONIC ASTHMA

The management of a chronic asthmatic will depend on how frequent the attacks are occurring and with what severity. If the attacks occur very infrequently such as once a month "rescue therapy" with bronchodilator drugs which relieve the bronchospasm immediately is all that is required. If the attacks are more frequent such as more than twice or thrice a week, then it is better to prevent the attacks (rather than respond to them) with drugs like inhaled steroids or sodium cromoglycate ("preventers"). The severity of the attack is going to dictate how aggressive the treatment is going to be and with what drugs. The following are the guidelines for the treatment of chronic asthma according to increasing severity and frequency:

Mild Intermittent Asthma

This means the attacks are occurring only occasionally *less than once a week* or so and are mild in nature. Rescue therapy with salbutamol preferably via the inhaled route is advocated. If the response is less, then adequate addition of inhaled ipratropium bromide using a metered dose inhaler (MDI) or a rotahaler is all that is usually required. Oral salbutamol alone or in combination with theophylline as and when required can be used if the attacks are far in between. Under the circumstances the patient many times prefers to and finds it convenient and economical to stock a few bronchodilator tablets rather than an inhaler.

Mild Persistent Asthma

Under this category are patients who have attacks *more than twice a week* but not daily. All patients with persistent asthma have extensive inflammation of the airways and hence treatment should be with regular anti-inflammatory drugs, either inhaled sodium cromoglycate or inhaled corticosteroids ("preventers").

- Inhaled SCG can be given through a rota haler at a dose of 20 mg four times a day. Compliance is less because of the high frequency of the doses used for prophylaxis and the irritant property of SCG.

- Low dose inhaled steroids are therefore preferred, e.g., beclomethasone diproprio-nate via a MDI. The dose of this steroid in adults should be 500–800 μg/day in two divided doses.
- If in spite of the above prophylactic treatment, breakthrough attacks occur, these should be treated by short-acting inhaled bronchodilator via a MDI or through a nebuliser.

Severe Persistent Asthma

In this category, the patients have attacks *daily,* affecting their lifestyle and their work. Hence, they require high dose inhaled steroids and long acting inhaled bronchodilators as daily prophylaxis.

- High dose of inhaled steroids like beclomethasone diproprionate 1500–2000 μg/day twice daily is recommended. At this dose suppression of hypothalamus–pituitary–adrenal axis is possible. Oral candidiasis and aphonia are common. The latter complications can be reduced by using a large spacer device along with a MDI and gargling after each dose.
- Long acting bronchodilators may be required daily depending on the severity. This will be in the form of inhaled salmeterol or a sustain release oral preparation or salbutamol or theophylline.
- Frequent use of short acting bronchodilator through MDI or nebuliser in case of exacerbations.
- Oral prednisolone 30–40 mg/day, the whole daily dose being given in the morning, may be required frequently to tide away crises.

For monitoring your asthmatic patients, the peak flow meter is extremely useful. First record the patient's "personal best" PEFR. This is done when the patient is asymptomatic. Every time the patient attends your asthma clinic for an exacerbation, record the PEFR by the peak flow meter. If the patient's PEFR is within 20% of his personal best reading, all is well. If not, increase the dose of the prophylactic medicine and reassess the trigger factors, compliance, etc., educate the patient about the peak flow meter and advise him to use it at home to monitor his condition, similar to a glucometer for diabetics.

Conclusion: Having now equipped yourself with the knowledge of various inhalation devices available in the market and the techniques to use them, the emergency management of a severe attack of asthma and your classic way of managing your chronic asthmatic, you are now fully dressed up to start an asthma clinic from tomorrow. Just buy a nebuliser, a peak flow meter, the drugs mentioned under "Inhalation devices & techniques" earlier in this chapter, and declare yourself as an '*asthma-specialist*'. In a few days time there will be a flow of asthmatics coming for nebulisation. Parents will bring children who have been prescribed nebulisation by paediatrician to your clinic. Patients newly diagnosed as having asthma by your neighbouring general practitioner will come to you for a higher opinion and probably remain with you for a lifetime. And in time to come, a chestful of asthmatic patients will be discussing in your OPD without panting for breath, the bad old yesteryears of asthmatics.

| **Table 25.7** Management of chronic asthma |

Category	Symptoms	Preventers	Relievers
Step I Mild intermittent	Less than once a week. Brief episodes	Nil	Inhaled salbutamol sos
Step II Mild persistent	More than twice a week but not daily. Prolonged episodes.	Low dose inhaled steroids daily	Inhaled salbutamol sos
Step III Severe persistent	Continual symptoms Limited physical activity Frequent exacerbations	High dose inhaled steroids + long acting bronchodilator daily	Inhaled salbutamol sos oral prednisolone sos

This chapter has been reviewed by ***Dr Himanshu Pophale****, MD, Chest Physician, Pune.*

GP Tip

How do you auscultate the child who refuses to take deep breaths?

Ask him to blow hard on the handkerchief held in front of his mouth. Auscultate during and after the blowing act for clear and loud expiratory and inspiratory sounds.

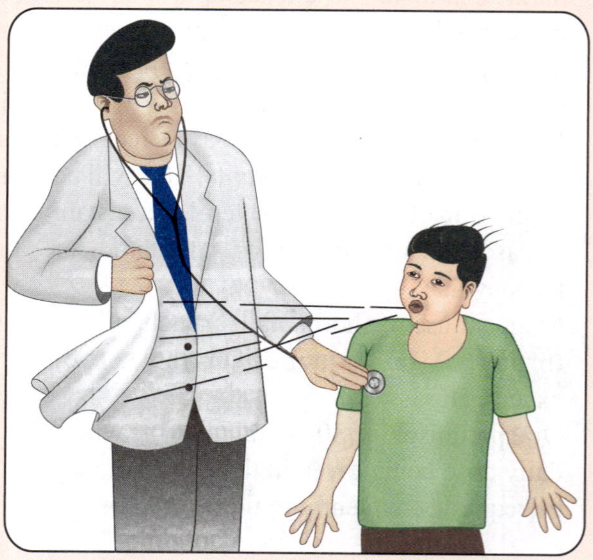

CHAPTER 26

ABC of Hypertension

- Definitions and Classification
- Symptoms of Hypertension
- Measurement of BP
- Confirmation of Hypertension
- Evaluation of Patient
- Drugs used to Control Hypertension
- How to Initiate Drug Therapy in Hypertension
- Continuation of Treatment
- Special Problems Faced by GPs

Hypertension has been rightly described as a "silent killer". Most of the patients with hypertension are not aware of its presence and therefore do not take any treatment. The result is that they suddenly land up with complications of hypertension (like myocardial infarction, stroke, renal failure, etc.) and ultimately die. Even in a rich country like USA, many cases remain undiagnosed and they have described this default as the "rule of halves". This means that in spite of their best efforts:

- Only half of the hypertension patients are ever diagnosed.
- Of these only half receive treatment.
- Of these only half will have adequate control of their blood pressure.

This effectively means that <15% of the total hypertensive patients will be correctly diagnosed and treated. This is the situation in USA, where almost the whole population gets a routine and free check up, whether they have any symptoms or not. In India, where the majority of the patients approach the doctor only, if they have symptoms, the situation must be disastrous and left best to imagination as there are hardly any systematic studies in this direction.

DEFINITIONS AND CLASSIFICATION

It is impossible to give a precise definition of hypertension, as there is controversy as to what constitutes "normal blood pressure". Logically speaking, normal blood pressure is that range of blood pressure where the person has virtually no chance of getting hypertensive complications in the long run. This line of demarcation between normal BP and high BP varies depending on different sources and different population surveys. For a long time, high BP included all values more than 140/90 mm Hg and according to severity, was classified as mild, moderate or severe. This definition has been subjected to changes in the last few decades. The recent classification (May 2003) as given by JNC-7 is given in Box 1. In contrast to classification given in JNC-6, a new category designated as pre-hypertension has been added and stage II and III hypertension have been combined.

The rationale of introducing the concept of "pre-hypertension" is the observation that these subjects of population have double the risk of progression to hypertension than do normotensives. According to JNC-7, normal BP is <120/80 mm Hg and pre-hypertension is systolic BP < 140 or diastolic BP < 90 mm Hg.

| **Box 1** Definition and classification of hypertension (Joint National Committee, May 2003) (simplified |

Classification	Systolic BP (mm Hg)		Diastolic BP (mm Hg)
Normal	<120	and	<80
Pre-hypertension	<140	or	<90
Stage I hypertension	<160	or	<100
Stage II hypertension	>160	or	>100

1. **Essential or primary or idiopathic hypertension**
   Terms used when the cause of raised BP is not known. Classically, both systolic and diastolic BP are raised. Common in young and middle aged.
2. **Isolated systolic hypertension (ISH)**
   Only the systolic pressure is raised above 160 mm Hg while diastolic BP is below 90 mm Hg. It is common in elderly because of stiffness of the arteries.
3. **Secondary hypertension**
   The cause of hypertension is known. Seen in <5% of patients.
4. **Accelerated hypertension**
   Patients in whom the BP has accelerated rapidly to severe levels from previously mild to moderate levels, but have not developed complications.
5. **Malignant hypertension**
   Patients with stage II hypertension having severe headache, vomiting, visual disturbance, convulsions, stroke or coma.
6. **Resistant hypertension**
   Hypertensive patients who do not become normotensive despite maximum doses of 3 drugs given for at least 3–4 months.

SYMPTOMS OF HYPERTENSION

How does the Patient Present?

It is of utmost importance to note that *most of the patients with hypertension do not have any symptoms at all*. They are most of the time detected on routine physical examination. The only symptom that hypertension (without complications) can cause is headache. The typical headache described is throbbing, occipital and is present in mornings and subsides by noon. But even this symptom is present only when diastolic BP is persistently above 120 mm Hg.

The popular symptoms of hypertension firmly embedded in the minds of the lay people all over in India (and probably all over the world) are dizziness, palpitations, fatigue, insomnia, etc. These are classical symptoms of anxiety and depression and whenever an anxious patient gets these symptoms, the patient feels that he must be having high BP and will demand and expect his GP to measure his BP. The positive side of this scenario is that many cases of hypertension are in this manner accidentally detected and treated. Of course, when a hypertensive patient gets complications, he has many symptoms and signs, e.g., he may have blurring of vision because of retinopathy, dyspnoea because of heart failure, etc.

MEASUREMENT OF BLOOD PRESSURE

This is a simple procedure but if carried out incorrectly often leads to inaccurate readings. As such many normotensives are wrongly diagnosed as hypertensive, unnecessarily treated, resulting in loss of money and undue side effects to the person. The correct technique is described below.

Positioning the Patient

Seat the patient on a chair comfortably (rather than on the examination table) with the bare arms supported on a table or resting comfortably by the side so that the midpoint of the upper arm is at the level of the heart. Ensure that the sleeve of the shirt is not rolled up above the elbow, which will then act as a tourniquet and give false readings. Ideally, clothing should be removed from the arm. If not, it is better to leave it as it is and BP measured over the clothing.

The Cuff and the Bladder

Cuff is the cloth that encloses the rubber bladders. Wrap the cuff snugly around the center of the patient's upper arm and secure it with the attached Velcro. The cuff should not be loose and its lower border should be 1 inch above the cubital fossa, where the diaphragm of the stethoscope is to be placed. The tubes from the bladder should emerge proximally, thus leaving the cubital fossa free for auscultation.

Taking the Reading

First take the systolic BP by the *palpatory method*. Inflate the cuff rapidly to a pressure of 20 mm Hg above the point when the radial pulse disappears. Then deflate slowly, all the while palpating the radial pulse. Note the level at which the pulse appears. This is the approximate systolic pressure. Diastolic pressure cannot be measured by this method.

Now the accurate systolic and diastolic pressure is measured by *auscultatory method*.

Place the diaphragm of the stethoscope firmly over the brachial artery, which is felt just medial to the biceps tendon in the cubital fossa. Inflate the bladder rapidly to a pressure 30 mm Hg above systolic pressure determined by the palpatory method. Partially unscrew the valve and deflate gradually while listening to the Korotkoff's sounds. Note the level at which the Korotkoff's sound first appears (phase I). This is the systolic BP. Continue deflating the bladder slowly and note the level at which the Korotkoff sounds disappear (phase V). This is the diastolic BP. It should be recorded to the nearest 2 mm Hg, i.e., do not record the reading as "95 mm Hg diastolic." Wait for 1 min. Repeat the BP reading and average the two readings. Phase III and IV sounds have no clinical significance. Occasionally, the sounds continue to be heard to a level of almost '0' mm Hg. In such a case, the diastolic BP should be recorded as a level at which the sounds get muffled (phase IV). Occasionally, the Korotkoff's sounds are not clearly audible. You can make these more audible by asking the patient to open and close the fist forcefully 5–6 times when the cuff pressure is above 200 mm Hg. After this, auscultation by routine method will give you louder sounds.

Which Type of Instrument should be Used?

It is best to use a mercury sphygmomanometer as it is accurate and requires little maintenance. If the aneroid instrument is used, calibrate it every 2–3 years as after this period, it starts giving false readings. The electronic instruments currently available are inaccurate and best avoided at present.

Lying, Sitting or Standing Position?

Ideally, the BP should be measured in the sitting position as described above, though the lying down position is a convenient alternative used by most doctors. In the standing position, the systolic BP may fall a little while diastolic BP remains unchanged in hypertensive patients without any complications. In patients complicated by autonomic neuropathy, in elderly patients and in patients on prazosin, postural hypotension can occur.

Under these circumstances, the BP should be taken in lying, sitting and standing positions. Also the BP reading should be taken in all the 3 positions in a newly diagnosed case.

Which Arm?

As some studies have demonstrated significant differences between BP readings in the left and right arm, it is advisable to record readings from both the arms at initial examination. If the difference is >20 mm Hg for systolic and 10 mm Hg for diastolic, the patient should be referred for further evaluation.

What are the Factors Affecting the BP Readings?

The BP is influenced by many factors such as emotions, exercise, tobacco, alcohol, severe pain, coffee intake, bladder distension, etc. It is usually lowest during sleep. It may not be possible to modify all the factors during BP recording, but weightage must be given to these factors while interpreting the readings.

CONFIRMATION OF HYPERTENSION

Once hypertension is suspected on initial readings, it has to be confirmed by repeated follow up readings. There is no hurry to institute antihypertensive drugs unless the patients have stage II HTN when the patient has to be evaluated immediately (see below). Pre-hypertensives should be re-checked every 6 months to 1 year, while stage I hypertension should be followed up every month and if found to be hypertensive in the follow up visits, should be evaluated and treated.

EVALUATION OF PATIENT

Once it is confirmed that the patient has hypertension, before the patient is put on antihypertensive drugs, the patient should be evaluated with the following objectives in mind:

1. **Rule out secondary hypertension** (Box 3). In <5% of patients with hypertension a cause of elevated BP can be found. Nevertheless, it is important to identify these patients, as with proper treatment, they can be cured permanently. So when do you suspect secondary hypertension?
   - Any newly diagnosed *young* hypertensive.
   - Patients whose BP is not controlled with drugs (resistant hypertension).

Box 2 What is the (so-called) "white coat hypertension"?

This is a condition where in a normotensive subject, the BP recorded by a doctor in his clinic is high because of extreme anxiety. This becomes normal outside the clinic or at the patient's home. Hence, no patient should be put on antihypertensive drugs on the basis of a single reading. The patient usually becomes less anxious with repeated visits to the doctor, and the BP comes down to normal. These patients may progress to sustained hypertension in the long run and should be therefore followed up at regular intervals. (In India, where GPs usually do not wear white aprons in their clinics, we can call this phenomenon as "*clinic or dispensary hypertension*!") In big cities, "*ambulatory BP measurement*" is available where BP is monitored throughout the day while the patient is doing his routine work. This solves the issue.

- Patients with *accelerated* or *malignant* hypertension.
- The most common causes of secondary hypertension are the various *renal* causes (3–4%). Usually, there are no symptoms or physical findings, but the presence of albumin, RBCs or casts in urine or abnormality of kidneys in USG of abdomen should alert the general practitioner about the presence of secondary hypertension.

| **Box 3** Causes of secondary hypertension |

1. **Renal** (3–4%)
   - Glomerulonephritis
   - Renal artery stenosis
   - Pyelonephritis
2. **Endocrine**
   - Cushing's syndrome
   - Pheochromocytoma
3. **Coarctation of aorta**
4. **Drugs**
   - Oral steroids
   - OC pills
   - Antidepressant
   - Decongestants
   - Analgesics

Coarctation of aorta is a rare cause. Majority of the patients would have been already diagnosed in childhood. A few patients are diagnosed when adults. They present with pain in the calf (claudication). If you palpate the radial and femoral artery simultaneously, there is a delay in the arrival of the femoral pulse, which will also be of low volume.

Pheochromocytoma should be suspected in young HTNve patients who get attacks of sweating, palpitation, tachycardia and raised BP.

Patients who are steroid dependent commonly get HTN. About 5% patients on *OC pills* get significant rise in diastolic BP. These patients need discontinuation of the pills.

2. **Find out** what are the chances your patient will develop **complications** of hypertension in the near future or has he developed these complications already?

   Luckily for a general practitioner this requires very few investigations.

   A thorough history and physical examination is most of the times all that is required, which should be done with the risk factors and possible complications in mind (see **Boxes 4 and 5**).

| **Box 4** Complications of hypertension |

Organ that can be damaged	Possible complications
Heart	Left ventricular hypertrophy Myocardial infarction Heart failure
Brain	Stroke
Kidney	Renal insufficiency
Retina	Retinopathy
Blood vessels	Peripheral vascular disease Dissecting aortic aneurysm

| **Box 5** Risk factors for developing complications of hypertension |

- Cigarette smoking
- Obesity
- Physical inactivity
- Hyperlipidaemia
- Excessive alcohol
- Diabetes
- F/H/O premature deaths due to MI

3. **Investigate the patient**

   Again with the above objectives in mind, certain **basic screening tests** are recommended for all patients:

   a) Urine analysis
   b) CBC
   c) Blood urea or creatinine
   d) Blood sugar

e) Serum lipids
f) Serum electrolytes
g) ECG

These tests will help in detecting secondary hypertension, possible renal damage that has already occurred, diabetes, hyperlipidaemia, etc. ECG will show whether left ventricular hypertrophy has developed, which is a major risk factor for development of cardiac complications. If these tests do not show any abnormality we can safely label the patient as having 'essential' hypertension and initiate treatment. More sophisticated investigations such as 2D Echo, plasma renin levels, etc., are not routinely required. These are to be done only, if BP control is not achieved with the maximum doses of 3 drugs given for at least 3 months (resistant hypertension) and are best done under the directions of a cardiologist.

DRUGS USED TO CONTROL HYPERTENSION

In order to use antihypertensive drugs correctly, a brief resume of the 5 classes of drugs that are commonly used is given below.

Thiazide Diuretics

These drugs are extremely useful in treating mild to moderate hypertension. They have been clearly shown to reduce incidence of stroke and heart attacks in long-term trials. In addition, they enhance the action of other hypotensive agents and are therefore used in combination with other hypotensive agents. They are first drug of choice in isolated systolic hypertension in elderly patients.

However, in recent years their use has diminished because of the fear of their side effects, which include adverse metabolic effects like hyperglycaemia, hyperuricaemia, hypocalcaemia, hyperlipidaemia and hypokalaemia.

Another problem with their use is that they decrease quality of life of the hypertensive patient by causing loss of energy, increased urination, loss of drive, nightmares, impotence, etc. Nevertheless in the long run, mildly increased uric acid levels do not cause symptomatic gout, serum cholesterol levels are only increased in the initial few months of therapy and potassium loss is not severe enough to warrant prophylactic supplement of potassium.

Thiazide diuretics like *hydrochlorthiazide*, *xipamide* or *indapamide* are used in low doses only. High doses increase the side effects without increasing the hypotensive effect. Frusemide is not used as it can cause severe electrolyte imbalance. *Spirinolactone*, *triamterene* and *amiloride* are potassium sparing diuretics (i.e., cause retention of potassium) and hence are used in combination with thaizide diuretics.

Beta Blockers

They decrease blood pressure by inhibiting cardiac contractility and heart rate, thus reducing the cardiac output and arterial pressure. Because of low incidence of side effects, low cost and once-a-day regime, they are the first choice drugs in *young hypertensives* and in those with *ischaemic heart disease*, especially post-myocardial infarction. They are very useful when used in combination with thiazide diuretics or calcium channel blockers.

However, these agents can precipitate heart failure in patients with cardiac enlargement as they decrease cardiac contractility, can precipitate bronchospasm in susceptible individuals and should be used with caution in diabetics as they can mask symptoms of hypoglycaemia. Like thiazide diuretics, these drugs can also affect the quality of life of the hypertensive individual.

Direct Vasodilators

The most commonly used vasodilator *hydralazine*, causes direct relaxation of the smooth muscles of the peripheral blood vessels and thus corrects the primary abnormality of hypertension. Unfortunately, it also causes sympathetic stimulation, which increases the cardiac output and heart rate, thus practically nullifying the hypotensive effect caused by vasodilatation. However, the efficacy of hydralazine can be increased by using it in combination with a beta-blocker, which blocks the sympathetic stimulation of the heart.

The side effects of hydralazine are mainly because of vasodilatation, i.e., facial flushing, throbbing headache, dizziness, palpitations, anginal pain and nasal stuffiness. Long-term use can give rise to SLE-like syndrome and therefore its use has declined. It is still used in severe hypertensive emergencies. Other vasodilator drugs like *minoxidil*, *diazoxide*, *nitroprusside* are also used only in hypertensive emergencies.

ACE Inhibitors

They decrease blood pressure by inhibiting the enzyme (angiotensin converting enzyme) that converts angiotensin I to angiotensin II. Angiotensin II is a powerful vasoconstrictor, which increases the blood pressure.

ACE inhibitors are now regarded as the first choice hypertensives as they can be virtually used in all cases of hypertension. They are as effective as beta-blockers or thiazide diuretics in young individuals, that too with fewer side effects. They do not affect the quality of life of the individuals. They are also the preferred agents in the elderly with heart failure or diabetes. Used alone, they control hypertension in 60–70% of the patients. Used in combination with low dose thiazide diuretics, their efficacy is enhanced to 90–95%. Here, the low dose diuretic does not cause metabolic side effects. These drugs are particularly effective in patients with heart-failure (where beta-blockers should not be used) and in type I DM to prevent progression of renal disease.

Captopril is getting out of use as it needs to be given at least three times a day and can cause first-dose-hypotension. It is better to use *enalapril or lisonopril* as they are to be given once a day and do not cause first-dose-hypotension.

The only side effect of ACE inhibitors is persistent dry cough. If this develops, *losarten* (which blocks the angiotensive receptors) can be used which causes cough in extremely small number of patients.

Calcium Channel Blockers (CCB)

These drugs modify the entry of calcium into cells by blocking the calcium channels. This results in vasodilatation and fall in BP. CCBs are now considered front-line antihypertensive agents. They decrease BP quickly. Unlike beta-blockers they are not contraindicated in asthma, diabetics, etc. They also do not cause metabolic side effects like diuretics. They have been shown to regress left ventricular hypertrophy. The only side effects are because of vasodilatation, i.e., flushing, dizziness, headache, palpitation, etc. They also cause ankle oedema, which does not respond to diuretics but responds to elevation of the feet. Like diuretics, they are particularly recommended for elderly patient with systolic hypertension.

There are three major classes of CCBs, which differ in their action on the heart:

a) *Nifedipine, felodipine and amlodipine* are peripheral as well as coronary vasodilators and hence used in hypertension as well as in angina. Nifedipine is rapidly absorbed. Hence it can cause rapid fall in BP, which can be dangerous in severe hypertension and in the elderly. It is also short acting and has to be given 3–4 times a day. However, slow release preparations are now available to circumvent this problem. Amlodipine has a slow onset of action, has to be taken only once a day and hence is now preferred. These drugs cause tachycardia and are hence usefully combined with a beta-blocker which causes bradycardia.

b) *Diltiazem* is again short acting and has to be given three times a day for treating hypertension. It has a better side effect profile.
c) *Verapamil*: It differs from the above in that it suppresses A-V conduction and therefore mainly used for atrial tachycardia and other arrhythmias. As beta-blockers also slow down the heart, verapamil should never be combined with a beta-blocker.

Angiotensin II Receptor Antagonists (ARBs)

These are a new class of drugs that block angiotensin II receptors. They have many features in common with ACE inhibitors. Like ACE inhibitors they are particularly useful in patients with heart failure. They have not been proved to be superior to ACE inhibitors, but absence of cough as a side effect is the biggest advantage they offer. Losartan was the first molecule to be approved and now other molecules like Irbesartan, Candesartan, Telmisartan have been introduced.

In the recommended doses given in Box 9, all ARBs have similar efficacy and none have been found to have distinctive advantage. All are potentiated by adding a diuretic. All can be combined with other antihypertensive agents for additive effects.

- ARBs are recommended in hypertensive patients to protect the kidneys. They reduce proteinuria.
- ARBs are also recommended in hypertensive patients with heart failure as significant regression of LVH is seen.

HOW TO INITIATE DRUG THERAPY IN HYPERTENSION

Once it is decided to initiate an antihypertensive drug in the patient, the selection of the drug will depend on two factors:

Age of the Patient

If the patient is young (below 55 years of age), the initial choice is an ARB. These patients also do respond to ACE inhibitors, diuretics or CCBs, but a smaller percentage of patients become normotensive.

If the patient is old (above 55 years), the initial choice is a CCB or ARB.

Again these patients also do respond to beta-blockers or ACE inhibitors, but a smaller percentage become normotensive.

Presence of Concomitant Disease (Comorbid Conditions)

If the patient is otherwise hale and hearty, not suffering from any other disease apart from hypertension, the initial drug of choice will depend on the age of the patient. However, if the patient has any of the concomitant diseases listed in Boxes 6 and 7, the choice will depend on the disease present. For example, even if the patient is young, never initiate the treatment with beta-blockers, if the patient is suffering from asthma, type I DM, peripheral vascular disease, heart failure or heart block. Similarly, do not use a diuretic in your elderly patient, if he is suffering from gout. Also, if your elderly patient has heart failure do not use a CCB. You can use an ACE inhibitor. Although they are probably second line choice to bring down the raised BP, they definitely do help in preventing infarcts.

| **Box 6** Which drug to use |

Indication	Drug preferred
▪ Diabetes with proteinuria	ACE inhibitors
▪ Isolated systolic hypertension	Diuretics, CCBs
▪ Myocardial infarction	Beta-blockers, ACE inhibitors
▪ Heart failure	ACE inhibitors
▪ Angina	Beta-blockers, CCBs
▪ Atrial tachycardia, fibrillation	Verapamil
▪ Essential tremor	Beta-blockers
▪ Hyperthyroidism with tachycardia	Beta-blockers
▪ Migraine	Beta-blockers
▪ Pregnancy	Methyl dopa

| **Box 7** Which drug to use with caution |

Indication	Drug to use with caution
▪ Asthma	Beta-blockers
▪ Depression	Beta-blockers
▪ Dyslipidaemia	Beta-blockers, Diuretics
▪ Heart failure	Beta-blockers
▪ Heart block	Beta-blockers, Verapamil
▪ Peripheral vascular disease	Beta-blockers
▪ Gout	Diuretics
▪ Diabetes	Diuretics, Beta-blockers

| **Box 8** |

Class of drug	Compelling indication	Compelling contraindication
Alpha-blockers	Prostate hypertrophy	Urinary incontinence
Beta-blockers	Post myocardial infarction Angina	Asthma COPD Heart block
ACE inhibitors	Heart failure Type I DM nephropathy	Pregnancy Renal artery stenosis
Calcium channel blockers	Elderly ISH Angina	Heart block Heart failure
Thiazides	Elderly ISH	Gout

Most physicians and cardiologists agree upon the guidelines suggested above. These guidelines have kept on changing over a period of years because of the new information gained from various clinical trials. The latest JNC-7 report strongly recommends initiation with low dose diuretics in most patients unless there is a specific contraindication for its use. However, the WHO International Society of Hypertension (WHO-ISH) report suggests somewhat a different approach. It says any drug can be used initially and adds, "*The degree of BP lowering is more important than the manner in which it is achieved.*"

CONTINUATION OF TREATMENT

Majority of the patients respond to the drug initiated in a matter of weeks without any troublesome side effects. If however the blood pressure does not come below 140/90 mm Hg with regular intake of drug and lifestyle modifications, a diuretic in a small dose may be added to the initial drug, whether it is a beta-blocker or an ACE inhibitor. If a beta-blocker was used as initial therapy, alternatively a CCB like *amlodipine* can be added, which also corrects the bradycardia induced by the beta-blockers, by its effect of producing tachycardia. If the initial drug is giving rise to troublesome side effects, the drug should be discontinued and another agent substituted.

If two-drug combination fails to achieve normotension in a few weeks, add one more drug. If even a combination of three drugs fails to achieve normotension in 2–3 months, it is a case of resistant hypertension. In such a situation:

1. Check if patient is taking drugs regularly.
2. Confirm that lifestyle modifications suggested have been implemented.
3. Investigate further with:
   a) Renal angiogram
   b) Urinary catecholamines
   c) Renin levels
   d) 2D Echo
   e) Transoesophageal 2D Echo to r/o coarctation of aorta.

Patients with resistant hypertension and malignant hypertension are better referred to and managed by competent cardiologists.

SPECIAL PROBLEMS FACED BY GPs

Cost of Treatment of Hypertension

As treatment of hypertension is life long, this becomes a very important issue for the poor patient. It is foolishness to prescribe a costly new drug to one who can ill afford it. He is bound to stop it after a few days. At the other end, we see GPs prescribing a cheap drug like 'Hydralazine', which is to be taken three times a day. Hydralazine does work, provided it is taken three

| **Box 9** Angiotensin II receptor blockers |

Drugs	Daily dosage (mg)
Losartan	50–100
Irbesartan	150–300
Valsartan	80–320
Candesartan	8–32
Telmisartan	40–80
Eprosartan	400–500

times a day. Fortunately, the situation is improving, as the commonly used drugs are now available at a lower cost.

Bad Drug Compliance

Many of the patients seen in general practice do not take the drug regularly or leave the drug after a few months because "they were feeling well." Educating the patient about his disease is of paramount importance.

The Highly-Strung Patient

The neurotic patient who thinks that his symptoms of palpitations, vertigo, tremors, etc., are related to his 'high BP' becomes a headache for the GP, because of frequent visits. Again, it is important to tell the patient that his symptoms are not due to 'high BP' and he is being given treatment to prevent heart attack, stroke, kidney failure, etc.

The Highly-Strung GP

This is another common scenario seen in general practice.

The GP is upset and irritable with BP readings like 160/96 mm Hg. He then prescribes a combination of more and more costly drugs without giving due attention to lifestyle modifications (such GPs probably become hypertensives themselves in the long run!). It is important to realize that the majority of cases that we see in general practice are mild to moderate hypertension and that hypertension is just one of the risk factors for development of MI and stroke. If the patient continues to be overweight, continues smoking, does not do proper exercise, even if his hypertension is controlled, the risk of getting MI or stroke is virtually the same.

Pseudo-Hypertension

Finally, starting antihypertensive drugs without proper confirmation is very commonly seen in general practice. The patient goes on taking antihypertensive drug for years without having hypertension at all! (I jokingly refer to this entity as 'pseudo-hypertension'!). When in doubt, it is better to withhold the drug and monitor the BP periodically. All GPs should know about the entity of '*white coat hypertension*.'

*This chapter has been reviewed by **Dr Parag Vaste**, MD, Consultant Physician, Pune.*

CHAPTER 27

ABC of Diabetes

- Management of Uncomplicated Type II Diabetes
- Role of Exercise in Type II DM
- Diet in Type II Diabetics
- OHAs in Type II DM
- Management of Type II DM with Insulin
- Types of Insulin

MANAGEMENT OF UNCOMPLICATED TYPE II DIABETES

It is estimated that every 7th patient in a GP's OPD in India is a diabetic, most of them type II diabetics. According to WHO, there are 35 lac diabetics in India. This number is increasing in leaps and bounds, so much so that it is projected that by the year 2025, there will be 55 lac diabetics in India. In a study in urban India in the year 2000, 14 out of a hundred urbanites had type II diabetes. With the dubious distinction of having the highest number of diabetics in the world, India has been declared the "*Diabetes capital of the world*" by WHO.

If then diabetes is such a common disease, every GP should be conversant with the management of diabetes, especially of type II uncomplicated diabetes. Type I DM and type II DM with complications are better managed by physicians or diabetologists. The next few pages focus mainly on management of type II DM uncomplicated diabetes. This will be dealt with under the following headings:

1. Role of exercise
2. Role of diet
3. Management with oral drugs
4. Management with insulin

| **Box 1** Laboratory criteria for diagnosis of diabetes |

- Symptoms of diabetes + Random plasma glucose > 200 mg/dL, **or**
- 8 hr fasting plasma glucose > 126 mg/dL, **or**
- 2 hr post glucose (75 g) plasma glucose > 200 mg/dL

Note:

- *Impaired fasting glucose* (IFG): Fasting BSL levels between 110 and 125 mg/dL.
- *Impaired glucose tolerance* (IGT): Post glucose plasma levels between 141 and 199 mg/dL

Patients with IFG and IGT are not labelled as diabetics but are at risk of developing diabetes and cardiovascular disease.

| **Box 2** Classification of Diabetes |

New name	Old name	Aetiology
Type I	▪ Juvenile onset DM ▪ IDDM	Autoantibodies destroy beta-cells. Therefore, there is insulin deficiency.
Type II	▪ Maturity onset DM ▪ NIDDM	Reduced insulin secretion or peripheral resistance to action of insulin.
Gestational	Gestational	Develops in pregnancy and disappears after delivery with increased risk of getting it later in life.

| **Box 3** Characteristic features of type I and type II DM |

Type I DM: Due to auto-antibodies against insulin

1. Commonly develops in children and young adults.
2. Acute or subacute in onset.
3. Tendency to ketoacidosis.
4. Insulin dependent.

Type II DM: Due to decreased insulin sensitivity and beta-cell failure.

1. Very common. Seen in 95% of total diabetics.
2. 80% are overweight.
3. Insidious onset.
4. Seen in individuals over 30 years of age.
5. Can be managed by oral drugs + diet + exercise. Insulin may or may not be required.

| **Box 4** Monitoring control in type II DM |

1. **Fasting BSL**: Ideal parameter. Should be done every month.
2. **PP BSL and random BSL**: Unreliable parameters. Can be used, if fasting BSL not possible. Do not make major changes in insulin or OHL based on PP or random BSL.
3. **Urine test with diastix**: Gives rough estimate of control.
4. **Home monitoring with glucometer**: Usually not required.
5. **Glycosylated Haemoglobin A_1C (GHb A_1C)** should be done every 6 months. Should be <7%.
6. **Weight record**: Good parameter.

| **Box 5** Complications of diabetes: A silent killer |

1. **Infections** like cellulitis, pulmonary Koch's, etc.
2. **Short-term metabolic complications**
   - Drug-induced hypoglycaemia
   - Ketoacidosis
3. **Long-term angiopathic complications**
   - Microvascular (small vessels)
     - Retinopathy
     - Nephropathy
     - Neuropathy
   - Macrovascular (large vessels)
     - Coronary artery disease
     - Cerebrovascular disease
     - Peripheral vascular disease

ROLE OF EXERCISE IN TYPE II DM

"Doctor, but I don't have any time for exercise because of my busy schedule". This is a common reply that we general practitioners get when we advise any patient to do exercises. Even after a lot of persuasion the patient ends up not doing the exercises recommended by us but instead buys a stationary fancy cycle or a treadmill. This instrument after a few months of initial enthusiasm remains as a showpiece in the drawing hall or is used as a hanger to dry wet clothes! So the major problem a GP faces is how to persuade the diabetic to do regular exercise. It is a difficult task, by any standards. In my initial days of practice, I used to present the patient with a "menu card of diseases". For example, I used to tell them "If you don't exercise, in a few years you might get a heart attack or a stroke, high BP, OA knee, etc". I have now realized that this is not working. So, now I have changed my strategy. Rather than putting the fear of diseases in them, I tell them the positive effects of exercise, e.g., "your heart will become strong and you will have a shapely body and you will be saving Rs 3 lac for a coronary bypass surgery." Such motivation usually yields better results (see **Box 6**).

Box 6 Benefits of exercise in a diabetic

1. Reduces blood glucose.
2. Reduces insulin and oral drug requirement to control BSL.
3. Helps in reducing weight.
4. In mild diabetics (type 2), exercise & diet alone will help in controlling blood sugar levels.
5. Increase in good (HDL) cholesterol level and decrease in bad (LDL) cholesterol.
6. Lots of other benefits like improvement of blood circulation in legs, increased stamina and improved quality of life.

Precautions

Proper exercises, no doubt enhance the quality of life of the diabetic. However, in diabetics with complications like neuropathy, nephropathy, retinopathy and CVS complications, exercises should be done with caution. Even in diabetics without complications, but on insulin, heavy exercises can induce sudden hypoglycaemia leading to collapse on the street or on the ground. To prevent this:

- He should always eat 2 biscuits before exercise and in addition carry glucose powder in his pocket.
- He should not take insulin on the moving part of the body, e.g., thigh.
- He should not exercise during peak insulin time, i.e., 3 hrs after intermediate acting insulin. The ideal time is to exercise in the morning after a light breakfast.

Which Type of Exercises should you Advise?

The common alternatives that the patient has are dynamic (or aerobic) exercise, static (or anaerobic) exercise, work up in a gymnasium or doing yoga. Yoga cannot be considered an exercise in the true sense, as it does not burn calories. Neither does it rapidly pump the heart. Nevertheless, it can be performed in addition to other exercises.

Dynamic exercises are best suited for the diabetic patients. There are prolonged repetitive movements, which use oxygen from the atmosphere, burn calories and give a workout for the heart, thus preventing cardiovascular complication. Walking, jogging, cycling, swimming, playing badminton or tennis are dynamic exercises. **Static exercises** like weight lifting do not offer the above advantages and hence should not be recommended. Fancy exercises in health clubs or gymnasiums are recommended as a last resort, if the patient fails to get motivated for outdoor aerobic exercises.

Ideally, the patient should do dynamic exercises up to 45 min a day at least 5 times a week. How fast should he walk, jog or cycle for optimum benefits? This is achieved by keeping the pulse rate within the **target heart rate zone**, which is 60–80% of the maximum heart rate (MHR). MHR = 220 minus the age of the patient, e.g., if the patient is 50-year old, his MHR is 170/min. To keep himself in the target heart rate zone, initially for a month or so, the patient should maintain his pulse during exercise at approximately 100/min (60% of 170) for at least 10–15 min. He can gradually increase it to about 135/min (80% of 170). It has been shown that at the lower end of this zone, calories are burnt and at the upper end of this zone, patient has a better cardiac profile.

If the GP or the patient finds this formula confusing, or keeping a tab on the pulse during exercise is difficult, tell him "You are below this zone if you can sing during exercise, and you are above this zone if you cannot talk a sentence without taking a breath." Rich patients can use a treadmill fitted with a minicomputer, which shows his pulse rate and also the number of calories burnt as he walks or runs on the machine.

And as a last resort, for patients who just won't do regular exercises, give them the following advice:

1. Avoid lifts—walk up the stairs.
2. Park your vehicle far away from your destination and then walk the distance speedily.
3. Do not use cordless phone or remote control for your TV.
4. Involve in household activities like cleaning, helping your partner, etc.
5. Whenever possible:

   "Sit, instead of lying down
   Stand, instead of sitting down
   Walk, instead of standing up
   Jog, instead of strolling down."

DIET IN TYPE II DIABETICS

10Diabetes is one of the few diseases where diet plays a very important role in the management. About 30% of type II diabetics can be managed only by diet and exercise. In the rest, it is an integral part of the treatment programme. In spite of this, I regret to add, a very superficial dietary advice is given by majority of GPs. I remember a prescription for a newly diagnosed diabetic, which ended with "No sugar. Avoid potatoes. Little rice." At the other extreme, we see young inexperienced dieticians chalking out a rigid diet plan, which makes life miserable for the diabetic. While giving dietary advice, the GP should strike a mean between these two extreme recommendations.

Principles

A fundamental knowledge of the principles of diet therapy is necessary in order to plan the diet in your diabetic patient.

1. Immediately after the diagnosis of diabetes is made, the general practitioner should give the patient a general idea about what foods he has to avoid and what foods he can take in plenty (see Box 7).

| Box 7 |

1. *Foods to be avoided*—sugar, sweets, chocolates, ice cream, soft drinks, fried foods, groundnuts, coconut, papad, pickles.
2. *Foods which can be taken liberally*— wheat, jowar, bajari, pulses, green leafy vegetables, salads.

2. Traditionally, Indians usually take 2 large meals in a day. This should be avoided, as this is likely to cause large fluctuations in the blood sugar levels. Hence, the patient should be advised to take **3 major meals** (breakfast, lunch and dinner) & **2 small meals** (afternoon and bed time). The cooking pattern

and the type of food the patient is taking for years, should not be changed radically, it should only be modified.

3. The patient's attitude towards diet need not be too rigid as long as his glycosylated haemoglobin is normal. Religious fasts can be observed provided the total caloric requirement is not exceeded and the fast is not total. If the patient wishes to have a sweet dish occasionally, he should be allowed to do so, preferably by using artificial sweeteners like saccharin or aspartame (Sweeter, Equal, etc.). Similarly, diet should be adjusted for receptions and tours.
4. **Carbohydrates** should form about 50–60% of the total calories. Simple sugars like common sugar, glucose, ice creams and cakes should be avoided as they are rapidly absorbed and cause postprandial hyperglycaemia. Complex sugars, which are present in pulses, dals, cereals, etc., on the other hand cause a gradual rise in blood sugar and should form an integral part of diet planning.
5. **Fats and oils**: Not more than 20% of the total calories should come from fats and oils and these should be in the form of oils that contain polyunsaturated fatty acids (PUFA), which prevents arteriosclerosis, heart disease and stroke. The controversies in the media and in scientific journals regarding which oil to use have confused patients as well as doctors. Patients who have not read about these controversies, innocently believe that 'desi ghee is the best.' This is far from true. Then, which is the best oil to use? Let us clarify the issue.

Fats are divided into three broad classes, viz., saturated fatty acids (SFA), polyunsaturated fatty acids (PUFA) and monounsaturated fatty acids (MUFA).

SFAs present in foods like butter, ghee, egg yolk, meat, beef, pork, etc., elevate bad cholesterol (LDL) that causes heart trouble and hence should be avoided. PUFAs are present in most of the vegetable oils like safflower oil, soyabean oil, til oil, kardi oil (except coconut oil). PUFAs lower the bad cholesterol, thus preventing arteriosclerosis. MUFA, present in groundnut oil also lowers the bad cholesterol. Essential fatty acids like Omega-6 (present in vegetable oils) and Omega-3 (present in fish) also lower the bad cholesterol.

Most of the animal fats are high in cholesterol and should be restricted. The exception is fish oil, which contains linolenic acid, which protects against arteriosclerosis.

So what should be our advice to our patients to reduce bad cholesterol in blood?

- Have any vegetable oil except coconut oil as cooking media.
- Avoid egg yolk, meat, etc.
- Avoid foods rich in saturated fats like ghee, butter, vanaspati, etc.
- Milk should be used after removal of the cream.
- Avoid deep fry foods like chivada, bhajia, papad, batata wada etc.

Planning the Diabetic Diet

Armed with these facts, we can now proceed in planning the diet of our diabetic patient. At the outset, the weight of the patient should be taken to find out whether the patient is overweight, of normal weight or underweight. This can be ascertained by referring to the standard life insurance tables. Alternatively, a simple method of determining the ideal body weight is to subtract the number 100 from the patient's height in centimeters, e.g., for a patient of 160 cm in height, the ideal weight is 160 – 100 = 60 kg. The dietary advice to your diabetic patient then depends on his weight and whether he has type I or type II diabetes.

1. Type I insulin-dependent diabetics are better managed by a diabetologist or a general physician.
2. For type II diabetics who are underweight or are of normal weight, there need not be any restrictions on the amount of intake, as long as he or she complies with the food, which is suggested to be taken in **Box 2**. In other words, there is simply the limitation of all simple sugars together with modest reduction of animal fat.
3. The major bulk of the patients seen in general practice are obese type II diabetics. Here, the aim is to decrease the body weight both by reducing the calorie intake and by burning the calories consumed by vigorous exercises. Properly followed, this should result in reduction in weight to approximately the ideal weight in a few months. If unsuccessful, a vigorous diet programme is required. This includes restriction of food intake according to a pre-calculated daily calorie intake.

   The method of calculation of the daily calorie intake for such patients follows. (The calculation of daily calorie intake is also done for normal weight patients who fail to control their blood sugar in spite of adequate exercise and oral hypoglycaemic drugs.)

Method of Calculating Daily Calorie Intake

First, the daily calorie requirement is calculated by referring to **Box 8**, e.g., in an overweight diabetic, with a sedentary job and of ideal weight 60 kg, the calories required per day is 60 × 20 = 1200 calories. However, in a normal weight diabetic, of 60 kg ideal body weight, doing heavy manual work, the calories required per day is 60 × 35 = 2100 calories.

Having calculated the calorie requirement of your patient, he is given the sample menu chart given in **Box 4**. The patient should be advised to follow this chart according to his calorie requirement. In addition, the patient should be provided with an exchange list (**Box 10**), which gives foods of approximately same calorie value and hence can be substituted. This will add variety to his diet.

| Box 8 |

Weight	Type of work	Cal/kg of ideal body weight
1. **Normal**	Heavy manual work	35
2. **Normal**	Sedentary	30
3. **Overweight**	Sedentary	20

Quantifying the Degree of Obesity of Your Patient

Many different scales are used for this purpose. This includes weight, waist circumference, waist to hip ratio, skin fold thickness, body mass index, etc. Obesity is just not "excess weight than stipulated". It is the distribution of fat in the body that matters. It is the waist circumference (central obesity) that predisposes the person to heart attacks, strokes, etc. Women have a lot of fat in the gluteal region or thighs (peripheral obesity). That does not predispose them to cardiovascular accidents. (Women with big "bums" live longer than men with big bellies!) How do you then calculate the degree of obesity of your patient? There are three indices used in clinical practice.

1. **Waist circumference**: Should be <94 cm (37") in men and 80 cm (32") in women.
2. **Waist hip ratio (WHR)** should not exceed 0.9 in men and 0.85 in women.
3. **Body mass index (BMI)**: The normal range is between 18.5 and 30. It is calculated according to the following formula.

| **Box 9** Sample menu chart |

Time	Calories				
	1200	1500	1800	2000	2300 cal
Morning					
Cup of tea without sugar	1	1	1	1	1
Breakfast					
Cup of milk without sugar & cream or one egg	1	1	1	1	1
Pieces of bread	2	2	3	3	4
Mid morning					
Marie biscuits	2	3	3	3	4
Lunch					
Chapattis (No)	1	2	3	4	5
Rice (wati)	1	1	1	1	1
Dal (wati)	1	1	1	1	1
Plenty of vegetables					
Mid afternoon					
Cup of tea or coffee without sugar	1	1	1	1	1
Marie biscuits	2	3	3	3	4
Dinner	Same as lunch				
Before sleeping at night	One fruit				

MI = weight in kg/height in meters square. e.g.: If your patient's weight is 70 kg and height is 160 cm (1.6 m) = 70/1.6 × 1.6 = 70/2.56= 27, which is normal BMI.

It is important that for proper control of diabetes and to prevent CV complications, your patient's weight, WHR, BMI, etc., should be maintained in the normal range with correct diet and exercise.

| **Box 10** Exchange list |

- 1 chapatti = 2 puris = ½ paratha.
- 1 wati dal = ½ wati usal.
- 1 wati of cauliflower, bhendi, cabbage, leafy vegetable = ½ wati of potato, gram, peas, onions.
- 1 apple = ½ mango = 12 grapes.
- 1 orange = ½ banana

ORAL HYPOGLYCAEMIC AGENTS (OHAs) IN TYPE II DM

In 1970, the University Group Diabetes Program (UGDP) in USA after 8 years of study presented findings that shook diabetologists & the diabetic patients on OHAs all over the world. It concluded that the deaths from heart attacks in diabetics were higher in patients treated with OHAs than in those treated with diet or with insulin alone. This report has not been universally accepted because of the methodology used. But, the fall out of this report is that indiscriminate use of these drugs should be stopped. OHAs should only be used in type II diabetes when:

1. FBSL is <200 mg/dL (mild diabetes)
2. Patients who have failed "diet + exercise" treatment
3. Obese adult diabetics
4. Diabetes of short duration without complications.

Nevertheless, general practitioners usually prescribe OHAs mainly because:

1. It is very difficult to persuade obese adult patients to follow strict diet and exercise.
2. Patients many times refuse insulin because it has to be injected.

Luckily for the GP, unlike antihypertensive drugs, hardly a dozen OHAs are available, of which he has to get conversant with less than half a dozen.

1. Sulphonylureas (SUs)

They stimulate insulin release from the pancreas and are therefore ineffective in the absence of a functioning pancreas like in type I DM. Here, they can only be used in addition to insulin. Please refer to 'Drugs Formulary' (p. 479) for the different sulphonylureas available in the market.

Which of the sulphonylureas will you use?
The choice is not clear-cut as there is hardly any difference in the clinical efficacy of different sulphonylureas dose to dose. The choice will depend on the propensity to cause hypoglycaemia and the need to give OD or BD dose. The following general guidelines will however help:

- *Tolbutamide* (Rastinon) is preferred in old patients who get frequent episodes of hypoglycaemia.
- *Chlorpropamide* (Diabenase) is going out of use because of the prolonged and sometimes fatal hypoglycaemia it causes. It is not generally available now.
- *Glibenclamide* (Daonil) and *Glipizide* (Glynase) are both very potent and cheap drugs. They are most widely used by GPs.
- *Gliclazide* (Diamicron) is said to prevent strokes and infarcts, but is costly.
- *Glimepiride* (Glypride) is long acting and is used when single daily dose is preferred.

Hypoglycaemia is less common with sulphonylureas than with insulin, but it is more severe and prolonged (especially with chlorpropamide) and may be fatal. An insulin induced hypoglycaemic patient may be given IV or oral dextrose and can be treated on OPD basis. However, an OHA-induced hypoglycaemic patient has to be hospitalized for prolonged IV dextrose administration (see Box 11).

2. Biguanides

Phenformin has been banned because it causes lactic acidosis, which may be fatal. *Metformin* (Glyciphage) is very widely used because it is safer and is particularly useful in obese type II diabetics as it causes weight loss. It can be effectively combined with other OHAs or insulin.

The only side effect is occasional diarrhoea or heartburn, which can be minimized by giving it with or after food. Unlike sulphonylureas, it has no action on the pancreas, but acts by suppressing the release of glucose from the liver.

| **Box 11** To avoid sulphonylurea induced hypoglycaemia |

1. Do not miss a meal.
2. Do not suddenly increase exercise.
3. Avoid alcohol.
4. Elderly patients can suddenly go into hypoglycaemia without warning symptoms. Prefer weaker OHAs like tolbutamide or glipizide.
5. Try to decrease dose of sulphonylureas from time to time.

3. Acarbose (Glucobay)

This drug is used to reduce postprandial hyperglycaemia in combination with other OHAs. It acts by reducing and delaying the absorption of glucose from the intestine.

4. Glitazones

Rosiglitazone and pioglitazone are new class of drugs and are called insulin sensitizers as they potentiate the action of insulin and hence reduce the dose of insulin. They are usefully combined with others OHAs and should never be used alone.

However, there are some problems in using these highly effective drugs in general practice:

- They are very costly.
- Most of the type II DM patients are already obese, and glitazones cause increase in weight.
- Pedal oedema and puffiness of face is common and frightening to the patients.
- Hepatotoxicity is another side effect, which prohibits its use. LFTs are to be done frequently, which is not always feasible in general practice.
- As these drugs are new, long-term side effects are not known.

The biggest advantage of pio- and rosiglitazone is that they can be used in patients on insulin to reduce the dose of insulin or in patients on maximum doses of sulphonylureas plus metformin and still blood sugar control cannot be achieved. They should never be used as monotherapy, but always be added to insulin or OHAs.

Practical Management of Type II Uncomplicated Diabetes with OHAs

If the patient's blood sugar levels are not under control after about a month of proper diet plus exercise, drug therapy is instituted. It is important to note that drugs are meant to supplement diet and exercise and not to replace them.

- **Initiation of treatment** (Fig. 27.1): Determine first whether the patient is underweight, normal weight or overweight. If the patient is **underweight** or is of **normal weight**, the patient is put on ¼th the maximum effective dose of a sulphonylurea, e.g., glibenclamide, whose maximum effective dose is 20 mg, is given 2.5 mg BD before food, i.e., 5 mg daily. If BSL values are still high after 2–3 weeks, the dose is increased to half the maximum effective dose, i.e., 10 mg daily. A further dose increase is unlikely to be useful. Even a change to another sulphonylurea may not help. This is then called primary failure, which is seen in 20% of the patients. Many of the patients who initially respond to sulphonylurea, do not do so after 8–10 years of sulphonylurea therapy. This is called **secondary failure**. This is mainly due to progressive deterioration of beta function. In such cases, metformin or glitazone or both (various combinations are available) should be added,

| **Box 12** Target values as recommended by American Diabetic Association |

Target blood glucose values	▪ Fasting ▪ 2 hrs PP ▪ GHb A_1C	80–110 120–140 <6%
Target cholesterol values	▪ LDL cholesterol ▪ HDL cholesterol ▪ Triglycerides	<100 mg/dL >45 mg/dL <200 mg/dL
Target blood pressure values	▪ Systolic ▪ Diastolic	<130 mm Hg <85 mm Hg

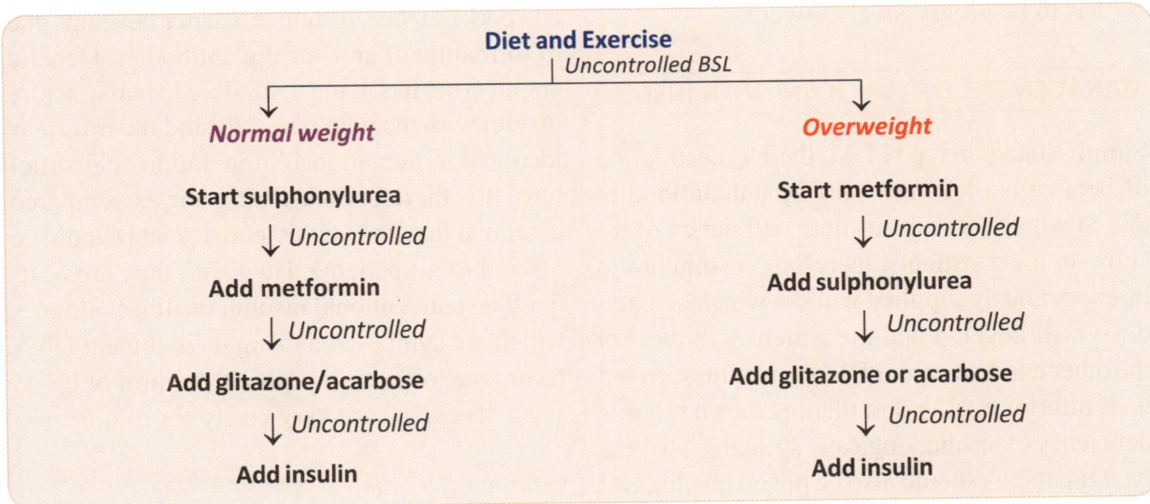

| **Fig. 27.1** Management of type II DM |

sticking to the same principle of starting with a low dose and titrating upwards every 2–3 weeks. In the event that the F-BSL is normal, but the PP-BSL is high, acarbose may be added. If all the combinations fail, then there is no option but to initiate insulin.

If the patient is **overweight**, metformin is the drug of choice as it causes weight loss, which is beneficial in these patients. Half to one tablet of 500 mg metformin BD is recommended after or during food to prevent gastritis. If BSL values are still high after 2–3 weeks, a sulphonylurea is added, either alone or with rosi- or pioglitazone. Again if these combinations fail, there is no option but to initiate insulin.

- **Maintenance treatment**: If the patient becomes euglycaemic with any of the above regimens, the corrected dose is continued and BSLs are monitored every 3–4 months along with glycosylated Hb. If these are satisfactory (FBS < 100 mg; PPBSL < 130; GHB < 6%) an attempt is made to **reduce the dose**

periodically. This is necessary because with the improvement of glycaemic control and decrease in weight, islet cell function improves and the patient may get repeated hypoglycaemic attacks.

In patients controlled on a small dose of OHA, the drug can be withdrawn abruptly. In a patient on a large dose of OHAs, the doses should be gradually tapered off. Similarly, in patients well controlled with <20 units of insulin, insulin can be stopped abruptly and the patient put on OHAs. However, if the dose of insulin is more than 20 units, the dose has to be progressively lowered.

MANAGEMENT OF TYPE II DM WITH INSULIN

Simply stated, in type I DM, there is destruction of beta cells of Langerhans by autoantibodies due to which there is absolute deficiency of insulin. In these patients, therefore, insulin has to be exogenously supplied without which ketoacidosis will develop and the patient will die. On the other hand, in type II DM the insulin secreted is of inferior quality and there is thus a relative deficiency of insulin. Logically speaking, all these type II patients should also be put on insulin. But because of the practical difficulties in giving injectable insulin for a lifetime, insulin is avoided. Nevertheless, under the following situations in type II DM, insulin use is mandatory:

1. When optimum dose of OHAs has failed.
2. During pregnancy.
3. To tide over stressful situations like major surgery, severe infections, myocardial infarction, etc.
4. Type II DM with complications.

TYPES OF INSULIN

There are five main types of insulin classified on the basis of their duration of action:

1. **Ultra short acting**: Insulin Lispro (analog) Humalog.
2. **Short acting**: Regular (soluble).
3. **Intermediate acting**: NPH isophane, Lente.
4. **Long acting**: Ultra lente
5. **Analogues**: Long acting (insulin glargine). Short acting (Lispro insulin).
6. **Premixed insulins**: Soluble + NPH; Lispro + NPH

Conventional and Newer Insulin

Conventional insulins are of animal origin (beaf and pork). Hence, insulin resistance develops due to formation of anti-insulin antibodies. Genetic engineering has made it possible to manufacture insulin with the help of *E. coli* and the insulin is identical to human insulin in amino acid structure. It is therefore least antigenic as compared to animal insulins, highly purified and should be offered to all patients. However, they are costlier than conventional insulin. Insulin analogues which are synthesized using recombinant DNA technique, offer a very smooth control of blood sugar levels but are very costly for routine use.

Initiation of Insulin

Patients who are severely ill with complications require rigid control of diabetes with 3 daily or even 4 daily insulin injections for which hospitalization becomes mandatory. Uncomplicated diabetic patients requiring insulin can be managed in general practice with once or twice daily insulin.

1. ***Twice-a-day dose***

   Most of these patients can be very well managed on this regime. Premixed insulin with 30:70 combination of soluble plus NPH (e.g., Mixtard) is used.

   The total daily dose is calculated as 1/3rd the weight of the patient. About 60% is given before breakfast and 40% before dinner, e.g.,

GENERAL PRACTICE AS SPECIALITY

in a patient weighting 60 kg, the daily dose is 20 units; 12 units are given before breakfast and 8 units before dinner. If after 4 days the FBS is still high, increase the pre-dinner dose by 4 units. If the PP BSL is high, the pre-breakfast dose is increased by 4 units.

Similar increments are made every 3rd day till both the fasting and PP BSL values are normal.

2. ***Once-a-day dose***
   Those patients who refuse 2 injections/day can be given 12–16 units either before breakfast or before dinner depending on the blood sugar levels, while continuing the oral drugs.

| **Box 13** Prevention of complications of diabetes |

1. Lifestyle modifications.
2. Strict control of blood sugar.
3. Optimum control of BP.
4. Drugs—aspirin, statins.
5. Screening for early detection of microvascular complications
   - Ophthalmoscopy
   - Urine exam for micro-albumins.
   - Regular foot examination

Conclusion: We are indeed fortunate to have OHAs acting at different levels, which ultimately results in smoother control of diabetes in majority of type 2 patients.

Sulphonylureas stimulate the pancreas to secrete more insulin, metformin reduces the release of glucose from the liver into the circulation and glitazones increase the uptake of glucose into the muscles and thus potentiate the action of endogenous insulin. In combination therefore, blood sugar is effectively lowered.

We are also fortunate to have highly purified human or porcine insulin, both short and intermediate acting. A combination of these insulins can go a long way in controlling diabetes.

The introduction of insulin analogues like short acting lispro insulin and long-acting glagine insulin will definitely add to the smoother control. Insulin has saved millions of lives in the past and will continue to do this in future. There is no parallel drug in medicine with such a track record. This wonder drug is very much under used by GPs. They readily accede to the demand of the diabetic to avoid pricks because they themselves fear initiating insulin therapy. This is understandable in type I DM, where a rigid control is required. But, there is no reason why a GP should not initiate and educate the patient to adjust the insulin doses in type II DM.

However, we are indeed unfortunate in the sense that achieving good glycaemic control is only half the battle won. Complications of diabetes can still occur, if concomitant BP is not controlled to below 130/85 mm Hg, obesity is not corrected and lipid levels remain abnormal (Box 12). Therefore, it is the duty of the general practitioner to stress the need for concomitant BP control, maintaining a good lipid profile, moderation of alcohol, cessation of smoking and a healthy life style.

*This chapter has been reviewed by **Dr Parag Vaste**, MD, Consultant Physician, Pune.*

CHAPTER 28

The Immunization Clinic

- Need for Immunization Clinic
- Important and Commonly Used Vaccines
  - BCG Vaccine
  - Polio Vaccine
  - DPT Vaccine
  - DTaP
  - Td
  - TdaP
  - Measles Vaccine
  - Mumps Vaccine
  - Rubella Vaccine
  - Tetanus Toxoid
  - Rabies Vaccine
  - Typhoid Vaccine
  - Varicella Vaccine
  - Hepatitis A Vaccine
  - Pneumococcal Vaccine
  - Meningococcal Vaccine
  - Hepatitis B Vaccine
  - Haemophilus Influenza B (Hib) Vaccine
  - Influenza Vaccine
  - Rotavirus
  - HPV Vaccines
  - Cholera Vaccine
  - Japanese Encephalitis (JE) Vaccine
  - Yellow Fever Vaccine
- Immunization Schedule
- Essential and Optional Vaccines
- Traveller's Vaccines
- Passive Immunization
- Adverse Reactions after Vaccination
- Cold Chain Guidelines for Storage of Vaccines

— **Madhu J Oswal**

NEED FOR AN IMMUNIZATION CLINIC

Don't you want to become a part of a Historical Event?

Small pox has been eradicated from the face of this planet. Now, it is the turn of the disease called poliomyelitis. In 1988, WHO decided to eradicate this disease by means of mass immunization. As a result WHO, UNICEF, Govt of India, Rotary International and other agencies came together and a record 88 million under-five children were newly vaccinated in a single day! The WHO congratulated the Government and NGOs for their supreme effort. Unfortunately it said, "the participation of private practitioners was less than adequate."

Age old diseases like measles, diphtheria, tetanus, pertussis, etc., have virtually been eliminated by extensive use of vaccines in the developed countries. In the underdeveloped countries, 2 million children die every year because of these diseases. One person dies every minute because of TB. And the cold fact is that, effective vaccines are available for these diseases for decades. One of the most important reasons for this failure of immunization is the indifference on the part of general practitioners. While GPs cater to a mammoth 70% of medical treatment in India, their contribution to disease prevention is a meagre 6%. Several studies have proved that lack of knowledge and lack of motivation on the part of general practitioners are major contributory factors for non-immunization.

My dear friends and colleagues, a little extra effort is required from us to help eradicate these diseases. Participation in mass immunization programmes will automatically make your clinic known to everybody in your locality. In addition your practice gets a big boost, as with the infant, the whole family usually gets enrolled with you. And how much do we require to start an immunization clinic? Simply:

1. A sound knowledge about vaccines,
2. A portable thermos flask,
3. A handful of vaccines and
4. A mindful of motivation!

A basic information of the important vaccines follows, without going into details of immunology and vaccinology, a subject though interesting, is probably not very useful for general practitioners.

IMPORTANT AND COMMONLY USED VACCINES

1. BCG Vaccine

There is hardly any necessity to explain how grave is the problem of tuberculosis in our country, more so in this HIV era. Every year 1.9 million children get primary infection. It is the single largest killer causing 5,00,000 deaths per year. The question is what is the role of BCG in tuberculosis prevention and control? The present consensus is that it provides 50–60% protection against childhood tuberculosis, more so against its disseminated forms, especially meningitis.

We as general practitioners are usually not required to give BCG, as it is usually given in the hospital at birth. But, we are many times consulted by parents for various queries and conditions related to BCG vaccination. The frequently asked questions are:

1. *When to give BCG vaccine*? Ideally at birth before a baby is exposed to the TB bacilli. If not at birth, then at any time at the earliest or at 6 weeks with DPT.
2. *Any child presenting before 5 years of age and with no history of BCG vaccination or no scar of BCG should be advised to take BCG?* Yes.
3. *If a baby was given BCG and 'failed' to produce a scar within 90 days, should we repeat BCG*? Yes.
4. *If a Mantoux test is done and shows induration < 5 mm, should BCG be given?* Yes. The basis of this is not very clear, but this is an accepted practice.
5. *What is the normal reaction and what is an abnormal reaction after BCG vaccination*? 2–3 weeks after a correct intradermal injection of a potent BCG vaccine, a papule develops at the site of inoculation. It reaches to a size of 4–5 mm in about a month's time after which it may subside or may break open to form a shallow ulcer—open or crusted. Healing usually occurs in 6–12 weeks leading to a permanant tiny scar of 4–8 mm size. Prolonged severe ulceration or suppurative adenitis can occur in 1–10% patients. Complications like osteomyelitis and disseminated BCG infection are very rare (1 in 1 million).

Available as *BCG* (*Serum Institute*) *at Rs. 80/- for 10 doses.*

2. Polio Vaccine

Small pox has become the disease of the past, so will polio. And with that, mankind will boast of eliminating two diseases. In 1988, the Global Polio Eradication Initiative was launched with the resolution of eradicating polio by 2005. And in 15 years, we have come a long-long way from 3,50,000 cases seen in 1988 to 14 cases in 2005. But 90% of these cases unfortunately were in India in our UP state. United States, Western Pacific region, Europe and Central Asia appear to be polio-free.

Two types of vaccines are available against polio—*live attenuated oral polio vaccine* (*OPV*) and *inactivated polio vaccine* (*IPV*).

Oral Polio Vaccine (OPV)

It gives both humoral and mucosal, i.e., intestinal immunity like the natural polio virus infection. Thus, it not only prevents paralysis of polio infected person, but it also prevents intestinal infection. This vaccine virus is excreted in the faeces and secondary spread occurs in the contacts by faeco-oral route. Thus, we get 'herd-immunity' in the community even if only 60% of children are immunized. This is utilized as a principle of pulse polio campaign to replace wild polio virus with the vaccine virus. Efficiency rate of OPV for unknown reasons has been different in developed and developing countries. The recommended three doses at 1 month intervals produced just 60–70% seroconversion in Indian population as compared to 88–100% in the American counterparts. Therefore, 5 doses were recommended: 1st dose at birth, 2nd dose at 6th week with DPT, 3rd dose at 10th week, 4th dose at 14th week and 5th dose at 9th month. Two booster doses – one at 18th month and second at 5 years of age – were recommended in addition.

Even when increasing the doses was not found enough, Pulse Polio Immunization (PPI) campaign was started in India, in 1995. The idea was to give two doses of OPV at 6–8 weeks interval every year for 3–4 years to all children below 5 years of age irrespective of their immunization status.

OPV is a safe vaccine. Vaccine-induced paralysis (i.e., polio within 6 months of OPV administration with recovery of viral strain in stool) is an extremely rare phenomenon in India. It is a major problem in countries where polio has been eradicated, where all paralytic poliomyelitis are vaccine induced! Therefore, these countries have stopped giving OPV and have started using IPV.

Storage is a major problem with OPV. It is an extremely heat labile vaccine and requires strict cold chain maintenance. It requires to be stored in freezer compartment (<-15°C) and vials in current use in vaccination should be kept in the central compartment (2–8°C). At the room temperature, it loses its potency in 48 hrs. Now, OPV vials are provided with vaccine vial monitor (VVM) which gives an idea, if the vial has been exposed to higher temperature for more than the allowed time and this gives a rough idea that the vaccine might have lost its potency and needs to be discarded.

Mild URTI, mild diarrhoea or other minor ailments are not contraindications for OPV. There is no need to withhold breastfeeding before or after the dose. If the baby immediately vomits after the dose, it has to be repeated.

Inactivated Polio Vaccines (IPV)

IPV is formaldehyde killed poliovirus and is highly immunogenic as seroconversion rates are 90–100%. Earlier, it was believed that in countries like India where wild polio virus is still endemic, IPV is of little use as it does not give mucosal and herd immunity. But, now it is known that IPV with its high immunogenicity and efficacy induces high levels of antibodies which spill over to the gut and thus prevent transmission potential of immunized individuals besides protecting them. Thus contrary to the earlier belief, IPV exhibits a demonstrable herd effect.

EPI recommends three doses at 6, 10 and 14 weeks with a booster at 18 months along with usual doses of OPV.

For polio eradication in India, it is recommended to introduce IPV in routine immunization in southern states free of wild polio, to facilitate OPV cessation. This should be followed gradually by universal use of IPV in regular immunization all over the country (when UP and Bihar are also polio free).

Available as *Imovax* (*Sanofi Pasteur*).

3. DPT Vaccine

Vaccines for diphtheria, pertussis and tetanus were all delevoped at very close intervals in mid 1920s. Naturally, they were soon combined as a 'DPT' vaccine.

DPT vaccine is used in Expanded Program of Immunization (EPI), since 1978 as aluminium phosphate absorbed vaccine. Three primary doses at monthly intervals are given IM starting at 6 weeks of age. Two booster doses are given at 18 months and 4–5 years of age. In an unimmunized child more than 2 years but less than 6 years of age, the same schedule of three primary and two booster doses is to be followed. For children older than 6 years, only two doses of DT at monthly interval are required. There is no change in DPT dosage recommendation in low birth weight, malnourished, preterm or immunocompromised babies. If a dose is delayed, there is no need to restart the schedule. Start from where it was left.

Adverse reactions after DPT consist of local pain, swelling or erythema and are seen in 30–50% of children, especially after booster doses. Other systemic symptoms like fever, irritability, crying and anorexia are also seen in 30–50% of vaccinated children. The pertussis component is responsible for severe but rare complications like convulsions, hypotonic-hyporesponsive state, persistent crying, encephalopathy, etc. But these complications are extremely rare, occurring in 1 in 1,40,000 vaccinated children.

DPT is contraindicated in infants with progressive neurological disease (not stable) or those with "uncontrolled" seizures. It should not be repeated in babies who showed severe adverse reactions to a previous dose. Mild upper respiratory tract symptoms with fever are not a contraindication, but DPT can be delayed till the baby is symptom free. Controlled epilepsy, febrile seizures, mental retardation or cerebral palsy are not contraindications for DPT. Though DPT vaccine is one of the earliest vaccines to be used in Expanded Program of Immunization, 25% of our infants still remain unimmunized; at some places this figure rises to 50%!! A lot needs to be done.

Available as *DPT* (*Haffkine*) *at Rs. 25/- for 10 doses.*

4. DTaP

(Tetanus vaccine with regular amount of diphtheria toxoid and acellular pertussis)

Popularly known triple vaccine of DPT vaccine, is composed of tetanus and diphtheria toxoids as well as killed whole cell pertussis bacilli . Now DTaP (acellullar) vaccine is available as an alternative to DPwT. The efficacy and duration of protection with DTaP vaccines against diphtheria/tetanus and pertussis is similar to that afforded by the whole cell vaccines. The DTaP vaccines score over the whole cell vaccines in terms of adverse effects which are reduced by two thirds with the acellular vaccines.

Available as *Infanrix* (*GSK Biologicals*).

5. Td

(Tetanus vaccine with low dose diphtheria toxoid)

Td: Studies show that diphtheria antibody levels decline over time resulting in increasing susceptibility of adolescents and adults to diphtheria. To regularly boost adult immunity against diphtheria, Td is recommended to be given every 10 years. Td contains the usual dose of tetanus toxoid with low dose of diphtheria toxoid to reduce reactions. It is stored at 2–8°C and is administered intramuscularly in a dose of 0.5 mL.

Available as *Tdvac* (*Serum Institute of India*)

6. TdaP

(Tetanus vaccine with low dose diphtheria toxoid and acellular pertussis)

Immunity against pertussis following primary/booster DTwP/DTaP vaccination wanes over the next 6–12 years. In those children who have received all three primary and the two booster doses of DTwP/DTaP, Tdap should be administered as a single dose at the age of 10–12 years. Catch up vaccination is recommended till the age of 18 years. A single dose of Tdap may also be used as replacement for Td/TT booster in adults of any age if they have not received Tdap in the past. It is also acceptable to use Tdap as a replacement for TT/Td in wound management of children aged 10 and above if they have not received Tdap in the past, and at least 5 years have elapsed since receipt of Td/TT vaccine.

Available as *Boostrix (GSK Biologicals).*

7. Measles

It is the most common vaccine preventable disease, killing more than two million children per year all over the world. About 30% of the survivors suffer severe complications. This is in spite of the fact that we have a vaccine with 95% efficacy, since more than 20 years.

The live monovalent vaccine against measles is available in dried powder form and has to be reconstituted with a diluent stored at 2–8°C. 0.5 mL dose is given subcutaneously either alone or in combination with rubella and mumps vaccine (MMR). The reconstituted vaccine is to be used within 4–6 hrs and never after one working day. It is contraindicated in pregnancy and immunosuppressive states. In HIV +ve infant, it is advisable to give measles vaccine at an earlier age. Mild adverse effects like fever, rash, upper respiratory catarrh, etc., are seen 5–12 days after vaccination and may last for 2–3 days. Severe complications like encephalitis, convulsions, SSPE are very rare and unnecessarily feared. The protection provided by measles vaccine far supersedes the rare adverse effects seen in some children.

Now, about the age of vaccine administration. There is a lot of controversy surrounding this issue. In countries like India, measles occurs rather early with almost 10–40% cases seen below 1 year of age. Maternal antibodies start waning by 7–10 months. If we give vaccine between 6–8 months of age, it will protect those children who might have suffered from measles but then seroconversion is just 85% because of interference with maternal antibodies.

A booster dose at 15 months (as MMR) is then required. And if we give at 9 months, the usual trend that we have been following in UIP (Universal Immunisation Program), we fail to provide protection to that substantial number of children who get infected with measles before 9 months of age. Of course, we get a good seroconversion of 95% and no booster is then required. Therefore, the Immunization Advisory Committee of Indian Association of Paediatrics has recommended measles vaccine at 8 months and with MMR vaccine at 18 months. This would give immunity for 15–20 years.

Measles is being considered as a potential disease that can be eradicated from the globe.

Available as *Rimevax at Rs. 25/- per dose.*

8. Mumps Vaccine

Mumps is predominantly a disease of school going children and adolescents, though not uncommon in adults. Clinical cases are seen throughout the year though more commonly in winter. Its most common manifestation is bilateral parotitis. Other manifestations include bilateral epididymoorchitis leading to sterility and meningoencephalitis. It is usually a mild disease. Complications may occur however, which include infertility, pancreatitis, deafness, etc.

A live attenuated vaccine is available against mumps since 1967, both as mumps vaccine alone and as a part of MMR vaccine. Two doses are recommended, one at the age of 12–15 months and second at school entry (4–6 years) or at any time 8 weeks after the first dose. The second dose of MMR vaccine is to protect children failing to seroconvert against primarily mumps and less commonly against rubella (primary vaccine failures). In a child aged 12 months or older, who has not received measles vaccine, 2 doses of MMR at 8 weeks interval suffices; monovalent measles vaccine is not required.

Adverse reactions after vaccination are few consisting of local pain, swelling or fever. MMR vaccine is contraindicated in pregnancy and the vaccinee should be advised to use contraceptive measures for at least 3 months after vaccination. A gap of at least 3 weeks should be kept between MMR and any other vaccines.

Available as *Trimovax at Rs.75/- per dose.*

9. Rubella Vaccine (German Measles)

The exact epidemiological data of incidence of rubella in India is not available. The disease is mild and benign in children and adults (milder form of measles). It is the congenital rubella that demands attention and prevention. Infection risk with rubella is highest in first and last trimester. The most devastating effects of congenital rubella infection are the permanent disabilities seen at birth or within first year of life like deafness (80%), retinopathy, cataract, cardiac disorders and mental retardation. In one Indian study, about 29% of deafness in children could be attributed to rubella.

Rubella vaccine in live attenuated form is available as a monovalent vaccine and as a trivalent MMR vaccine. A single dose of 0.5 mL given subcutaneously gives a protective immunity in 95% of vaccinees and this immunity is life long at least in countries like India. In India, this vaccine is given to children above 15 months of age. Rubella immunisation not only prevents the disease in the recipient, but in females it protects the unborn babies from congenital infection and that is its primary aim. Fever, rash, arthralgia or arthritis and lymphadenopathy are seen 2–3 weeks after vaccination but are self-limiting. It is contraindicated in pregnancy and vaccinated women should not conceive at least for three months following vaccination.

Similarly, being a live vaccine, it is to be avoided in those on immunosuppressive therapy. Although it is not a part of NIP (National Immunisation Program) in India, its inclusion is highly recommended considering its complications in congenital infections. Total elimination of congenital rubella is seen in those countries who have adopted rubella vaccination in their programme.

Available as *Trimovax at Rs. 75/- per dose.*

10. Tetanus Toxoid (TT)

This is the most frequently used and misused vaccine. When any patient presents with any type of injury, we ask—have you taken TT in last 6 months? If the answer is no, we give TT. This is unscientific. Where has this '6 months' come from?

Let us understand what the primary immunization schedule of tetanus prophylaxis is. If a child has taken five doses of TT (i.e., in the form of DPT) and a TT at 10 years of age, then a booster every 10 years is enough. If an adult presents with no history of childhood immunization, then two doses of TT 4–8 weeks apart with a third dose 3–7 months after the first dose gives protection against tetanus for the next 10 years.

When a patient presents with an injury, when should we give TT and when should we give human tetanus immunoglobulin (HTI)? It depends upon the type of injury.

- For tetanus prone wounds (i.e., contaminated, penetrating, with significant tissue damage), only one dose of TT is required if the patient has taken booster within 10 years.
- If more than 10 years have elapsed, then we have to give human tetanus immunoglobulins (250–500 IU).
- If the immunization status of the patient is not known, then we should be giving complete course of TT (as described above) along with HTI.
- In non-tetanus prone injuries, there is no need to add HTI.

TT is not without side effects. Locally pain, redness and swelling lasting for almost 10 days is not uncommon. Systemic symptoms like fever, myalgia, headache, arthus-type of reactions, etc., are often seen. Observation of the patient for anaphylaxis for 10 min after TT injection is advisable, though this is extremely rare.

As 30% of the cases of tetanus are seen in neonates, preventing neonatal (perinatal) tetanus and death is of utmost importance. For this, two doses of TT any time after the first trimester should be given at one month interval. The timing should be adjusted such that the second dose is given at least 15 days prior to the expected date of delivery. In subsequent pregnancies, a single booster dose is enough. One should not lose any chance of providing TT to a pregnant woman, irrespective of her month of pregnancy. For those practising in rural areas, where most deliveries are home deliveries, just training the 'dais' about 'clean hands, clean delivery surface and clean cord' can reduce the rate of neonatal tetanus substantially (to the tune of 90%).

Available as *Tetanus toxoid (Hafkine) at Rs. 6/- per 10 doses.*

11. Rabies Vaccine

In contrast to the progress made by most other Asian countries, rabies continues to be a major problem in India. We earn the dubious distinction of harboring 50% of the global rabies cases! This is in spite of the fact that rabies vaccine is available in India for more than 50 years. The main elements of rabies prevention are—control of rabies in dogs and cats, control of stray dogs in human habitats, post-exposure prophylaxis of persons after animal bites and pre-exposure vaccination of persons at risk. Stray dogs need not be destroyed to control rabies; they could be caught and sterilized or vaccinated, preferably both.

Rabies, an ancient disease, is still having 100% mortality. And it causes one of the most painful and horrifying death. The only option remaining for its control is prevention. Fortunately, we have very safe and effective preventive tools in the form of vaccines and immunoglobulins/ anti-rabies serum.

Tissue Culture Vaccines

Three types are available in the market. In all the three types, cell-lines of non-nervous tissue origin have been utilized. These are HDCV (human diploid cell vaccine), PCEC (Purified chick embryo cell vaccine) and PVRV (Purified verocell rabies vaccine). All the three vaccines are extremely safe and give excellent protective immunity and there is little to choose in between them.

Five doses are recommended on day 0, 3, 7, 14, 30 where day "zero" indicates the day on which vaccination is started and not the day on which the person was bitten. The sixth dose (D-90) is optional to be used in extremes of age or those with poor immunity. The dose of vaccine per injection is 1 mL in HDCV and PCEV vaccines and 0.5 mL in PVCV irrespective of the age of the patient. These injections are to be given in deltoid or in lateral thigh, as fat present in the gluteal region prevents proper absorption.

The incubation period of rabies in humans varies from 5 days to 1 year (average 2 months). The vaccine must be given at the earliest before the virus invades CNS. But seeing the long incubation period, complete PEP should be offered even if the patient presents one month after the bite. Now the question arises—do all types of bites need same type of prophylaxis? It depends on two things—first on the severity of the injury and second on the state of the biting animal (Table 28.1).

Passive Immunization

The *horse* antirabies serum that is available is recommended for all class III exposures at a dose of 40 IU/kg. Sensitivity testing is a must to avoid severe reactions. Half the dose is infiltrated around the wound and half is given IM in the gluteal region. Giving *human* anti-rabies immunoglobulins is a safer but costlier option. Dose is 20 IU/kg and does not require sensitivity testing.

Pre-exposure Immunization

This is recommended in those who are at risk of getting exposed to rabies virus because of their hobby or profession. These include laboratory staff workers handling rabies virus, veterinarians, animal handlers, wild life officers and postmen. Three injections are given on day 0, 7 and 21 with a booster dose after 1 year. This gives immunity for 3 years, after which it has to be repeated.

Re-exposure Immunization

What if a previously immunized individual is again bitten by a stray dog? Two doses 1 week apart are administered. If the previous exposure is beyond 3 years, the complete 6 doses schedule is recommended (Table 28.1).

The most important part is local treatment of the wound. Thorough washing and cleaning of the wound with plenty of soap and water is required. Reducing viral load in the wound greatly reduces the chances of rabies. The wound should be left open. Antiseptic should be applied. Avoid suturing. If essential, infiltrate with RIG before suturing.

Available as *Rabipur or Verorab at Rs. 300/- per dose.*

12. Typhoid Vaccine

Typhoid fever, caused by *Salmonella typhi* continues to be a major public health problem in many developing countries of the world.

Lack of safe water supply and proper environmental sanitation on one hand and emergence of multi-drugs resistant strains on the other hand has made prevention of typhoid fever a need of the hour.

| Table 28.1 Postexposure prophylaxis |

Class	Nature of exposure	State of biting animal	Treatment
I	Licks on intact skin	▪ Remain healthy after 10 days ▪ Not known	No vaccine required Complete course (0, 3, 7, 14, 28, 90)
II	Licks on uncovered skin, minor superficial scratches	▪ Remain healthy after 10 days ▪ Not known	3 doses (0, 3, 7), then stop Complete course (0, 3, 7, 14, 28, 90)
III	Deep bites and scratches, or contamination of mucous membranes	▪ Remain healthy after 10 days ▪ Not known	3 doses (0, 3, 7), then stop Complete course (0, 3, 7, 14, 28, 90) + Immunoglobulin

Types

1. ***Parenteral killed whole cell vaccine*** (Acetone killed or phenol inactivated): It is prepared from Ty-2 strain of *Salmonella typhi*. The vaccine efficiency is about 51–76%. Children above 6 months can be given this vaccine. Two doses (0.5 mL in those above 10 years and 0.25 mL for 6 months – 10 year age group) are to be given subcutaneously, 4 weeks apart. A booster dose is to be repeated every 3 years. It should be stored in dark at 2–8°C and should not be frozen. Local pain and swelling with fever, severe headache and malaise lasting for 2–3 days of the injection, are the common adverse effects and make this vaccine not a favoured vaccine. For the same reason, it was discontinued from NIP in 1987.
2. ***Ty-21a oral vaccine*** is an oral vaccine. It mimics the exact course of natural infections with typhoid bacilli. Therefore, it provides all the three types of immunity, i.e., gut (mucosal), cell-mediated, as well as humoural immunity. There are evidences to suggest that this may lead to herd immunity. It is prepared from the mutant of S typhi-21a strain and is available as enteric coated capsules. One capsule is to be taken on an empty stomach on alternate days for 3 days (within a week) to complete the course. Booster dose after every 5 years is required. It cannot be used below 6 years of age. Efficiency rate varies between 52–61%. It is to be stored at 2–8°C. Minor side effects like vomiting and abdominal pain are seen in <1%.
3. ***Purified Vi polysaccharide vaccine*** is prepared from the Vi-capsule antigen of *S typhi*. A single dose of 0.5 mL IM gives protective immunity for 3 years. As compared to whole-cell vaccine it has less local and systemic side effects. It cannot be used in children below 2 years. As against oral vaccine it can be stored at room temperature. A single dose has protective efficiency of 60–65%.

A vaccine having the combined plus points of both Ty-21a vaccine (oral, herd immunity) and that of Vi polysaccharide vaccine (single dose, lower age limit) is badly awaited. Though, at present there are no hopes of including it in NIP, it is worth offering typhoid vaccine to all those who can afford it—adults and children.

Available as *Typhim Vi (injectable) at Rs. 150/- per dose and Typhoral (oral) at Rs. 290/-* for one course.

13. Varicella Vaccine

Varicella (chickenpox) is an acute, highly contagious viral disease with a worldwide prevalence. It is caused by the varicella zoster virus (VZ virus). The primary infection by the virus causes chickenpox while reactivation at a later stage causes herpes zoster. Due to its extremely contagious nature, varicella is experienced by almost every child below 10 years or even by adults. Though in older children and adults, this disease can manifest in a severe form, essentially chickenpox is a benign disease with extremely low case fatality rate and thus never considered as a major public health problem. With the advent of HIV epidemic, the incidence of herpes zoster, a re-activation disease of varicella virus, has increased exponentially. Even the cases of chickenpox in adults are on the rise.

A live attenuated 'oka' vaccine against varicella is available, since 1994. For children below 13 years of age a single dose is required, while for those above 13 years, two doses at 4–8 weeks interval are needed for protective immunity. It is contraindicated in pregnancy and in immunocompromised state. Adverse effects are mild and local. Storage temperature for vaccine is below –15°C for the freeze-dried form and after reconstitution, it has to be used within 30 min. If to be given in children, preferred age is between 12–24 months of age.

Who should be Offered this Vaccine?

If its use is made extensive and in a sustained manner in children, we can achieve a significant reduction in incidence of chickenpox and this disease might disappear. But, its partial coverage in children can have a negative effect on the epidemiology of varicella—it may shift to older children and adults in whom it manifests in a severe form with complications. Therefore, especially in developing countries like ours where there are other vaccines in the waiting list, vaccine for varicella should be recommended for those above 12–14 years of age who have not been infected with chickenpox in the past. This will protect that individual and there would be no negative impact on the epidemiology of the disease as natural infection in children would remain unaffected.

Apart from preventing varicella, can varicella vaccine be given to prevent zoster in those who have already been exposed to the VZ virus? This has yet not been established. This would have great utility especially in HIV+ patients.

Varicella-zoster immunoglobulins can be given to a contact (1.25–5 mL IM) within 72 hrs of exposure to a case of chickenpox. This can modify or prevent the disease and can be given in newborns or immunosuppressed contacts.

Available as *Varilex at Rs. 1250/- per dose.*

14. Hepatitis A Virus Vaccine (HAV Vaccine)

In India, HAV infection is holoendemic and most (90%) of our children are infected before 10 years of age. But, this infection is asymptomatic or mild with only 10% of those infected manifesting clinical jaundice. As against this, 70–80% of the adults infected with HAV develop jaundice but chronic hepatitis is not known. Though HAV is endemic in India, most of the epidemics are caused by HEV and not HAV.

A number of inactivated viral vaccines are available from various HAV isolates. The dosage schedule is like that of hepatitis B, i.e., two primary dosages 1 month apart with a booster dose at 6 months after the first primary dose. In adults 1440 IU per dose and in children 720 IU per dose has to be given IM. Two doses give seroconversion rate of 99.8% and a protective immunity level for 10 years. It is not proved to prevent sub-clinical infection or clinical attack in those with subclinical infection. Storage is to be done at 2–8°C. Safety profile is quite good. Live attenuated vaccine has been developed requiring only one dose, but it is not available in India.

As far as the use of HAV vaccine in India where the disease is holoendemic and most of the infections are subclinical, its regular use is not recommended.

Available as *Havrix at Rs. 1250/- per adult dose.*

15. Pneumococcal Vaccine

In developing countries like India, bacteria still play a major role in acute respiratory tract infections as compared to viruses in developed countries and *Streptococcus pneumoniae* is a culprit in 25–80% of these bacterial infections especially in lobar pneumonias. It selectively affects infants (a major cause of infant mortality is pneumonia), elderly, alcoholics and those with chronic diseases. Other than pneumonia, it is also considered as a major cause of neonatal meningitis. It is estimated that by the time children are of 6 years of age, 25% of these must have had an attack of pneumococcal otitis media. In 90% cases of occult bacteraemia in infancy, pneumococcus and *H influenzae* type B are the causative agents.

A pneumococcal vaccine was therefore urgently required and efforts were made in this direction. In 1983, a polyvalent pneumococcal vaccine containing capsular polysaccharide of 23 subtypes of pneumococci was licensed in USA. A single dose of 0.5 mL IM or SC gives a protective immunity for 5 years in 60–90% of the vaccinees. No major adverse reactions are seen. It cannot be used for children below 2 years (the most susceptible age group). Its safety has not been established in pregnancy and in patients on chemotherapy or radiotherapy for malignancies. It is to be stored at 2–8°C and freezing should be avoided. It should be specifically emphasized that this pneumococcal vaccine is not to be repeated as revaccination is met with severe reactions. At present, when it cannot be used below 2 years age group, its usage is restricted to at risk individuals—chronic pulmonary disease, CCF, CRF and in immunocompromised individuals.

Conjugated pneumococcal vaccines are now available in India, which can be given in babies from 6 weeks onwards. Two types are available: 7-valent pneumococcal conjugate vaccine (PCV7) and 13-valent conjugate vaccine (PCV13). While PCV-13 offers wider serotype coverage, PCV-10 promises to provide better protection against otitis media.

The vaccination schedule of PCV13 and PCV7 is the same, i.e., 4-dose schedule as followed for PCV7, administering doses at ages 6, 10, 14 weeks and a booster at 12–15 months. Routine use of PCV13 is not recommended for healthy children aged more than 5 years.

Following points are to be remembered:

- Minimum age for administering first dose is 6 weeks.
- Minimum interval between two doses is 4 weeks for children vaccinated at age <12 months whereas for those vaccinated at age >12 months, the minimum interval between doses is 8 weeks.

Available as *Pneumo 23 at Rs. 750/- per dose.*

Pneumococcal Vaccine for High-risk Children

Children aged 2 years with underlying medical conditions (chronic heart disease, chronic lung disease, including asthma if treated with prolonged high-dose oral corticosteroids, sickle cell disease, haemoglobinopathies, congenital or acquired asplenia, HIV infection, diabetes mellitus) should receive 1 dose of PPV (polyvalent pneumococcal vaccine) at age ≥ 2 years. This is in addition to recommended doses of PCV13. A second dose of PPV is recommended 5 years after the first dose. No more than two PPV doses are recommended.

Available as *Prevenar 13* (*Pfizer-Wyeth*)

16. Meningococcal Vaccine

Meningococcal meningitis has a worldwide distribution and major epidemics are usually superimposed every 5–10 years on a background of endemic disease. It is caused by the Gram -ve diplococci *Neisseria meningitides*, a commensal of the human oropharynx. Many different subgroups are found, but most of the epidemics are caused by Gr A and Gr C, while the endemic cases are due to Gr B. It is usually a disease of children between 6 months and 2 years in endemic regions, but in epidemics older children and even adults are affected. Case fatality rate is high—about 10–15%! Between epidemics, 2–30% of individuals carry meningococci in their throats which rises to 40% during epidemics.

In India, meningococcal A and C vaccine, containing capsular polysaccharides of subgroups A and C responsible for the epidemics, is available. A single dose of 0.5 mL given SC gives protective immunity in 75–90% of vaccinees for 3 years. Children below 2 years cannot be given this vaccine (who incidentally require it the most).

Only in an event of contact with a patient suffering from meningococcal meningitis, can an infant above 3 months be given this vaccine. It is available as lysophilised powder and has to be reconstituted with distilled water before use. It can be stored at 2–8°C for 2 years, but after reconstitution it has to be used within 4–6 hrs. No major local or systemic adverse reactions are seen. It has no effect on the established nasopharyngeal carrier state, though it can prevent acquisition of carrier state. As the time taken for seroconversion is more than the average incubation period of 5 days, it is necessary to provide chemoprophylaxis to household contacts during epidemics along with the vaccine.

Sulphadiazine (500 mg BD for those <12 years) and 1 g BD (>12 years) for two days is recommended. Alternatively, rifampicin 10 mg/kg/dose bd may be used for 2 days.

A vaccine for Gr B strains which is responsible for almost 50% of meningococcal meningitis cases is much awaited. Also Gr A and Gr C vaccine which can be used in children below 2 years need to be developed. At present the available vaccine is recommended in the close contacts of a meningococcal meningitis case during an epidemic (especially in schools, orphanages, army, etc.) Also, the health care providers caring for a case of meningococcal meningitis need to take this vaccine. Safety of this vaccine is not established in pregnancy.

Available as *Meningococcal A and C vaccine (API) at Rs. 280/- per dose.*

17. Hepatitis B Vaccine

Hepatitis-B is a world-wide problem with around 300 million carriers of Hepatitis-B globally. About 75% of these are in Asia. The international task force has divided the world into three divisions according to the prevalence of the carrier state of hepatitis B (>7%, 7–2%, <2%). India is believed to fall in intermediate risk group with carrier rate of 4.7% (42.5 million carriers). But, there is a lot of controversy about this figure and many believe that we have carrier rate < 2%. At least 25% of the carriers develop chronic progressive liver diseases such as chronic hepatitis, cirrhosis or hepatic carcinoma. But, what is the chance of acquiring carrier state after infection with hepatitis B virus? It depends upon the age at which the infection is acquired. Thus an adult if infected with HBV has 2.5% chances of developing a carrier state; while in comparison the chances in a newborn baby are 90–95%, if perinatally acquired from an HBV infected mother. In India, 30–50% of the HBV carriers are due to perinatal transmission.

HBV can be transmitted by three routes, i.e., sexual, parenteral and perinatal. But, seeing the preponderance of latter in India, strategy of prevention ought to be directed at this route of transmission. Therefore, HBV vaccine should be given at birth (ideally within 1 hr and maximum within 6 hrs) to all the newborn babies. This acts as a postexposure prophylaxis. The second dose should be given ideally at 4 weeks but not later than 6 weeks and the 3rd dose at 6th or 8th month. This gives protective immunity in 90–99% vaccinees. Normally no boosters are recommended but preterm babies, HIV infected, drug addicts, etc., require a booster dose every 2–3 years depending on the antibodies levels.

Two types of hepatitis B vaccines are available—*plasma derived vaccine* and *recombinant vaccine*. *Plasma derived vaccines* are based on the surface antigens (HbsAg) which are harvested and purified from the plasma of human carriers of HBV. It has a good safety profile and has an efficiency of 95% after three doses. Its limitations are the inadequate availability of sera and variations in potency among different batches.

These limitations are overcome in *recombinant vaccines* in which HBsAg DNA sequence from HBV is isolated and integrated in the genome of the common baker's yeast. Safety and efficacy wise it is as good as plasma derived. Apart from minor local side effects like pain and induration and minor systemic side effects like headaches, myalgias or transient rash, this vaccine is absolutely safe.

HBV vaccine need not be given in HBsAg carriers and in those with anti-HBs antibodies in their serum. Apart from universal immunisation of infants, those at risk like drug addicts, haemophiliacs, medical personnel, laboratory technicians, sexual contacts of hepatitis B carriers, etc., should be given HBV. It is advisable but not mandatory to give anti-HBs immunoglobulins in post-exposure prophylaxis of HBV.

HBV vaccine is on the topmost position in the priority list of vaccines to be included in NIP.

Available as *Revac-B at Rs.80/- for adult dose or as Engerix-B at Rs. 275/- for adult dose or as Tritanrex (DPT+Hep.B) at Rs.210/-per dose.*

18. Haemophilus Influenzae B Vaccine (HiB)

Haemophilus influenzae is the most common cause of bacterial infection in 0–5-year age group. About 95% of serious infections are caused by this bacterium alone causing 4 lac deaths per year worldwide. It is the most common causative agent of meningitis. Other manifestations are epiglottitis, septic arthritis, pneumonitis, cellulitis and bacteraemia. It affects children between 3 months to 6 years of age group with maximum infections occurring in infancy.

The first vaccine developed in 1970s against Hib was prepared from capsular polysaccharide.

It gave protective immunity to those above 18 months of age. Thus, it proved useless for the most susceptible age group. The conjugate vaccine developed in 1980s enhanced the immunity and most important, it could be used as early as 6 weeks. The vaccine is given IM.

The number of doses required differs with the age group and is as shown in Table 28.2.

| **Table 28.2** Schedule for the Hib vaccine |

Age group	No. of doses	Timing
0–6 months	4	6 wk, 10 wk, 14 wk, 15 months
6 months to 1 year	3	2 doses 1 month apart. Booster at 15 months.
1–5 years	1	Any time 1 dose

Hib vaccine has an excellent safety profile. Local reactions like pain and swelling may occur. It is available in combined form with DPT, reducing the total cost and increasing compliance.

Introduction of this vaccine in NIP in United States has virtually eliminated invasive Hib infection in their country. Except for the high cost, there is no reason why Hib should not be included in our NIP.

Available as *Hibtiter at Rs. 300/- for single dose or as Tetra ACT HiB (DPT+HiB) at Rs. 380/- for single dose.*

19. Influenza Vaccine

'Flu' is a layman's term for any trivial fever. But, influenza virus is a major cause of severe morbidity and mortality all over the globe. Major epidemics occur at intervals of 2–3 years and pandemic every 10–15 years.

Influenza vaccine is a unique vaccine in the sense that it is newly prepared every year, as influenza virus strains go on changing all the time. Influenza strains are isolated worldwide, their antigens identified and on this basis WHO recommends the composition of the vaccine to be used in that year.

Influenza vaccine is a killed inactivated vaccine to be stored at 2°C. 0.5 mL, single dose is given in adults. Children between 4–12 years may require two doses. It is contraindicated in children below 4 years and in pregnancy. Protective immunity develops in 1 week in 60–80% in the vaccinees. It causes severe local reaction and fever, rash, etc.

Currently, it is recommended for at risk individuals—in renal failure, chronic cardiac or pulmonary disease, or immunosuppressed.

Available as *Vaxigrip (0.5 mL) at Rs. 525/- per dose.*

20. Rotavirus

Rotavirus is a major cause of diarrhoea related morbidity and mortality in children worldwide. India alone accounts for 25 million diarrhoeal episodes and over a lac of deaths in the under five children per annum due to rotavirus disease. Is rotavirus infection as cause of diarrhoeal infections increasing? Improvements in hygiene and sanitation have had a great impact on the prevention of diarrhoea caused by bacterial and parasitic agents over the past 2 decades, but rotavirus infection is spread mostly through person-to-person contact rather than poor hygienic or sanitary conditions. Therefore, it is turning out to be major cause of diarrhoeal disease. So, effective vaccination will be the most promising prevention strategy against the rotavirus disease.

In India, **human monovalent live vaccine** is available which is administered orally in a 2-dose schedule to infants of approximately 2–4 months of age. The first dose can already be administered at the age of 6 weeks and should be given no later than at the age of 12 weeks as there is a higher risk of intussusceptions, if vaccines are given to older infants. It should never be given to child older than 32 weeks, i.e., 8 months. It is not necessary to restart the series or add doses because of a prolonged interval between doses.

Vaccination should be avoided if age of the infant is uncertain. The vaccine and the diluents should be stored at 2–8°C and must not be frozen and should be administered promptly after reconstitution as 1 mL *orally*. Re-administration need not be done to an infant who regurgitates, spits out, or vomits during or after administration.

Available as *Rotarix (GSK Biologicals) at Rs.925/- for single dose.*

21. Human Papilloma Virus (HPV) Vaccines

Prevalence of HPV infection in general population of India is about 7.9%. Whereas, most HPV infections are transient and benign, persistent genital infection with certain viral genotypes can lead to the development of anogenital and oral cancers. Cervical cancer is responsible for significant morbidity/mortality in Indian women and affects women of all socio-economic strata. Compliance with cervical Papanicolou (PAP) smear screening is low in India. The HPV vaccines are thus of public health importance.

Two vaccines have been licensed globally; a quadrivalent and a bivalent vaccine.

The bivalent vaccine is of HPV serotypes 16 and 18 which gives protection against cervical intraepithelial neoplasia (CIN) 2/3 and adenocarcinoma *in situ* (AIS). Quadrivalent vaccine has HPV serotypes 16, 18, 6 & 11. It gives protection against cervical intraepithelial neoplasia (CIN) 2/3 and adenocarcinoma in situ (AIS) and also, protection against genital warts, vaginal intraepithelial neoplasia (VaIN) and vulvar intraepithelial neoplasia (VIN).

The vaccines should be stored at 2–8°C and must not be frozen. The dose is 0.5 mL intramuscular in deltoid. The recommended age for initiation of vaccination is 10–12 years. As of current licensing regulations in India, catch up vaccination is permitted up to the age of 45 years. Three doses at 0, 2 and 6 months are recommended with the quadrivalent vaccine (minimum interval between 1st and 2nd dose is 4 weeks and 2nd and 3rd dose is 12 weeks) and 0, 1 and 6 months with the bivalent vaccine.

Local adverse effects include pain and swelling at the injection site. Systemic adverse effects as such are rarely seen.

Since protection is seen only when the vaccine is given before infection with HPV, the vaccine should preferably be given prior to sexual debut. Vaccines are not 100% protective against cervical cancer and not a replacement for periodic screening. Hence, screening programmes should continue as per recommendations.

Available as *HPV quadrivalent Gardasil (MSD) and HPV bivalent Cervarix (GSK Biologicals).*

22. Cholera Vaccine

Cholera caused by the bacterium *Vibrio cholerae*, is known to be the cause of epidemic diarrhoeal disease for more than two centuries. Spread by faeco-oral route, it has been responsible for millions and millions of deaths and still continues to cause diarrhoea and deaths where safe drinking water and proper sanitation facilities are not available. The drug resistant strain 0139 of *Vibrio cholerae* has compounded the problem. Many candidate vaccines have been and are being tested, but none has proved adequately efficient. Therefore, since 1973, WHO has stopped recommending cholera vaccine prior to entering endemic areas.

The available vaccine is a killed whole cell vaccine to be stored at 2–8°C. Two doses (0.2 and 0.5 mL) are required to be given which gives immunity for 3–6 months. A booster has to be given every 6 months. Although no major side effects are seen, protective efficiency is just 60% of vaccines. It fails to prevent asymptomatic infection or carrier stage. Newer vaccines like non-living oral vaccines, live oral vaccines and CVD-103-HSR vaccine have been developed but none has proved to be satisfactory.

23. Japanese Encephalitis (Je) Vaccine

It is basically a zoonotic disease. In India, the first serologically diagnosed case was detected in 1958, in Tamil Nadu. Subsequent surveys carried out by NARI, Pune, indicated that half the population of South India had neutralizing antibodies to JE virus. Now, JE is found in many Indian states. The arbovirus causing JE infects many animals (like pigs, horses, etc.) and birds. Humans are infected by mosquitoes of culicine species which transmit the virus from birds/animals to man. Acute encephalitis results after an incubation period of 5–15 days. It has a mortality of 20–40%.

The vaccine that is available against JE is prepared from killed mouse brain. It is available in freeze-dried form. Two primary doses of 1 mL each given at 1–2 weeks interval are required for those above 3 years of age. A booster dose before first year after the first dose gives immunity for 3 years. In endemic areas, a three yearly booster is recommended. It takes about a month for protective immunity to develop after the second dose—a point to be remembered. No major side effects are seen and seroconversion is 100%.

24. Yellow Fever Vaccine

Yellow fever is called so not because it causes jaundice but because of the yellow quarantine flag that was used by the ships to give warning of the highly infectious fatal disease. Though found rarely in Asian population, yellow fever is endemic in African and American countries. It is caused by arbovirus and transmitted by mosquitoes. It causes symptoms like other viral haemorrhagic fevers but with severe hepatic and renal involvement and death. It is especially seen in children below 15 years. In endemic countries, yellow fever vaccine is now included in EPI (Expanded Programme of Immunisation) to be given at 9th month after birth. For others, it is required for international travel to these countries.

The first vaccine against yellow fever, 17D vaccine, was developed in 1938 by Max Theiler which saved lives of millions of British and American troops in the Second World War. The vaccine is available in freeze-dried form which is to be stored at sub-zero temperatures. A single dose of 0.5 mL SC of reconstituted vaccine gives protective immunity for more than 10 years when it has to be repeated. It has to be taken at least 10 days before travel to endemic countries.

No major side effects are seen. Reactions may occur in those sensitive to egg as this vaccine is prepared in developing eggs. It should not be given to pregnant ladies and in children below 6 months. Cholera and yellow fever vaccines given together or within 3 weeks, interfere with each other. Whenever possible they should be given 2 weeks or more apart.

THE IMMUNIZATION SCHEDULE

| **Table 28.3** Immunization schedule recommended by Indian Paediatric Association |

Age	Vaccines	Trade names
Birth	BCG OPV-0 HepB1	Engerix-B
6 weeks	DTwP1/DTaP1 OPV1*/OPV1 + IPV1 Hib1 HepB2 Rotavirus**# PCV2	Infanrix + Hiberix Hiberix Rotarix Synflorix
10 weeks	DTwP2/DTap2 OPV2*/OPV2+IPV2 Hib2 Rotavirus2 PCV2	Infanrix
14 weeks	DTwP3/DTaP3 OPV3*/OPV3+IPV3 Hib3 Rotavirus3 HepB3** PCV3	
9 months	Measles	
12 months	HepatitisA1	Havrix
15 months	MMR1 Varicella PCV booster	 Varilrix
16–18 months	DTwP B1/DTaP B1 OPV4*/OPV4+IPVB1 HibB1	
18 months	Hepatitis A 2	
2 years	Typhoid 1#	
5 years	DTwP B2/DtaP B2 OPV5 MMR2$ Typhoid2 Varicella2$$	 Priorix
10–12 years	Tdap/Td& HPV^	Boostrix Cervarix

*OPV alone if IPV cannot be given.

**#Rotavirus vaccine (2/3 doses depending on the brand at 4–8 weeks interval.)

**The third dose of Hepatitis B can be given at 6 months.

$The second dose of MMR vaccine can be given at any time 4–8 weeks after the first dose.

$$Varicella (2nd dose may be given any time 3 months after the 1st dose.)

#Typhoid revaccination every 3 years.

&Tdap preferred to Td, followed by repeat Td every 10 years.

^Only females, three doses at 0, 1–2 (depending on brands) and 6 months.

| **Table 28.4** Immunization in an unimmunized child |

Visit	Less than 5 years	More than 5 years
1st visit	DPT + OPV + BCG	DT or TT, Mantoux test
2nd visit (after 1 month)	DPT + OPV	DT or TT & BCG (if Mantoux -ve)
3rd visit (after 1 month)	DPT + OPV + Typhoid Vi + Measles/MMR	Typhoid + Measles/MMR
1 year later	DPT + OPV	Nil

ESSENTIAL AND OPTIONAL VACCINES

The National Immunization Schedule includes BCG, DPT, OPV and measles with DT and TT. Many more vaccines are now freely available in the market. The Indian Academy of Paediatrics (IAP) has considered most of these vaccines as 'optional' and not included them in the National Immunization Programme (NIP). But, who has to exercise this option—the physician or the patient? And thus 'optional' suggests that they are not 'essential'? Are HBV or Hib or typhoid vaccines not essential? Unfortunately, affordability makes them 'optional'. But when affordable, should the child be given all vaccines that are available in the market? We must think beyond mere availability and affordability. A physician should recommend to the parents that the vaccines under NIP are given routinely, but when it comes to 'optional' vaccines, there should be dialogue in which the pros and cons are presented to the parents and a joint decision made. Parents rely heavily on their physician to help them make a decision. However, the physician makes such decision more on personal bias than on scientific knowledge. This needs to be changed.

| Table 28.5 |

- *Vaccines contraindicated in pregnancy and lactation*: MMR, measles, chickenpox, cholera
- *Vaccines safe in pregnancy and lactation*: TT, yellow fever, HBV, influenza, pneumococcal, rabies
- *Vaccines in pipeline*: Malaria, tuberculosis, Shigella-induced dysentery, Rota virus, *E. coli* induced diarrhoea, leprosy

VACCINES FOR TRAVELLERS

1. Those that are routinely used especially in children—DPT, OPV/IPV, Hep B, Hib, measles/MMR.
2. Those that in some situations are mandatory —yellow fever, meningococcal meningitis.
3. Others that may be advised before travel—cholera, influenza, hepatitis A, JE, tick borne encephalitis, BCG, typhoid. These are for individual protection and optional.

Vaccine for Yellow Fever

This is the only vaccine that is mandatory for international travel as authorized by International Health Regulation. It is to be taken at least 2 weeks before the travel and revaccination is recommended after 10 years.

Vaccination against meningococcal diseases is required by Saudi Arabia for pilgrims visiting Mecca for the Hajj and also required by some countries for some pilgrims returning after the Hajj.

Travellers should be provided with a written record of all vaccines given. An International vaccination certificate is required for yellow fever vaccination.

Booster doses of the regular vaccines (Group I) are to be taken if primary immunization schedule has not been properly followed. A full course of primary immunization is required (as shown in Table 28.4) for those who have never been immunized.

Important thing to remember is that one should consult the physician or travel clinic at least 4–6 weeks before the departure, as protective immunity takes some time to develop. Also, vaccines do not always give 100% immunity against the diseases for which it is taken. Hence, additional precautions against these infections should be followed carefully.

PASSIVE IMMUNIZATION

Passive immunization is required when there is no time for antibodies to form and preventing or controlling the infection with 'readymade' antibodies is required. Passive immunity against many infections can be conferred with immunoglobulins or antisera. Immunoglobulin can be 'general' or 'specific'. In general practice, immunoglobulin for rabies, tetanus and hepatitis B infection are usually required. Other infections where passive immunization with immunoglobulin can be given are rubella, measles, varicella, gas gangrene and botulism.

Allergic reactions are a major concern when using immunoglobulin and antisera.

Rabies	Berirab.P	Rs. 2250/-
Tetanus	Tetglob	Rs. 100/-
Hepatitis B	Hepabig	Rs. 800/-
Gammaglobulin	Bharat Serum	Rs. 600/-
Antisnake antisera	Bharat Serum	Rs. 35/-

ADVERSE REACTIONS AFTER VACCINATION

One of the common reasons why we general practitioners avoid giving vaccines is because of fear of adverse reactions to vaccines. But, is this fear justified? This issue of reactions is blown out of proportion. Probably, the reason is that vaccination involves babies and that too healthy babies. And so, if something goes wrong with this baby who had entered your clinic absolutely healthy and smiling, the parents as well as yourself are bound to panic. But, we have to consider risks and benefits of our every act. And the act of immunization is associated with much benefit of reducing disease morbidity and mortality compared to the very small risk of adverse reactions. So, we should first reassure ourselves and then our patients.

Some symptoms and signs seen after immunisation are taken to be as 'normal' reaction. This includes mild to moderate fever, irritability, refusal to eat, drowsiness, local pain and swelling. 'Abnormal' reactions are local or systemic. In 15–20% of the babies, a painless nodule lasting for several weeks may develop especially after adsorbed vaccines like DPT, TT, etc. Reactions seen locally after BCG vaccination are given under the 'BCG vaccine'. The general reactions though rare are more common after DPT and measles. These include prolonged crying spells, convulsions, encephalopathy or shock after DPT. In such a case, DPT should be halted and a dose of DT should be given subsequently. Reactions to rabies, measles and OPV have already been described.

In any case of reaction, the most important thing to do is NOT TO PANIC. Remain calm or at least show that you are in a position to handle the situation. Do not ignore the parent's complaints or run away from the scene. You should always be prepared to handle the possible adverse reactions. Keep Inj. adrenaline and Inj. hydrocortisone at hand before giving any vaccine. If the child develops any sign of anaphylaxis, give Inj. adrenaline 1:1000 aqueous in a dose of 0.01 mL/kg per dose subcutaneously. Refer the baby to the nearest hospital having facility of endotracheal intubation. Such reactions are very very rare and not a reason for not starting an immunization clinic!

COLD CHAIN GUIDELINES FOR STORAGE OF VACCINES

It is a well established fact that the immunogenicity of vaccines is affected when exposed to the extremes of temperatures during storage, transportation or administration. Vaccines given with lost potency will not protect the individual and will only give false sense of security. And potency once lost cannot be restored. Therefore, care should be taken to store vaccines as per the temperatures recommended by the manufacturer.

And doing this is termed as maintaining the 'cold chain'. The components of the cold chain are storage, transportation and administration.

Storage

In clinical practice, vaccines are usually stored in ordinary freeze at home or at the clinic. The different shelves in the freeze have different temperatures. In order to obtain a correct temperature in all the shelves of the refrigerator, the thermostat switch should be turned to its maximum. Once this is done, the inner freezer compartment will cool to nearly -10°C. And the temperature in the shelves will range from 2°C to 8°C, cooler in the upper shelves and less in the lower shelves. The vaccines should be stored in the relevant compartments as given below:

- Freezer/chiller tray—*MMR, BCG, Measles and OPV*
- Upper shelf—*Hepatitis B, Typhoid, Hepatitis A, Rabies, Meningococcal and Pneumococcal vaccines*
- Lower shelf—*DPT, DT, TT, Hib vaccines*

Optimum care should be taken that *DPT, DT, TT or Typhoid vaccines* are never frozen. Vaccines should not be stored in the door compartments or other trays of the refrigerator where the temperatures are relatively high.

In the event of a power failure, essential vaccines can be kept along with frozen *ice packs* available in medical stores. Ice packs can be prepared at home by neatly placing ice cubes in a polythene bag and sealing it. They help in absorbing the heat and maintaining a required level of temperature.

Transportation

Thermocol box or thermos flask can be used. They should be wide mouthed. Adequate amount of ice in the form of ice packs should be kept in them for transportation. Care should be taken that vials of vaccines, especially DPT, TT and Typhoid do not come in direct contact with the ice. This will also prevent damage to the vaccine labels by avoiding possible soaking.

Administration

Preferably 1 day in a week should be fixed up as 'vaccination day'. This will avoid daily transportation of vaccines.

During administering vaccines, a cup with ice cubes should be kept at hand to keep the vaccines in it. Vaccines should be kept in the hands for the shortest possible time.

Checking for Potency

Unfortunately, there is no way one can know, if the vaccine had been exposed to temperatures above the recommended temperature and lost its potency, except with OPV vial which has a 'vaccine vial monitor'. But, if the vaccine had been frozen, granular or flaky particles are seen in the vial. Such vaccines should be discarded, not only because they may have lost their potency but also because such vaccines have more chances of causing a septic abscess at the site of injection.

The 'cold chain' maintenance is not a 'Herculean' task as is usually feared by general practitioners. This is one reason which most physicians give for not practising immunisation. (Only 6% of the total immunization is catered by private practitioners.) It requires just a little motivation with some basic precautions for running a successful 'immunisation clinic'.

This chapter has been reviewed by ***Dr Rahul Khade****, MD, Paediatrician, Pune.*

CHAPTER 29

Acupuncture

— **Madhu J Oswal**

INTRODUCTION

Most of us know of acupuncture as some Chinese therapy of needling, to be used in cases of non-remitting painful conditions or paralysis. But, this is too much an underevaluation of one of the oldest forms of healing, as old as mankind. The history of acupuncture can be traced for more than 2000 years in the past and the fact that it is still in vogue in itself proves it to be an effective and scientific mode of treatment. For people in China and other eastern countries, it is as much a norm to see an acupuncturist as it is here to visit a general practitioner for any ailment. And in the Western world, it has been accepted as the most favoured 'alternative therapy'—rather it has been streamlined into mainstream medicine in many developed countries. The scope of application of acupuncture therapy is enormous in our practice, if we learn about its principles and techniques. This chapter is a good beginning for a novice, providing basic concepts of acupuncture, its theory and practical aspects. Finer points of this therapy can be acquired by attending some crash courses or attending an acupuncturist clinic.

SCOPE OF PRACTICE

The scope and limitations of any medical discipline depends upon the training, orientation and practice environment of the provider. In China, acupuncture is the mainstream medicine, so, acupuncture is a primary therapy and one seeks additional therapies only if acupuncture proves insufficient as the sole treatment. In most other countries including India, acupuncture is basically regarded as 'alternative' therapy and sought when everything else fails. Acupuncture therapy yields good results in well selected early cases. It is less successful in chronic and complicated cases.

In general, acupuncture has found its greatest acceptance in treating musculoskeletal pain. Acute musculoskeletal lesions such as soft tissue contusions, acute muscle spasms, musculotendinous sprain and strains, pain of acute nerve entrapments, etc., are among the problems most frequently and succesfully treated with acupuncture as a primary therapy.

Chronic musculoskeletal pain problems like lumbar spondylosis, cervical spondylosis, carpal tunnel syndrome, tennis elbow, plantar fasciitis, frozen shoulder, postherpetic neuralgia, peripheral neuropathic pains, etc., are commonly treated with acupuncture with benefit.

Other than pain, acupuncture has been proved very valuable for managing substance abuse. It has gained the acceptance in all rehabilitation programmes internationally and is currently used in 300 de-addiction programmes in US alone.

Other than this, acupuncture has its role to play in many respiratory, gastrointestinal, gynaecological and genitourinary complaints. WHO has identified 41 ailments that can be effectively treated with acupuncture. Some of these are listed below:

- Migraine
- Neuralgia
- Insomnia
- Anxiety neurosis, depression
- Chronic diarrhoea
- Gingivitis/gum problems
- Post-tooth extraction pain, toothache
- Respiratory conditions like bronchitis, asthma, sinusitis, allergic rhinitis
- Infertility
- Premenstrual syndrome
- Menopausal symptoms
- Impotence
- Backache
- Sciatica
- Disc problems
- Sports injuries
- Musculoskeletal sprains, strains
- Muscle cramping
- Arthritis
- Colitis
- Hyperacidity
- Aphthous ulcers
- Obesity
- Hypertension
- Poststroke paralysis
- Addictions to cocaine, heroin, alcohol, tobacco, etc.

PHILOSOPHY OF TRADITIONAL CHINESE MEDICINE AND ACUPUNCTURE

1. Concept of 'Qi' or 'T-chi'

The traditional Chinese medicine states that the vital or life force in the body, called 'Qi' or 'T-chi' controls the working of all main organs and systems of the body. The concept is similar to the concept of 'Prana' of Hindu philosophy or 'Spirit' of Christian philosophy. Balanced flow of 'Qi' is essential for health and any excess, deficiency or block of 'Qi' along the meridians, the channels through which it flows, results in disease. The role of acupuncture is basically to restore the balance.

2. Concept of 'Yin' and 'Yang'

The idea of harmony and balance are the basis of 'Yin' and 'Yang'. Everything in the Chinese view of the world and the life is related to a dynamic balance of these 'Yin' and 'Yang'. These are two opposing but complementary forces governing our lives. Their proper relationship is 'health' and any imbalance between them results in a 'disease' state.

Traditionally, 'Yin' is weak, dark, negative, cold, feminine; while 'Yang' is strong, light, positive, warm, male like. One can be predominantly 'Yin' type or of 'Yang' type depending upon the characteristics one possesses. But, one cannot exist without another and they always flow into each other. A little 'yin' is always present within 'yang' and little 'yang' is always present within 'yin'. This continuous intermingling of 'yin' and 'yang' is beautifully illustrated by the 'Tai-Ji' symbol.

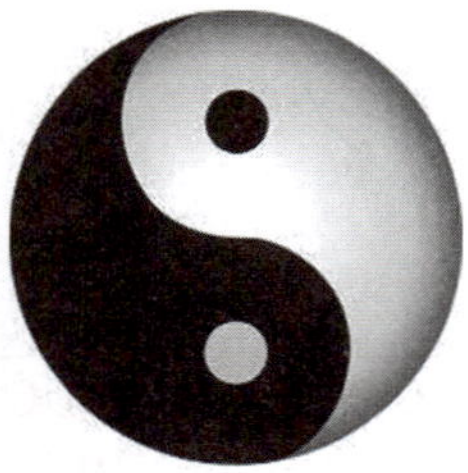

'Tai-Ji' Symbol

This concept of 'Yin' and 'Yang' should not be difficult to grasp for one who is familiar with the Ayurvedic concept of 'Tridosha', i.e., 'Vata-Kaffa-Pitta', which also believes in proper harmony of these forces for maintenance of health and treatment aims at restoring the balance of these forces.

3. Concept of 'Organs'

The Chinese medicine has a different concept of 'organs'. They divide all the body organs into two types, namely the 'Zang' organs and 'Fu' organs. The 'Zang' organs are solid organs which are predominantly 'Yin' type, namely, heart, lungs, kidneys, liver, spleen and pericardium. The 'Fu' organs are hollow organs, predominantly 'Yang' in origin, namely, stomach, gallbladder, large intestine, small intestine, urinary bladder and tripple warmer. The 'Zang' organs are meant for storing and preserving various substances while Fu organs do the absorbing and eliminating functions.

4. The Five Element Theory

As in Ayurveda, there is a concept of 'Panch-Maha-Bhuta', the traditional Chinese medicine also has the concept of 'five elements', viz., Wood, Fire, Earth, Metal & Water. Just as 'Yin/Yang' represents a *spinning unit* of rest/activity, dark/light, etc., so the five elements represent five different movements or aspects of energy.

5. Concept of Meridian (Jing-Luo)

According to traditional Chinese medicine, there is a network of channels inside our body which connects the internal organs with the surface of the body, known as 'Jing-Luo' or 'Meridians'. The life energy 'Qi' flow through these channels and acupuncture points are the locations on these meridians where the 'Qi' of the channels rises close to the surface of the body. They are places of lowered resistance and high conductance. The balance and harmonious flow of the 'Qi' energy can be influenced by the insertion of fine needles into these acupuncture points, dispersing where it is in excess and tonifying in deficiency.

There are 12 main meridians, each connected with an 'organ' and are the means of spreading the influence of each organ over the body surface. Out of these, six are 'Yin' meridians which are related to solid organs of the body, namely, heart, lung, pericardium, kidney, spleen and liver. 'Yin' meridians are on the ventral surface of the body and have a centrifugal route, i.e., they start centrally and end peripherally. As against this, the 'Yang' meridians are related to hollow organs of the body namely small intestine, large intestine, gall bladder, stomach, urinary bladder and triple warmer (related to pleural, peritoneal and pelvic cavities). They run on the dorsal surface of the body and have centripetal route, i.e., start peripherally and end centrally.

Other than these 12 main meridians, there are 8 extra meridians and many minor ones. Out of these, the 'Du Mai—governing vessel' meridian which runs vertically on the midline of the back and 'Ren Mai—conception vessel' meridian, running vertically on the midline anteriorly, are of clinical significance.

Along these meridians are more than 2000 acupuncture points out of which WHO has classified 400 points for various ailments.

Any scientific explanation of the concept of meridians has not been accepted yet. The meridian network is very similar to the nervous system network in our body but does not correlate exactly. The acupuncture points were thought to be points of nerve insertion on the muscles, but this theory has been refuted. Some believe that there is a relation between electromagnetic fields in the body. Meridians and acupuncture points have certain electrical properties, which when stimulated alter neurotransmitters in the body.

ACUPUNCTURE NEEDLES AND NEEDLING TECHNIQUES

Acupuncture Needles

In the ancient days when people had no knowledge of metal, the so-called needles were pointed stones termed as 'bain'. In the later years, they were replaced by needles made of bones and bamboo. During the Shang dynasty (16th century), it became possible to manufacture bronze needles. In the course of evolution, needles of iron, copper, silver, gold and steel came into use. In practice, filiform needles made of stainless steel are used most frequently.

Needles are available in variable sizes and thickness ranging from 0.5″ to 6″ in length and 26–32 gauge in thickness. Choice depends upon the thickness of area to be needled, e.g., for face, half inch needles are sufficient; while for areas on back and thigh, needles of 3″ are required. But for general use, 1″ needles of 30 gauge are most commonly required.

A typical filiform needle consists of a handle and a so-called needle body, the part to be inserted. The tip of the needle is 20 times thinner than the usual hypodermic injection needle. Other than this, there are different needles called 'staying needles' or 'press needles', which are to be kept for prolonged periods or for ear acupuncture. Disposable needles are widely used in affluent countries.

Technique of Insertion

The patient should preferably be in a lying down position with the areas to be needled properly exposed and disinfected with antiseptic solution. Proper hand washing by the acupuncturist is a must. The needling should be swift in order to minimize pain. Distraction of patient during needling and reassurance also help in pain-free needling.

The angle of insertion depends upon the area where the needle has to be inserted. Needles can be inserted vertically where the muscle is quite thick like buttocks, back, thigh, etc.

An angle of 45° is preferred in needling of relatively thin areas of extremities and abdomen. More horizontal needling (15%) is desirable in face, chest, etc.

One can hold the skin fold between thumb and forefinger for thin areas and then insert the needle or one can stretch the part before inserting if the part is thick. Common sense helps more than anything else in proper needling technique. The needle is to be inserted in the direction of the meridian for tonification and in opposite direction for sedation.

Stimulation Techniques

After needling, the needle has to be stimulated to get the 'De-qi'. De-qi is a subjective sensation of soreness, heaviness, numbness and distension which one gets after needle insertion. It can be done in various ways as follows:

1. ***Manual stimulation***: Manual rotation in clockwise and anticlockwise direction (20–30 times/min) or lifting it up and then again

thrusting it down rhythmically (20–30 times/min). This is a traditional and effective method but time consuming.

2. ***Electrostimulation***: It is done by a device (Fig. 29.1) which delivers an electrical stimulus to the point in varying intensity, frequency and wavelength. In 1953, Dr Reinhold Voll, an accomplished acupuncturist, developed his own system of electrodermal testing that enhanced the theoretical understanding and practical application of modern acupuncture. Using a very sensitive voltmeter called **Diatherapuncteur**, he diagnosed functional and structural changes in the organs by measuring the change in voltage potential on points of corresponding meridians of those organs. This instrument which was basically designed for locating acupuncture points was later modified for therapeutic purpose of giving electrical stimulations to acupuncture points, as these points were found to have low resistance and high conductance. In this instrument, we have a choice of different pulse waves like adjustable/continuous for anaesthesia, paralysis, etc., dense and disperse for analgesia and discontinuous type for flaccidity. Frequency of 50–100 Hz are used for analgesia, more acute the condition, more the frequency. Drug addiction treatment requires frequency of 250–350 Hz while surgical anaesthesia requires frequency of 1500–2500 Hz. Once the selected points are needled, small wires are attached by tiny clamps to the needles. The wire with black clamp is always to be attached to distal and outer points. Never connect 'Yin' and 'Yang' meridian together or points on opposite sides by one wire. Once connected, the pulse and frequency is selected and electrostimulation is given for 20–30 min. Increase & decrease of electrical impulse has to be gradually done.

Electrostimulation is to be avoided in those with cardiac arrhythmias, epilepsy, patients with pacemakers and in pregnancy.

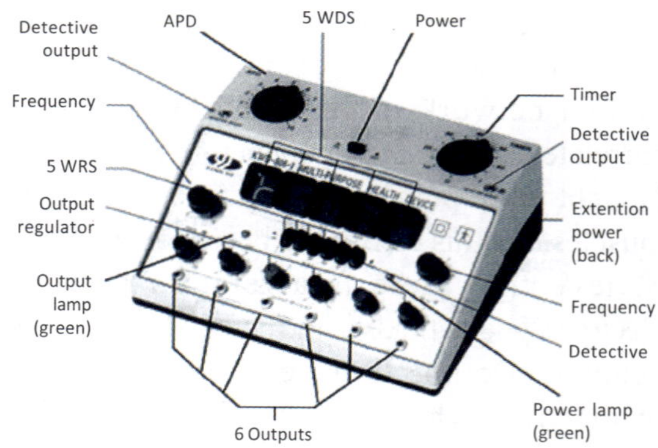

| Fig. 28.1 Electrostimulation device |

Stimulation is to be given for 22–30 min in each session of acupuncture. The number of sessions required will depend on the presenting complaint. Acute complaints may respond in 3–4 sessions each per day though they may require up to 10 sessions. Chronic ailments may require treatment for many months with one session of acupuncture each week.

FREQUENTLY USED ACUPUNCTURE POINTS

WHO has listed more than 400 acupuncture points for treating innumerable conditions. In general practice, acupuncture is used for treating mainly acute and chronic musculoskeletal disorders, for which we require hardly 50 points, which are given below.

Different Types

1. *Ah-Shi points* → These are reflexly tender points.
2. *Xi-Cleft points* → Points to be used in acute disorder of respective organ (Table 29.3).

3. *Yuan-Source points* → Points to be used in chronic disorder of respective organ (Table 29.3).
4. *Jing-well points* → Used in emergencies like convulsions, syncope, etc.
5. *Back-Shu points* → Alarm points on the back that become tender when the respective organ is affected (Table 29.1).
6. *Front-Mu points* → Alarm points on chest and abdomen that become tender when the respective organ is affected (Table 29.1).
7. *Distal analgesic points* → These are the points used for pain relief in respective areas (Table 29.4).
8. *Influential points* → For influencing the concerned organ or tissue (Table 29.4).
9. *Physiological effect points* → Affects the physiological functions (Table 29.2).
10. *Symptomatic points* → Specific points for various symptoms.

| Table 29.1 |

Zang-Fu organ	Back-Shu point	Front-Mu point
Lung	UB13	L1
Pericardium	UB14	CV17
Heart	UB16	CV14
Liver	UB17	L14
Gallbladder	UB18	GB24
Spleen	UB19	Liv13
Stomach	UB20	CV12
Triple warmer	UB21	CV5
Kidney	UB23	GB25
Large intestine	UB25	ST25
Small intestine	UB27	CV4
Urinary bladder	UB28	CV3

| Table 29.2 Physiological effect points |

1.	**Analgesic**	: Li-4, St-44
2.	**Sedation**	: GV-20, P-6, H-7
3.	**Homoeostasis**	: Li-11, St-36, Sp-6
4.	**Immunological point**	: Li-11, St-36, Sp-6, GV-14, Sp-10
5.	**Psychological effect**	: GV-20, H-1, P-6
6.	**Motor effect**	: GB-34

| Table 29.3 |

Meridian	Yuan-source point	Xi-cleft point
Lung	Lu9	L6
Large intestine	Li4	Li7
Stomach	St42	St348
Spleen	Sp6	Sp
Heart	H7	H6
Small intestine	Si14	Si6
Urinary bladder	UB64	UB63
Kidney	K3	K5
Pericardium	P7	P4
Triple warmer	TW	TW7
Gall bladder	GB4	GB36
Liver	L3	L6
Governing vessel	–	–
Conception vessel	–	–

| Table 29.4 Influential points: For influencing the concerned organ system or tissues |

1.	**Bone and cartilage**	: UB-11
2.	**Muscle and tendons**	: GB-34
3.	**Respiratory system**	: CV-17
4.	**Blood vessels**	: Lu-9, Sp-6, Sp-9
5.	**Hollow organs**	: CV-12
6.	**Solid organs**	: Liv-13

PRINCIPLES OF POINTS SELECTION

1. All acupuncture points of a meridian treat diseases occurring along that meridian and also diseases of the corresponding internal organs.
2. All acupuncture points treat diseases of the local and adjacent area.
3. For local disorders, a combination of Ah-Shi points, local points on the affected or adjacent meridian and distal analgesic points on that meridian are selected. One may add influential point or physiological effect point to it.
4. For internal disorder of organs, a combination of local points, Front-Mu, Back-Shu, Xi-cleft, Yuan-Source points, etc., is required.
5. Needling should be restricted to maximum 10 points in one sitting.

LOCATION OF ACUPUNCTURE POINTS

Best results are assured, if one properly localises the acupuncture points to be used. Proper knowledge of surface markings is a must to locate acupuncture points, as most are described in relation to some surface landmark. A special unit of measurement used in acupuncture called '**cun**' is described as the distance between the palmar creases across the proximal and distal interphalangeal joints of the middle finger of the patient. It is also measured as the width of the thumb at its widest part. An instrument called '**cunometer**' is available to facilitate this measurement. Points can also be located with the help of point detectors that are provided with electrostimulation machine.

| **Table 29.5** Distal analgesic points (These points are very useful for pain relief in respective areas) |

In upper limbs	
1. **Li-4**	: Face and special sense organs, ventral surface of head and neck
2. **Lu-7**	: Dorsal surface of head, neck and chest.
3. **P-6**	: Ventral surface of chest and upper half of anterior abdomen wall. Internal organs of chest, diaphragm and internal organs in the upper half of the abdomen
In lower limbs	
1. **St-36**	: Internal organs of the abdomen and abdominal wall below umbilicus
2. **Ub-40**	: Low back, urogenital organs
3. **Sp-6**	: Perineum, pelvic organs and external genitals

TWELVE MAIN MERIDIANS AND TWO EXTRA MERIDIANS

1. Lung meridian

Lu-5 : *Position* : In elbow crease, lateral to bicipital tendon.
Indications : Any type of skin disorder. Pain in elbow.

Lu-7 : *Position* : 2 cun proximal to distal wrist crease, on styloid process of radius.
Indications : *Distal analgesic point* of back of neck, head and thorax. Therefore used in occipital headache, cervical spondylosis, torticollis, neck pain, facial palsy.

2. Heart meridian

H-3 : *Position* : Just anterior to the medial epicondyle of the ulna.
Indications : Tennis elbow, elbow joint arthritis.

H-7 : *Position* : On the wrist joint crease medial to the tendon of flexor digiti minimi muscle.
Indications : *Sedating point*, wrist joint arthritis.

3. Pericardium meridian

P-3 : *Position* : In the elbow crease medial to biceps tendon.
Indications : Elbow joint arthritis, tremors, palpitation, angina pectoris.

P-4 : *Position* : 5 cun above centre of anterior wrist joint crease, between palmaris longus and flexor carpi radialis.
Indications : *Xi-cleft point* useful in mental disorders, psychosis, suicidal tendencies.

P-6 : *Position* : 2 cun above centre of anterior wrist joint crease.
Indications : *Distal analgesic point* for area of chest and upper abdomen. Costochondritis, postherpetic neuralgia, angina, hiccough, upper abdominal pain, specific point for vomiting, tranquilising point, insomnia.

4. Small intestine meridian

Si-3 : *Position* : Proximal to head of 5th metacarpal bone on the ulnar palm border (where the transverse crease of the palm ends)

Indications : Occipital headache, cervical spondylosis, acute low backache, bronchial asthma, ear disorders.

Si-6 : *Position* : On the styloid process of the ulna.
Indications : Acute bronchial asthma, ulnar neuritis, eye disorders, deafness, vertigo. *Distal analgesic point, Xi-cleft point.*

contd.

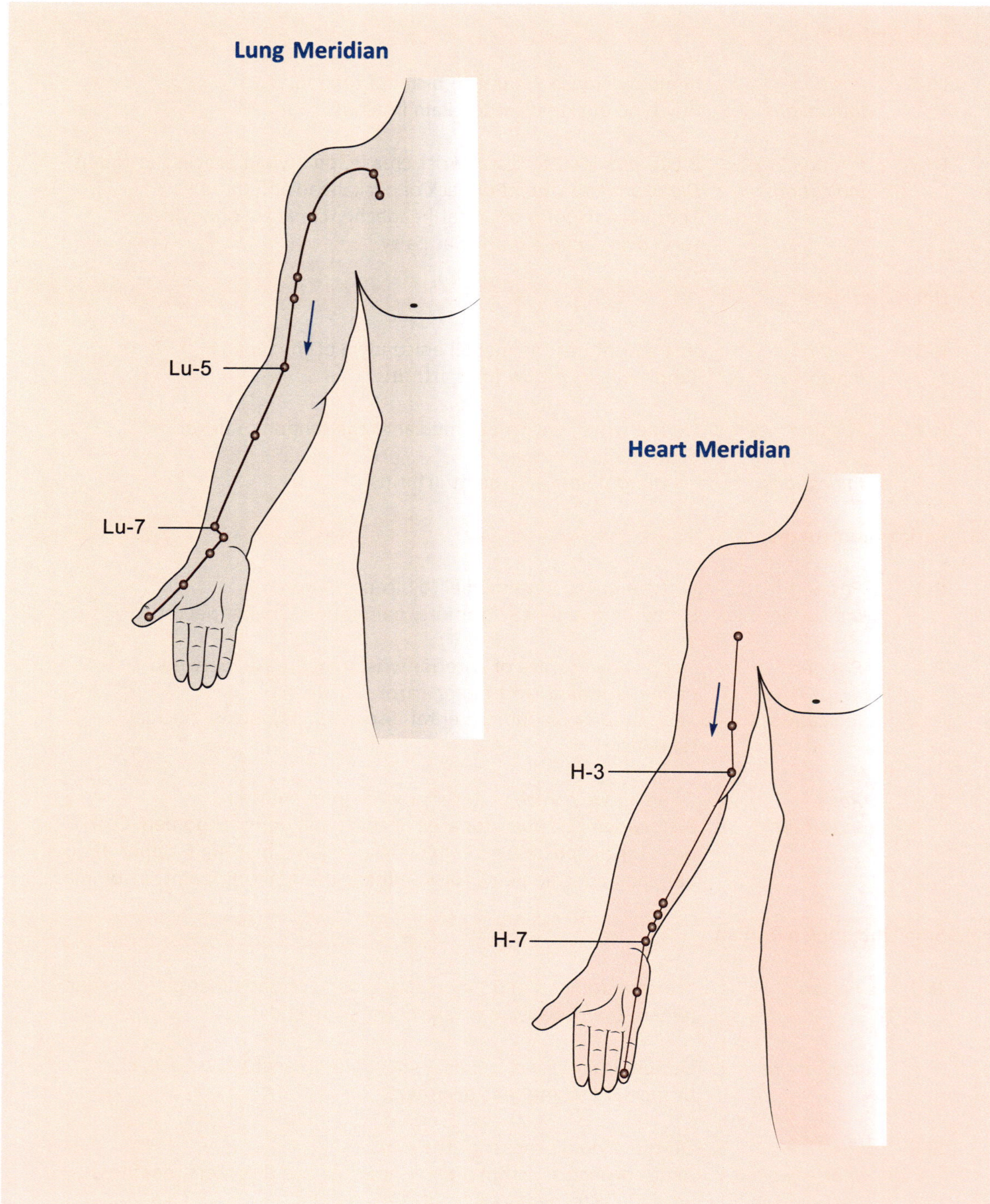
Lung Meridian
Lu-5
Lu-7
Heart Meridian
H-3
H-7

Si-8	: *Position*	: Between medial epicondyle and olecranon process.
	Indications	: Ulnar neuritis, tennis elbow, elbow joint pain.
Si-9	: *Position*	: 1 cun above the posterior axillary fold.
	Indications	: Frozen shoulder, shoulder joint pain, cervical spondylosis, paralysis, hemiplegia.
Si-10	: *Position*	: At a point vertically above Si-9, just below the spine of the scapula.
	Indications	: Same as Si-9.
Si-11	: *Position*	: On a point on scapula that is equidistant from Si-9 and Si-10.
	Indications	: Same as Si-9.
Si-12	: *Position*	: On the point just above scapular spine, equidistant from Si-10 and Si-11.
	Indications	: Same as Si-9.
5. **Large intestine meridian**		
Li-4	: *Position*	: In the web space between thumb and the index finger on the highest point of interosseous muscle.
	Indications	: *General analgesic point* for pain anywhere in the body, anaesthesia for any surgical procedures, e.g., tooth extraction. *Distal analgesic point* for frontal headache, face and neck and sensory organs of the face. '*Yuan*' *source point* for large intestine, therefore used in chronic complaints like constipation, colitis, diarrhoea etc. It is called '*Hegu*', i.e., great elimination of many disorders.
Li-5	: *Position*	: Centre of anatomical snuff box.
	Indications	Headache
Li-9	: *Position*	: 3 cun below Li-11 on the line (Li-5 ® Li-11)
	Indications	: Headache, flatulence, dyspnoea, stomach pain.
Li-10	: *Position*	: 2 cun below Li-11 on the line (Li-5 ® Li-11)
	Indications	: Tennis elbow, elbow arthritis, polio, paralysis of upper extremity frontal headache.
Li-11	: *Position*	: On the lateral end of elbow joint crease when elbow is semiflexed and pronated.
	Indications	: Immunological point: e.g., in immunodeficiency & autoimmune disorders Haemostatic point: e.g., hypertension, hyperpyrexia, etc. Paralysis, polio, tennis-elbow, elbow joint arthritis

contd.

Pericardium Meridian

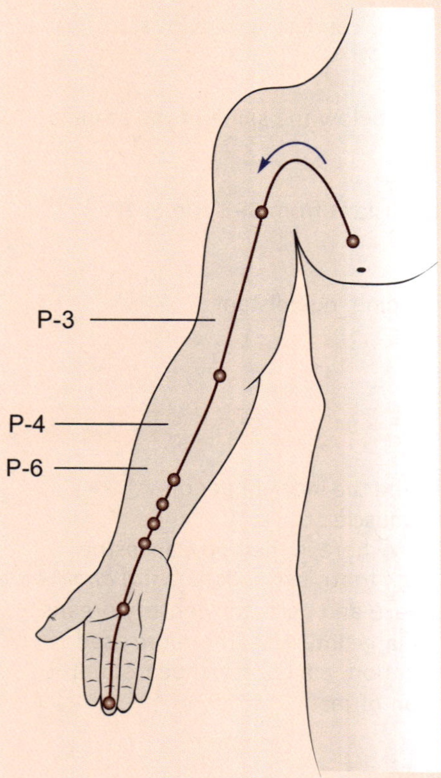

Small Intestine Meridian

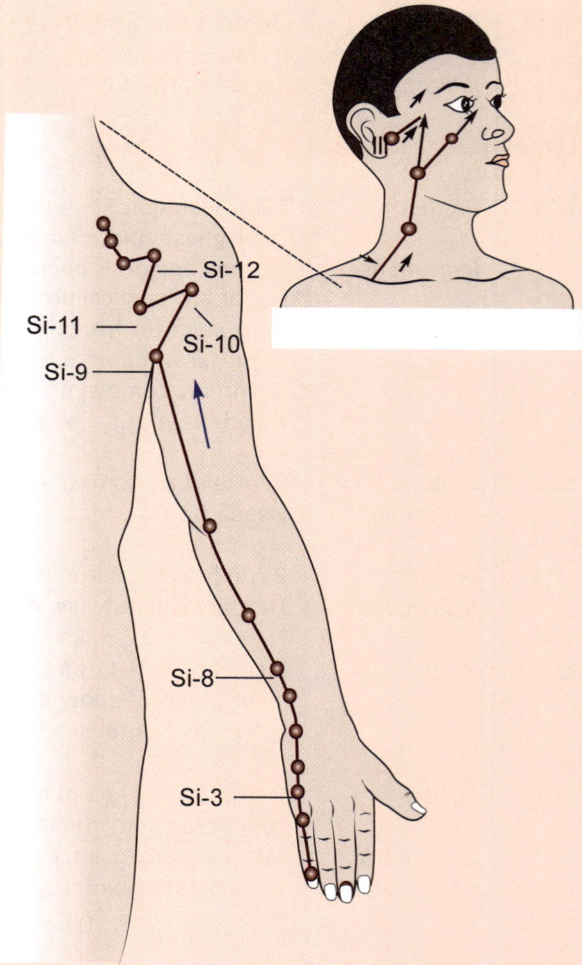

Li-15 : *Position* : On the point in the depression formed on the shoulder joint when the arm is abducted, just medial to the medial margin of deltoid muscle.
Indications : Frozen shoulder, shoulder joint arthritis, cervical spondylosis, paralysis, polio.

Li-16 : *Position* : Superior to shoulder joint between the acromial end of the clavicle and the spine of the scapula.
Indications : Same as Li-15.

Li-19 : *Position* : 0.5 cun lateral to the line joining middle of the nose to middle of the lips.
Indications : Facial palsy, trigeminal neuralgia.

6. Triple warmer meridian

Tw-4 : *Position* : Centre point of dorsal wrist joint crease.
Indications : *'Yuan' source point*, wrist joint arthritis, wrist drop, migraine.

Tw-14: *Position* : The point of depression on shoulder joint posteriorly when shoulder joint is abducted.
Indications : Frozen shoulder, arthritis, cervical spondylosis, brachial neuralgia.

Tw-21: *Position* : Above the head of the mandible in front of the ear.
Indications : Ear disorders like deafness, tinnitus, vertigo, otitis externa, facial palsy, trigeminal neuralgia.

Tw-23: *Position* : On lateral end of eyebrow.
Indications : Eye disorders, facial palsy, sinusitis, frontal headache.

7. Gallbladder meridian

Gb-14: *Position* : 1 cun above the centre of midpoint of eyebrow.
Indications : Frontal headache, sinusitis, migraine, eye disorders.

Gb-20: *Position* : Lies on the point below occipital prominence where sternomastoid muscle and trapezius muscles meet.
Indications : Occipital headache, cervical spondylosis, torticollis, neck pain, rigidity, frontal headache, rhinitis, common cold, facial palsy. Very important point for eye disorders, eyestrain. Sedative point. Drug addiction. Epilepsy, fibromyositis.

Gb-21: *Position* : Midpoint between GV-14, i.e., point between C-7 & T-1, vertebral spines and acromial head of the clavicle.
Indications : Occipital headache, torticollis, hiccough, spasmodic croup, influential point and alarm point for the gallbladder. Menstrual disturbances. Frozen shoulder.

contd.

Large Intestine Meridian

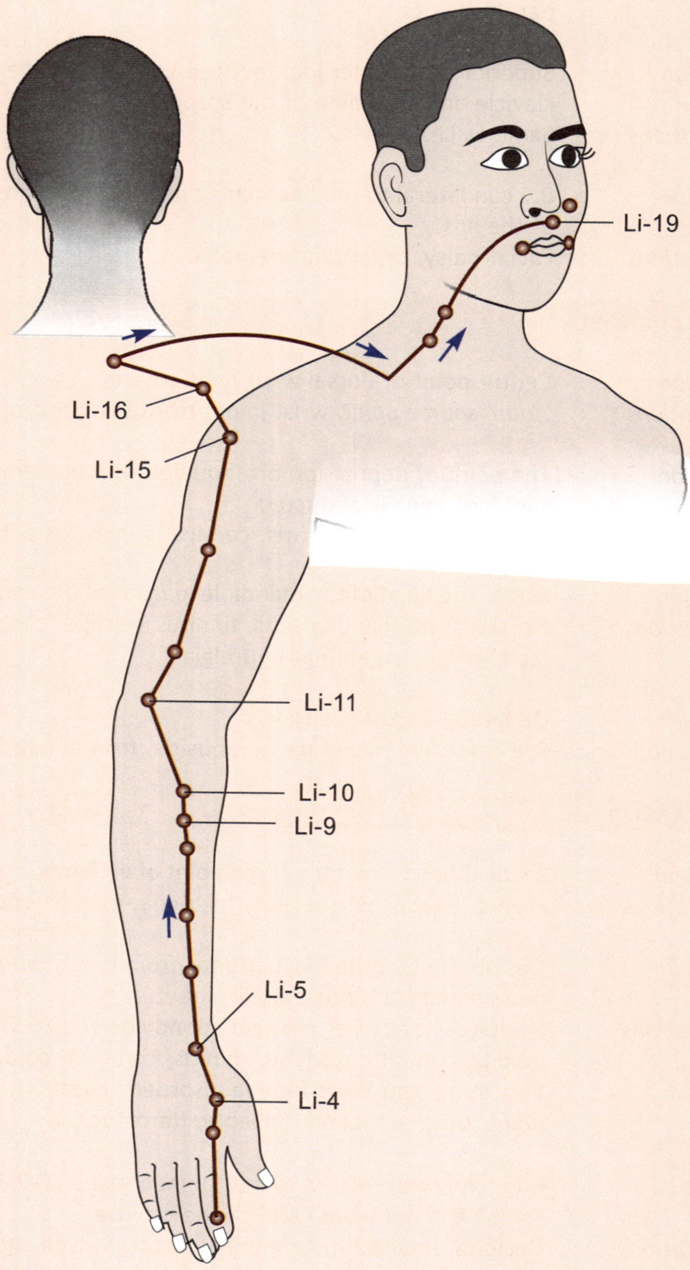

Gb-29:	*Position*	:	Midpoint between anterior superior iliac spine and greater trochanter.
	Indications	:	Any low backache, spondylosis, ankylosing spondylitis. Hip joint arthritis. Sciatica.
Gb-34:	*Position*	:	Lies just in front of and under the fibular head.
	Indications	:	Influential point for muscles and tendons. Migraine, tension headache, knee joint arthritis, epilepsy, insomnia, foot drop, neuritis.
Gb-40:	*Position*	:	Draw a line perpendicular from anterior border of lateral malleolus and a line passing through its base—the point where the two lines intersect is GB-40.
	Indications	:	Sprain, foot drop, ankle joint arthritis.

Triple Warmer Meridian

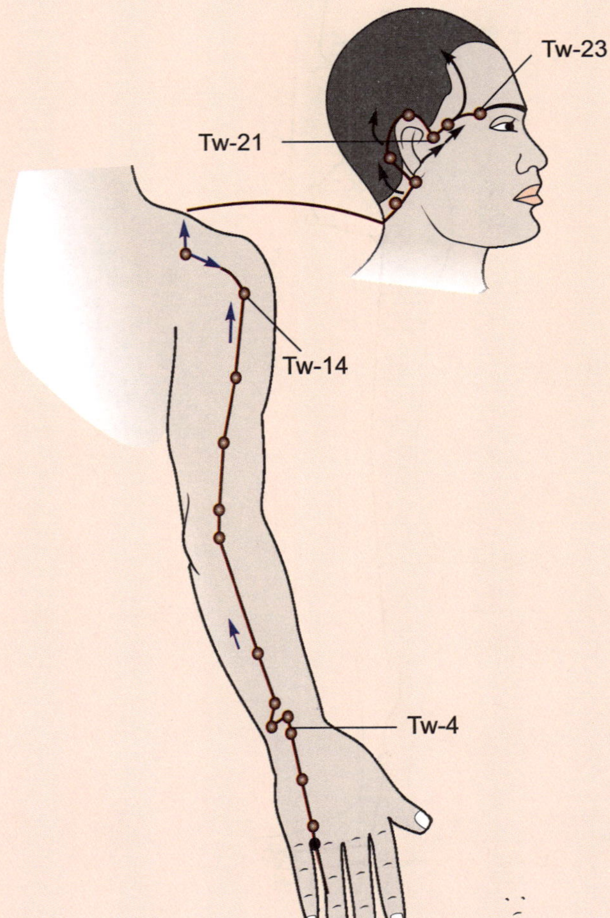

Gallbladder Meridian

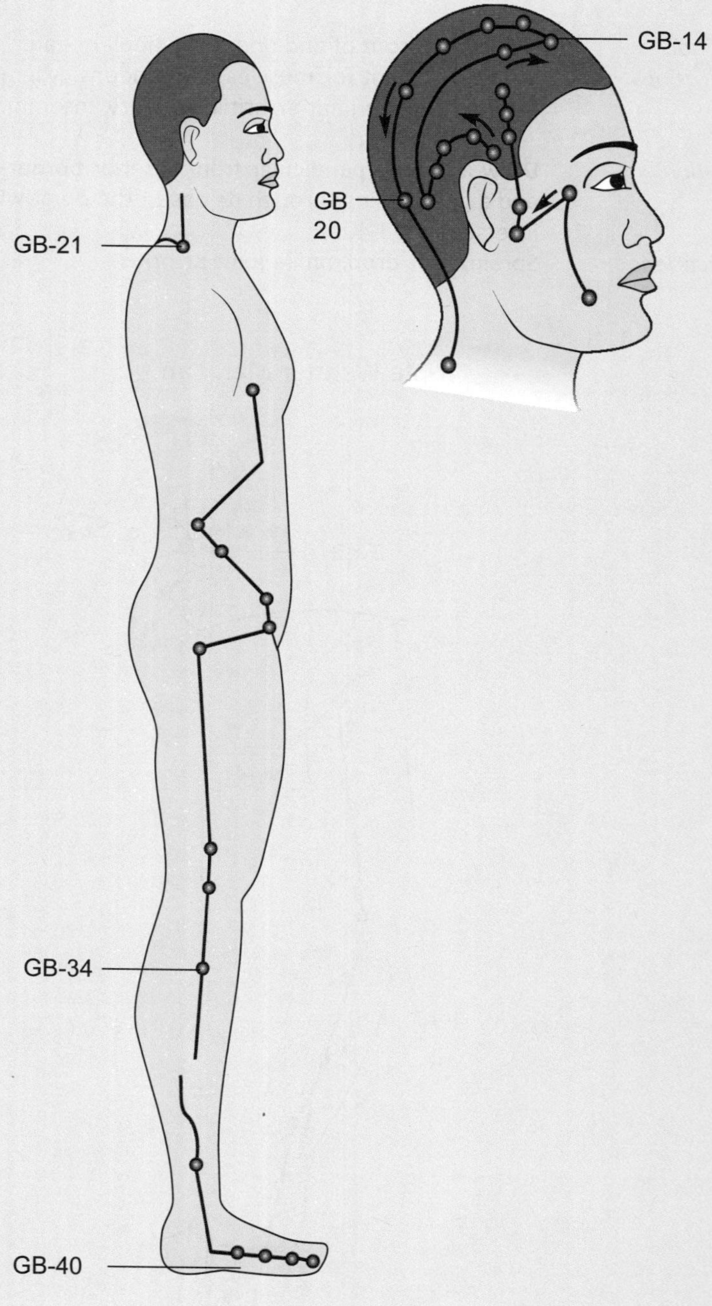

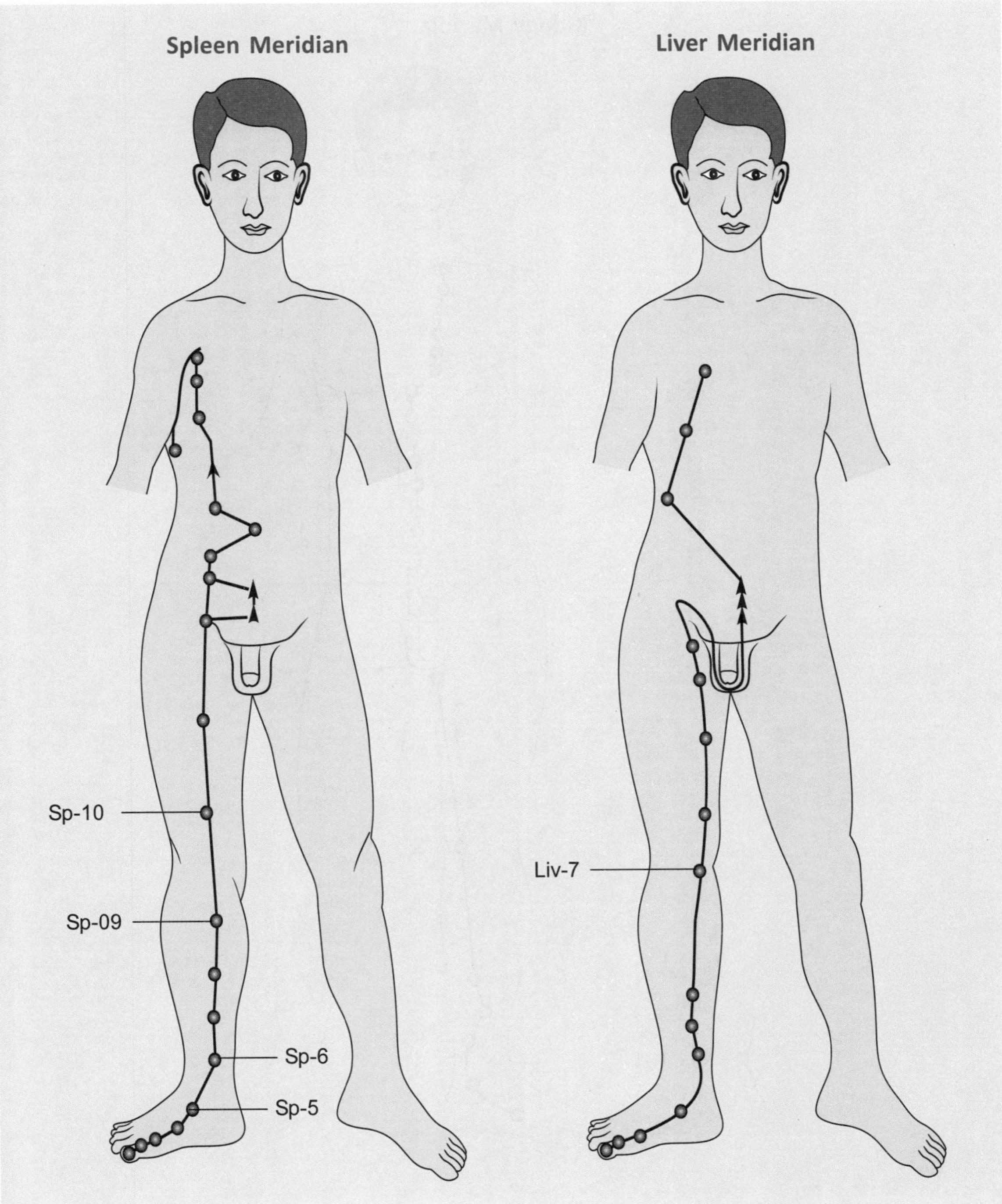
Spleen Meridian
Liver Meridian
Sp-10
Sp-09
Sp-6
Sp-5
Liv-7

Kidney Meridian

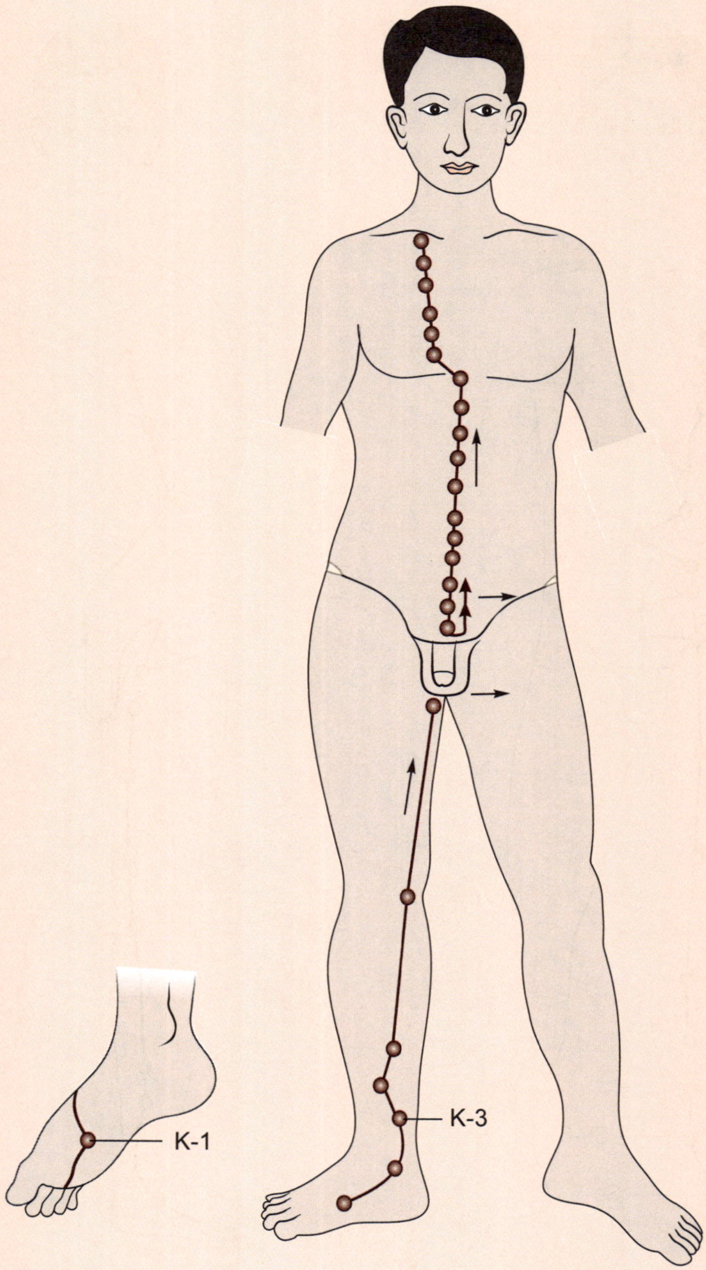

8. Spleen meridian

Sp-5 : *Position* : Just in front of and below the medial malleolus.
Indications : Ankle joint arthritis, sprain in medial ligaments; sedating point, ankle oedema, gastritis.

Sp-6 : *Position* : 3 cun above medial malleolus on posterior border of the tibia.
Indications : Distal analgesic point for pelvic organs, perineum and genitourinary organs. Antidiabetic point. Influential point for blood. Immunological point, insomnia.

Sp-9 : *Position* : On the medial condyle of tibia at the level of tibial tuberosity.
Indications : Gynaec disorders, oedema, knee joint arthritis.

Sp-10 : *Position* : 2 cun above mediosuperior angle of patella.
Indications : Antiallergic point, immunological point, knee joint arthritis, quadriceps weakness.

9. Liver meridian

Liv-7 : *Position* : Medial end of the popliteal crease between semimembranous and semitendinous tendon in semiflexed knee position.
Indications : Migraine, dysmenorrhoea, oligospermia, external genital organs pain, leucoderma.

10. Kidney meridian

K-1 : *Position* : At the point of deepest part on the sole.
Indications : Jing-well point, hysteria, cyclical vomiting, epilepsy, vertex head ache, deep boring type of pain anywhere in the body, plantar fasciitis, sweating of soles, etc.

11. Urinary bladder meridian

Ub-10: *Position* : 1 cun below the occipital protuberance.
Indications : Cervical spondylosis, neck pain, torticollis, eyestrain, refractory errors, vertigo.

Ub-11: *Position* : 1.5 cun lateral to T1 spinous process.
Indications : Influential point for bone and cartilage, cervical spondylosis, cough.

Ub-31–Ub-34
Position : In each sacral foramen.
Indications : Genitourinary disorders, dysmenorrhoea, enuresis, dribbling, low backache, sacroiliac joint arthritis.

contd.

Urinary Bladder Meridian

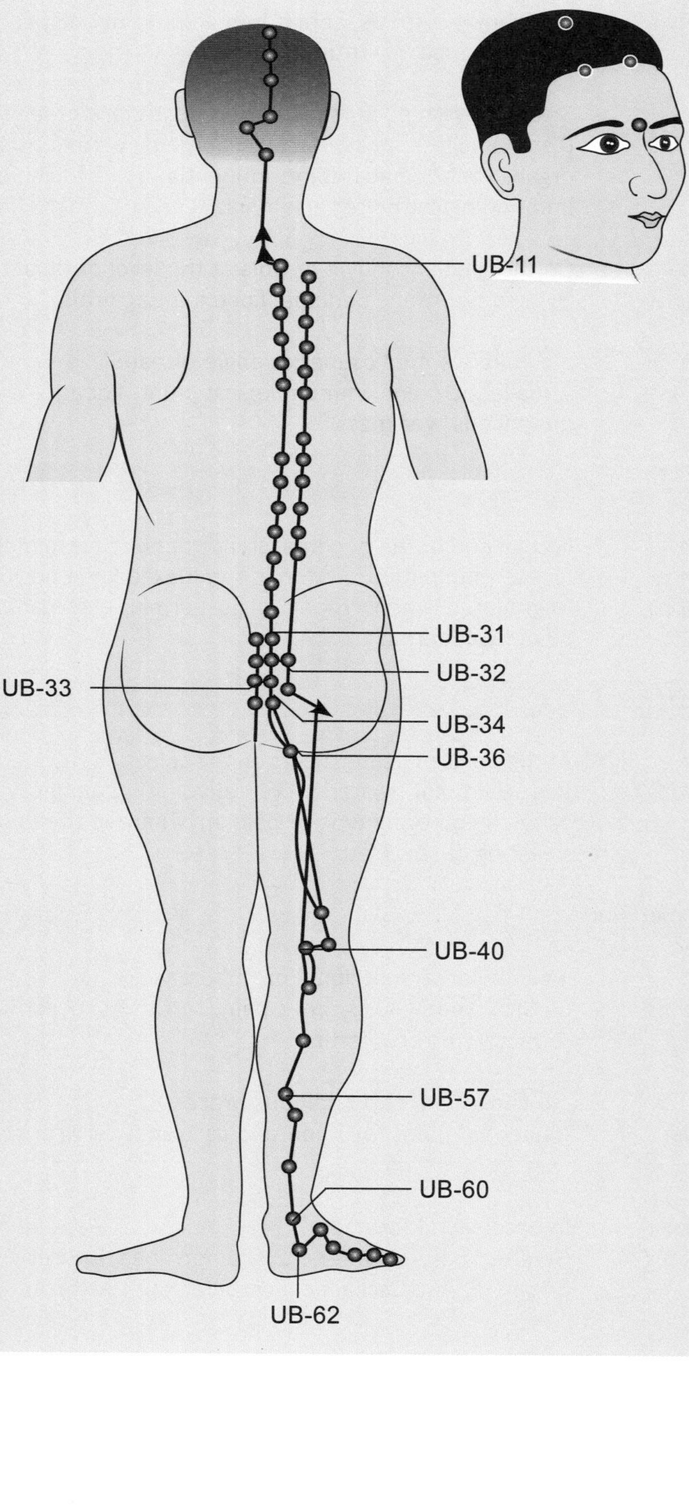

Ub-35:	*Position*	:	0.5 cun lateral to coccygeal tip.
	Indications	:	Coccidynia, sciatica, perineal pain, fissure, fistula.
Ub-36:	*Position*	:	Midpoint of gluteal fold.
	Indications	:	Sciatica, low backache, lumbar spondylosis, sacroiliac joint arthritis, fissures, fistula, piles.
Ub40 :	*Position*	:	Midpoint of popliteal crease.
	Indications	:	Distal analgesic point for pelvic organs and lower back. Knee joint arthritis, leg cramps, paralysis, calcanean spur, plantar fasciitis, skin disorders of any kind.
Ub-57:	*Position*	:	Point where 2 bellies of gastronemius muscle meet.
	Indications	:	Sciatica, muscle cramps, knee joint arthritis, calcanean spur, plantar fasciitis.
Ub-60:	*Position*	:	Midpoint between lateral malleolus and tendoachilles tendon.
	Indications	:	Ankle joint arthritis, lateral ligamental sprain, occipital headache, cervical spondylosis, low backache.
Ub-62:	*Position*	:	0.5 cun below lateral malleolus.
	Indications	:	Sedative point, insomnia, drug addiction, epilepsy, anxiety neurosis. Ankle joint arthritis, calcanean spur, ankle sprain, occipital headache, cervical spondylosis.

12. Stomach meridian

St-6 :	*Position*	:	On the most prominent part of masseter muscle, just superior to angle of mandible.
	Indications	:	Temporomandibular joint arthritis, toothache, mumps, tooth extraction (lower molars), facial palsy.
St-34 :	*Position*	:	2 cun above superiolateral angle of patella
	Indications	:	Xi-cleft point of stomach, i.e., used in acute stomach disorders. Knee joint pain, osteoarthritis, polio, paralysis.
St-35 :	*Position*	:	In the point of depression lateral to the ligamentum patellae in a semi-flexed knee position.
	Indications	:	Knee joint osteoarthritis, knee pain, polio, paralysis.
St-36 :	*Position*	:	1 finger lateral to tibial tuberosity.
	Indications	:	Distal analgesic point for abdominal complaints, immunological point, haemostatic point. Tonification point for depression, anxiety, fatigue, obesity (it controls craving for food), chronic diarrhoea, sprue.

contd.

Stomach Meridian

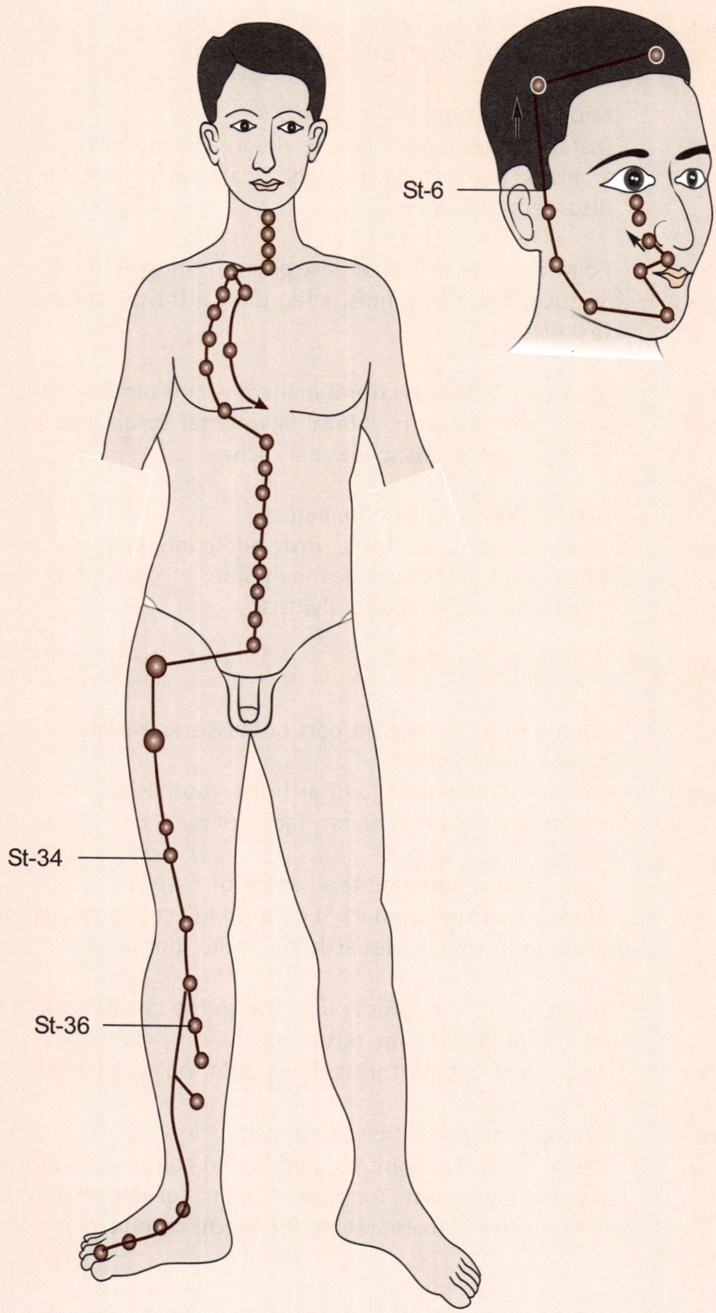

13. Conception vessel meridian

CV-6 : *Position* : 1.5 cun below umbilicus.
Indications : Diarrhoea, malabsorption syndrome, depression, fatigue, weight loss, impotence, hypertension. Tonification point.

14. Governing vessel meridian

GV-3 : *Position* : Between 4th and 5th lumbar vertebrae in the midline.
Indications : Low backache, sciatica, hip joint arthritis, urinary incontinence, menstrual disorders, impotence, painless labour.

GV-4 : *Position* : Between 2nd and 3rd lumbar vertebrae in the midline.
Indications : Same as GV-3.

GV-14: *Position* : Between C7 and T1 vertebrae in the midline.
Indications : Tranquilliser point, epilepsy, insomnia, drug addiction, immunological point, torticollis, cervical pain

GV-20: *Position* : On the point on the vertex in the midline of the line joining both the earlobe tips.
Indications : Most important tranquilliser point. Insomnia, drug addiction, epilepsy, acute low backache, pain in perineum, painful piles.

GV-26: *Position* : On a point at the upper most $1/3^{rd}$ part of the philtrum of the nose.
Indications : Most effective Jing-well point, nasal disorders, facial palsy, trigeminal neuralgia.

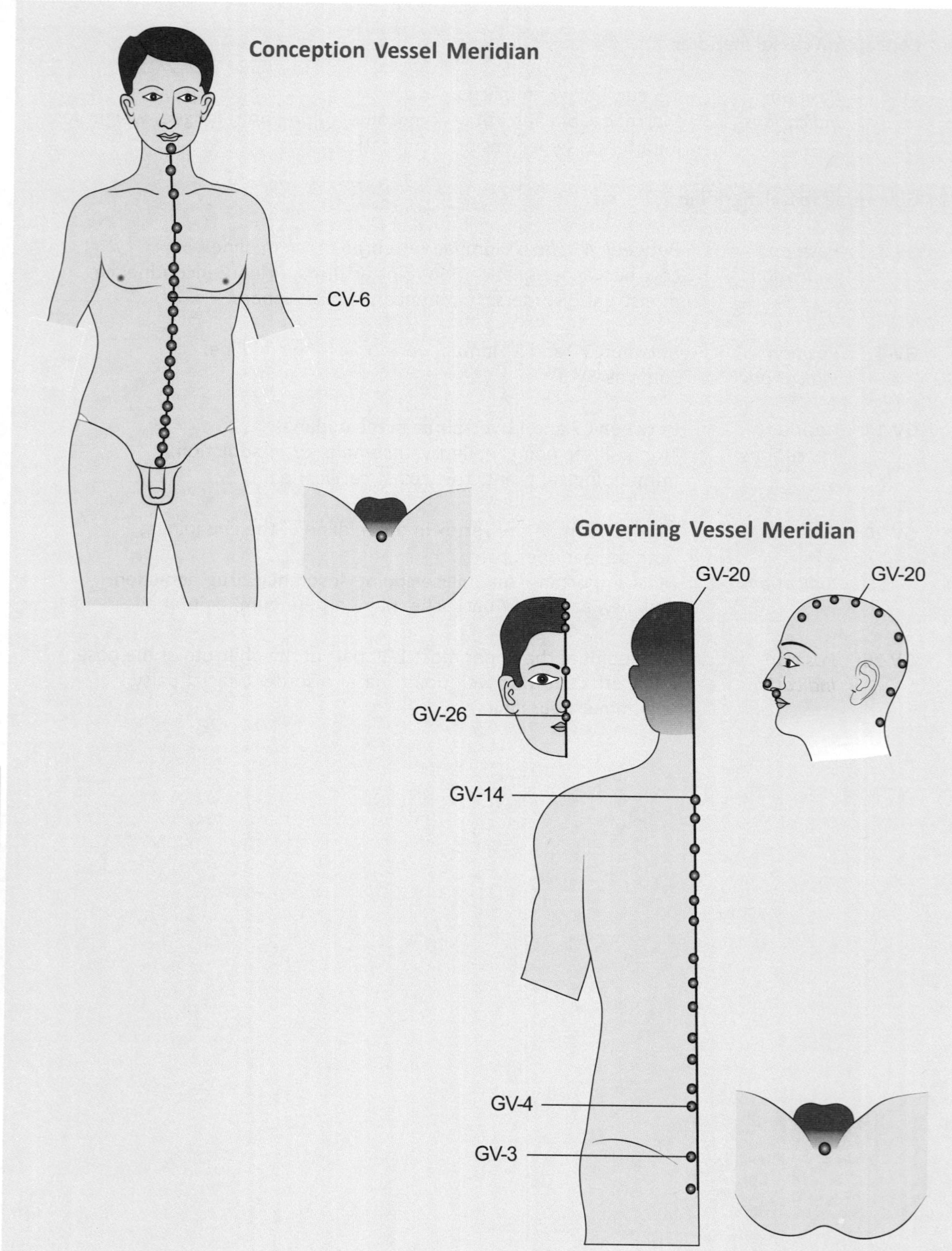
Conception Vessel Meridian
CV-6
Governing Vessel Meridian
GV-20
GV-20
GV-26
GV-14
GV-4
GV-3

THERAPEUTICS

Acupuncture points required for treating common conditions seen in general practice and where acupuncture gives good results, are given below. In the beginning till you have memorized the locations of different points, you will need to refer to the point charts. We have to follow the principle of point selection given above while choosing the points.

- **Cervical pain**—Ashi points, Ub-10, Ub-11, Ub-62, Gb-20, Si-3, Si-9, Si-10, Si-11, Si-12.
- **Shoulder pain**—Ashi points, Li-4, Li-10, Li-15, Li-16, Si-9, Si-10, Si-11, Ub-11, Tw-14.
- **Elbow pain**—Ashi points, Li-4, Li-10, Li-11, Li-12, Tw-5, Tw-10, H-3, Lu-5, Si-8.
- **Wrist pain**—Ashi points, Si-6, Tw-4, Li-5, Tw-5.
- **Low backache**—Ashi points, Ub-23, Ub-25, Ub-31, Ub-37, Ub-40, Ub-57, Ub-60, Ub-34, GV-4, Si-3, GV-20.
- **Hip pain**—Ashi points, Gb-29, Gb-30, Gb-31, Gb-34, Ub-40, Ub-60, St-36.
- **Knee pain**—Ashi points, Gb-31, Gb-34, Ub-40, Liv-6, St-34, St-35, St-36, Sp-9, Sp-10, Sp-6.
- **Sciatica**—Ashi points, Ub-27–34, Ub-6, Ub-40, Ub-57, Ub-60, Gb-29, GB-34, GV-3, GV-4.
- **Neurodegenerative disorders**—P-6, GV-3, Sp-6, Lu-5, Ub-40, Li-4, Gb-20, Ub-10.
- **Nasal complaints**—Li-4, Li-20, Li-11, GV-14, Li-19.
- **Gastritis**—P-6, St-36, CV-12, Ub-21, St-25, Sp-6.
- **Toothache**—Li-4, Li-11, St-6, St-44.
- **Cough**—Lu-7, Sp-6.
- **Hiccough**—St-36.
- **Insomnia**—H-7, Sp-6, GV-20.
- **Nausea, vomiting**—P-6, St-36.
- **Trigeminal neuralgia**—Li-19, Li-20, Tw-21, GV-26.
- **Facial palsy**—Tw-21, Tw-23, GV-26, Li-19, Li-20.
- **Drug addiction**—UB-62, GB-20, GV-20
- **Migraine, sinusitis**—Gb-14, Gb-34, Ub-2, Tw-4.
- **Hemiplegia**—K-6, Ub-62, Li-4, Li-11, Si-6, Ub-36, Ub-40, Ub-58, Ub-60, Gb-30, Gb-33.
- **Most commonly used points**—St-35, St-36, Sp-6, H-7, UB-23, UB-40, P-6, GB-20, GB-34, Li-4, CV-12, GV-4, GV-24, GV-20, GV-26.

ADVERSE EFFECTS

In the hands of a well-trained practitioner, acupuncture is fairly safe, devoid of any risks or complications. 'Does acupuncture hurt?' is probably the most frequently asked question by people seeking acupuncture treatment for the first time.

The question is simple, but the answer is difficult. Some people show very little sensitivity to the needles, others don't. Needling in some areas might be painful while in other areas it is not. A patient may feel more pain on one occasion than on another. In general, however, treatment should not cause significant pain. Slight bleeding after removing the needle is not very uncommon but innocuous. A very sensitive individual might have a vasovagal syncope after needling, which can be prevented by always needling the patient in lying down position. The risk of local infection can be minimised by scrupulous disinfection of the part to be punctured.

Blood-borne infections are a theoretical risk only if one pays proper attention to sterilisation technique of the needles, i.e., boiling for 20 min or keeping them in a box containing formalin tablets. Disposable needles can be used in affording patients. Having a fair idea of internal anatomy will avoid complications like pneumothorax, haemothorax, cardiac tamponade, penetration of kidney or bladder, injury to nerves, etc. Care must be exercised while treating the very young or the very old and debilitated patients.

FUTURE

Acupuncture is now quite widely used in Europe and North America, both as a method of therapy and in many centres as a method of anaesthesia, even in major surgeries like those of heart and brain. Acupuncture clinics and training centres have come up in large numbers in many countries like France, Australia, Germany, Russia, Japan, etc. In the last 20 years, there has been a lot of research in understanding the mechanism of acupuncture and in its application. New concepts like electro-acupuncture, laser acupuncture, needleless acupuncture are a fall-out of the western interest in this eastern science. In this comparison, acupuncture is in its infancy in India. The Acupuncture Research and Training Centre established at Raipur is amongst the few centres which provides training to doctors and has a good patient turnover. It is surprising that the science whose origins can be traced to all Vedas and Shrutis, is still in the dark, and neglected here. It is ironical that acupuncture, which is the most ancient and oldest medical technique, is considered 'alternative' even till today. It is hoped that the future will see acupuncture as one of the 'main stream' medicine with wider application than just a means of analgesia and anaesthesia.

*This chapter has been reviewed by **Dr Nitin Bidkar**, Pune.*

CHAPTER 30

Skills in Practice Management

- Your Clinic
  - Area selection
  - Design of the clinic
  - Drug stock
  - Management of staff
- Prescription Writing
- Maintaining Records
- Time Management
- Continuing Medical Education (CME)
- Research in General Practice
- The General Practitioner and the Law

A family practice these days demands that this profession is managed in a professional way. Family practice has to be compared with a small-scale industry, which delivers the goods to its customer in an efficient manner, within prescribed time and with the best of quality. A family practice also requires proper planning, organization of the clinic and the staff, time management, finance management, etc. All the foregoing is part of the '*practice management skills*' and will be discussed under the following headings.

'YOUR CLINIC'

Make Proper Choice of the Area of Your Practice

This fast world of competition requires proper selection of the place of practice and I feel no GP should start a practice in a place merely because a premise is already available to him from his forefathers, ready to use. This can be one of the factors in failure of a practice. Time spent in selecting the area of your prospective practice is time well spent (I know one GP who has changed seven clinics in 14 short years!).

Gone are those days when the patient used to walk long distance to take treatment from the doctor of his choice. The life today is fast and most of the patients want nearby service. They will compromise even on quality, especially for trivial illnesses, if the clinic is inconvenient or the waiting time is long.

Hence, the aim should be to make quality care available at the doorstep. At the least, it should be easily reachable by public or private transport. It should be preferably on the ground floor for the convenience of the seriously ill or the aged patients. See that parking facilities are available, especially if you are opening the clinic in a metropolis or in a crowded market place. Neighbouring business activity should be such that, especially old patients or ladies should have safe and easy passage (e.g., see that your neighbour's business is not a two wheeler repair shop, who will in all probability, place all his vehicles at your doorstep).

With health and hygiene at their low profiles, it may appear that the low socio-economic class residing locality is ideal to start your practice. However, it is very difficult to develop the ideal ethical practice style in such localities. This is because of ignorance and negligence (mind you, never the poverty) on the part of the patients and therefore improper obeyance of the commands of the GP.

There is no such place as 'a virgin area of practice' today, where no doctor is practising, except the remotest areas, in the deep rural interiors. Hence competing with the already practising doctors is the call of the day. If 10 GPs are doing fine, you could be the 11th GP doing the finest amongst them.

Design Your Clinic Properly

This is important due to scarcity of space available and its increasing cost. The minimum stipulatory requirement of clinic space by some health organizations like CGHS or ESIS, is 250 sq ft. This is rightly the bare minimum, considering the easy movement of the patient and the doctor. A family clinic ideally should have 3 rooms.

1. ***Doctor's room***: This includes the doctor's table and chair, examination table (2′ × 7′), 2–3 chairs for the patient's relatives, partition for the examination table and a proper place for instruments like BP apparatus, ophthalmoscope, dressing material, etc.
2. ***Reception area***: Ideally, this should have comfortable sitting arrangements, a receptionist's cubicle, a dispensing cubicle and an additional space for storing drugs, old record books, etc.
3. ***Additional service area***: Family practice in recent years has widened its horizons and limits as family physicians are 'grasping' more and more specialization areas in medi cine and surgery. This requires additional space for additional instruments like the ECG machine, nebuliser, short wave diathermy, cervical traction apparatus, laboratory instruments, etc. An additional room if available can be a boon. It can be used as "multipurpose room" for patients who are severely ill, putting emergency IV fluids, suturing wounds, etc. As the patients are going to spend a couple of hours at your clinic sitting idle, make your clinic agreeable with comfortable sitting arrangements, entertainment facilities (like soft music, a TV set, magazines, dailies, etc.), projection boards (displaying notices, information articles, services available), a weighing machine, etc. All these go long way in keeping the patients engaged and make the long uneasy wait bearable!

Drug Stocks and Inventory

A general practice can be purely consulting or dispensing or a mixture of the two. Still in most of the areas in India, dispensed drugs are valued much by the patients due to their tremendous faith in the doctor. Hence, stocking of drugs is an essential feature in general practice.

Some hints on how to handle these stocks:

1. The drugs are generally purchased in bulk quantities. The purchases should therefore be streamlined as per the requirements only.
2. The stocks must have a register. Separate inward and outward registers can give proper idea of drug usage, the drugs in stock and the drugs required to be ordered.
3. Sudden rise in the purchase of drug indicates some pilferage by the staff or theft.
4. Storing of certain drugs requires a refrigerator. This is also required to maintain the cold chain for vaccines.
5. The unnecessary stocking of the drugs and drug samples leads to drugs expiry. Hence,

periodic check-up of the stock, especially of injections is very much essential.

Management of Staff

Gone are the days when the family doctor used to run the whole show singlehandedly. Now, it is essential to have helping hands to smoothen your work process. The salient features of staff selection and management are given below:

1. The staff members usually required are a trained assistant, a receptionist, a sweeper and a compounder to dispense drugs.
2. The staff is either pre-trained or should be trained at your clinic.
3. The staff should be qualified to read and write simple English. The receptionist should have the knowledge of computers.
4. Salaries should be according to minimum wage scale.
5. Dispensaries are covered under the Bombay Shops and Establishment Act, 1948. Hence, proper attendance and leave records should be maintained.
6. Each of the staff members must be assigned specific duties. Their performance should be subject to periodic evaluation.
7. Regular staff meetings can provide a good feedback and increase the rapport with them.
8. The staff should never feel indispensable.
9. Insurance coverage: The staff mistakes, which can be problematic medicolegally, can be covered under your indemnity by addition of little extra premium. The social and medical security of the staff can be achieved by taking out their insurance (mediclaim or life insurance).

THE ART OF PRESCRIPTION WRITING

A prescription is a document, which the patient takes from you and goes to the chemist for "filling in". He keeps the prescription paper with himself. He might go to other doctors and show them your prescription. Needless to add that this important document is going to make or mar your reputation. Hence, while writing a prescription, observe the following ground rules:

1. Write the prescription on a proper printed-paper, which contains your name, address, telephone number, etc.
2. Inscribe the symbol 'Rx' on the left hand corner. This is equivalent to 'Om' in the Indian context. It symbolizes a prayer to the God of medicine that "may the following prescribed drugs help my patient".
3. Write down the patient's name, address and date on which the prescription is written.
4. Legibility is important. Don't force the chemist to pass a remark that he cannot read the doctor's handwriting. A good doctor–chemist relationship is helpful.
5. Write the important items first, followed by the less important items, e.g., start with antibiotics and end up with B-complex.
6. The instructions to the patient should be clear as to how to take the medicines. Do not write short-forms like tds, bd, stat or sos, which the patient will not understand.
7. Check the availability of the drug before prescribing. Do not create a situation where the patient has to move from shop to shop for a B-complex preparation of your choice. More hazardously, the patient suffering from typhoid should not land up in a hospital with toxicity just because the ciprofloxacin you have prescribed is not available.
8. In case of uneducated patients, ask them to show the medicines prescribed. Instruct them properly as to how to take them.
9. Prescribe proper dosages to children and beware of drug toxicity in elderly.

10. Finally, consider before prescribing "Is this drug really necessary?" Some patients believe that there is a "drug solution to every discomfort" and "there is pill for every ill". Good counselling is any time better than a fancy coloured placebo.

MAINTAINING RECORDS IN GENERAL PRACTICE

Under the Bombay Nursing Home Act, it is compulsory for every doctor to keep records of his patients, which contains the details about their illnesses. It is an important confidential document and no doctor can disclose it without the consent of his patient.

It is essential and useful to keep records for the following reasons:

1. Because it is legally compulsory.
2. For proper treatment of the patient—Records give F/H/O hereditary diseases like hypertension, diabetes, etc. H/o drug allergies can be recorded which could occasionally save a life. For a difficult case, such records are a great help in following the evolution of the case.
3. For medicolegal use, if and when required. Ideally, it is expected of a GP to maintain records for 21 years!
4. For research or practice audit—the data available in family practice is huge. If documentation is done in a proper way, there is tremendous scope for using this material for research.
5. For computing the income and the income tax.
6. For health department records, as and when demanded during epidemics. Or for knowing the incidence and prevalence of various diseases.
7. For remembering the names of your patients.

Nevertheless, it is surprising that an average GP refrains form keeping records. What could be the reasons behind this attitude and trend?

Name: **Age:**

Address: **Sex:**

Known case of: Allergic to:

Family history of:

Past history of:

Date	Clinical	Treatment		Bill	
		Dispensed	Prescribed	Cash	Balance

Summary

Sample Case Paper

1. Record keeping is a time consuming and clerical job and most of the GPs consider this as a waste of time.
2. Many of their patients are "wanderers" shifting their loyalty from one doctor to another, and hence may visit the GP once in their lifetime.
3. Most of the patients come for minor complaints like headache for which keeping records is hardly of any value.

How to Keep Records?

There are hardly any write-ups in the literature of how to keep records in your clinic. A few references will explain to you about family folders with family genograms or problem oriented medical records (POMR) where records are kept according to major class of diseases like diabetes, hypertension, heart diseases, etc.

But in practice, most GPs gradually evolve their own system and case paper sheets over a period of years. Broadly speaking, doctors can be categorized into 3 subsets according to the case paper record they maintain. A few have case paper system, which they maintain and keep with them. Others prepare the case papers and hand it over to the patients to be brought to the clinic on every visit. The third category of doctors, the majority of them, have no case paper system at all! The ideal format of a case paper sheet is shown above.

The system of handing over the case paper sheet to the patient has its own pros and cons. For the doctor, it saves him the headache of filling the records. But, there are many pitfalls in this system:

- The case paper might get lost or the patient forgets to bring the paper at each visit.
- The GP has to write the details properly as the paper might land up in another GP or consultant's hands. The treatment given there is exposed to criticism.
- The papers are handled by the patients very frequently and hence can get torn or spoilt. Hence, a good quality paper has to be used or a protective plastic folder supplied. Few government hospitals circumvent this problem by asking the patient to keep a hardcover notebook. It is a good, economical system for poor patients.

How to Preserve Records?

- *Alphabetic filing system*: Here, the case papers are preserved surname wise, alphabetically.
- *Numeric system*: The case papers are numbered and the patient has to remember his number (like a bank account number) and give it to the receptionist, whenever he visits the GP.
- *Colour coding* helps in identifying special categories, e.g., all diabetics with a red mark at the corner of the case paper or each year case papers can have different colours.
- *Inactive records,* i.e., records of patients who have not attended for the past 5 years, should be purged periodically to avoid burdening of the record system.
- *Case referral records*: The details of the patients who have been referred to hospitals, specialists or diagnostic centres can be compiled separately.
- *The register system*: Here, the names of the patients can be in a register each day. When the patient comes back again the patient is asked the date of his last visit, and the record found. The problem comes when the patient does not remember this date.

A number of GPs have started using computers for keeping records. In time to come, computers may become a necessary part of a GP's set up.

Computers in Family Medicine

Introduction

Until quite recently, family physicians (F.Ps) seemed to be apprehensive in accepting the recent technological advances, especially use of computers in their day to day practice. But now, many family physicians have become conversant with the use of computers including maintaining records of their patients. Previously, it was justified to manage the record manually on hard paper format. However, now the expectations of the patients from the family physicians are increasing and fast recording and retrieval is the order of the day; resorting to this modality of record keeping has become essential.

Advantages

1. Computers can store huge data in a very short space. This reduces the paper work and space occupancy required by huge paper files.
2. Various user friendly softwares are available which can be used by the family physician very easily.
3. Variety of parameters like details of investigations, immunisations, of drug allergies, family history, etc., can be recorded in the software along with the routine record of patients.
4. All these parameters can be retrieved at a fingertip instantly. This helps to give accurate and in depth planning of patient's treatment.
5. Perfect prescription writing is possible which reduces confusion and gives clear cut instructions to the patients. Charts about diet, exercise, post-operative/preoperative instructions, etc., can be easily provided as print out, as and when required.
6. The computer records can be economical and help a lot in perfectly maintaining the balance sheet of the clinic.
7. Telemedicine is the subject of the decade and F. Ps should also take the advantage of the same. Broadband and Internet are now giving quite reliable services. In the hours of emergency, an immediate help in the form of tele-consultation is possible, e.g., evaluation of critical ECGs or even routine ones can also be reported with the help of cardiologist's colleagues. For routine initial first-aid consultations or for follow-up, this can be a good tool.
8. Research in Family Practice is still at quite a rudimentary stage, at least in our country. Computerisation will be very much useful in data collection/analysis interpretation/and even better presentation.
9. The clinical audit of one's practice would become most easy and can be done at regular intervals.
10. With the use of Internet, the knowledge updating process becomes easier and the free time can be used to update the knowledge available from all over the world.

Thus, to improve the quality of the services, computers can become a good tool.

Disadvantages

1. The basic problem at least in the present scenario is the non-availability of the trained staff. However, in the near future, this will not be the problem.
2. Time required to discharge the patients may take longer.
3. The cost of hardware and software, the staff salary and the maintenance costs presently are adding to the overheads. But those can be managed by escalation of fees reasonably

in lieu of superior quality provided to the patients.

Few Suggestions

Day by day family physicians are expected to expand their services beyond the 'Disease and Cure' approach. They should offer extra services as time has become costlier than money. Hence, by appointing assistants and use of fast acting gadgets, maximum care should be provided to the patients under one roof. This will save the time and at the same time, update the clinic.

HOW TO DIGITALISE YOUR CLINIC?

As a part of 'Digital India' and 'Digital Transformation' going all over the World, it is high time for all individual medical practitioners to digitalise their clinics also. For the last 30 years, we have seen 'Digital Disruption' taking over each industry and it has already taken over most of the Healthcare Industry. All big players in the industry have made changes to their infrastructure and processes to keep up with the rest of the World. Now, it is the time for all professionals to match the pace to remain in line with everyone in their industry.

While getting into the details of digitalisation, let us understand a few concepts and advantages to make the decision easy for each one of you.

Advantages of Digitalisation

Computerisation and Digitalisation are synonyms and they both mean entering, storing and processing the data into the electronic form. Indians are doing this for many years and we have tons of pages of data already converted into electronic form. We are trying to replace or reduce the use of paper and at the same time control the use and access of this data as required. As we all know, when the data is stored on computers, it is extremely easy for us to retrieve the same, filter it, sort it or analyse it and create meaningful reports from the same.

Exchange of data through the internet, email and chat applications has become extremely easy with all the innovations in this field. If almost every Doctor in the country is using Smart Phone (which I will call a mini version of a Computer), it should not be a challenge to use a Desktop or a Laptop for your official/clinical work.

It will soon become a mandate to keep all medical records in Electronic Format only and compliance will become an important factor in this journey.

Which Data do you need to Store as a Doctor?

- **EMR** – Electronic Medical Record – The patient record created by you as a Medical Practitioner.
- **EHR** – Electronic Health Record – Collection of patient's health data from various clinicians.
- **PHR** – Personal Health Record – Comprehensive medical data maintained by the patient himself/herself.

As we know it all, most of the patients from India do not maintain their medical records meticulously, so as a Doctor or as Family Physician, it is more important for a Doctor to maintain the same.

As a part of maintaining your clinic, apart from the Patient Records, you may also need to maintain invoices, payment receipts and stock/inventory of any medicines you maintain in your clinic.

Once you have a Computer in your Clinic, you will find more ways of utilising the same in improving the efficiency of all tasks. Taking that 'First Step' is most important!

Use of Electronic Devices & Internet by Medical Practitioners & Healthcare Staff

In general, most doctors do not make much use of Computers at their Clinics as it is not a mandatory device to carry out their work. At the same time, involved in the below activities:

- Using *Smart Phone* for all personal and professional use.
- Most of them use *email* and do various other subscriptions.
- For study and research, they search *Medical Journals* and Databases.
- They attend online training sessions, *webinars*, conferences.
- Everyone *watches videos* on YouTube and other sites.
- Most Practitioners use *Social Media*, Read Blogs, visit Medico sites.
- *Exchange of lab reports*, X-ray and other documents also happens through email.
- Because of the pandemic, *Medical consultation* started through video calls.

With so much familiarity with electronic data, it should not be difficult to use Computers in the clinic.

We have to see where our industry is moving. So let us see, how the large players in Healthcare Industry are already digitalised. Some examples:

- Insurance Companies who are computerising very fast and all policy-related services are available online. Entire claim processing is also digitalised long back.
- Hospitals are also computerising fast and from registration to billing to all Administrative services are already computerised in big cities & all western countries. There are large Hospital Management Systems (HMS) already in place.
- Pharmacies have computerised stock management and billing & now medicines are sold online also.

Considering the Digital Disruption all over the World, we should also see **the future technological trends in Healthcare Industry** and try to align ourselves with the same:

- *On-Demand Healthcare* availability of all healthcare services wherever needed.
- *Big Data* to improve Healthcare (gathering and analysing large data will help get the analysis better).
- Most organisations are not interested in managing their own IT infrastructure now, so the data is stored in Cloud.
- The use of *Virtual Reality* is increasing in Training and Care delivery.
- *Robotic Surgery* (Robots being used for complex tasks) with remote control is no longer sci-fi!
- *Wearable Medical Devices* (health status monitoring) connected to the Internet is coming to the common man's reach.
- The use of *Artificial Intelligence* (*AI*) has already started in Medical Field for chatbots, virtual assistants, etc.

What Immediate Benefits Doctors & Society are going to Derive from this Digitalisation?

- User/Patient need to benefit from the Computerisation for sure!
- One-Stop Solution/Convenience!
- Ease of diagnosis, increase in efficiency and Revenue Growth for Doctor.
- Ease of Use (Readymade/Customised software).
- Impact – A Doctor becoming Digital is equivalent to hundred patients becoming Digital!
- Advantages to Patient: No manual forms, no Xerox, no queue, no need to carry cash, single point treatment, not much travel and no tension!

There can be different scenarios of Medical Practitioners who are at various stages in the journey of Digitalisation:

Pre-requisites for All:

Familiarity with computer and basic knowledge of Windows and MS Office (Word, Excel and PowerPoint), use Google or any other email. The use of the internet is known to everyone due to smartphones, so that is assumed.

Recommended set-up:

Buy any new/used Laptop and/or Desktop with Internet connectivity. Use a ready-made/customised Clinic Management System and start capturing data of patients. The data will be entered by the Doctor/Assistant. In case you still don't have software in place, you can even start entering the data in an Excel sheet but taking that first step towards digitalisation is important.

An economical option is the main Doctor in the clinic should have his/her Laptop which they should carry to the Clinic every day and take home while leaving. The receptionist/Assistant should have another Desktop or Laptop (permanent) at the Clinic.

Scenario 1 – A Practitioner who has never used a Computer in the Clinic/has set up a New Clinic:

Process: Start entering new patient data first and in the background, ask someone to do data entry for all old patients provided you have their paper-based records available with you. Give a unique 'Patient Number' to each patient and so that every time the patient re-visits, you can search patient record with that number. You can create a standard format for the prescription on your Computer. Use the same to fill in the prescription and hand over the printout to the patient.

Assuming the Main Doctor is in the Clinic:

- The patient enters your clinic.
- Receptionist/Assistant/Doctor asks for Patient Number/Patient ID/Registration Number/Patient Name and pulls out the EMR on her computer. If the patient is new, a new record (EMR) is created.
- Any previous laboratory report details are entered into the EMR.
- Patient meets Doctor.
- Doctor adds notes, types Prescription and next appointment & hand-over print out to the patient.
- The patient goes out with a prescription and next appointment as well.
- The patient will have a paper record and the Doctor will have an electronic record.
- 2 Computers and 1 Printer. Computers are connected through the Internet.

Scenario 2 – A Practitioner who is already using a Computer in the Clinic:

Process: Make sure you have some Clinic Management System in place and existing patient data is already entered into the System. The system should have a provision to create prescriptions also.

Assuming the Junior Doctor is in the Clinic and the Main Doctor is at some other location:

- The patient enters your clinic.
- The Receptionist/Assistant asks Patient Number/Patient ID/Registration Number/Patient Name to pull out the EMR on her computer. If the patient is new, a new record (EMR) is created.
- If the patient has got any reports, the details are entered into the EMR.
- Patient meets Junior Doctor.

- Junior Doctor calls the main Doctor who also opens the EMR on his Laptop. They discuss and finalise the treatment. Junior Doctor adds notes, types prescription and next appointment & hand-over print-out to the patient.
- The patient goes out with a prescription and next appointment date as well.
- We are not trying to make patients high-tech but Doctors will be more high-tech.
- 2 Computers, 1 Printer. Computers are connected through the internet.

Scenario 3 – A Practitioner who is well-versed with Digitalised Systems and want to use them more:

Process: You can have a cloud-based Clinic Management System in place where the data is stored at a central location. Any other devices in the Clinic should also be connected to computers and printers.

Assuming the Main Doctor is in the Clinic:

- The patient enters your clinic.
- The Receptionist/Assistant asks Patient Number/Patient ID/Registration Number/ Patient Name and pulls out the EMR on the Clinic computer. If the patient is new, a new record (EMR) is created.
- If the patient has got any reports, the details are entered in the EMR.
- Patient meets the Doctor.
- Along with medical notes and prescription, Doctor may have ECG machine connected to ECG Printer & Digital X-ray machine (in case of Dentists) connected to the Computer.
- Doctor takes ECG (if required).
- Accept Digital Payment (POS/UPI/Cash) and give a printed receipt.
- The patient goes out with a prescription and next appointment date as well.
- 2 Computers, 2 Printers (one to print prescriptions and another to print ECG) and other Medical Instruments connected to the net. Consultants send their reports, images through email. Some ECG machines have an in-built printer, in which case you do not need an additional printer.

Scenario 4 – A Practitioner who is at the advanced stage of using Computers in the Clinic:

Process: Doctor and Staff are well-versed with Clinic Management System and able to use it from Clinic and any remote place. They can analyse the data and can get customised reports also. All medical devices are connected to Computers and Printers. Medicines stock also can be maintained in the inventory.

Assuming the Main Doctor is in the Clinic:

- The patient has taken an online appointment.
- A patient comes and shows any reports which are entered into Clinic Management System at the reception.
- Any other Doctor reports, notes are shared with your Doctor by email.
- Patient meets the Doctor.
- Doctor adds notes; type prescriptions and next appointment & hand-over print out to the patient.
- Doctor takes ECG (if required).
- The receptionist sends a photo of the prescription to the nearby medical shop and they deliver the medicines to the clinic (optional)/ Doctor gives medicines (optional).
- Accept Digital Payment (POS/UPI/Cash) and give a printed receipt.
- The patient goes out with a prescription and next appointment date as well.
- Patients can also get a SMS reminder a day before appointment (need to integrate SMS Gateway into the Clinic Management System).

- 2 Computers, 2 Printers (One to print prescriptions and another to print ECG) and other Medical Instruments connected to the net. Consultants send their reports, images through email. Some ECG machines have an in-built printer, in which case you do not need an additional printer.
- Ensure that the data backup is taken regularly, since you are having a lot of data now!

Summary

The below points play an important role in the *Digitalisation of your Clinic*:

- Taking the first step towards Digitalisation is important.
- Trust, Time and Technology give a Wow effect! 2 Computers and 1 Printer can be a sufficient set-up to digitalise your clinic.
- Patients are likely to get one-stop services, also increasing Doctor's revenue.
- Economical and easy to implement solutions will last longer.
- Latest Clinic Management Systems are Web-based, so you can connect as many computers as you want to the data stored at a central location/cloud.
- You will have 'data', which is the most important asset to any profession/business today.
- Convenience to patients matters the most! Satisfied patients are like to re-visit and refer others.

TIME MANAGEMENT IN GENERAL PRACTICE

Especially for GPs, the importance of time cannot be undervalued. This is because as compared to specialists, who charge hefty consultation fees per patient, the GP has to depend on the rapid turnover of his patients. This is because the per patient income for a GP is proportionately less.

Understandably, restlessly waiting in crowded waiting room, especially for a patient who is suffering is quite a tiring proposition. But, majority of the patients even though not seriously ill are not patient enough to wait for long hours in the waiting room. They are ready to pay more elsewhere in order to save time (as for them, time is money). They will opt for an unknown doctor, if their regular family doctor is busy.

You cannot change patient's attitude. So, how can you change your style of functioning and save time in your clinic without compromising on the quality of your health care?

1. *Ensure your presence in your clinic at the declared timings*: Coming late or closing too early must be avoided. This ensures the availability of the doctor in his clinic and helps the patient to plan his visit.
2. *Give adequate time to your clinic*: This suggestion especially applies to doctors who have more than one establishment.
3. *Give adequate time to each patient*: The time required per patient varies. However, about 6–9 min/patient is considered adequate enough in general practice for patient's satisfaction and at the same time ensuring proper quality of your health care. Provide only essential slot of time required for history taking, examination and management. No irrelevant questions, no unnecessary detailed examination.
4. *Find out areas where your expertise* is not required and pass on these areas to your assistant, e.g., writing notes or prescriptions, maintaining case paper, giving injections, etc.
5. *Use a competent assistant*: Doctors who have just passed out will readily help you in your work in the hope of gaining experience for their future practice.

6. *Use a computer*: However, worldwide it has been found that in a GP's clinic, computers are helpful only for record maintenance or data entry rather than in minute-to-minute management.
7. Design convenient movement of the patient in the clinic. This saves much of the transit time of the patient. Make provisions for accepting two patients at one time in the examination room.
8. Instruct the receptionist to pass on only the most essential phone calls.

As a result, if you have managed time properly in your clinic, you will have enough time available at hand for personal development, for relaxation, for family and friends and for research and reading. This refreshes the mind and in turn improves the quality of patient care.

CONTINUING MEDICAL EDUCATION (CME)

The medical scene is growing, developing and changing every day. With newer and newer diagnostic aids and therapeutic modalities becoming available, it is very much essential for a GP to update himself. Also, many medical associations have opined that periodic medical updating should be made compulsory as a prerequisite to renewing the license of a general practitioner to practise. A new law has been introduced in Maharashtra and in a few other states which require 6 CME credit points (certified by respective Medical Council) per year and 30 credit points per 5 years for renewing the registration of all medical practitioners. If introduced as a law all over India, this would definitely help to upgrade the quality of practice in India.

What are the opportunities available to a general practitioner to medically upgrade himself periodically?

1. *Medical workshops, conferences and symposia*: These are arranged by various medical associations and provide a platform to impart knowledge.
2. *Peer group formation*: Small groups of interested doctors can be formed. They can have periodic meetings where they can have discussion on various academic subjects and also on various aspects on practice management. They can also take up bigger research projects by pooling the individual data.
3. *Training programmes*: Considering that the present undergraduate training system is grossly inadequate to be of any practical value to a GP, special general practice training courses have now been designed, e.g., DNB in family practice or the FCGP course conducted by the IMA. Many universities also conduct certificate course examinations.

RESEARCH IN GENERAL PRACTICE

One of the few ways by which a GP can become a "master in general practice" is by doing research. The number of patients seen by a GP is quite large and the clinical presentation varied requiring immaculate management skills.

A GP has therefore a large choice of subjects to choose from. This could include simple questions that we ask patients or simple queries that come to our mind during day-to-day clinical work. Or the subject could be on practice management or doctor–patient relationship. Typically, the subject of research could be something like:

- Does recurrent cough without associated bronchospasm in children be associated with asthma?

- Is suicidal tendency in teenage boys precipitated by sexual misbeliefs?
- Is there any association of migraine with cervical spondylosis?
- What is the response of different antibiotics given for acute bacillary dysentery or chronic otitis media.
- Is alcohol abuse related to impotency?
- Is osteoarthritis of the knee related to depression?
- Do patient education leaflets kept in consulting room lead to increased rate of vaccination, blood sugar estimation or Pap smear?
- Are your patients satisfied with your services? A review.

The list is endless. With the present development of primary health care all over the world and the increasing use of the Internet, many foray/conferences/discussion media are available for presentation, in addition to the platform offered by your local IMA body.

The exact methodology for doing research is a comprehensive topic, beyond the scope of the present chapter. The interested researcher is referred to longer essays on the subject.

THE GENERAL PRACTITIONER AND THE LAW

In order to prevent himself from getting entangled in a troublesome suit, the GP has to know the duties of a doctor as regards to his patients in the eyes of the law. Flouting these may place the GP in a difficult situation in the court of law.

To Prevent Medicolegal Cases

1. ***Listen attentively***
   Listen to the patient's complaints and take the proper history. If the history of drug sensitivity is missed and the patient dies of drug reaction, the doctor is held responsible.
2. ***Always examine thoroughly***
   If the diagnosis is missed just because the doctor has not examined the patient properly, he will be held liable, e.g., the diagnosis of peritonitis is overlooked and the patient disposed off, the doctor will be held responsible. Similarly, in case of meningitis if the neck stiffness is overlooked and the patient dies, the doctor will be held responsible.
3. ***Take pains to explain***
   If the GP does not explain to the patient and his relatives important aspect of the disease he is suffering from and complications that arise the GP will be held responsible, e.g., if the patient is an 'open' case of pulmonary TB, explain to the family members about the infectious nature of the condition. If this is not done and if any family member gets infected, the GP could be held responsible.
4. ***Always explain the side effects*** of the prescribed drugs and to caution the patient accordingly, e.g., while prescribing a sedative antihistaminic the patient must be cautioned against driving a vehicle. Failing this, if a mishap occurs, it will amount to negligence on the part of the GP.
5. ***Timely refer*** to a hospital or to a relevant consultant, if the GP thinks that the case is beyond his capabilities. A GP has to know his limits and that he is a bachelor of medicine and bachelor of surgery and not a master of medicine and master of surgery. Refer the patient in time. If the patient becomes critically ill because of delay in referring, the GP will be held responsible, e.g., referring a patient of enteric fever after toxicity has developed or perforation of the gut has taken place, will be seen as negligence.
6. Keep only a **qualified assistant** or qualified locum.
7. Do not issue false **medical certificates**.

8. Keep proper **records** of the patients. Every physician is required to maintain and preserve records of his/her patients for a period of 3 years from the commencement of treatment in a standard format laid down by MCI (see p. 291).
9. **Investigate** whenever necessary, e.g., not ordering an X-ray chest in case of more than one-month cough. If the patient is ultimately diagnosed as having pulmonary TB, it will amount to negligence.
10. **Always update his/her knowledge**. The GP must remain in tune with the developments in the medical field by attending CME activities, etc. Ignorance cannot be held as a defence.
11. **In case of emergency**, the GP must treat the patient.
12. **In case of a road traffic accident (RTA)**, the GP must give emergency treatment. If he does not give first aid like dressing the wound, suturing a bleeding laceration, give a splint to immobilise a fracture, he can invite MCI rules being imposed on him.
13. Do not write degrees and qualifications which are not recognised by MCI on your letter heads, sign boards, etc.
14. Always attend summons for cases given to you in the respective courts. It is a professional obligation.

The GP has a right to collect his fees or refuse a visit.

Conclusion: It is heartening to know that litigation against family physicians are far less in comparison to other specialities. There are two chief reasons for this.

The first is that the family physician gives only basic primary treatment. Hence, mistakes committed by him are usually not serious enough or fatal to invite litigation. Secondly, the family physician treats the family under his care as a whole. His advice is called for even in domestic or social problems of the family. Hence, he is considered as a respected family member.

Still, it is prudent policy for all of us to have an insurance cover in order to ensure financial relief and mental peace.

*This chapter has been reviewed by **Dr Anil Panse**, MD, Family Physician, Pune.*

Topic on "How to Digitalize Your Clinic" has been written by Mr Chittaranjan Deo, MSc (Physics), ADCSSAA, IT Consultant, Pune.

CHAPTER 31

Certificates in General Practice

1. Sickness
2. Fitness
3. Indoor patients
4. Fitness for Employment
5. Vaccination
6. Will
7. Weapon License
8. Life
9. Thumb Impression
10. Character
11. Job Fitness
12. Death

INTRODUCTION

This is one of the most important areas where a family doctor is involved. It is an important source of evidence in the court of law and is liable for confirmation by cross-examination.

Hence, it has the potential of putting the family doctor in a lot of trouble, if proper care is not taken while issuing the certificate.

Essentials of Medical Certificate

1. Preferably should be on the doctor's printed letterhead.
2. It must also have the date, time, place of issue, identification-marks of the patient with his signature or his left thumb impression.
3. It should be issued for a legitimate purpose only.
4. It should be based only on facts examined by the doctor and never on the history provided by the patient.
5. It should be handed over to the patient himself and preferably an acknowledgement of the receipt obtained.
6. A duplicate copy of every certificate issued must be maintained.

Salient Features of Different Types of Certificates

Sickness and Fitness Certificate

This is the most commonly required certificate in general practice. It is required to be given under the following circumstances:

1. Employers need it for the confirmation of the sickness of their employee and for his physical fitness to rejoin the job.
2. Worker needs it in order to secure compensation for his sickness or liability.
3. For declaration of fitness of the individual for a particular occupation.
4. For declaring that the person is physically and mentally sound before signing an important document, e.g., signing a 'will'.

SICKNESS CERTIFICATE

Dr Prakash V Mahajan
MBBS, DDV (CPS), FCGP
Reg No. 38735
Skin–VD Specialist
HIV Specialist

Clinic address:
Deep Bunglow Chowk
Model Colony, Chinar Heights,
Shivajinagar, Pune
Timing:
Ph no:

I, Dr _______________ after careful personal examination, do hereby certify that Mr/Mrs/Miss __________________ (whose signature is given below) is treated as OPD patient. He is suffering from ______________ and I consider that a period of absence from duty of about ___________ days /weeks/months with effect from _____________ is absolutely essential for the restoration of his health.

Identification marks: 1. .... 2. ....

Signature/Left hand impression of Mr/Mrs/Miss ....

Signature of Doctor **Date:** **Time:**

FITNESS (RECOVERY AFTER ILLNESS) CERTIFICATE

This is to certify that I have examined Mr/Mrs/Miss............................ whose signature is given below, as on today and find that he/she has recovered from his/her illness and in my opinion he/she is physically fit to resume his/her duties from today/tomorrow, i.e. ....

Identification marks: 1. .... 2. ....

Signature/Left hand impression of Mr./ Mrs./Miss................................

Signature of Doctor **Date:** **Time:**

(Note: It is advisable to issue illness /unfit certificate and fitness certificate separately)

5. For declaring fitness of the persons for obtaining a driving license.

To avoid getting entangled in legal tangles, never issue a false certificate, as it is a criminal offence punishable under Criminal Law Procedures section no. 197. Issue the certificate only when the patient is under your care and issue it only for the period under which the patient is under your care. Avoid giving back-dated certificates. However, it can be issued after confirmation of previous documented records.

Death Certificate (DC)

Whenever the cause of death is not certain, give only a 'death declaration certificate' on a prescribed form available from the local municipal corporation. Advise the relatives to ascertain the cause of death by a postmortem examination performed in the local government hospital.

When the cause is suspicious, do not issue the certificate and inform the police. However, if under unforeseen pressure situations the general practitioner has to issue the death certificate, inform the police about the situation as early as possible. Note the details of the police authority registering your complaint.

Life Certificate

This certificate, usually requested by an elderly person's relative to receive pension, is always to be given after verifying that the person to be certified is truely alive by making a house call to avoid medico-legal case. In most cases, the relative demands the certificate claiming the inability of the elderly person to come to the clinic as he or she is bedridden or crippled.

The GP is usually not called upon to issue the following certificates. However, a fundamental knowledge about the issue of these certificate is essential to guide the patient and the relatives properly.

Fitness Certificate for Driving Licence

Snellen's chart evaluation for colour blindness and checking for refractory error are essentials before issue of a driving licence. It would be taking a risk for the lay public and your own profession if the patient is myopic and colour blind.

Age Certificate

This is required in employment or while taking out insurance or in offences of rape, child marriage, etc. While determining the age, the physician takes into consideration the general built, teeth eruption, secondary sexual characters and finally radiologist's opinion for skeletal age.

Certificate of Lunacy

Only authorized government doctor can issue this certificate after having ascertained the mental status of the individual by a psychiatrist. Direct the patient's relatives to the local civil hospital.

Disability Certificate

Again, this certificate can only be issued by an authorized government doctor along with a certificate of the extent of disability from an orthopaedic surgeon.

Birth Certificate

The maternity home where the baby was delivered informs the municipal authorities about the birth, which then issues the birth certificate.

Certificate of Infectious Diseases

This can be issued by a GP under certain conditions, e.g., a student suffering from chickenpox. Certificate for absence of infectious diseases are required by food related industries (e.g., hotels, sweet shops, etc.) for their employees. This can be issued by the GP after relevant detailed examination.

Certificate of Fitness for Surgery

Ophthalmologist demands this from the referring doctor before cataract surgery. Otherwise, in a hospital set up, a physician with the qualification of an MD is required to issue the certificate.

Vaccination Certificate

This is required before international travel and is usually issued by a designated authority.

CERTIFICATE FOR INDOOR PATIENTS

Certificate No. : ....
Date :
IPD No. : ....
MLC No. and Date : ....

To whomsoever, it may concern

This is to certify that Mr/Mrs/Miss ....is admitted in this hospital on ....as an emergency/routine patient and is suffering from ....He is under care of Dr ....

He/She was treated as IPD patient. He/She was discharged on .... and advised to have bed rest/ light duty for a period of .... days from .... till ....
He/She was operated for .... on ....
He/She is advised to undergo .... by Dr ....

He/She is fit to resume his/her duties again from ....
He/She is not in a position to give any statement or sign any papers as of now .

Signature of the Doctor

Name of the Doctor

FITNESS CERTIFICATE FOR EMPLOYMENT

This is to certify that I have examined Mr/Mrs/Miss. ....today. In my opinion at the time of examination he/she is physically fit to work as .... He/She is not suffering from any contagious disease.

Identification marks: 1) ....
2) ....

Signature/Lt. hand thumb impression of Mr/Mrs/Miss ....

Signature of the Doctor

Date:

Time:

VACCINATION CERTIFICATE

This is to certify that I have vaccinated Mr/Mrs/Miss .... as per the details given below:

1. Name of the vaccine administered:
2. Name of the pharmaceutical company:
3. Batch no:
4. Manufacturing date:
5. Expiry date:
6. Route of administration:
7. Dose:
8. Date & time of administration:

Identification marks: 1) ....
2) ....

Signature/Lt. hand thumb impression of Mr/Mrs/Miss:

Signature of the Doctor **Time**: **Date**:

Note: Take consent in local language for vaccination. The consent form should mention the advantages and side effects and complications of vaccination.

CERTIFICATE FOR WILL

This is to certify that I have examined Mr/Mrs/Miss .... today. In my opinion at the time of examination he/she is mentally in a sound state of mind to take decisions to depose his/her assets in his/her will.

Signature/Lt. hand thumb
impression of Mr./Mrs./Miss ....

Signature of the Doctor

Date: **Time:**

MENTAL FITNESS CERTIFICATE FOR WEAPON LICENSE

This is to certify that I have examined Mr/Mrs/Miss .... today. In my opinion at the time of examination he/she is in a mentally sound condition.

Signature/Lt. hand thumb
impression of Mr/Mrs/Miss ....

Signature of the Doctor

Date: **Time:**

LIFE CERTIFICATE

This is to certify that I have examined Mr/Mrs/Miss .... today. He/She is alive today on .... at .... a.m./p.m.

Identification marks: (1)..........................
(2) ....

Signature/Lt. hand thumb
impression of Mr/Mrs/Miss ....

Signature of the Doctor

Date: **Time:**

FORMAT OF LEFT HAND THUMB IMPRESSION

This is to certify that the left hand thumb impression of Mr/Mrs/Miss .... is taken in my presence.

Signature/Lt. hand thumb
impression of Mr/Mrs/Miss ....

Signature of the Doctor

Date: **Time:**

CERTIFICATE OF CHARACTER

Certified that I have known Shri .... son/daughter of Shri .... for the last* .... years .... months and that to the best of my knowledge and belief he bears a reputable character, does not have irregular or extravagant habits and has no antecedent bad or immoral behaviour which renders him unsuitable for employment.

The above Shri . ... is not related to me.

Signature: ....

Name: ....

Place: ....

Date: ....

Designation: ....

**At least 6 months at the time of signing the certificate.*

JOB FITNESS CERTIFICATE

This is to certify that I have examined Mr/Mrs/Miss .... as on today. I further certify that:

1) His eye sight is good and that any minor defect therein can be overcome by means of suitable glasses.
2) His constitution is sound.
3) He has no disease or bodily infirmity unfitting him now or likely to unfit him in the near future from the job of a ....

Identification marks: (1) ....
(2) ....

Signature/Lt hand thumb impression of Mr/Miss ....

Signature of the Doctor

Date: **Time:**

DEATH CERTIFICATE

Medical Certification of Cause of Death

FORM NO.4A (See Rule7)
(For non-institutional deaths. Not to be used for still births)

To be sent to registrar along with form No.2 (Death Report)

I, hereby certify that the deceased Shri /Smt/Kum/........... son /wife/daughter of ....resident of .... was under my treatment from .... to .... and he/she died on .... at .... am/pm

Name of deceased: ....
Sex: M/F
Age at death: If 1 year or more age: .... in years
If less than 1 year: .... in months
If less than 1 month age: .... in days
If less than 1 day age: .... in hours

Cause of Death

1. A) Immediate cause:
Due to (or as a consequence of)

State the disease, injury or complication which caused death, not the mode of dying such as heart failure, asthenia, etc. ....

B) Antecedent cause:

Due to [or as a consequence of]

Morbid condition, if any giving rise to the cause, stating underlying condition last

....

C) ....

....

2) Other significant condition contributing to the death but not related to the disease or conditions causing it ....

Interval between onset and death approx ....

If deceased was a female, was the death associated with pregnancy? Yes/No

If yes, was there a delivery? Yes No

Name and signature of the medical attendant certifying the cause of death: ....

Date of verification: ....

Certified that Shri/Smt/Kum ....

Son/wife/daughter of Shri .... R/O ....

was under my treatment from .... to .... and he/she expired on .... at .... am/pm

Doctor: ....

Medical Superintendent: ....

Name of the Hospital: ....

Directions for completing the form

Name of deceased: To be given in full. Do not use initials. If deceased is an infant, not yet named at time of death, write son of (S/O) or daughter of (D/O), followed by names of mother and father.

Age at death: If the deceased was over 1 year of age, write age in completed years. If the deceased was below 1 year of age, write age in months, if below 1 month, give age in completed number of days and if below 1 day, in hours.

Cause of death:

This part of form should always be completed by attending physician personally.

The certificate of cause of death is divided into two parts, 1 and 2. Part 1 is divided into three parts, lines (a), (b), (c). If a single morbid condition completely explains the death, then this will be written on line (a) of part 1 and nothing more need to be written in the rest of part 1 or 2. For example, lobar pneumonia is sufficient cause of death and usually nothing more is needed.

Often, however, number of morbid conditions will have been present at death and the doctor must then complete the certificate in the proper manner so that the correct underlying cause will be tabulated.

First, enter in **Part 1 (A)** the *immediate cause* of death for example 'lung cancer'. Never write down here the mode of dying, e.g., heart failure, cardiorespiratory arrest, etc. These terms should not appear on the certificate at all since they are modes of dying and not causes of death.

Next, consider whether the immediate cause is a complication or a delayed result of some other cause. If so, enter the *antecedent cause* in **Part 1 (B)**. In the above example, this could be 'chronic bronchitis'.

Sometimes, there will be three stages in the course of events leading to death. In the above example in **Part 1 (C)**, you can enter 'chronic smoker' as this, though not directly related to the chain of events causing death but has contributed to the fatal outcome.

If the other diseases contributing to the death but not related to the disease causing it, are entered in **Part 2**, for example 'severe anaemia'.

Please note: Do not write two or more conditions on a single line. Write the names of the diseases (in full) in the certificates as legible as possible to avoid the risk of being misread. Convulsion, diarrhoea, fever, ascites, jaundice, debility, etc., are symptoms which may be due to a number of different conditions. Sometimes nothing more is known, but whenever possible, give the disease which caused the symptom.

Onset: Complete the column for interval between onset and death whenever possible, even if very approximate e.g., from birth to several years.

Maternal deaths: Be sure to answer the questions of pregnancy and delivery. This information is needed for all women of child bearing age, even though the pregnancy may have had nothing to do with the death.

Old age or Senility: Old age should not be given as a cause of death, if a more specific cause is known. If old age was contributory factor, it should be entered in **Part 2**.

Completeness of information: A complete case history is not wanted, but if the information is available, enough details should be given to enable the underlying cause to be properly classified.

For example:

- *Anaemia*—Give type of anaemia, if known.
- *Neoplasms*—Indicate whether benign or malignant and site with site of primary neoplasm, whenever possible.
- *Heart disease*—Describe the condition specifically, if congestive heart failure, chronic corpulmonale, etc., are mentioned, give the antecedent conditions.
- *Tetanus*—Describe the antecedent injury, if known.
- *Operation*—State the condition for which the operation was performed.
- *Dysentery*—Specify whether bacillary, amoebic, etc., if known.
- *Complications of pregnancy and delivery*—Describe complications specifically.
- *Tuberculosis*—Give organs affected.

CHAPTER 32

The De-Addiction Centre

- Alcohol
- Tobacco (Nicotine) Dependence
- Prescription Drug Abuse

This is one more speciality you can add to your clinic. The advantages are:

- Hardly any investment is required to begin with.
- The results of counselling and drug treatment are good with perseverance and dedication.
- Any severe addiction destroys the family socially as well as financially and it is the duty of the family physician to look after the family health.
- Finally, the family becomes addicted to you, if de-addiction is successful with your efforts!

The World Health Organization (WHO) lists substance use disorders for the following classes of substances: alcohol, tobacco, opioid, cannabis, sedative hypnotics, cocaine, caffeine, hallucinogens and volatile solvents.

In this chapter, three common addictions (alcohol, tobacco and addiction to medications) which can be dealt with at a general practitioner's level are described. But, before you read on be convinced that addiction is a neurological disease like parkinsonism, dementia, etc.

ADDICTION IS A DISEASE

Till the recent past addiction was considered as *a bad habit, a lack of will power, a fault in character, lack in morality, etc. The addict was morally a bad character and the treatment was punishment.*

With the amazing development in psychiatry and neuroscience, **NIDA (National Institute on Drug Abuse)** has also come out with a new definition of addiction: *Addiction is defined as a chronic, relapsing disorder characterized by compulsive drug seeking, continued use despite harmful consequences and long-lasting changes in the brain.*

With these new definition from a competent authorities, addiction has acquired a new meaning:

- Addiction is a primary disease.
- Addiction is defined as a *chronic, relapsing disorder like diabetes and has to be managed life long.*

- It does not depend on a person's will, morals, weaknesses or character.
- It is primarily a neurological disease which affects the physical health, mental health and social life.
- Addiction causes permanent irreversible changes in the brain of the affected person.

Let us now try to understand now, why addiction has been called a disease and not a consequence of a bad moral character.

THE LIFE HISTORY OF AN ADDICT

1. The Genes the Addict is Born with

Many studies have found that genes are responsible for a significant part that someone will become addicted to any kind of substance, if he or she inherits that gene. However, it should be noted that *there is no such thing as a gene for alcoholism or a gene for opium addiction*. Numerous genes are involved in substance addiction.

Genetic influences are variable depending on the type of substance used. Genetic influences appear to account for about half (50%) the risk of becoming an alcoholic, more than half in case of heroin and opium and less than half in case of cannabis.

Some genes predisposes someone to *certain aspects of addiction*. For example, certain genes may make some people less likely to get a hangover after drinking large amounts of alcohol. On the other hand, some genes make people release a large amount of dopamine, a neurotransmitter associated with pleasurable feelings, from drinking a small amount of alcohol.

People might be genetically predisposed to thrill-seeking or risk-taking behaviour.

2. Environmental Influence on Addiction

Environment plays a very important role in developing an individual's brain, making the individual more or less susceptible to addiction. In humans, most of the brain development takes place after birth giving the environment an important role in physically shaping the various neurological systems in the brain.

The best attempt to separate these genetic and environmental factors was done by the study of identical twins who were raised in different environments. Since identical twins share all their genes, any differences between them with regard to substance addiction would be the result of differences in their environments and personal experiences. These studies found that roughly the half risk of becoming an addict is due to genetics and the other half can be attributed to environmental factors.

3. Addiction is a Progressive Disease

Another important characteristic of addiction is that it **Progresses**!

On repetitive use of a substance, the brain develops *tolerance* for the substance making him/her need more and more of the substance each time to experience the first high as he did on the first use. This leads to intake of more and more intake of the drug and the addiction progresses. More receptor sites keep on developing progressively. More the empty receptor sites more the craving.

4. Addiction Gradually Becomes a Bad Habit

The person will also prefer the drug to other healthy pleasures and may lose interest in normal life activities. Eventually, it is only the addictive behaviour that brings the addict any sense of joy or freedom from pain – not family, friends, a good meal or a pleasure trip. In the most chronic form of the disease, addiction can cause a person to stop caring about himself and his own well-being or survival.

5. Brain Chemicals and Addiction

People feel pleasure when basic needs such as hunger, thirst and sex are satisfied. In most cases, these feelings of pleasure are caused by the release of certain chemicals in the brain. Most addictive substances cause the brain to release *very high* levels of these chemicals that are associated with pleasure or reward. Over time, continued release of these chemicals causes structural changes in the brain systems involved in reward, motivation and memory. When these changes occur, the individual may also experience intense desires or cravings for the addictive substance and will continue to use it despite the harmful or dangerous consequences.

There are four major chemicals in the brain that influence our happiness (**DOSE**):

1. **D**opamine
2. **O**xytocin
3. **S**erotonin
4. **E**ndorphins

Each plays a different role in happiness.

- *Dopamine* is responsible for causing excitement and euphoria. Unfortunately, it is also associated with addictions, such as taking drugs, gambling, viewing pornography, etc.
- *Oxytocin* is the neurochemical that makes us feel empathy which helps us feel close and bonded to others when it is released. It has also called as a love chemical.
- *Serotonin* is responsible for regulation of mood. If you're in a good mood, you've got serotonin to thank. And if you're in a bad mood, you've got serotonin to blame. It is a regulator.
- *Endorphins* are responsible for masking pain or discomfort. It also will give you stimulus for achieving goals.

These neurochemicals are released in the synapsis of the nerve fibres and on repeated release create a neurological pathway (called "neuroplasticity", as explained below). Experiences that release the DOSE neurochemicals make us happy, which makes us want more and more. People suffering from addiction related problems usually have impairment in one or more of these circuitries and turn to the substance of abuse to fulfill this impairment. These substances then take the place of the deficient natural chemical.

The effects of these identical chemicals are far much stronger than our naturally existing chemicals.

6. Neuroplasticity

The term 'Neuroplasticity' is derived from the words 'Neuron' and 'Plastic'. The word *neuron* means the cell in our brain. Each neuron is made up of an axon and dendritis which are linked to each other by small spaces called synapsis. The word *plastic* means to mold or to modify. *Neuroplasticity* means that our brain can modify itself structurally and functionally and create new neural pathways as a result of our repeated actions or behaviour.

It was believed until recently that the human brain, which consists of around 100 billion neural cells, could not generate new ones. Now, it has been proven that certain areas in the brain can generate fresh cells (neurogenesis). New studies have shown through the use PET and MRI brain scanning technology that new neural cells as well as new neural pathways are generated throughout life.

How does this Theory of Neuroplasty help in the Treatment of Addiction?

In treatment, we can *re-train* the brain to develop a new pathway that helps the patient to recover. With intensive psychotherapy, we can retrain the brain and we can rebalance the addict's biochemistry, by doing activities that can rewire their brain. The brain then learns to enjoy recovery.

Conclusion: With this new definition the whole addict family has come from the clutches of the police and the law to the care of the medical fraternity. *Addiction will be gradually decriminalized gradually medicalized!*

A glaring example: 15 years back, 1% of the whole adult population of Portugal was affected by Heroin. These "criminals" were sentenced to life long imprisonment! Result? Addicts increased and there was no place in jails. A high power meeting between the president, the leader of the opposition and deaddiction specialists from all over the world decided to decriminalize addiction in Portugal. They released the addicts, rehabilitated them in the society and gave them medical treatment. Result? Addictions came down by about 50% in 2 years!

CLASSIFICATION OF PSYCHOACTIVE SUBSTANCES

In all, there are six classes of psychoactive substances.

1. Central Nervous System Depressants

- They slow down central nervous system function. Effects depends on the dose and duration of drug use.
- *Low doses*: Feelings of relaxation and calmness.
- *Mid-level doses*: Muscle relaxation, disinhibition, impairment in motor coordination.
- *High doses*: Slurred speech, bradycardia, hypotension, coma and death.
- Alcohol and Benzodiazepines are examples of CNS depressants.

2. Central Nervous System Stimulants

- A **stimulant** is a type of psychoactive drug that stimulates the activity of the central nervous system. These drugs are taken by people to feel stronger, faster & more confident.
- *Low doses*: Increases alertness
- *Mid-level doses*: Agitation, euphoria.
- *High doses*: Convulsions, myocardial infarction, stroke.
- *Chronic use*: Paranoid schizophrenia.
- Examples of CNS stimulants are Amphetamines & Methamphetamine, Caffeine and Nicotine.

3. Cannabinols

- It has both mild stimulant and depressant effects.
- In the short-term, cannabis use results in an increased heart rate, blood pressure and appetite.
- It also produces a slow reaction time, problems with memory and learning.
- Examples of cannabinols include Marijuana and Ganja.

4. Opiates

- Also called narcotics, opioids are used to relieve pain.
- They fit into the receptor cites of natural pain killer endorphin and dopamine to create a dream-like state of well being.
- At high doses, they can cause slow breathing, hypotension, bradycardia, coma and death.
- Examples of opiates include Morphine, codeine and Heroin (Brown sugar).

5. Hallucinogens

- They produce an altered state of consciousness including altered sensory perceptions (visual, spatial, auditory, etc.).

- Examples of hallucinogens include LSD and MDMA.

6. Inhalants

- An inhalant is a drug containing volatile substances that once inhaled has mind-altering capabilities.
- Examples of inhalants include: Gasoline, kerosene, nail polish remover and paint thinner.

ALCOHOL

By far the most common addiction is due to alcohol and is dealt with here in some details.

Terms Used in Alcohol Addiction

We should never use the term 'alcoholic' as this term is derogatory and we are suggesting a behaviour that is morally bad. We as doctors should not be judgemental. For clinical purposes, it is better to use more specific terms. So let us start by understanding the various terms used while talking about alcohol and other substance abuse.

The following is a brief description of the six terms used while talking about alcohol in the increasing order of alcohol intake (**Use → Misuse → Excessive use of alcohol → Abuse → Problem drinker → Dependence syndrome**).

Use: 'Use' is simply the ingestion of alcohol or other drugs without experiencing any negative consequences. It may be social use, like in parties; recreational or experimental use, or maybe religious ritual. For example, if a student had drunk beer at a party and his parents had not found out, we could say he has 'used' alcohol.

Misuse: When a person experiences negative consequence from the use of alcohol or other drugs, it is clearly misuse. For example: A 40-year-old man uses alcohol occasionally, his boss throws a party and the man drinks more than usual and on the way home he is arrested by police. This man has clearly 'misused' alcohol.

Excessive use of alcohol: This is the amount of alcohol intake which has potential of developing alcohol dependence and related complications. The guidelines given by National Institute of Alcohol Abuse and Alcoholism refer to 'safe' levels as *less than 14 standard drinks per week for men and 7 for women.* This holds true provided the whole amount is not taken in one bout and not more than 4 drinks are taken in a day, provided there are drink free days, provided the women is not pregnant, and provided the age is below 65 years. It further adds that no drinking level is absolutely risk free and that any drinking level is risky for vehicle driving.

One standard drink is equal to 360 of Beer or 45 mL of Brandy/Whisky/Rum/Vodka/Gin. In other words, men are less likely to develop alcohol related problems, if the daily limit is reduced to <2 standard drinks (i.e., 90 mL) or <14 standard drinks per week, defined as 'moderate consumption of alcohol' by US dietary guidelines. For women, this is <1 standard drink per day or <7 standard drinks per week. (*A 'quarter' bottle of whisky/rum, etc., contains 180 mL, i.e., 4 standard drinks. 'Half' bottle contains 8 standard drinks and 'full' bottle [750 mL] contains more than 17 standard drinks.*)

Abuse: Abuse refers to a pattern of use resulting in physical, social, legal harm or continued use in spite of negative consequences. For example: the same 40-year old man continues drinking alcohol even after the incident and continues to experience physical and psychological problems.

Diagnostic criteria: One or more of the following occurring in the past 1 year:

- Failure to fulfill role at work or at home.
- Recurrent drinking in hazardous situations like driving a car.
- Recurrent legal problems related to alcohol.
- Continued use despite physical or social problems.

The Problem Drinker

This refers to that person whose excessive drinking has already caused alcohol related complications [harmful use], but has not advanced to dependence.

A problem drinker has high potential to develop dependence. If these people are identified at this stage and timely therapy instituted, there are good chances that dependence on alcohol can be avoided (which is very difficult to treat).

So, How do you Recognize a Problem Drinker?

- The problem drinkers are predominantly men in their 2nd or 3rd decade of life. The risk is more in barmen, army personnel, executives, salesmen and lastly but not the least, amongst doctors!
- If the person is abusing alcohol, the person will have alcohol related physical problems such as unexplained gastritis, hepatitis, pancreatitis, peripheral neuropathy, repeated infections, tremors, etc.
- Having suspected alcohol abuse, he should proceed to take a proper history of the amount of alcohol consumed. Both the patient and the spouse should be involved in the interview. A careful face-to-face interview for few minutes is all that is required. The patient should be asked in a matter of fact manner, two simple questions: How often he drinks in a week and what is the maximum number of drinks he has on a single day? If the patient is exceeding 'safe levels' or consuming more than 4 standard drinks on a given day, he is a problem drinker.
- However, patients usually conceal the right amount they drink and doctors too do not ask the right questions. Hence, screening tests have been advised. A simple 25-item form, called the Michigan Alcohol Screening Test [MAST] is available, but is too elaborate for a GP's use. A simpler CAGE questionnaire is practical for a GP's set up and hardly takes few minutes.

'CAGE' Questionnaire

- Have you ever had to CUT down on alcohol?
- Have people ANNOYED you by criticizing your drinking?
- Have you ever felt GUILTY about your drinking?
- Have you ever had an 'EYE OPENER' drink to steady your nerves or to get rid of hangover?

Two or more positive replies identifies 'problem drinkers'.

- Problem drinkers can be identified by certain laboratory tests also:
  - *GGT—Gamma glutamyl transpeptidase* is raised. GGT returns to normal rapidly after stopping alcohol.
  - *MCV* is more than 96 [normal 76–96] in heavy drinkers. MCV takes several weeks to return to normal after abstinence from alcohol.
  - *Blood alcohol concentration*—A high level means either a single episode of heavy drinking or a problem drinker.

Dependence Syndrome

This condition is seen in persons who have resorted to prolonged and heavy alcohol drinking.

There are seven essential elements in alcohol dependence syndrome:

- An overpowering desire to take alcohol [*craving*].
- Priority is given to alcohol drinking with *neglect of family*, career and health.
- *Tolerance*: Increased quantities of alcohol are required in order to achieve the same euphoric and psychological effects originally produced by lower quantities.
- A *stereotype pattern of drinking* from day-to-day and always. There is no variation to the amount and pattern of drinking as is the case of non-dependant person.
- The development of *withdrawal symptoms* (see below) when alcohol intake is reduced or stopped.
- *Relief drinking*, i.e., the person requires drinking to reduce the withdrawal symptoms. Early morning drinking is almost diagnostic of dependency.
- *Reinstatement after abstinence*: The dependent person restarts drinking again after a period of abstinence.

Withdrawal Syndrome

When a person who has taken alcohol in excessive amounts, stops or even decreases intake he experiences a wide range of psychological and physical symptoms. All these symptoms are relieved by taking alcohol [relief drinking].

The mildest, probably is "*hangover*" seen next day morning for which the patient does not approach the GP and this is associated with episodic drinking.

Features of withdrawal seen after severe alcohol abuse include tremors, generalized anxiety, irritability, vomiting and epigastric pain and autonomic nervous system dysfunction such as tachycardia, tachypnoea and fever. Symptoms begin within 8–10 hrs after stopping alcohol, begin maximum after 2 days, and reduce within 4–5 days. This is called the *tremulous state* [the shakes] and is seen most commonly in general practice. More severe withdrawal symptoms are seen with even more severe alcohol abuse. These include in addition to the above symptoms a state of confusion accompanied by hallucinations, usually visual. This state is called as "*tremulous hallucinatory state*" [or the '*horrors*'].

A small percentage of patients also developed generalized seizures usually 48 hrs after stopping alcohol. These are called "*rum fits*".

The most serious withdrawal syndrome is called '*delirium tremens*'. This is an organic brain syndrome characterized by clouding of consciousness with disorientation of time and space, frightening visual hallucinations, marked autonomic disturbances with tachycardia, sweating, fever, dehydration, etc. The patient is highly agitated and frightened. Untreated, the mortality rate is around 25%.

Treatment

The patient in tremulous state can be managed on out patient basis. All patients must be given B complex in large doses [vitamin flooding] along with 50–100 mg of thiamin daily for at least a week. Majority of the symptoms can be alleviated by given chlordiazepoxide [Librium] 25 mg QID till the symptoms subside, then gradually tapered off over a period of 3–5 days. Patients with any of the clinical features of Wernicke's syndrome must be treated immediately with intravenous thiamine, 100 mg twice in a day, for the first five days. The hallucinating/convulsing and the delirious patients require hospitalization as they require injection haloperidol or phenytoin, as well as correction of dehydration or metabolic disturbances.

Management

1. An important aspect is to decide to aim at total abstinence as against limited consumption of alcohol [controlled drinking].
   - ***Total abstinence*** is advised to those:
     i) Who are heavily dependent.
     ii) Who have physical damage due to alcohol.
     iii) In whom controlled drinking has failed.
   - ***Controlled drinking*** is advised to those:
     i) Who are not heavily dependent.
     ii) Who have not incurred physical damage.
     iii) Who are responsible enough to avoid Disulphiram Ethanol Reaction (see below).

   If the aim is controlled drinking, the patient should be properly informed about the "safe levels".
2. The next step is to *anticipate* '***withdrawal symptoms***' and a plan to control the withdrawal.
3. ***Drugs***: Drugs have an important role to play in the management of alcohol abuse. It is important in the acute phase (detoxification—2–4 weeks), in withdrawal state and also in the long term management (relapse prevention—deterrent and anti-craving agents—3–12 months). Drugs along with brief intervention counselling help in achieving long term remission. Two types of drugs are used—deterrent agents and anticraving agents.
   - *Disulfiram* (*Esperal*) acts as a deterrent. The symptom complex which develops when an individual who has taken disulfiram consumes alcohol, has been termed as **Disulfiram-Ethanol Reaction (DER)**. Disulfiram blocks the oxidation of alcohol so that acetaldehyde accumulates. When on disulfiram, if the patient drinks alcohol he experiences sensation of heat in the face and neck, headache, flushing, nausea, vomiting, hypotension and anxiety due to rapid accumulation of acetaldehyde. This acts as a deterrent to the patient for further intake of alcohol. Disulfiram should always be given after obtaining informed consent as occasionally, DER can result in cardiac arrhythmias and collapse. The usual dose is 250 mg/day; some patients may require a higher dose of 500–750 mg/day. Hepatic dysfunction, peripheral neuropathy and psychosis are the common relative contraindications. Patients taking disulfiram must be advised to avoid alcohol in all forms (including, for example, that found in some cough syrups). In many cities in India, disulfiram is given by unauthorized agencies camouflaged as ayurvedic medicine for commercial reasons. This is illegal and not without risks.
   - Acamprosate, naltrexone [costly] and SSRI [fluxetine or sertraline] are useful anticraving agents. Acamprosate decreases alcohol craving. The dose is two 333 mg pills t.i.d. (total dose of 1998 mg). Both naltrexone and acamprosate are to be given for 3–6 months.
   - Naltrexone (Naltima) 50 mg/day, is thought to act by preventing the euphoric and rewarding effects of alcohol. It is effective but costly.
4. ***Self help groups***: *Alcoholics Anonymous* for problem drinkers, *Al-Anon* for spouses of excessive drinkers and *Al-Ateen* for the children.

Despite the above intensive and combination treatments, there will be patients who will continue to drink alcohol but more than 70% have demonstrated at least a reduced intake when followed up for more than 2 years and that is heartening!

TOBACCO (NICOTINE) DEPENDENCE

Tobacco use among men and women is widespread in all regions of India and among all sections of society. It has been estimated that more than 50% of males and 15% of women currently use tobacco.

Tobacco use is the single most preventable cause of morbidity and mortality. The World Health Organization estimates that globally every 8 sec somebody dies from tobacco related disease. In India, tobacco use results in one billion deaths every year, which is more than the combined deaths due to malaria, TB and HIV! Three out of every five tobacco users, use tobacco within half an hour of waking up, indicating dependence on tobacco.

Ways in which Tobacco is Used

In India, tobacco is used in a wide variety of ways. Beedi smoking is the most popular form of smoking, while cigarettes form the second most popular form of tobacco smoking. Chewing *paan* (betel leaf) with tobacco and areca nut (supari), applying *mishri*, sucking dry tobacco with lime and using products such as paan masala, gutka and mawa are the major forms of smokeless-tobacco (SMT) used in India.

Harmful Effects

- *Cancers* of the oral cavity, oesophagus, pharynx, cervix and penis.
- *Vascular diseases*, cardiovascular diseases, peripheral arterial obstructive diseases leading to deaths at a younger age.
- *COPD*. Children and women who are exposed to passive smoking are prone to respiratory infections and worsening of asthma.
- *Oral precancerous lesions* such as leucoplakia, erythroplakia and submucous fibrosis. In fact, oral submucous fibrosis (OSMF) is emerging as a new epidemic. This disease does not regress, has no known cure and has a very high potential for cancer development.
- *Low sperm count* and poor sperm quality. It can lead to spontaneous abortions, fetal deaths, preterm delivery and IUGR.

Why Tobacco is so Addicting?

Nicotine is the chemical in tobacco that causes addiction. It acts like a stimulant by triggering release of dopamine—which causes feeling of pleasure, mood elevation, memory improvement and reduction of anxiety.

Other factors like easy availability, no legal and social consequences of tobacco use and the rampant advertising used by tobacco companies—all contribute to widespread abuse of tobacco.

How to find who is Nicotine Dependent and needs Treatment?

The *Fagerström Test for Nicotine Dependence* is a standard instrument for assessing the intensity of nicotine physical addiction. The higher the score on this questionnaire, the higher the level of dependence. This test, although used widely by professionals in this field, need not be referred to by general practitioners as they should advise all tobacco chewers and smokers to stop the habit. This is so because development of the above harmful effects of tobacco is not necessarily dose dependent.

Symptoms Experienced by the Patient on Nicotine Withdrawal and Treatment

Common symptoms include: Cravings (irresistible urge for tobacco), feeling irritable, insomnia, fatigue, inability to concentrate, headache, in creased cough with postnasal drip, sore throat and constipation.

There is no specific medication for treatment of nicotine withdrawal symptoms. Use of nicotine chewing gum makes the detoxification easier.

Drugs Used to Treat Nicotine Dependence

Drug treatment should be strongly recommended to all persons with severe dependence.

Bupropion (*Nicotex*), a new antidepressant agent which reduces craving for nicotine. It is a first-line drug for smokers who want to quit smoking. After discussing with the patient, a date is fixed approximately 2 weeks away for quitting tobacco use (the Quit Date) and bupropion treatment is started immediately. It is to be given at the dose of 150 mg/day in the morning. The side effects associated with bupropion are headache, jitteriness, insomnia and gastrointestinal symptoms. If these side effects are not severe, the dose is increased to 150 mg bd after a week.

This dose is continued for 3 months after the quit date and may be given for 6 months. Bupropion can also be used in combination with nicotine replacement therapy (NRT) which is started on the 'Quit Date' when the user is advised to absolutely stop all tobacco products and use NRT instead.

Nicotine replacement therapy (***NRT***)—Nicotine gum, nicotine inhaler, nicotine nasal spray and nicotine patch is used to relieve withdrawal symptoms in tobacco users by substituting the nicotine in tobacco with nicotine in relatively safer form. The nicotine gum, patch, etc., do not contain all the dangerous chemicals present in tobacco.

Nicotine gum (***Nicorette***) is available in strengths of 2 and 4 mg of nicotine that can be released by chewing. Patients should chew the gum slowly until a peppery taste appears, then "park" the gum in the cheek until the taste disappears. Chew and park again—continue for 30 min. One piece of 2 mg gum/hr for light smokers and 4 mg gum/hr for highly nicotine-dependent smokers is recommended. Maximum of 30 pieces of 2 mg or 20 pieces of 4 mg are allowed per day. The gum is weaned off subsequently by tapering the frequency and strength of the gum over 2–3 months or less.

NRT is only available as gum in India. However, other forms may be available soon.

Role of Family Physicians in Reducing Tobacco Use

We as family physicians are in a unique position to influence the many smokers who are not ready to quit as well as to aid the ones who are ready. GPs see patients who smoke at many moments when they are concerned about their health and this can be used as an opportunity. The general practitioner should make it a habit to use *brief interventional therapy* (*BIT*) which is given in the box. This does not take more than a few minutes. Most general practitioners are already using this method. It is a matter of polishing their method. Combined with pharmacologic treatment, it can motivate many patients to quit and this goes a long way in preventing the harmful effects of tobacco.

Brief Interventional Therapy (BIT)

- Ask every patient on every visit about his or her tobacco use status. Record tobacco use status prominently in your case paper, along with signs of tobacco ill effects.
- Advise strongly all users to quit. Tailor the advice towards the patient's current medical problems and concerns.
- Assess the patient's willingness to quit. Ask every user, if he or she is willing to make a quit attempt. If the patient is not yet ready to make a quit attempt, motivate him/her to quit by stating medical reasons.
- Assist patients in their efforts to quit. Plan a 'Quit Date' within the next 2 weeks. Provide nicotine replacement and/or bupropion as well as teach behavioural strategies to quit. Deal with withdrawal and prevent relapse. The patient should be made aware about relapse triggers and skills to deal with them.
- Arrange a follow-up close around the quit date and regularly later on to provide continuous support.

PRESCRIPTION DRUG ABUSE

It is the use of a prescription medication in a way not intended by the prescribing doctor. It is the abuse of drugs prescribed by the doctor.

We have a huge population that knowingly or unknowingly is hooked on to prescription drugs. What are the reasons?

- Anxiolytics (benzodiazepines) are prescribed without giving patient enough warning about its dependence potential.
- There is rampant unlawful selling of these drugs without prescription.
- Prescription drugs are also difficult to detect by laboratory investigations. When caught, one just needs to feign a cough or headache convincingly and explain the need for possessing that drug.

Commonly Abused Prescription Drugs

Opioids like morphine, codeine, propoxyphene (Darvocet), pentazocine (Fortwin) injections, fentanyl (Duragesic), dextropropoxyphene (Proxyvon), dextromethorphan (Dexcof) and buprenorphine (Tidegesic) are prescribed to treat pain. Cough syrups such as Corex and Phensedyl have opiates, and antihistamines as well as alcohol. Opioid drugs cause euphoria leading to addiction and dependence.

Drugs used in psychiatry: Commonly used are diazepam (Valium), chlordiazepoxide (Librium), alprazolam (Restyl), lorazepam (Larpose) and nitrazepam (Nitravet). Benzodiazepines should not be taken for more than 2–3 weeks as dependence develops.

Stimulants like dextroamphetamine (Dexedrine) and methylphenidate (Ritalin) are drugs causing an increase in alertness, attention and energy and are therefore abused especially by students during examination times. Actually stimulants are prescribed for the treatment of only a few conditions like narcolepsy, attention-deficit hyperactivity disorder and as appetite suppressants for short-term treatment of obesity. However, their use has become rampant because of the above reasons.

Steroids like prednisolone (Wysolone), dexamethasone (Decadron), betamethasone (Betnelan) are rampantly used in India by patients without the knowledge of their physicians. The prescription once given is repeated over and over again and finally the patient presents to the practitioner with a moon face, buffalo neck, weight gain and other side effects of steroids.

Anabolic steroids like nandrolone (Durabolin), testosterone (Testoviron depot) are demanded by patients and prescribed by doctors to enhance performance both sexual and competitive games. Patients on these drugs feel a sense of well being. However, mood swings can also occur with these drugs, including maniac-like symptoms that could lead to violence. Users may also suffer from paranoid jealousy, irritability, delusions and impaired judgement. Hence, these drugs should be used with caution.

How to Diagnose this Disorder?

We need to have a high level of clinical suspicion to diagnose prescription drug abuse disorder in our busy practice. We should take notice if a patient demands to increase the dose of these prescribed drugs or comes frequently to us for refills.

We can also identify these patients if we are aware of withdrawal symptoms of these abused prescription drugs. Many patients are brought by relatives for the withdrawal symptoms which should be promptly recognized by the general practitioner.

Symptoms of *opiate* withdrawal include restlessness, muscle and bone pain, insomnia, diarrhoea, vomiting, cold flushes with goose bumps ("cold turkey") and involuntary leg movements.

Benzodiazepines in withdrawal state cause sleeplessness, restlessness, tremors of the hand, slurring, irritability, vomiting, sadness, altered appetite and abnormal behaviour.

Withdrawal symptoms of *anabolic steroids* include mood swings, fatigue and restlessness, loss of appetite, insomnia, all of which may contribute to continued abuse.

Our Role as Doctors

We are in a unique position to identify prescription drug abuse and manage the problem. Discussing and motivating our neighbouring chemists about this issue can play a key role in preventing prescription drug abuse. They should be vigilant about false or altered prescriptions and should not unlawfully refill prescriptions.

Other alternative could be dispensing from our clinics the drugs that can be potentially abused, instead of prescribing them.

Treatment

Opioid withdrawal is best managed by a psychiatrist specialized in de-addiction medicine. Suffice it to mention here that for withdrawal symptoms of *opioid*, buprenorphine (Tidigesic) 6–12 capsules of dextropropoxyphene (Proxyvon) are given initially and tapered off after the third day. Methadone (60 mg/day) or buprenorphine (4 and 8 mg/day) are used as maintenance therapy.

In cases of mild to moderate *benzodiazepine dependence*, an outpatient detoxification by tapering of the drug, with weekly reduction in doses can be carried out. In patients with severe dependence, particularly with dependence on short acting benzodiazepines, indoor detoxification is preferred. In patients dependent on short or intermediately acting benzodiazepine (oxazepam, alprazolam, etc.), risk of withdrawal seizures should be kept in mind and to prevent the seizures, detoxification is started with equivalent doses of long acting benzodiazepines (diazepam, chlordiazepoxide), which then should be tapered off as usual. Usually, detoxification in indoor setting is over within 2 weeks.

For *steroids*, if withdrawal symptoms are severe or prolonged, and if the patient is unable to stop steroids, hospitalization may be needed.

Cannabis

Cannabis is derived from the plant *Cannabis sativa*. This grows all around the world including India. Cannabis is available in various forms:

- *Bhang* is used in various religious festivals, is legal in India.
- *Ganja*
- *Charas* (or *Hashish*) also used in various religious festivals in India can be smoked in cigarettes, or in clay pipes or in water pipes like the traditional hookah. Charas and Ganja are illegal in India.

At low dose, cannabis causes a state of well being and a dreamy state of enjoyment. This is generally followed by a period of drowsiness.
At higher doses, confusion and mental/behavioural problems may occur.

Chronic cannabis use is not associated with any significant medical complications. However, regular use of cannabis must be discouraged as there is greater likelihood that the individual might come into contact with drugs with far greater health consequences such as heroin.

But, having knowledge about something is not enough. You have to make your patients know that you offer treatment for substance abuse. Display a poster on your notice board that yours is a DRUG DE-ADDICTION CENTRE!

CHAPTER 33

The Hair Loss Treatment Clinic

- Structure of Hair

Patients with hair loss will often consult their family physician first. Hair loss is not life threatening, but it is distressing and significantly affects the patient's quality of life.

As with most conditions, the physician should begin the evaluation with a detailed history and physical examination. As a first step, the family physician should determine whether the patient has diffuse hair loss or patchy hair loss. This greatly narrows down the differential diagnosis. Next, it is helpful to determine whether the hair loss is *nonscarring* (also called *noncicatricial*), or *scarring* (also called *cicatricial*). Nonscarring alopecia is reversible. Scarring alopecia is permanent. Scarring alopecia is rare and is due to a variety of conditions including autoimmune diseases such as discoid lupus erythematosus. If the follicular orifices are absent in the patch, the alopecia is probably scarring. Scarring alopecia is best evaluated by a dermatologist.

Nonscarring alopecias can be readily diagnosed and treated by the family physician.

Hair Types

1. **Terminal hair**: This is the hair of *scalp*, *eye brows* and *eye lashes*. Terminal hair is thicker and more pigmented than villous hair. At puberty, it also develops in axillae and pubic area of both sexes and the bearded area and body in males. If it occurs in bearded areas in females, it is called hirsutism.
2. **Vellous hair**: This is the fine hair covering the *whole skin* surface except the palms, soles and penis.
3. **Lanugo hair**: This is present in *the foetus* and is shed in the 8th month of pregnancy in utero. Therefore, lanugo hair are seen only in premature babies. Lanugo hair is soft and fine.

STRUCTURE OF HAIR

Skin consists of little pocket-like structures called 'follicles'. The hair follicle is an invagination in the skin. It has a bulb at the base of the follicle from which the new hair grows.

Hair structure (see figure) can be described in two parts:

1. The structure inside the follicle **(Fig. 33.1)**.
2. The structure of the hair shaft outside the hair follicle that is present above the epidermis **(Fig. 33.2)**.

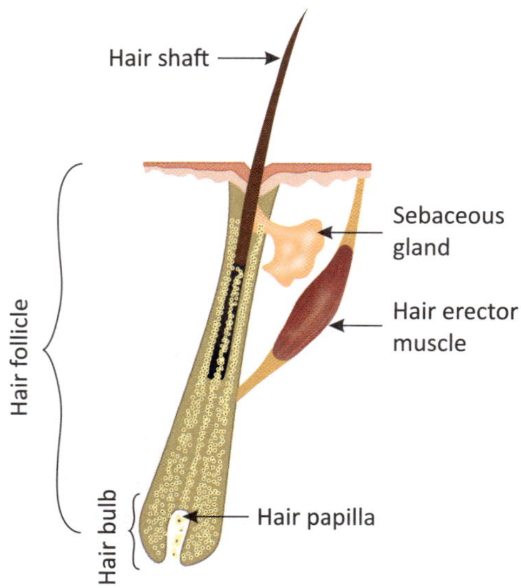

| **Fig. 33.1** Hair structure inside Follicle |

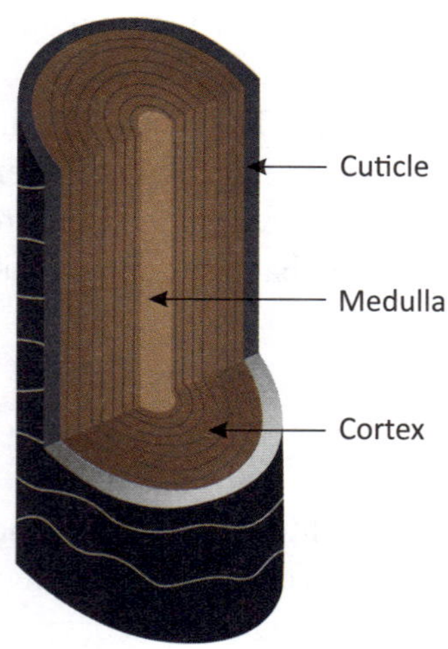

| **Fig. 33.2** Structure of hair shaft outside hair follicle |

1. Structure Inside Follicle

A. Hair Bulb

It is the bulb shaped lowest part of the hair. It is attached to the skin by the hair papilla.

B. Hair Papilla (or dermal papilla)

It is the cone-shaped elevation which is present at the base of the hair follicle inside the hair bulb.

It fits into the hair bulb and holds it. Dermal papilla is supplied by the blood vessels of the scalp which supply essential nutrients to the roots.

C. Arrector Pili Muscle

It is an involuntary muscle present at the base of the hair follicle. When arrector pili contracts we get goose pimples.

D. Sebaceous Glands

These are the oil glands that are connected to the hair follicles. Sebaceous glands secrete sebum which gives lustre to the hair.

2. Structure of Hair Shaft Outside Hair Follicle

The hair shaft consists of several layers. There is a central medulla, surrounded by a cortex, which in turn surrounded by a cuticle.

A. Cuticle

It is the outermost layer of the hair shaft. It is responsible for the elasticity and colour. It acts as a protecting layer to the inner hair structure and gives shine and smoothness to the hair.

B. Cortex

It is the middle layer of the hair strand. The protein present in the cortex is responsible for the elasticity and colour of your hair.

C. Medulla

It is the innermost layer. The purpose of medulla has not been identified yet.

Normal Hair Growth

People who live with pets notice that some animals and birds shed their skin or feathers in certain seasons. This is called **moulting**. After losing its feathers or skin the animal or bird look unattractive, but later leads to a beautiful new coat to survive the winter or to attract a mate. Human hairs don't moult at one time but are shed daily throughout life.

Life Cycle of a Hair

All body tissues follow a simple cycle of growth, rest and death. This tissue is then replaced by a healthy new tissue. Likewise, hair undergoes a natural cycle of growth, rest and fall, only to be replaced by a new healthier shaft.

Skin consists of little pocket-like structures called 'follicles'. The base of each follicle contains the root of the hair from which the hair begins to grow. The blood vessels in scalp supply essential nutrients to the roots. As the hair grows, it gets pushed up through the layers of the skin and pokes out. The oil glands attached to the follicles provide natural lubrication, softness and shine to hair.

Human hair growth happens in the follicles in a cyclical process. The cycle consists of four phases – anagen (growth), catagen (transition), telogen (rest) and exogen (shedding). To understand the hair cycle with clarity, I compare it with the life cycle of humans (child, adult, retired and death).

During the **anagen phase** (which is also called the **growth phase**), hair starts growing from the root of the follicle underneath the shrivelled follicle of the last hair. The new hair grows up alongside the old one, peeping out of the same orifice, until the old rootless hair finally falls out.

The scalp hair grows approximately 6 inches per year. The life of a single hair varies greatly, anywhere from 2 to 6 years. This is the reason why some people cannot grow their hair past their shoulders, while others can grow it out long enough to sit on. It is not more than 6 years, which explains why hair growth usually to waist or buttocks, but not down to the ground.

At any one time, approximately 85–90% of scalp follicles are in the anagen phase of hair growth.

After the anagen phase comes **the catagen** or **transitional phase**. The hair stops growing.

The follicle begins to shrink. The hair strand gets separated from the dermal papilla. However, the hair shaft does not shed off immediately in the catagen phase as the hair is attached to the hair follicle. This phase lasts for about 2–3 weeks.

At any one time, approximately 2–3% of hair follicles are in catagen phase.

By the end of the catagen phase, the hair strand becomes a club and the **telogen (resting) phase** begins. In this phase, hair follicles undergo a rest period for about 3 months still remaining attached to the hair follicle. At any one time, approximately 10–15% of hair follicles are in telogen phase.

Finally, in the **exogen phase** of the hair growth cycle, the hair strand completely detaches from the scalp and sheds off naturally.

The scalp sheds approximately 100 hairs per day. This is normal hair loss. This cycle is then repeated.

The growth is short for body hair like eyebrows and eyelashes, but can last for years in scalp hair.

Examination of Hair in Clinic

Physical scalp examination is done in every patient. This will reveal whether the hair loss is localized (patchy alopecia) or diffuse (diffuse alopecia) or has a typical pattern of distribution of hair loss (patterned alopecia). It is also done to determine the area most affected (i.e., vertex, occiput, etc.).

Simple clinical tests including the tug and pull test should be done on all patients complaining of hair loss.

- ***The Hair Pull Test*** is a simple screening test to assess the *degree of hair loss*. Grasp approximately 40–60 hairs at their base using the thumb, index and middle fingers and firmly but not forcefully apply gentle traction away from the scalp. A positive result is when more than 10% of hairs (more than six) are pulled from the scalp. This means there is active hair shedding. If less than six hairs can be easily pulled out, this is considered normal physiologic shedding. In general, resting telogen hair comes out easily, whereas growing anagen hair remains rooted in place.

  This test is subject to false interpretations, is neither standardized or nor diagnostic. This is because the pulling force is variable, it is difficult to judge the number of hair grasped, the count of 60 is arbitrary and also depends on when the patient had shampooed hair before coming to the clinic. The patient must not shampoo for at least 1 day before the pull test.

  A positive pull test indicates following conditions: telogen effluvium, anagen effluvium, or advanced alopecia areata.
- ***The Hair Tug Test*** is used to get information about a *hair shaft abnormality*, the brittleness or fragility of hair strands. Grasp a section of hair and holds it with fingers of two hands, one near the scalp and one near the tip of the hair. Then, tugs to see if any of the strands break in the middle.
- ***The Card Test*** to *examine the hair shafts* and to evaluate the number of *new hair* strands that are growing. The procedure is simple. Hold a small rectangular card covered against a section of the scalp hair. The colour of the card should contrast with the colour of the hair. New hair strands can be counted and examined.
- ***Trichosopy*** uses of a dermatoscope to directy visualize the scalp and hair at various regions of scalp. In scarring alopecia, no follicular openings are seen. In non scarring alopecia, the follicular openings are preserved and visble. Trichoscopy is the term coined for dermoscopic imaging of the scalp and hair. This novel diagnostic technique, both simple and non-invasive, can be used as a handy bed side tool for diagnosing common hair and scalp disorders. Trichoscopic observations can be broadly grouped as hair signs, vascular patterns, pigment patterns and interfollicular patterns.

  It is essential for a general practitioner aspiring to practice trichology as a speciality in his clinic to buy a good trichoscope.
- ***Light Microscopy***: Used to diagnose infections, shaft abnormalities and hair loss. It is always important to evaluate roots of pulled hair under a microscope to definitively distinguish telogen from anagen hairs.
- ***Biopsy***: Used to diagnose different types of cicatricial alopecias.

| **Box 1** Common causes of hair loss |

Common	Uncommon
▪ Alopecia areata	▪ Discoid lupus erythematosus
▪ Traction alopecia	▪ Lichen planus
▪ Trichotillomania	▪ Fungal or bacterial infection
▪ Tinea capitis	▪ Injury or burn

Alopecia Areata

Here, we see well-defined round or oval bald patches which have developed rapidly, sometimes even overnight. The scalp is the most common site, but patches can be encountered also in bearded area, eye lashes and eye brows. The condition is common in young adults and in children. All the scalp hair can be lost (alopecia totalis). In addition, there can be near complete loss of body hair (alopecia universalis). The hallmark of alopecia areata is that there is *complete loss of hair in the patch*. The patch is smooth with no scaling, no itching, no scarring and no signs of inflammation. As opposed to this in tinea capitis, itching is present and the skin can look slightly scaly and erythematous, and there may be occipital adenopathy.

It is believed that alopecia areata is an autoimmune disorder as it is commonly seen in other autoimmune disorders such as diabetes and Hashimoto's thyroiditis and also because there is lymphocytic infiltrate around hair follicles.

Treatment

In the majority, there is spontaneous re-growth of hair in about 6–9 months, especially who have one or two patches. A few do not.

Features of poor prognosis are:

- More than 3 patches
- Patches in occipital and temporal areas
- Loss of eyebrows and eye lashes
- Totalis/universalis
- Children
- Relapsing cases

These could be resistant to treatment and should ideally be referred to a dermatologist.

There are several treatment options available:

- Give a trial of local irritants like anthralin (Derobin) or psoralens which are supposed to stimulate hair growth.
- PUVA therapy. Local application of psoralen lotion followed by sun exposure for 5 min.
- Topical minoxidil 5% solution.
- Potent steroids locally.
- Systemic steroids in case of alopecia totalis or universalis. Hair do regrow, but they usually fall off on stopping steroids.
- Intralesional steroids (triamcinolone, Kenacort) is the best option. Dilute 10 mg of triamcinolone with 1 mL of xylocaine. Inject 0.1 mL with insulin syringe at 1 cm interval to cover the whole patch. Repeat after 6 weeks and 3 months. Appreciable growth is usually seen by this time. If at 3 months no hair growth is seen, investigate for autoimmune diseases or refer.

  As patients recover, fine white hairs appear which gradually become pigmented to normal colour.

Trichotillomania (TTM) (Hair Pulling Disorder or Compulsive Hair Pulling)

It is a rather fanciful name to describe a condition which is a psychological disorder characterized by irresistible urges to pull out hair from scalp, eyebrows or other areas of the body, despite trying to resist the temptation. Efforts to stop pulling hair typically fail and results in distress.

A brief positive feeling may occur as hair is removed. It is regarded as a form of obsessive compulsive disorder. The milder forms could be just a habit tic like nail biting.

Local examination will reveal stubs of broken hair of unequal length with an underlying normal scalp. Trichotillomania most commonly begins in childhood or adolescence. Women are affected about 10 times more often than men.

Treatment is typically with cognitive behavioural therapy (CBT). The medication clomipramine and clipping fingernails may be helpful. In patients not responding to counselling, psychiatric assessment should be done from a psychiatrist.

Scaring (Cicatricial Alopecia)

Scarring alopecia is permanent hair loss in scalp secondary to a disorder of skin like DLE, few fungal infection of scalp skin or lichen planus. It could also result from scarring due to injury. It results in bald patches on scalp due to permanent destruction of hair follicles. The underlying tissues in and around the hair get destroyed or scarred and replaced by fibrous tissue. The hairless skin on the scalp becomes fixed to the underlying subcutaneous tissue, so that it cannot be pinched or picked up.

Once the hair follicles get destroyed, the hair cannot be regrown. These patients should be referred to a dermatologist.

Traction Alopecia

Traction alopecia is localized hair loss usually secondary to unsuitable method of hair styling. For example, if the hair is pulled back tightly in a hair style like a tight ponytail, a recession in frontal hair line will result. In infants rubbing of the occiput on the bed will result in loss of hair in the region. Traction alopecia can be reversed, if the traction is corrected early. If hair follicles are damaged, the loss can be permanent.

Tinea Capitis

It is rare in adults and in urban areas but is encountered in children belonging to low socioeconomic strata in rural areas. Two kinds of presentations are seen. The non-inflammatory type presents as one or more patches on the scalp. There is loss of hair in the patch, but as opposed to alopecia areata, the patches are not completely bald, contain broken-off hair and the scalp surface is scaly with minimal inflammation. In the inflammatory variety there is a boggy mass called '*Kerion*' which is studded with broken hair and oozes purulent material.

Common causes of DIFFUSE hair loss
▪ Female pattern hair loss
▪ Male pattern hair loss
▪ Diffuse alopecia areata
▪ Alopecia totalis or universalis
▪ Telogen effluvium
▪ Anagen effluvium
▪ Iron and Nutritional deficiency
▪ Thyroid disorders
▪ Drugs

Androgenic Alopecia (AGA)

This is a common disorder affecting genetically predisposed men and women. Genetic factors determine age of onset and also the severity. In AGA, there is *progressive miniaturization* of the hair follicle which means the hair becomes thin, short and sparse. There is progressive transformation of thick, pigmented terminal hair into short, thin, non-pigmented villous hair. Hair loss occurs very slowly, presenting as thinning rather than shedding.

The prevalence increases with age in both sexes and there is a characteristic *pattern* of distribution in males and females. Hence, AGA is also called male pattern baldness and female pattern baldness.

Male pattern baldness is characterized by fronto-parietal recession beginning above both temples with thinning of the frontal hair. Over time, the hairline recedes to form a characteristic "M" shape. This is followed by thinning of the hair of the vertex (crown). However, in most cases the parietal and occipital hair is retained and only in severe cases all hair is lost. Men with this condition can begin suffering hair loss as early as their teens or early 20s. Androgenic alopecia in men has been associated with several other medical conditions including coronary heart disease, diabetes, obesity and hypertension.

Female pattern baldness differs from male-pattern baldness. In women, the hair becomes thin all over the head, with the most extensive hair loss at the crown and the hairline does not recede. Androgenetic alopecia in women rarely leads to total baldness. Women with this condition do not experience noticeable thinning until their 40s or later. It is seen commonly in women with polycystic ovary syndrome (PCOS). PCOS is characterized by a hormonal imbalance that can lead to irregular menstruation, acne, excess hair elsewhere on the body (hirsutism) and weight gain.

Treatment Options for AGA

When discussing treatment options for this form of hair loss, it is important to emphasise that *no treatment will completely reverse the process.* Response to treatment is quite variable. Some people will not respond to particular treatments. Expectations need to be realistic.

Management Options

- No treatment: Some people accept baldness gracefully as a "sign of maturity".
- Treating with: Topical minoxidil 2–5% and Oral finasteride 1 mg daily.
- Oral dutasteride 0.5 mg daily.
- Use of a hair wig.
- Surgery.

The safest option is a hair wig, and this will be suitable and acceptable for some patients. The next safest option is topical treatment but this is less effective than oral medication. Topical and oral treatments combined gives better results. It needs to be emphasized to the patient that response is not seen for at least 3 months, and treatment is lifelong.

Surgery is an option for some, but is highly dependent on the skill of the surgeon. Small pieces of scalp with hair follicles are taken from the back of the head and moved to slits in the areas of baldness. Potential problems with this treatment include the usual risks of surgery, folliculitis and the hair falling out from the transplant area. In cases where the bald areas are large, there might be trouble trying to find enough hair to transplant. In addition, the surgery can be costly and is usually not covered by insurance.

Anagen Effluvium

This refers to hair shedding that arises during the anagen or growth stage of the hair cycle. Drugs used in cancer chemotherapy are probably the most common cause of anagen effluvium.

Anagen hairs have long roots covered with the inner and outer root sheaths and are pigmented.

Anagen effluvium is due to an acute injury to the hair follicles, resulting in sudden diffuse shedding of damaged hairs.

Diffuse alopecia may occur over a period of days. The alopecia is non-scarring and reversible.

Alopecia develops within 2–4 weeks of chemotherapy. It affects most parts of the scalp, but other sites may be affected, such as eyebrows, armpits and genital area. In anagen effluvium, the end of the hair that comes from the scalp is tapered, narrowed, irregular or broken off.

The patient will recover but clearly requires to be warned in advance about this side effect of chemotherapy.

The hair follicle resumes normal activity after any toxic agent is withdrawn. Complete regrowth occurs after 3–6 months after chemotherapy in most cases.

Acute Telogen Effluvium

In contrast to anagen effluvium, hair shedding occurs during the telogen or resting stage of the hair cycle after some shock to the system. Diffuse hair loss occurs 2–5 months after a major medical or sugical event. There is excessive shedding of resting or telogen hair. Because of this shock, as many as 70% of the anagen hairs can be precipitated into telogen, which are then shed excessively. The condition is usually self limiting and spontaneous recovery occurs within 9 months in 95% of cases. Approximately 5% of cases may experience persistent, episodic shedding as some follicles may not revert to previous growth pattern. They might develop chronic telogen effluvium or patterned hair loss. However, complete alopecia is not seen. In contrast to anagen hair root, telogen hair root is a roundish bulb or club.

Typical triggering events include:

- Childbirth (post partum)
- Certain fevers
- Major surgery
- Major accident
- Psychological stress
- Physiological neonatal hair loss
- Crash dieting
- Hypothyroidism, hyperthyroidism
- Discontinuing the contraceptive pill
- Overseas travel

Postpartum hair loss usually is reversed after a few months or may lead to chronic telogen effluvium or female pattern alopecia. Causative medications include retinoids, beta blockers, anticoagulants, anticonvulsants and antithyroid drugs.

The resting scalp club hairs remain firmly attached to the hair follicles at first. The new hairs coming up through the scalp push out the resting club hairs abruptly and alarmingly. Increased hair fall is noticed 2–5 months after the triggering event. New hair continues to grow. Thus, paradoxically, with this type of hair loss, *hair fall is a sign of hair regrowth.*

Because nail and hair growth are under the same influences, an arrest in hair growth is often mirrored in the nails by a groove across them coinciding with the time of the shock to the system — a Beau line. The time of the shock can be estimated from the fact that a fingernail takes 5 months to grow from the posterior nail fold to the free edge. So if the groove in the nail is halfway down the nail, the shock must have been two and a half months ago.

Treatment

- Counselling and reassurance: This is a spontaneously recovering condition.
- Correct anaemia, hypothyroidism, if present.

- Stop drugs which induce hair fall like retinoids, oral contraceptive pills, etc,
- Topical minoxidil can be used to prolong the anagen phase. This can decrease hair loss.

Chronic Telogen Effluvium

Chronic telogen effluvium is hair shedding lasting longer than 6 months. The onset is often slow, and it can be difficult to identify a triggering medical event as is observed in acute telogen effluvium. Because of the duration of the hair shedding, patients are more likely to complain of decreased scalp hair density, or they may note that their hair appears thin and lifeless. This is diagnosis of exclusion as there are no pathological tests to confirm the diagnosis.

It affects usually a middle aged women and the entire scalp is involved. Patients lose as many as 400–500 hairs daily as compared to about 100 hairs in a normal person. Usually, the patient comes with a bunch of hair in hand, displaying the profuse loss of hair and expresses their fear of going completely bald. Hair pull test is positive in all parts of scalp. No widening of the parting of hair is seen, which is a typical feature of androgenic alopecia. Trichoscopic findings show increase distance between hair follicles.

Treatment is difficult and depends on whether a cause can be found on investigations.

Topical minoxidil solution, biotin, protein rich diets, peptides, vitamins are used commonly, but are lacking extensive studies.

Iron Deficiency Anaemia

There is not enough evidence to say for sure that iron deficiency anaemia can cause hair loss in men or women. While some studies have found that people experiencing hair loss were deficient in iron, there is little evidence to suggest that an iron deficiency is the cause. If iron studies confirm iron deficiency anaemia, it is worthwhile treating anaemia which may lead to regrowth of hair.

Thyroid Disorders

Severe and prolonged hypothyroidism and hyperthyroidism can cause loss of hair. The loss is diffuse and involves the entire scalp rather than discrete areas. The hair appears uniformly sparse. Regrowth is usual with successful treatment of the thyroid disorder, though it will take several months and may be incomplete.

Drugs which cause hair loss:

- Anticoagulant medications such as heparin and warfarin.
- Oral contraceptive pill.
- Anticonvulsant medications, such as valproic acid, carbamazepine.
- Retinoids (e.g. isotretinoin).
- Antithyroid drugs.
- Levodopa.
- Tricyclic antidepressants (e.g. amitriptyline).

Drugs Used for Treating Alopecia

Minoxidil: The antihypertensive vasodilator drug '*minoxidil*' was found to produce hypertrichosis in many patients of hypertension. Hence, this drug was formulated for local use in concentration of 2%, 5% and 10% topical solution. It is not known how minoxidil causes hair growth.

It has to be applied continuously 1 mL, two times a day till good hair growth is seen, which takes about 1 year and then 1 mL/day daily lifelong as maintenance. This has to be explained to the patient before starting treatment.

Topically applied minoxidil is generally well tolerated, but common side effects include itching of the eye, irritation at the treated area and unwanted hair growth elsewhere on the body. Exacerbation of hair loss/alopecia has been reported. Temporary hair loss is a common side effect of minoxidil treatment after starting treatment and after abruptly stopping treatment. Manufacturers note that minoxidil-induced hair loss is a common side effect and describe the process as "shedding".

***Finasteride* (*Finast*)**: 1 mg/day od, if given orally improves the results when given in combination with topical minoxidil.

Hair follicles convert testosterone (the main male hormone) into another hormone called dihydrotestosterone (DHT). In male pattern baldness, affected hair follicles have become more sensitive to DHT. This causes the hair follicles to shrink (called miniaturized) and the hair becomes thin, short and sparse. Finasteride works by stopping the conversion of testosterone to DHT by inhibiting type II 5-alpha-reductase, which is the enzyme responsible for the conversion. DTH levels are reported to be reduced by 60% when the drug is taken, which prevents the susceptible follicles from being affected by the hormone.

Finasteride does not work in female patterned baldness.

Dutasteride: It works similarly to finasteride, but it is claimed to be more effective. Like finasteride, dutasteride inhibits the activity of type II 5-alpha reductase. However, dutasteride additionally inhibits type I 5-alpha reductase enzyme. Blocking both types of the enzyme lowers DHT even more and reduces the risk of damage to hair follicles.

Platelet Rich Plasma* (*PRP*) *therapy is now the latest trend in hair loss treatment and is proving to be effective in correcting hair loss when done correctly. It is a therapy that utilizes the growth factors from the patient's own platelets to trigger the growth of hair follicles. (It is also used to accelerate the healing of injured tendons, ligaments and joints.)

About 20 cc of patient's blood is withdrawn and centrifuged for 15 min.

The centrifuge will separate the platelets from the rest of the blood. This plasma is then set aside and gravity allows the platelets to collect at the bottom of the tube.

The *platelet poor plasma or PPP* is usually collected from the top of the tube and discarded; or, in some cases saved for micro-needling treatment post PRP injection.

The denser area of platelets in the plasma from the bottom of the tube called *platelet rich plasma* or *PRP* is injected back into the scalp eighter subcutaneously or intradermally. This has to be usually repeated after 3–6 months.

PRP therapy is not yet FDA approved for hair growth.

Other unproved drugs used for hair loss:
- Capixyl, Redensyl, Procapil, Anagain, Baicapil
- Peptides Acetyl Tetrapeptide-3 & Biotinoyl Tripeptide-1
- Saw Palmetto Extract

Hair Loss in Women: Special Comments

As a vast majority of patients approaching the family physician are females, a short overview of hair loss in women is in order here. Girls from the Indian subcontinent who want long hair will persistently come to the doctor complaining loss of a few hairs daily. Examination will not show any objective evidence for it and there is a magnificent head of hair. Explain that loss of 50–100 hairs is normal, if it has not lead to thinning or shortening of the hair. In the Indian subcontinent abundant hair is particularly desirable and expectations are high! As stated previously, the anagen phase lasts maximum up to 6 years and grows average of 6 inches in a year which is 3 feet. It is then shed off, and hence scalp hair will never grow to touch the floor!

In *telogen effluvium*, which is caused by stressful conditions like pregnancy or high-fever, the growing anagen hair will prematurely enter the telogen phase and shed profusely. As the telogen phase lasts only up to 3 months, the hair fall will stop spontaneously within that period. Counselling and reassurance that yes, there is hair fall but the fall is replaced at the same rate, is all that is needed.

Anaemia is more common in women. Request for serum ferritin (which shows iron stores) even if the haemoglobin is within normal range.

Traction alopecia is more common in women because of a peculiar hair style that pulls the hair roots, like tight ponytails.

Dieting (rapid weight loss) and fancy crash diets are resorted to by girls in order to remain thin.

Processing scalp hair, more commonly undertaken be women, can cause breakage. Processing involves treating hair chemically to remove the cuticle before being styled in a particular way.

Alopecia – When to refer?

- Alopecia areata patches in the temporal or occipital region are resistant to treatment. Don't try your luck for too long!
- Alopecia areata patches which have not responded to 2 injections of triamcinolone.
- All scarring alopecia
- Androgenic alopecia which has not responded to minoxidil + finesteride for 6 months.

Myths about hair loss are widespread. Nothing in the following list is true:

- Shampooing or colouring hair causes hair loss.
- Applying hair oil promotes hair growth.
- Dandruff causes permanent hair loss.
- Stress causes permanent hair loss.
- Shaving head completely causes hair to grow back twice as thick.
- Standing on head (in Yoga called "Shirsasan") increases circulation and stimulates hair growth.
- Brushing hair with comb continuously will make hair healthier.

Is hair coming out by the roots, or is it breaking?

Hair coming out by the roots include:

- Telogen effluvium
- Androgenic alopecia
- Alopecia areata
- Drug induced alopecia

Broken hairs in alopecia suggest possible:

- Tinea capitis
- Structural hair shaft abnormalities
- Breakage due to improper use of hair-care cosmetics
- Anagen arrest

Laboratory investigations in alopecia:

- Complete blood count
- ESR
- Iron profile
- Thyroid function tests
- Liver function tests
- Renal function tests
- Vit B_{12} and D_3 levels
- RA factor/CRP/ANA
- Scalp skin biopsy

Pearls of Practice:

- Androgenic alopecia (AGA), alopecia areata and telogen effluvium are the most common causes of nonscarring alopecia.
- In diffuse hair loss, ask if the loss is predominantly hair thinning or shedding. The patient who presents with gradual hair thinning most likely has male or female pattern hair loss, recognized by the typical distribution patterns. Increased shedding is a characteristic feature of telogen effluvium.
- In all patients with diffuse hair loss, serum ferritin and thyroid function tests should be requested for.
- Patients with scarring alopecia should be referred to a dermatologist.

Table 33.1 Summary of findings in alopecia

Diffuse	
Female pattern hair loss	Hair thinning; frontal hairline intact; negative pull test
Male pattern hair loss	Hair thinning; M pattern; negative pull test
Diffuse alopecia areata	Distribution more patchy; positive pull test
Alopecia totalis or universalis	Total hair loss on the scalp and/or body
Telogen effluvium	Hair loss 3 months after precipitating event; positive pull test
Anagen effluvium	Sudden hair loss of up to 90% 2 weeks following chemotherapy
Focal	
Nonscarring	
▪ Alopecia areata	Normal scalp with surrounding exclamation point hairs
▪ Tinea capitis	Scaly scalp patch with itching and broken hair
▪ Traction alopecia	Patchy; related to hair practices/styling.
▪ Trichotillomania	Patchy; may be associated psychological disturbance
Scarring	Scarring and atrophy of scalp. No follicles seen

Newer Hair Loss Treatments

- **Scalp micropigmentation**, or tattooing, is used most often for recreating eyebrows lost to alopecia.
- **Low-level laser therapy (LLLT)** is one of the few FDA-cleared medical devices for the treatment of hair loss. How it works is not well understood, but LLLT may trigger the hair follicle stem cells to stimulate new hair growth.
- **Microneedling** is another technique that uses an FDA-cleared medical device for treating hair loss. Small needles are used to puncture the outer layers of the skin. This procedure is thought to promote hair regrowth by causing a release of factors into the tissues that encourage hair growth.
- **Stem cell therapy** is a promising area of hair loss treatment where the stem cells are injected into the scalp. More studies are needed in this field, and stem cell therapy is not FDA-approved for the treatment of hair loss.

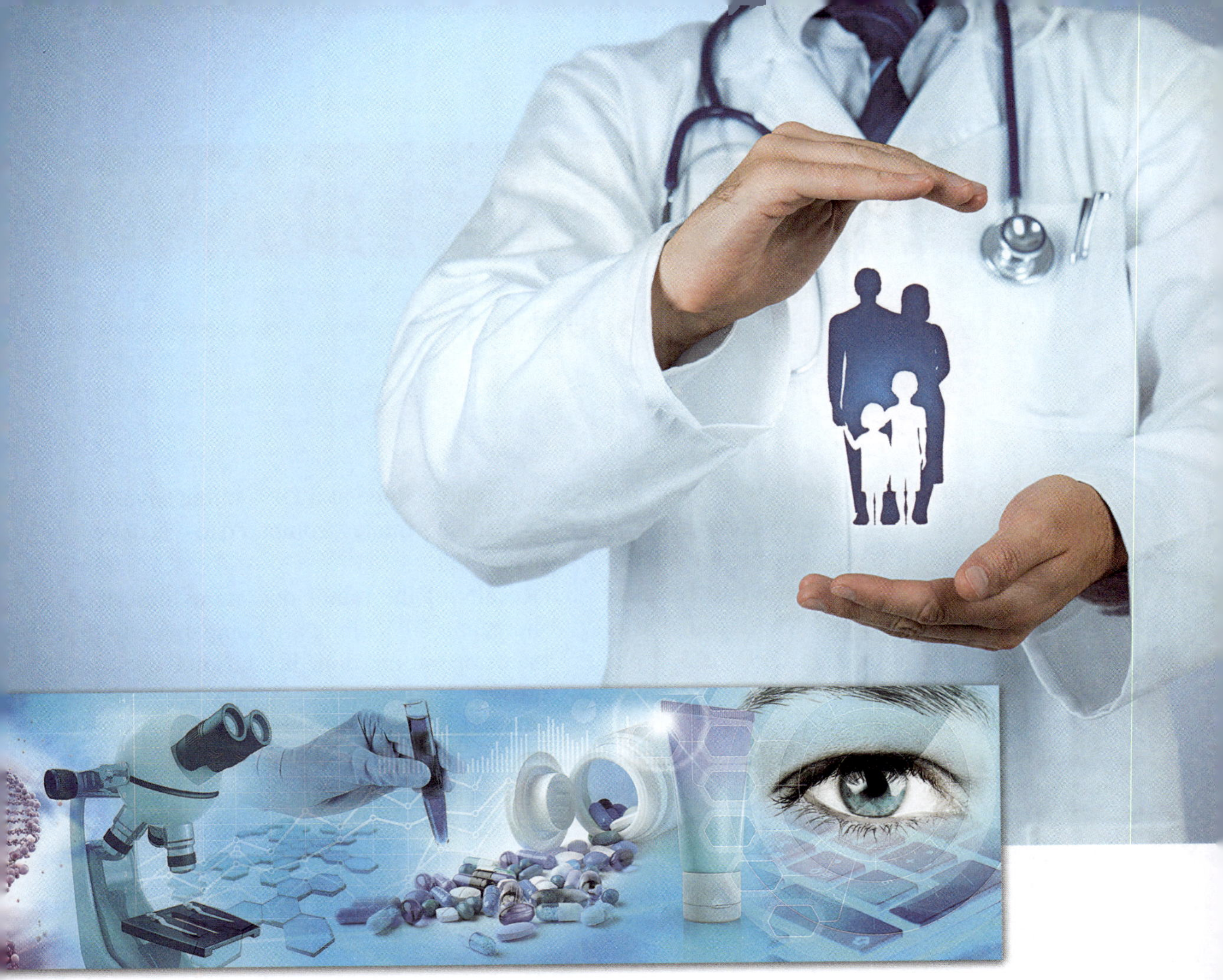

SECTION 3

SPECIALITY SURGICAL GENERAL PRACTICE

CHAPTER 34

Introduction

Around 25 years back, when I was doing my internship at Dound, a sleepy township in Western Maharashtra, I asked my mentor Dr CT Shah, MBBS, **What contributed to his success in general practice?** Mind you, I was asking a person who had an OPD of 300 patients daily, had two MD physicians and one MS surgeon as his assistants, a 70-bedded hospital, a blood bank and much more! All except an obstetric unit. "*I don't deliver babies, I deliver results*", he used to say. The answer to my question was immediate and forthright.

"A good doctor–patient relationship and a burning desire to develop".

"An in-depth knowledge of medicine must be the next pre-requisite?" I queried.

"No" he replied vehemently. "*The most fundamental knowledge of very basic surgery is more important than anything else, to boost one's practice.*"

Taking a cue from that same advice, I have over the years always tried to learn new and newer operations which can be performed in the clinic itself and I have discovered the following advantages:

1. It is the most challenging, gratifying and rewarding. The sigh of relief that you see on the face of a newly married boy after you have reduced his paraphimosis, is most satisfying.
2. Operations done at a GP's clinic save a lot of patient's money, compared to one done in a hospital.
3. Results of the minor operations described here, at a GP's clinic are comparable to the same operations done in a hospital by a surgeon.
4. An added advantage to the patient is that, he is not suddenly faced with a new doctor and a new environment. In the family physician's clinic, he is in familiar surroundings, with familiar staff and a familiar physician.
5. In rural India, doctor who performs surgery is a 'big' doctor, not withstanding his qualifications.
6. Last and not the least, it is financially rewarding for the doctor.

And is it so difficult? Mind you, there is no such animal, two legged or four legged, as a born surgeon. All surgeons are surgeons, because they have trained themselves in surgery. So can a GP. Any GP with a normal intellect, topped with a burning desire to acquire knowledge, can learn this "art of surgery", which is probably more rewarding than the "Science of Medicine". You don't even require a trained nurse to assist you.

Before Embarking on this Voyage with Purpose

1. Get Yourself Trained in Surgery

- Medical students should work as apprentice in private hospitals and get exposed to the operation theatre, very early in their career.
- Doctors doing internship, should jump at the opportunities to do operations themselves or at least assist surgeons. I know a doctor, who got a government award for doing 300 vasectomies during his internship.
- A practising doctor can join a government hospital, where he is usually allowed to attend surgery, as an observer. The medical officer gives opportunities once you have gained his confidence. (*Don't be shy in asking for help and advice. He will love it*!)
- You can also get adequately trained at a private surgical hospital, from a competent surgeon.
- You should not miss opportunities to attend refresher courses arranged by medical associations and local private hospitals.

2. Play Safe

- Always take a *written consent* before surgery, to avoid medicolegal complications later on. This is especially true about operations like vasectomies, piles, etc.
- Always inform the patient about the *complications*, if any, to be anticipated. Master the management of such complications. A surgeon once said "*I can teach you in 5 min how to remove the appendix. But, it will take me 5 years to teach you what to do if something goes wrong.*"
- Always inform the patient about the chances of *recurrence*, e.g., ganglion and piles surgeries have high rate of recurrence.
- *Never operate if the diagnosis is not certain.* We have heard of surgery being done for piles in a patient who was actually suffering from anal carcinoma.
- Always take *biopsy for HPE*, if in doubt. An excision of a 'benign' melanoma was done. The patient in a few days time, landed up with secondaries.
- *Don't cut* any structure *which you cannot identify*. It could be an important vessel or nerve.
- Always start with small operations, like excising a corn. Then, gradually graduate yourself to bigger operations, like circumcision.
- *Don't be overconfident*. Some operations, e.g., vasectomy, look simple when observed, but can be extremely tricky, if done without experience.
- Minor surgery requiring *general anaesthesia* automatically becomes a *major surgery*, because of the associated anaesthetic risks and specialized equipments and facilities required, e.g., circumcision in an infant is to be always done under GA. Always refer.
- *When not to operate* is equally important, e.g., never remove a keloid. It will surely come back and will be almost twice its original size. Do not remove a strawberry haemangioma in a child. It will resolve spontaneously without leaving tell-tale signs, but if operated upon, it may leave a permanent scar. Advise the patient against removal of 15–20 harmless lipomas. It is ridiculous!

Play safe! Refer if not confident! Do not be adventurous! Know your limitations!

Safety for All

- *Make the operation safe for the patient*: E.g., take good aseptic precautions.
- *Make the patient safe for the operation*: E.g., operate on diabetics only after his blood sugar has been brought under control.
- *Make the doctor safe for the operation*: Take universal safety precautions against HIV, HBV, etc.
- *Finally, make the doctor safe for the patient*: Train yourself properly, never miss an opportunity to operate and become a specialist surgical GP.

3. Sterilize your Instruments in a Proper Manner

This is a mandatory and a very important step. If not properly done, the suture site gets infected, giving sepsis to the patient and a bad reputation to the operator and the operation.

A **sterilization** procedure is one that kills all microorganisms (bacteria, viruses and fungi) including spores, rendering it free of all living microorganisms. This can be achieved by means of an autoclave.

Disinfection kills all microorganisms but not spores. This is achieved by chemical germicides.

- ***Autoclaves***: This is the method of choice and is used in most of the hospitals. Here, the instruments are sterilized by steam in an autoclave, by heating them for 15 min at 120°C.
- ***Modified pressure cookers***: Though autoclaves are ideal, cost is prohibitive and hence generally not used in a GP's clinic. Hence, especially for developing countries like India, WHO and UNICEF have collaborated in developing an inexpensive modified pressure cooker. It is fitted with a rack, where needles, syringes and other instruments, commonly required by a GP, can be kept.
- ***Disinfection by boiling*** in an electric "sterilizer" (or in an appropriate steel container on a gas stove) for 20 min, will kill all bacteria, viruses but not spores. If sterilization by autoclaving or by a pressure cooker is not possible, this is an acceptable procedure for minor operations described in this book.
- ***Disinfection by soaking in chemicals***: This method is not usually preferred as the chemical may get inactivated by blood, have to be freshly prepared every time, and may be corrosive to the instruments. Hence, this method should be employed as a last resort, if neither autoclaving nor boiling is feasible.

The instruments should be thoroughly cleaned of all blood and then disinfected by immersing them for at least 30 min, in one of the following solutions:

i) *Household bleach*: Prepare solution by putting 2 tsf in one litre of water. Costs about Rs. 30/L. The solution is unstable and has to be freshly prepared daily.
ii) *Povidone iodine* (*Betadine*) solution is more stable. Before immersing the instruments, it is to be diluted by adding 1 part to 3 parts of boiled water.
iii) *Formalin solution* (*Formaldehyde*): Commercially available as 40%, this should be diluted 10 times in boiled water, to make it 4%. Cost is about Rs. 100/L.
iv) *Hydrogen peroxide*: Available as 30%, it should be diluted to 4% by adding 1 part to 4 parts of boiled water. It is corrosive to the instruments. Costs about Rs. 160/L.
v) *Ethanol* and *Gluteraldehyde* (both Rs. 400/L) are costly and do not have any advantage over the above.
vi) *Disinfection by formalin tablets*: Previously boiled and washed instruments are kept in an airtight container (e.g., a bread box) in which 3–4 formalin tablets are kept (formalin chamber). Advantages in this method are that the solution need not be

prepared every time, it is not corrosive to the instruments and the disinfected instruments are kept in stock, ready for use. This method of preserving the instruments is highly recommended.

CHAPTER 35

Safety Precautions in the Clinic and During Minor Surgery

- Transmission Risk to Health Care Workers
- Universal Precautions in a GP's Setting
- Management of Occupational Exposure to HIV
- Antiretroviral Drugs for PEP for HIV

Minor surgery is very lucrative. Also performing any kind of surgery gives a 'big' reputation to a GP practising in India. Still surprisingly, very few GPs routinely do minor surgery in their clinics. There can be only two reasons for this:

1. ***Lack of adequate knowledge & experience***: Minor surgery is not routinely taught in the medical curriculum. Hence, acquiring basic skills about minor surgery depends on the practitioner himself, his desire to do so and the opportunities available to him. Both the knowledge and the skill can be easily obtained by a little extra effort on his part.
2. ***Fear of acquiring infection*** through exposure to blood during surgery, e.g., hepatitis B, (HBV), hepatitis C (HCV) and other viruses, but especially the human immunodeficiency virus (HIV). These fears are exaggerated and can be dispelled by a proper knowledge about the transmission of these viruses.

FACTS ABOUT TRANSMISSION RISK OF HBV, HCV AND HIV TO HEALTH CARE WORKERS

A health care worker (HCW) is defined as *a medical personnel whose activities involve contact with blood and other body fluids*. These include doctors, nurses, laboratory technicians, or even 'aayas', and 'dais'. All HCWs have increased risk of acquiring these viruses because of exposure to blood and body fluids.

Hepatitis B Virus (HBV)

Approximately 4%, i.e., 4 persons will become infected when percutaneously exposed to blood from 100 patients with hepatitis B infection. Asymptomatic HBV carriers are the greatest risk to HCWs, because there are no specific clinical features to identify them. Approximately 1% of the patients admitted to large hospitals are HbsAg positive, but 90% of these are not recognized as Australia antigen test is not done routinely. Most of these occupational exposures go unnoticed and forgotten only to be detected at a later date.

The most common route of transmission obviously is through contamination of blood in a health care setting, although HBV is also found in high concentration in other body fluids (like breast milk, saliva, semen, synovial fluid, etc.)

Hepatitis C Virus (HCV)

Although HBV and HCV are transmitted through similar routes, the risk of HCV infection to HCWs is substantially low (1.8%) as compared to HBV infection. This is due to the low viraemia associated with HCV infection. Most of the documented cases have been due to needle stick injuries of hollow bore needles during haemodialysis and very few because of mucous membrane exposure.

Human Immunodeficiency Virus (HIV)

Although HIV has been isolated from almost all body fluids, in a health care setting the important fluids are CSF (highest concentration), pleural, peritoneal or pericardial fluids and blood. In these settings, transmission of HIV from an HIV infected patient to HCW is extremely low (only 0.4% as compared to 4% with HBV infection, i.e., only 4 persons in 1000), but still it has generated a kind of fear psychosis amongst practitioners because the disease carries a stigma and is always fatal. This is unfortunate and is based on inadequate scientific information about the transmission of the virus coupled with inadequate information about the methods of protection. Let us examine the facts.

Till December end 1994, 42 "documented" cases and 91 "possible" cases were registered by Centre for Disease Control (CDC) in the United States. By "documented", we mean that the health care worker was proved to be HIV negative by ELISA test at the time of occupational exposure but seroconverted within 3–4 months. By 'possible', we mean that the initial negative status could not be documented for various reasons. Out of the documented 42 cases, 36 (i.e., 80%) became seropositive after an injury with a hollow bore needle and the rest after mucous membrane exposure. Of these, 17 were laboratory technicians, 13 were nurses and 6 were doctors. *None of these were surgeons.*

The statistics outside USA or in India or the whole world is not known and is not likely to be known in the near future. Many more obviously might have been infected with HIV occupationally, but these cases are not reported by the HCWs because of the fear of the HIV status becoming known. Nevertheless, the above data is representative sample, which tells us that surgeons are least at risk of getting infected with HIV in occupational setting, laboratory technicians and nurses are highly exposed while general practitioners are at risk because of hollow bore needles (and not due to scalpel blade or the suturing needle). But given the fact that lakhs of general practitioners are treating millions of HIV positive patients, with or without their knowledge, these figures are electron microscopic.

In short, the risk of transmission of HBV, HCV or HIV through minor surgery is extremely low and this can be made negligible by observing the "Universal precautions" described below. The HIV epidemic has assumed pandemic proportions and the virus is all over the world. It is folly to try to avoid the virus. It is wisdom to learn to live with the virus and take measures to prevent from getting infected (occupationally!).

UNIVERSAL PRECAUTIONS IN A GENERAL PRACTITIONER'S SETTING

In 1987, after 3 HCWs accidentally got infected in occupational set up, CDC published guidelines to reduce the occupational exposure to HIV.

These guidelines are called "**Universal precautions**" **(UP)**, which recommend that *all patients should be considered potentially infectious and precautions should be taken for all patients regardless of their HIV serostatus.* This means that blood and certain other body fluids (semen, vaginal secretions, CSF, pleural, peritoneal, pericardial and synovial fluids) and all body fluids contaminated with blood are to be treated as being potentially infectious and precautions taken in handling them. UP does not apply to saliva, tears, sweat, urine or vomitus as chances of HBV, HCV or HIV transmission from these fluids is virtually nonexistent.

Routine or mandatory testing for HIV preoperatively has its inherent pitfalls. A negative ELISA antibody test does not rule out HIV infection as the patient could be in the window period. In this period, the plasma viral load of HIV is very high, making the patient highly infective.

A negative test may therefore lead to failure to observe precautions, thereby increasing the risk of transmission during surgery.

A positive antibody test on the other hand, could lead to refusal by the GP to perform the planned surgery on the helpless HIV victim, a decision based on improper knowledge about the low transmissibility of the virus and about the fact that the lipid coated virus can be easily inactivated by washing the hands with soap and water for 2 min.

The **elements of UP** to avoid exposure to these viruses in a clinical setting are as follows:

1. Hand Washing

This is the single most important measure to prevent transmission of infection. Ideally, hands should be washed after examining each and every patient but necessarily after contact with blood and other body fluids mentioned above. Hand washing should also be done after removal of gloves following surgery because it is difficult for the HCW to know whether a leak in the gloves has taken place or not. Soap should be used for washing which should be done vigorously and thoroughly for at least 10 sec. Soap dissolves the lipid wall of the virus, rendering it inactive. There is no evidence to suggest that germicidal soaps (e.g., Dettol soap) are more effective in preventing the transmission of viruses.

2. Gloves

Using gloves is another important measure which provides a protective barrier, thereby preventing contamination of hands with blood and body fluids. However, the following aspects should be kept in mind:

- Wearing gloves is not a substitute for handwashing because gloves may have small leaks invisible to the naked eye or might have got torn during the procedure, both of which can lead to contamination of hands with blood.
- Gloves cannot prevent injury due to needles and other sharp instruments like scalpel blades.
- Surgical gloves (vinyl or latex) are meant for single use only and should be discarded after use. Occasionally, however there will be situations where gloves have to be reused. The method of reprocessing gloves under these circumstances is given in Table 35.2.
- Gloves cannot give absolute protection, but when used with other measures suggested under UP the effectiveness is enhanced to a great extent.
- It is not necessary to wear gloves when blood contact is unlikely, e.g., while examining a HIV positive patient or giving IM or SC injection to cooperative patient. Gloves are made of latex rubber, which is a natural

product obtained from trees; availability is therefore limited. Indiscriminate use may ultimately lead to shortage of gloves; use only when indicated (see Table 35.1).

3. Protective Shields

Gowns, plastic aprons, face shields or goggles, waterproof shoe covers (available as "ZED kits") are required only for major surgery and during delivery, where splashing of blood is likely.

4. Protection from Needle and Sharp Instruments

Most of the injuries sustained by a surgeon during surgery are by solid bore suture needles and sharps. These inject only a small quantity of blood and hence transmission of HIV or HBV is less likely. Hollow bore needle injuries usually sustained by physicians, laboratory technicians and nurses are associated with injection of larger quantities of blood and hence increased risk of transmission of these viruses. Hence, injections should be given only when absolutely necessary.

Disposable needles and syringes are ideally meant for single use only. Recapping, bending or breaking of needles should never be done. Maximum number of occupationally acquired infections with HIV and HBV have been due to hollow bore needles while doing recapping of needles. When this has to be done because disposable needles are not available, the cap should be placed on the table and the needle

| **Table 35.1** Gloves should be worn while performing the following |

- Giving IV injection or starting an IV drip.
- Suturing and dressing wounds.
- Genital examination of a patient having STD.
- P/V, P/R or even per oral examination (which may contain blood stained saliva).
- Insertion of urinary catheter or feeding tube.
- Cleaning contaminated instruments or blood spills. Thick gloves known as household gloves or utility gloves should be worn for this purpose.
- Any other condition where there is likelihood of exposure to blood or bloodstained fluid.

| **Table 35.2** Reprocessing of gloves |

1. After the procedure/operation is over, do not remove the *gloves* immediately. Wash them properly with a hypochlorite solution. Since hypochlorite solution may cause deterioration of the glove material, wash the hypochlorite solution with soap and clean tap water. Now remove the gloves.
2. Since *hands* could have got contaminated with blood, wash your hands properly with soap and water for 2 min.
3. Finally *test for holes* in the gloves by filling them with water till fully inflated and then turning them through 360° at the base. If holes are present puncture sites will leak. If so, discard the glove. If not, hang them up for drying for subsequent reuse after sterilization.

Summary

- Gloved hands: Hypochlorite followed by soap and water.
- Ungloved hands: Soap and water.
- Test for holes in the gloves.

should be inserted without touching the cap. Needles should not be removed from the syringe but thrown directly into a puncture-resistant container, which contains freshly prepared 1% hypochlorite solution. Using clippers to cut the needle increases the possibility of accidental injury but has to be occasionally resorted to, because disposing the needle along with the syringe *in toto* requires a large puncture proof container, not easily available. For similar reasons, the puncture resistant container should be located as close as possible to the area of administering injection.

Using double gloves in which the outer pair is half size larger than the inner pair can give added protection against injury with suture needles and sharps, without significantly affecting the tactile sensation. Another way of giving added protection is by applying a sticking plaster to the index finger and the thumb of non-dominant hand inside the gloves, as most of the injuries sustained during surgery are on this area.

During surgery, sharp instruments like scalp blades should never be passed on, hand to hand. Instead, a kidney tray should be used for the purpose. The person disposing off sharps should use thick utility gloves and place them in thick puncture resistant plastic bags, before disposal.

5. Precautions Under Special Circumstances

- HCWs who have *open wounds* should cover these wounds with water-proof adhesive tapes and also use double gloves during surgery.
- HCWs who have *weeping lesions* on the skin of the hand, which are difficult to cover up, should avoid operative procedures as far as possible.
- Pregnant HCWs should take extra precautions as exposure to infected blood may result in immediate transmission of the viruses to the expectant mother and subsequently to the foetus or the baby.
- When gloves are not available in an emergency, a gauze soaked in sodium hypochlorite may be used to hold blood-stained material.
- In case of *accidental spillage of blood* on the floor or table, the spill should first be covered by a blotting paper or a newspaper. Sodium hypochlorite solution should be poured on the paper and left there for 10–15 min. This is then removed by the gloved hand. The all purpose disinfectant sodium hypochlorite solution or household liquid bleach, which is cheap and very effective against liquid viruses like HIV and HBV, should be kept in all clinics and hospitals.

MANAGEMENT OF OCCUPATIONAL EXPOSURE TO HIV

As discussed above, most of the occupational exposure to blood and other body fluids are preventable but accidents do occur. The HCW then can get exposed to known HIV infected blood or blood of unknown HIV status, in one of the following manners:

1. Needle puncture
2. Injury by a sharp instrument like scalpel blade
3. Mucous membrane inoculation
4. Contamination of a wound
5. Contamination of an oozing dermatosis

Under the circumstances, as a doctor in-charge, what advice do you give to the HCW?

1. Do not panic. Know the facts. The risk of acquiring HIV infection after a pinprick to the skin sustained from a needle containing blood from an HIV positive patient is very low, i.e., 4 persons in 1000 (0.4%), which also

means that 99.6% of the times HIV is *not* transmitted. The risk is 0.1% for mucous membrane exposure and again 0.1% for non-intact (e.g., eczematous) skin exposure (1 in 1000). The HIV status of most patients is not known to the HCW at the time of exposure. If the prevalence of HIV infection amongst patients attending to the clinic (not in the community) is assumed to be about 1% (survey rates vary widely), the above rates get diluted 100 times. So, do not panic.

2. Do not stop the bleeding by pressing the wound, let the blood flow freely.
3. Wash the puncture wound thoroughly with soap and water for 2 min. If oral or nasal mucosa is exposed it should be vigorously flushed with water. Eyes should be irrigated with plain water or saline.
4. Dip the puncture wound in undiluted savlon for 15 sec, if possible. Although there is no scientific evidence of its efficiency,there is no contraindication of its use.
5. If the HIV status of the patients is not already known, explain the position to him and do a "rapid Tridot test" for HIV on his blood.

   If the rapid test is positive: Do the HIV ELISA test on the HCW on day 1 (as baseline), 1 month, 3 months and 6 months.

   If the rapid test is negative: He could still be positive because of the window period. Ask the patient in confidence about h/o unprotected sexual exposure in past 3 months. Even if there is no h/o exposure, it is better to repeat the HIV test after 6 weeks on both the patient and the HCW.
6. If desired, similar protocols can be followed for HBV and HCV.
7. Ask the HCW to report back to you if there is an acute febrile illness with lymphadenopathy and a rash (seroconversion illness?)
8. Ask the HCW to refrain from sexual intercourse or blood donation till the final HIV test is negative.
9. Counsel him about the various aspects of prophylactic antiretroviral treatment, keeping in mind the pros and cons as explained below.

| **Table 35.3** Methods of inactivating HIV/HBV pre and postoperatively |

1. **Physical methods**: For syringes, needles and surgical instruments
   - Autoclave for 20 min at 120°C (or)
   - Pressure cooker (or)
   - Boiling for 20 min
2. **Chemical disinfectants**: For surgical instruments only.
   - Sodium hypochlorite—for stainless steel equipment only and household liquid bleach for cleaning blood spills.
   - Formaldehyde or Gluteraldehyde solution—used for sterilizing endoscopes.
   - Undiluted savlon—for scalpel blades, scissors, etc.

ANTIRETROVIRAL DRUGS USED FOR POSTEXPOSURE PROPHYLAXIS (PEP) FOR HIV

The following information should be given to the HCW about PEP for HIV:

- The facts and figures pertaining to the risk of acquiring HIV infection as stated above.
- To be effective, the drugs should be started immediately, preferably within 1–2 hrs after exposure when the virus is in the dendritic cells of the skin and mucous membrane. However, their effectivity is doubtful if started after 72 hrs as the virus may already be replicating in the blood.
- The protection offered by antiretroviral drugs is not 100% (though in one study the risk reduction was shown to be 81% with AZT).

- Treatment is costly and has to be taken for at least 1 month.
- The drugs have side effects, e.g., AZT can cause severe nausea, vomiting, epigastric pain, headache, polyarthralgia and weakness although serious toxicity is rare. AZT can also cause haematological toxicity like anaemia and thrombocytopenia requiring blood count monitoring. Lamivudine can cause gastric upsets while indinavir can cause kidney stones. Hence, drugs like tenofovir and lamuvudine are preferred because of their low side effect profile.

If then the HCW opts for starting PEP, institute the following regimen depending on the transmission risk:

1. ***Low transmission risk***
   - Contamination of intact skin with HIV positive blood or body fluids.
   - Very superficial needle prick without bleeding.

> Advise HCW against starting antiretro-viral drugs.

2. ***Recognised transmission risk***
   - Injury with exposure to small amount of HIV positive blood or body fluids.
   - Superficial injury.
   - Solid bore needle.
   - Mucous membrane exposure.
   - Asymptomatic HIV positive patient.

> Advise "*basic PEP regimen*":
> AZT (Zidovir) 200 mg tds or Tenofovir 300 mg od
> **Plus**
> Lamivudine (Lamivir) 150 mg bd or 300 mg od for 4 weeks.

3. ***Increased risk of transmission***
   - Exposure to larger amounts of HIV positive blood or body fluids.
   - Deep percutaneous injury.
   - Hollow bore needle.
   - Patient in preterminal or terminal AIDS.
   - Patient on antiretroviral drugs.

> Advise "*expanded PEP regimen*":
> Basic regimen (AZT + Lamivudine)
> **Plus**
> Atazanavir 400 mg od + Ritonavir 100 mg od

During the PEP for HIV, the HCW should be followed-up by doing the ELISA antibody tests or rapid Tridot tests as recommended above. He is asked to report back in case of acute febrile illness. As the antibody tests are negative in the window period, it is tempting to advise viral load test (HIV RNA or DNA PCR) or HIV P24 antigen tests. These are more sensitive methods for detecting early HIV infection and are many times requested by the HCW in order to cut short the 'window of anxiety'. It is not advisable to use these tests, as false positive tests are seen in 2–3% of cases, which results in virtual panic for the already tensed HCW and further complicates matters.

GP Tip

A simple and economical way of preventing HIV transmission through needles in your clinic—make a hole on the lid of an empty plastic container. Insert the used needle in this hole and cut it at the shoulder with a wire cutter available in any electric shop.

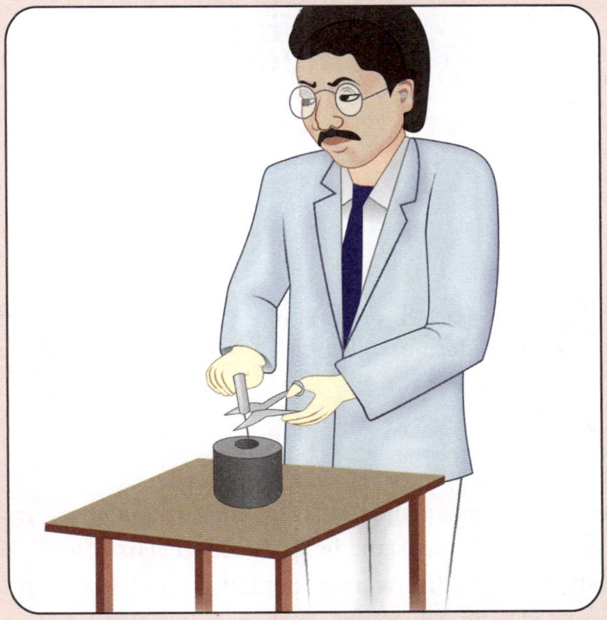

CHAPTER 36

Injections in General Practice

- General Considerations
- Intradermal Injection
- Subcutaneous Injection
- Intramuscular Injections
- Injection Practice & the Indian GP

Administering an injection is the most frequently used (and misused!) medical procedure. Historically, until the discovery of penicillin, only doctors used to give injection. Then, nurses took over this task in hospitals. It is estimated that more than 12 billion injections are administered throughout the world every year. In India alone 4.2 billion injections are administered annually, many of these judged to be unfortunately unnecessary. And surprisingly, this procedure is not taught in the medical colleges mainly "because they are too simple to be taught". The technique is passed on by a senior GP to a new GP by virtue of tradition, not necessarily based on strict scientific principles. Though a simple procedure, it is not benign without complications. Hence, this concise essay, describing the correct technique of giving various types of injections, viz., intradermal, subcutaneous, intramuscular, intravenous, etc.

GENERAL CONSIDERATIONS

Remember, giving injections is an invasive procedure and needs sterile technique.

The following basic steps are to be followed:

1. Wash your hands.
2. Use only new disposable syringes and needles every time.
3. Reassure the patients that the injection is not going to be very painful. Explain the procedure.
4. Disinfect the skin area to be injected by a spirit swab using a circular motion from centre outwards.
5. If there is aspiration of blood after inserting the needle, withdraw the syringe, dispose off the contents of the syringe, take fresh medication and inject at another site. Don't inject the bloody solution (not applicable to IV injections).

6. Observe "*Universal Precautions*" as laid down by WHO before and after giving any injection.
7. After the injection is completed, never recap the needle. Instead cut the needle in a special container especially meant for this purpose.
8. **Filling the syringe with medication**:
   - In case of a multidose vial, e.g., lignocaine: First push air into the bulb through the syringe equal to the volume of the medication to be withdrawn. Due to positive pressure the medication will then run into the syringe or can be forced into the syringe by pulling on the plunger.
   - In case of powdered drug to be prepared freshly, e.g., streptomycin: Aspirate distilled water into the syringe, push it into the vial, withdraw the syringe, shake the vial gently till the powder is dissolved completely and then withdraw the dissolved solution into the syringe.
   - In case of single dose ampoule which contains a liquid drug, e.g., B_1, B_6, B_{12}: Rub the ampoule's neck with a file and then snap it off by holding the top with a cotton swab soaked in spirit, directing the force away from body. Withdraw the solution with the needle and syringe, keeping the needle tip below the level of the solution.

INTRADERMAL (ID) INJECTION

This is usually required in general practice for testing sensitivity to injectable drugs like penicillin, streptomycin, B_1, B_6, B_{12}, etc., or for performing a tuberculin test. The test is done on the ventral aspect of the forearm. Occasionally, BCG vaccine is required to be given, which is to be given on the left deltoid.

Fill the tuberculin or insulin syringe with the solution to be tested. Stretch the selected area of skin between the thumb and the forefinger. With the needle bevel facing upwards and the needle at an angle of 5–15° to the skin, insert the tip of the needle into the superficial skin. Next, release the stretched skin and press on the plunger. If in the correct plane, a small pale wheal will appear (looking like a mosquito bite). If the wheal does not appear, you have given the injection too deep, in which case withdraw the needle slightly and push the plunger. Finally, draw a circle around the wheal with a ball-pen and write down the time of administering the injection on the side of the circle.

SUBCUTANEOUS (SC) INJECTION

Subcutaneous injections are used mainly for giving insulin, measles and MMR vaccines. It is to be given either on the upper arm, thigh or anterior abdominal wall (Fig. 36.1).

After the preliminaries are completed, attach a no. 25 or no. 26 needle to the syringe or else use a disposable insulin syringe. Pinch a fold of skin, insert needle at the base of the skin fold at an angle of 20–30°. Then, release the skin fold. Aspirate to see if you are in a vein. If not, inject slowly and withdraw the needle. For insulin injections, as they are to be given daily probably lifelong, rotate the sites every time in a fixed sequence. Then, return to the first site at least 2.5 cm away from the previous injection site in that area.

INTRAMUSCULAR (IM) INJECTIONS

Gently stretch the skin flat with the thumb and index finger of your non-dominant hand. Hold the syringe in your dominant hand as you hold a pen. Then, quickly and firmly thrust the needle through

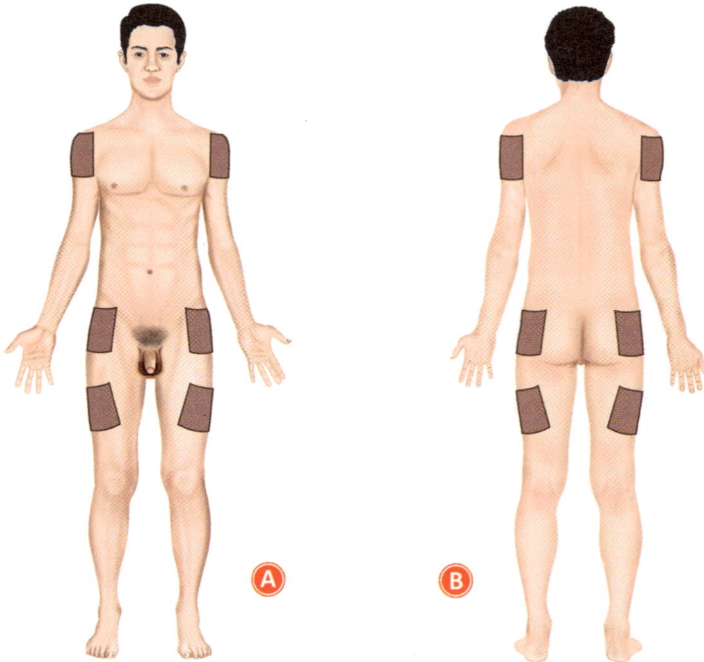

| Fig. 36.1 Sites for intramuscular injections

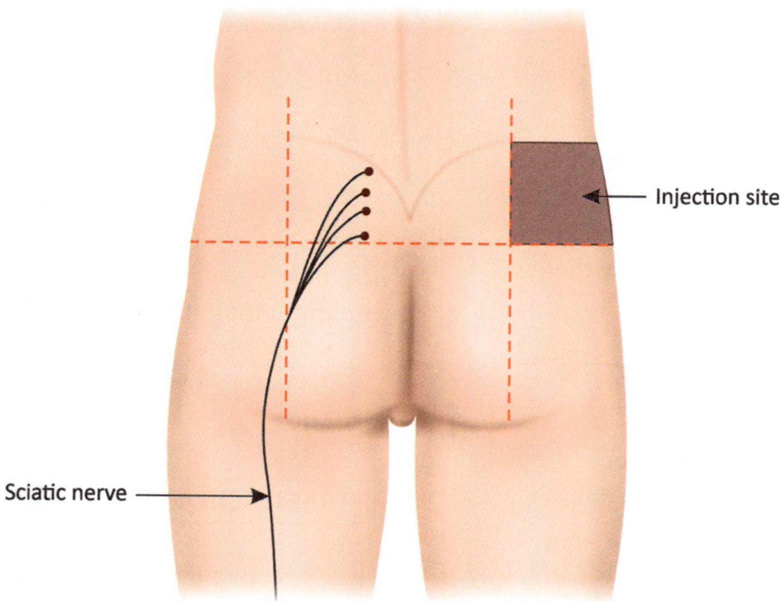

| Fig. 36.2 Upper and outer quadrants of gluteus region |

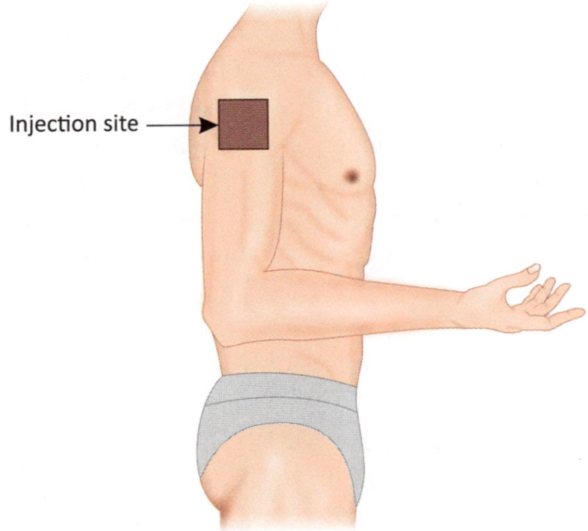

| **Fig. 36.3** Deltoid region for IM injection |

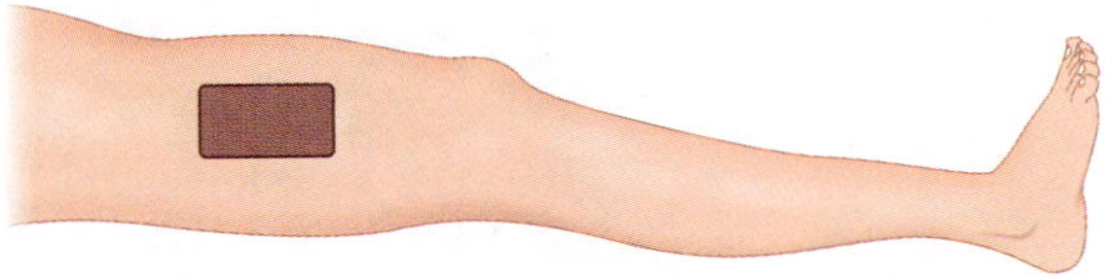

| **Fig. 36.4a** Anterio-lateral aspect of thigh: Side view for IM injection |

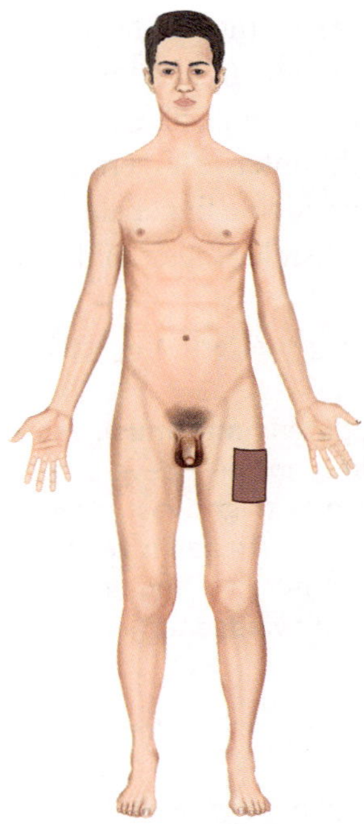

| **Fig. 36.4b** Anterio-lateral aspect of thigh: Front view for IM injection |

the skin and subcutaneous tissue, deep into the muscle mass (dart technique) at 90° to the skin.

Now support the syringe with your non-dominant hand and pull back slightly on the plunger with your dominant hand to aspirate for blood. If no blood appears in the syringe, push the plunger slowly till the whole medication is delivered into the muscle mass. Massage, stop capillary bleeding if present and watch for post injection syncope.

Locating IM Injection Sites

1. ***Gluteus area*** **(Fig. 36.2)**
   This area is bounded by the iliac crest above, anterior superior spine laterally, the natal cleft medially and the gluteus folds below. Divide this area into 4 quadrants. The injection is to be given in the upper and outer quadrant in order to avoid damage to the sciatic nerve.
   Another method is to place the heel of your non-dominant hand on the greater trochanter of the femur. Then, place your index finger on the anterior superior iliac spine and stretch your middle finger along the iliac crest as far as possible. Inject in the centre of the 'V' of the fingers about 2″–3″ below the iliac crest.
2. ***Deltoid area*** **(Fig. 36.3)**
   The selected site should be 2–3 finger breadths below the acromion process or midway between the acromion process and the deltoid insertion.
3. ***Anteriolateral thigh*** **(Figs. 36.4a & b)**
   Inject in the middle third of the thigh on the anterior-lateral aspect. This is the area in a child a handbreadth below greater trochanter to a handbreadth above the knee. You may have to bunch the muscle before injecting.
4. ***Triceps***
   Not recommended site as the radial nerve and branches of radial, brachial and ulnar nerves are under the triceps muscle. But, this area is used by many GPs in India for giving injections in women reluctant to remove blouse or expose their buttock.

Z-Track Technique

Some drugs like iron dextran are irritating to the subcutaneous tissue. Hence, when iron dextran is given by the conventional IM method, it may

Box 1 Selecting site for IM injection

1. **Gluteal (gluteus maximus)**: Preferred site for larger volume, painful or depot injections. This muscle does not fully develop until the child is walking for at least 1 year. So avoid in children.
2. **Anteriolateral thigh (vastus lateralis)**: Preferred site for children < 2 years. This muscle is well developed at birth and is relatively free from major nerves and vessels.
3. **Deltoid**: For non-oily and non-painful injection of <2 mL.
4. **Triceps**: Best avoided for fear of injury to the radial nerve.

Box 2 Positioning patient for IM injection

1. **Gluteal region**: Lay down the patient on side. Relax gluteus muscle by flexing upper leg and knee at 20°.
2. **Deltoid region**: Make patient sit and place his hand on the hip or thigh to relax the deltoid muscle.
3. **Anterolateral region in child**: The adult should hold child on his chest with his left arm around the child and holding the outside arm. The child's inside arm should be tucked against the adult's body. The adult's right arm holds the child's leg firmly.

leak into the SC tissue causing pain, staining and even sterile injection abscess. To prevent this, the Z-technique is used.

Displace laterally, the skin and subcutaneous tissue of the gluteal area by pulling it away from the injection site by the thumb of your non-dominant hand. Insert the needle at 90° to the skin and deposit the drug into the muscle. Now withdraw the needle slowly and release the skin and subcutaneous tissue. The needle tract is thus separated from the area of the drug, preventing its leakage into the SC tissue.

Complications

1. **Injection abscess**: This can be 'infective' if less than adequate aseptic precautions have been taken. It can be a "sterile abscess" if irritating drugs are given in the SC tissue where they cannot get absorbed.
2. **Muscle fibrosis**: This results from repeated injections given at the same site. In such cases, the sites should be rotated in turn.
3. **Nerve injury**: The commonest nerve to be injured is the radial and sciatic nerve.
4. **Post injection syncope** can be caused by painful injections.
5. Hepatitis B, hepatitis C and HIV transmission.

INJECTION PRACTICE AND THE INDIAN GP

Especially in rural settings in India, giving injections to patients as part of a 'package cure' by GPs is a norm. So much so that, if the GP does not administer an injection, albeit a placebo, the doctor is not considered a doctor at all by the patient! In India, over 4.2 billion injection are given per year, according to a study conducted in Hyderabad in 2004 by PATH, an international NGO. Out of these, only 3% are for vaccination purposes. These are absolutely necessary. The rest are given for so-called curative purposes. The study concludes that out of these, 2/3rd are un-indicated, as oral drugs can be used instead.

Why these Un-indicated Injections?

Box 3 gives the very few indications when injections are absolutely necessary. But in the scenario of general practice, such a situation is rare and most of injections administered are not necessary. Then why do GPs resort to "injection practice"?

| **Box 3** Indications for giving injections |

1. When patient is not retaining oral drugs because of severe vomiting, dysphagia, etc.
2. When the patient is suffering from life threatening illness, which requires high dose of antibiotics intravenously.
3. The drug is not available in oral form, e.g., streptomycin.
4. To correct dehydration by IV fluids.

The reasons are:

1. ***Patient factors***
   - *Placebo injections*: To satisfy the psychological needs of the patient.
   - *Demand injections:* Many patients demand injections because they wrongly believe that injections work faster and are more potent than oral drugs.
   - *Traditional injections*: People request for injections because they have taken injections since childhood.
2. ***Doctor factors***
   - Some GPs wrongly believe that injections are more effective and rapid in action than oral drugs.
   - GPs can charge higher fees and patients are ready to pay more, if an injection is administered.

Why a GP should avoid Un-indicated Injections?

Because administering injections poses problems to the doctor himself, to his patient and to the community at large.

1. ***Occupational risk to the GP***: Accidental needle stick injury, i.e., injury caused by the used needle to the GP can result in transmission of Hep. B, Hep. C and HIV infection. The transmission of HIV is feared the most, because the disease is invariably fatal in the long run, although the chances of Hep. B transmission is 100 times more. Let us compare the transmission rates.
   - Hepatitis B = 30%, i.e., 300 out of 1000 may get infected.
   - Hepatitis C = 3%, i.e., 30 out of 1000 may get infected.
   - HIV = 0.3%, i.e., 3 out of 1000 may get infected.
2. ***Risk to patients***: It has been estimated by WHO that across the globe in the year 2000, the number of new persons getting infected because of unsafe injection practices is a whooping 23 million!

   The split up is approximately 96,000 for HIV, 2 million for HCV and 21.7 million for HBV. This includes transmission by intravenous drug users. Add this to the already 5–7% of the population suffering from Hep. B, 2% from Hep. C and 0.5% from HIV and we have a big epidemic at hand.

   Apart from these risks of virus transmission, the additional risks to the patient is given under complications of IM injections.
3. ***Risk to the community***: If the needles and syringes are not disposed off correctly, these syringes may be recycled, i.e., they can be repacked and resold by unscrupulous elements. In addition, rag pickers may get accidental needle stick injuries. In urban areas, the syringes are to be destroyed by incineration. The syringes are to be dispatched to the authorities in a red plastic bag. In rural areas, these are to be sent to district hospitals for destruction by autoclaving. Plastic syringes cannot be burnt because they emit poisonous chemicals called "*furans*" into the atmosphere.

CHAPTER 37

Administering IV Fluids in Clinic

Intravenous therapy is giving medicines and fluids through a vein into the blood. This is commonly referred to as “drip” because most IV sets contain a “drip chamber” to regulate flow of fluid and to prevent air from going into circulation and causing air embolism. The administration of IV fluids is the most common intervention in medicine.

Advantages of Fluid Therapy

- Accurate, controlled administration of fluids can be given.
- Due to direct delivery of fluids in intravascular compartment, there is prompt correction of fluid and electrolyte disturbances.
- This results in faster clinical response.

Disadvantages of Fluid Therapy

- More expensive than oral.
- Needs strict aseptic precautions.
- Needs supervision.
- Improper fluid selection, volume and rate of infusion can lead to complications.

KNOW THE RISKS OF IV THERAPY

Giving IV therapy is not without risks. The complications could be mild or life threatening. They are always life threatening to the patient. Many of these are preventable, if proper care is taken. Always read labels on IV bottle to avoid mistakes. Examine each bottle against light to check clearness. Discard if cloudy or shows particles in suspension.

Local Complications

- ***Infiltration (or extravasation) of fluids***: This is caused by dislodgement of the needle from the vein (the needle has come “out”). Hence, the IV fluid leaks into the surrounding tissues. Look for coldness, swelling and blanching. It is usually not painful. The IV fluid has probably stopped or at least slowed down. This can be largely prevented by tapping the needle securely in place and providing boards for stability. In case the needle has come out, remove the needle and fix it at different site.

- ***Phlebitis***: This is inflammation of the vein in which the needle is inserted and is caused by either infection or by the mere presence of foreign body (IV catheter or needle) or by the medication given. Symptoms are warmth, pain and a cord like swelling at the site. The IV cannula must be removed and reinserted in to a different limb. Apply warm moist compresses and Thombophob ointment. Do not massage the area as this can lead to dislodgement of a thrombus.

Systemic Complications

- ***Pyrogenic reactions*** occur if the infusion is contaminated with microorganisms or due to allergy or sometimes due to IV fluid given too fast for the body temperature to adjust. Discontinue IV and give intravenously injection of dexamethasone or antihistaminic or injection tramadol. Restart at another site using all new solutions and equipment.
- ***Pyrogenic reactions due to sepsis*** can occur which are more serious in nature. This causes fever with rigors, headache, and abdominal cramps and may lead to hypotension & shock. Usually, this occurs about half an hour after the infusion has been started. Discontinue IV. Check vital signs and in case of hypotension, tachycardia or bradycardia, transport the patient to the nearest hospital.
- ***Air embolism***: This is a very serious complication of IV therapy. It occurs if sizeable amount of air gets into circulation. The air bubble can block a vessel so that tissue supplied by the vessel is unable to get oxygen. The air bubble can cut off cardiac, pulmonary or cerebral vessels leading to hypotension, tachycardia and unconsciousness. Air embolism can be prevented by removing all air from the IV set and by never allowing the IV line to run dry before discontinuing. Always check to see that the IV set is full with IV fluid before adding another bottle. One reason veins are preferred over arteries for IV administration is because flow will pass through right ventricle and lungs before passing through body. Air bubbles can leave blood through lungs.
- ***Electrolyte imbalance***: Administering too dilute or too concentrated a solution can disrupt patient's sodium, potassium, magnesium and other electrolytes. Patients admitted in hospital, given IV fluids are usually monitored with serum electrolyte levels and the infusion adjusted accordingly.

TYPES OF IV CATHETERS

- ***A hypodermic needle***: Here, the hollow of the needle is passed directly through the skin into the vein and the needle is directly connected to the IV line. It is cheap and easily available. The main problem is dislodgement and infiltration of fluid into the skin as the needle does not have a grip.
- ***Butterfly needle (Scalp vein)***: It has a stainless steel needle to which plastic wings are attached. The wings are tapped to the skin which prevents movement of the needle.
- ***The Intra-cath (Over-the-needle catheter)***: Here, there is a flexible catheter over a hollow, stainless steel needle. The needle and catheter are inserted in the vein and the needle removed leaving the catheter in place. This remains smugly in the vein without causing infiltration for a number of days.

TYPES OF IV FLUIDS THAT CAN BE GIVEN IN YOUR CLINIC

IV fluids come in many different forms and act differently in different situations in the body. Depending on the indication for the IV therapy, the type of fluid to be administered is to be selected. Some IV fluids are designed to stay in the intravascular space, increase the blood volume and therefore increase the fallen blood pressure. Other IV fluids are designed so that the fluid leaves the intravascular space and diffuses into the surrounding space. Still others are created to distribute equally between intra and extravascular spaces. Accordingly, IV fluids come in two different forms:

1) Colloid solutions;
2) Crystalloid solutions.

1. Colloid Solutions

These are solutions which are solutes in the form of large proteins which cannot pass through the walls of the capillaries. They remain in the blood vessels for long periods, increasing the blood volume and blood pressure. Their usefulness in an outpatient clinic is limited as they are expensive, have short shelf life and have specific storage requirements. Hence, they are more useful in a hospital setting. Examples of colloid solutions are Haemaccel or Plasmion.

2. Crystalloid Solutions

Of the different types of solutions used in outpatient clinic, crystalloids are the most frequently used fluids. They contain electrolytes (e.g., sodium, potassium, calcium and chlorides) but not the large proteins provided in colloids. Crystalloid IV solutions contain small molecules that flow easily across semi permeable membranes by a process called osmosis. In osmosis, molecules of a solvent tend to pass through a semi permeable membrane, from a less concentrated solution into a more concentrated one. When water moves out of the cell it can lead to shrinking in the size of the cell. When water moves into the cell, it can lead to swelling in the size of the cell.

Crystalloid solutions are either isotonic, hypertonic or hypotonic.

- *Isotonic solution*: When the solution contains the same amount of electrolytes found in the plasma (fluid surrounding the cells), it is referred to as isotonic. When a crystalloid isotonic solution is administered, they do not cause a significant shift of water between the blood stream and extra vascular space as there is no osmosis occurring. Normal saline, Ringer lactate and dextrose are examples of isotonic solution (see **Box 2**).
- *Hypertonic solution*: When the solution contains more amount of electrolytes than found in the plasma, it is referred to as hypertonic. Hypertonic solutions cause shift of water from extracellular space to blood stream because of osmosis. Sodium bicarbonate 8.4%, glucose 10% are examples of hypertonic solution.
- *Hypotonic solution*: When the solution contains fewer amounts of electrolytes than found in the plasma, it is referred to as hypotonic. Hypotonic solutions cause water to shift from blood stream into the surrounding tissues because of osmosis. Dextrose 5% in water (D5W) is an example of an isotonic solution.

INDICATIONS FOR IV THERAPY IN A CLINIC

- To correct dehydration following gastroenteritis or prolonged fever.
- To correct electrolyte disturbances.
- To give intravenous medications, esp. antibiotics.
- To keep vein open (TKVO) for use when a collapsed patient is shifted to a hospital. In such a situation, finding a vein becomes very difficult.

- In a patient of anaphylaxis, to give rapid IV therapy before shifting patient to hospital.
- In case of acute hypersensitivity to injection or oral drugs given in the clinic, to give steroid and antihistaminic drugs.
- To give intravenous iron therapy, e.g., injection Iron-sucrose (Orofer S) in a patient of severe iron deficiency anaemia. Instill 200 mg in 100 mL of normal saline and give over a period of 20–30 min. This can be repeated 2–3 times a week depending on the severity of anaemia.
- Hypoglycaemia where 25% dextrose is life saving
- To give Total Parental Nutrition.

CONTRA INDICATIONS OF FLUID THERAPY

Never administer to patients at risk for increased intracranial pressure as the potential fluid shift may cause cerebral oedema. Avoid in patients with liver disease, congestive heart failure and chronic renal failure.

PREPARING THE IV BAG AND SET

- Wash your hands with soap and water.
- Remove the tube from the plastic wrap and stretch it straight.
- Close the roller clamp.
- Invert the bag and hang it on the stand.
- Remove the cap on the port of the bag. Remove the covering on the spike of the IV tube and insert the spike in the port till it becomes flush with the port. Ensure not to contaminate the port or the spike.
- Squeeze the drip chamber with your fingers and release. Ensure that the chamber is half full with fluid.
- Ensure that there is no air in the tubing as air embolus can be a disastrous complication.

To do this, open the roller clamp and allow the fluid to pass through the tubing into the tray. This will push the air out. If air bubbles are still present in the tube, flick the line at the site of the bubbles with your fingers. The air bubbles will move up into the chamber.

SELECTION OF IV SITE

Time Spent on Selecting a Vein is Time Well Spent

Always first select a vein at distal end of patient's arm. If the IV needle displaces out of the vein, you can use a vein up the extremity. If a vein is selected down the extremity, the IV fluid can leak from the previously punctured site. Select a vein that is well fixed, not "rolling" and one that is fairly straight.

The best veins are on the dorsum of the hand and the forearm. However, avoid veins over a joint such as the cubital fossa and wrist as the needle can be displaced by movements of the joint.

Box 1 Finding a vein: Hints

1. Time spent on selecting a vein is time well spent: Do not hurry.
2. The best veins are on the dorsum of the hand or on the forearm of the non-dominant arm.
3. Always apply a tourniquet 5–6″ above the puncture site. You may use a BP instrument instead.
4. Tap on the vein with spirit swab to distend it.
5. Ask the patient to alternately clench and release the fist to make the vein prominent.
6. It is easy to enter a vein, which can be felt but not seen. It is difficult to puncture a partially collapsed vein, which is seen but not felt. Hence, locate such a vein by palpation.

contd.

7. If you still do not get the vein, release the tourniquet, ask the patient to sit up and hang his arm. This will make the veins fill up with blood & distend.
8. As a last resort, find a vein on the dorsum of the foot.

Avoid puncturing "Y" of a vein, i.e. where veins are bifurcating, as valves are present at these sites. Valves can get permanently damaged by the catheter needle.

Always ensure that it is a vein that you have selected and not an artery. Palpate the vessel selected by you to confirm that there are no pulsations which are felt in an artery and not in a vein. If an artery is punctured, blood will flow up the IV line and cause alarm to the patient and the doctor.

To make the vein prominent, tap on the vein with a spirit swab and ask the patient to alternately clench and release the fist. Also apply a tourniquet 5–6″ above the puncture site. You may use a BP instrument instead.

INSERTION OF CATHETER/NEEDLE

- Disinfect the selected site with a spirit swab.
- Apply the tourniquet above the selected site and ask the patient to clench his fist. This will make the vein prominent.
- Fix the vein by making the skin overlying it taut. This also straightens and reduces the curvature of the vein.
- Insert the needle and catheter in to the vein at an angle of 15–30° to the skin and towards the direction of the heart.
- Ensure that the bevel of the needle is facing upwards for adults and downwards for children and elderly.
- Now advance the needle, puncture the vein and push the needle tip inside the vein for about 2–3 mm.
- Now, lower the angle of the needle to skin to about 15° and push the catheter over the needle in the vein to about 1–2 cm.
- Connect IV tube to the bevel of the needle or end of the catheter.
- Release the tourniquet and check, if the flow has been established.

WHAT IF THE IV FLUID DOES NOT FLOW?

- Make sure that the tourniquet has been removed.
- Ensure that the needle has not been displaced from the vein.
- Check clamp to see if it is open or closed.
- Ensure that there is fluid in the IV bag.
- Make sure that IV line is not kinked in any place or that the patient's body is not on the IV line.
- Occasionally, the needle is not 'out' completely but the needle is at an angle where fluid cannot flow. Adjust the needle at a position so that the fluid is re-established. You might have to keep a small gauze piece under the needle to maintain the flow.
- Raise the bag still higher. Gravity pressure might re-establish the flow. Try compressing the bag.
- If the chamber is full, it is difficult to see if the fluid is flowing. Close the clamp, invert the IV bag, and squeeze the chamber until it is about half empty. Now open the clamp to re-establish the flow.

MONITORING THE IV DRIP

- Periodically check the flow of fluid in the drip chamber. Adjust rate of flow according to indication.

- Check site of needle for infiltration or phlebitis.
- Ensure that the fluid has not run out and that air has not entered the IV line. If so, this has to be removed while changing the bag.
- To change the IV bag, close the roller clamp on the IV line, remove the spike out of the empty bag and pierce the spike in the port of the new bag after removing the cap.
- If there is air in the tube, you have to remove it before it flows into the patient. This can be done by piercing the tube with a small bore needle distal to the air.

HOW TO REMOVE IV SET

- Keep 2 gauge pieces and 2 sticking plasters ready.
- Close down the clamp.
- Remove the sticking plaster stuck on the skin carefully, ensuring that the needle does not come out with the sticking plaster.
- Place the gauze piece on the insertion site, if a hypodermic needle is used; apply gentle pressure and then pull the needle straight out. When removing the needle, in case of an intracath, apply pressure over the catheter (and not at the puncture site) to prevent bleeding.
- Keep the pressure of the gauze piece on the skin till the bleeding stops (about 1 min).
- Place the second gauze piece and apply sticking plaster. Ensure that there is no bleeding.
- Dispose off IV set/IV bag as per guidelines.

FEW IV FLUIDS WHICH CAN BE USED IN YOUR CLINIC

Sodium Chloride 0.9% (NaCl, Physiological solution)

- Isotonic solution of sodium chloride.
- It is called *normal saline solution* because the percentage of sodium chloride dissolved in the solution is similar to the usual concentration of sodium and chloride in the intravascular space.
- Used for fluid replacement in case of dehydration and hypovolaemia.
- It is also used to replace large sodium losses such as in burn injuries and trauma.
- Used topically to clean wounds, eyes, etc.
- As it contains sodium, use with caution in patients with sodium retention like hypertension, heart failure, oedema, renal impairment or any other conditions that cause sodium retention as it may risk fluid volume overload.
- May cause pulmonary oedema, if too rapid infusion is given or if given in excessive amounts.
- Does not contain potassium or lactate. In case of severe dehydration use ringer lactate. If ringer lactate is not available, add 1 ampoule of KCl to a bottle of 5% glucose.
- It does not provide calories.

Glucose or Dextrose 5% (D5W)

- It is an isotonic crystalloid that contains sugar.
- It is useful in supplying energy in the form of sugar. However, the sugar is rapidly consumed and a hypotonic solution remains. This causes shift of water from blood stream to the cells.
- Indicated mainly for administration of Intra venous drugs.
- It should not be used for fluid resuscitation because hyperglycaemia can result.
- Not indicated in treatment of dehydration as it does not contain electrolytes.

Ringer Lactate (RL)

- It is an isotonic crystalloid that contains sodium chloride, potassium chloride, calcium hloride and sodium lactate in sterile water.
- It is the most physiologically adaptable fluid because its electrolyte content is most closely related to the composition of the body's blood serum and plasma. It is designed to be the near-physiological solution of balanced electrolytes.
- Used for correcting severe dehydration, hypovolaemia or correction of mild hypotension.
- Provides appropriate amounts of sodium, potassium, calcium and calcium. It contains lactate which is converted into bicarbonate for correction of metabolic acidosis if it exists.
- It does not provide calories.

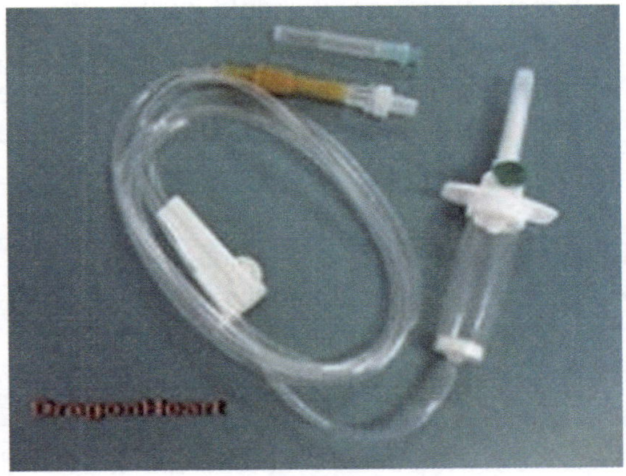

Fig. 37.1 IV set

Glucose 10%

- Hypertonic crystalloid solution.
- Used for emergency treatment of *severe hypoglycaemia.*
- For administration of loading dose of IV quinine to prevent hypoglycaemia.

Sodium Bicarbonate 8.4%

- Hypertonic crystalloid solution.
- Indicated to correct severe *metabolic acidosis.*
- Available as 10 or 20 mL ampoules.
- Contains high concentration of bicarbonate and sodium ions. Its use is rarely justified in case of metabolic acidosis caused by dehydration.

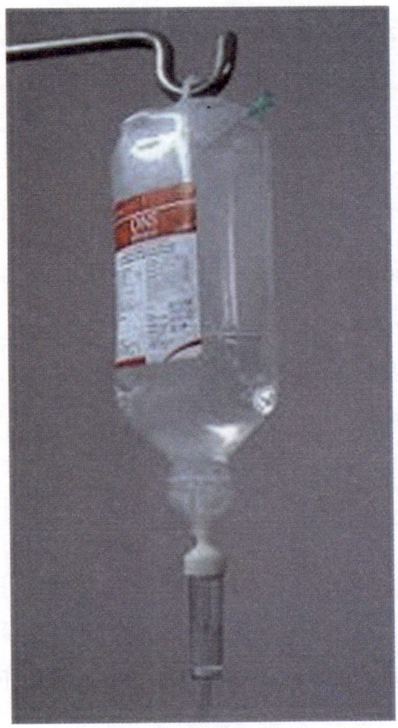

Fig. 37.2 IV bottle

Haemaccel/Plasmion

- Colloidal plasma substitute or expander.
- Used for fluid replacement in *hypovolemic shock* (haemorrhagic, septic).
- May cause allergic reactions, possibly anaphylaxis.
- Contraindicated in pregnancy.
- When a plasma expander is not available, use Ringer lactate (giving 3 times the lost blood amount).
- Lactated Ringer's solution is metabolized in the liver, which converts the lactate to bicar-

bonate, therefore, it should not be given to patients who cannot metabolize lactate (e.g., liver disease, lactic acidosis). It should be used in caution for patients with heart failure and renal failure.

Ringer's Solution

- Ringer's solution is another isotonic IV solution that has content similar to Lactated Ringer's Solution but does not contain lactate.
- Indications are the same for Lactated Ringer's but without the contraindications related to lactate.

| **Box 2** Chatacteristics of types of IV fluids |

Characteristic	Type of fluid
Most physiological	Ringer lactate (RL)
Rich in sodium	Isotonic saline, DNS
Rich in cholorides	Isotonic saline, DNS, Isolyte G
Rich in potassium	Isolyte M,P,G
Corrects acidosis	Ringer lactate , Isolyte E, P, M
Correct alkolosis	Isolyte G
Cautious use in renal failure	RL, Isolyte M, G, P, E
Free of glucose	Isotonic saline, RL
Free of sodium	Dextrose
Free of potassium	Isotonic saline, DNS, Dextrose fluid

SIMPLIFIED WAY OF CALCULATING THE AMOUNT OF FLUID TO BE GIVEN

"**Sensible loss**" is loss that can be perceived by the senses and can be measured and **insensible fluid** loss is the amount of body fluid lost daily that is not easily measured, from the respiratory system, skin, and water in the excreted stool. The exact amount is immeasurable but is estimated to be between 400 and 800 mL/day (about 700 mL) in the average adult.

Daily Fluid Requirement

- Urine output about 1.5–2 L (more in summer/less in winter) plus
- Loss by skin (500 mL) lungs (400 mL) stools (100 mL) = 1000 mL minus
- Amount of fluid produced by oxidation from glucose = 300 mL

Add for Abnormal Fluid Loss

- Mod fever with moderate sweating: 500 mL
- High fever with sweating: 1–1.5 L
- Burns: 500–3000 mL
- Diarrhoea: 100–200 mL/loose motion
- Vomiting: 100–200 mL/episode

Please remember: Oral route is always preferred over intravenous route when oral route is feasible.

CHAPTER 38

Instruments for Minor Surgery

- Instruments
- Suture Materials

INSTRUMENTS

The following instruments (Fig. 38.1) are required to be kept ready at hand for the operations described in this book. Be sure you buy good quality instruments. The cost of the whole minor surgery instruments should not exceed Rs. 1000/-, which should be recoverable from 2 or 3 minor operations. Buying cheap inferior quality instruments is a bad economy, as the instruments then do not last long.

Big and blunt *scissors* is required routinely in all minor procedures. Small pointed scissors are required for delicate surgery. Select only a Bard Parker No.3 scalpel *handle*. Along with this handle ***scalpel blades*** no. 10, 11 and 15 are a good combination for a variety of procedures. The no.10 blade is used to take a large incision, as it has a large cutting edge. The no.11 blade is used to stab abscesses, as it has a sharp pointed tip. The no.15 blade is useful in all minor surgeries because of its small curved cutting edge.

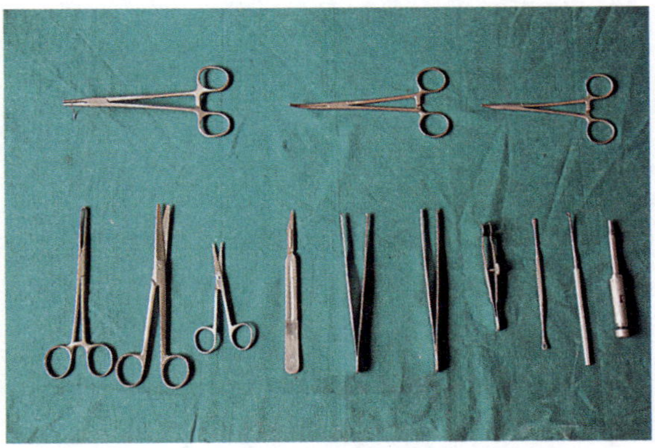

1. Needle holder with needle; 2. Artery forceps; 3. Mosquito forceps; 4. Allis forceps; 5. Scissors – big, blunt; 6. Scissors – small, pointed; 7. Scalpel handle with blade; 8. Toothed forceps; 9. Blunt forceps; 10. Chalazion forceps; 11. Chalazion spoon; 12. Biopsy punch

| Fig. 38.1 Instruments for minor surgery |

Fine toothed and non-toothed ***forceps*** are used for most of the procedures described here. Medium non-toothed forceps are used to hold cotton for skin preparation before surgery.

- Two scissors
  - One big and blunt.
  - One small and pointed.
- One scalpel handle size no. 3
- Scalpel blades no. 10, 11 and 15.
- Forceps
  - Fine (toothed and non-toothed).
  - Medium (toothed and non-toothed)
  - Mosquito
  - Large artery forceps
- Sutures
  - Absorbable: 3/0 Plain catgut, Vicryl
  - Non-absorbable
    - 5/0 and 3/0 Nylon, Prolene.
    - 3/0 and 4/0 Mersilk.
    - Linen No. 60
- Needle holder and needles
- Allis tissue holding forceps
- Chalazion forceps and spoons
- Curette
- Sinus forceps
- Splinter forceps
- Blunt probe
- Double ended retractor
- Biopsy punch
- Gabriel syringe
- Rubber-band applicator

Medium toothed forceps are used during suturing of large incisions. A large artery forceps (or clip) can be used for a variety of purposes like removing a thickened toe nail, holding a tourniquet, as a needle holder or as a dressing forceps. Mosquito forceps are tiny forceps used to catch bleeders, e.g., during circumcision.

Needle holders have serrated jaws and a ratchet lock and are used to grip the needle lightly. A medium sized needle holder is sufficient for minor procedures. *Needles* are either straight or curved. Straight needles can be used for suturing skin, though curved needles are usually preferred. They may have triangular bodies with cutting edges or are round bodied. Only cutting types should be used on the skin.

Allis tissue holding forceps is conveniently used during vasectomy for holding the vas, the *curette* for scraping the abscess cavity and the *chalazion forceps* for holding the Meibomian cyst in place.

The ***sinus forceps*** is useful for packing abscess cavities after drainage, the *splinter forceps* for removing splinters, a *blunt probe* for exploring a pilonidal sinus and *retractors* to get a clear view of deeper structures during dissection. A punch biopsy is extremely useful to simplify a skin biopsy procedure.

A ***Gabriel syringe*** or a ***rubber band applicator gun*** is to be stocked by a GP interested in managing 1st and 2nd degree piles.

Phenol can be easily obtained from a chemical shop (not a chemist shop). It is readily available as crystals (95%). On request this can be supplied diluted to 80% (for warts, ganglion, pilonidal sinus or in-growing toe nail) or 10% (for treatment of hydrocele) or 5% (for piles).

The 95% concentrated phenol can also be diluted in your own clinic by plain water.

SUTURE MATERIALS

These are of two types:

1. Absorbable, e.g., catgut and vicryl; and
2. Non-absorbable, e.g., cotton thread, silk, nylon, prolene, etc.

Absorbable Sutures

1. *Catgut* is made from the gut of the goat (not from the cat). Since plain catgut is absorbed in the tissue in less than 5 days, it is therefore hardened by chromic acid, which then remains in the tissue for more than 3 weeks. They are sterilized and supplied in sealed foils, ready for use instantly. The numbering of the catgut is done according to its thickness.

The extra-fine 5/0 or 6/0 size is used for delicate ophthalmic operations. The thick 1/0 size is used to tie firm structures like muscles. For minor surgeries done by a general practitioner, 3/0 catgut is ideal. Catgut is used for suturing mucous membrane, e.g., suturing a wound inside the lips or for circumcision or for subcutaneous sutures. They dissolve spontaneously.

2. *Vicryl* is a synthetic absorbable suture. It is a costly but superior option to catgut, as it provokes a very mild tissue reaction.

Non-Absorbable Sutures

These are used for skin closures and are to be removed after a variable period of about one-week.

1. ***Cotton or Linen thread*** (No. 60) is very popular amongst GPs, because it is cheap and can be easily sterilized by boiling.
2. ***Silk*** (e.g., Mersilk) is obtained from the cocoon of the silkworm and has good strength and knot tying properties.
3. ***Nylon*** (e.g., Ethilon) is a synthetic non-absorbable material, which produces little tissue reaction.
4. ***Prolene*** is also a synthetic non-absorbable material and is superior but costlier than nylon. It produces the least tissue reaction.

Although there is a large choice of sutures available, for the majority of minor surgical procedures expected to be done by a GP, only a few need to be stocked. For example, 5/0 and 3/0 nylon sutures and linen no.60 are sufficient for skin sutures. 3/0 Plain catgut is perfectly sufficient for all subcutaneous or mucous membrane sutures and 4/0 catgut is required for tying bleeders during circumcision surgery. Keeping the costly, luxurious but superior vicryl or prolene sutures will depend on the preference of the operator and the affordability of the patient.

CHAPTER 39

Local Anaesthesia

- Local Anaesthetic Drugs
  - Lignocaine
  - Bupivacaine
  - Adrenaline
- Local Anaesthetic Techniques
  - Surface Anaesthesia
  - Local Infiltration Anaesthesia
  - Regional Anaesthesia

Many minor surgical procedures can be safely performed by using a limited number of local anaesthetics and a few simple anaesthetic techniques in the clinic of the general practitioner. The minor surgeries described later can be done by using these techniques and do not require the facilities of an operation theatre. A few patients however, prefer general anaesthesia because they fear to remain conscious during the period of the operation.

LOCAL ANAESTHETIC DRUGS

The drugs that are commonly used are procaine, lignocaine (either plain or with adrenaline), amethocaine and bupivacaine. Procaine (Novocaine) and amethocaine (Tetracaine) are less potent and are associated with more frequent hypersensitivity reactions than lignocaine and are hence not recommended.

- ***Lignocaine (Xylocaine)***

  It is the most commonly employed anaesthetic agent in general practice. It is stable and can be stored at room temperature. The onset of action is rapid and the duration of action varies between 30 and 60 min depending on the local vascularity and the site. Addition of adrenaline (1 in 2,00,000) prolongs its action for more than 2 hrs. It is available as 2% solution with or without adrenaline. The maximum amount of plain lignocaine permissible in adults is about 20 mL of 2% solution.
- ***Bupivacaine (Marcaine, Sensorcaine)***: It has a more prolonged action and is four times more potent as compared to lignocaine. These properties have made it very popular for spinal anaesthesia and for painless labour. But these properties are of no benefit in minor surgical procedures done at a general practice level.
- ***Adrenaline***: Adrenaline is usually combined with lignocaine to obtain the following advantages:
  - Adrenaline produces local vasoconstriction, so that less amount of lignocaine is

absorbed. The drug therefore remains in the tissues longer, thus prolonging the local anaesthetic effect.

- The combination is particularly useful in highly vascular areas like the face and the scalp, where it gives a dry operative field in 5–10 min.
- By reducing the absorption of lignocaine, the maximal permissible dose will increase to approximately 30–40 mL, though it should not exceed 80 mL because of risk of adrenaline toxicity.

| **Table 39.1** Making local anaesthetics safe |

- Always enquire about H/o allergy to anaesthetic drugs.
- Avoid accidental intravenous injection.
- Do not exceed the toxic dose.
- Use minimal effective dose preferably with adrenaline.
- Do not be in a hurry to repeat the dose in case of failure of anaesthesia. Remember the latent period.
- Use cautiously in the presence of heart disease.
- Select proper site of nerve block. This way, repeated injections will be avoided.
- Watch pulse for bradycardia and face for twitching (early signs of toxicity).

Despite the above advantages, there is one risk though. Because it causes local vasoconstriction, if it is used around end arteries, e.g., around the digit or penis, it can cause gangrene. Although in one such study, the incidence requiring amputation of the part was as low as one case in 1,32,000 cases, there is no justification in using lignocaine with adrenaline in the situations given in Table 39.2. An equally dry operative field in the finger can be produced more safely by plain lignocaine plus a properly applied tourniquet.

In case of accidental injection into the digit, warming the part may increase the blood supply. To prevent such accidents, both plain lignocaine and lignocaine with adrenaline are available in different colour bottles, letterings or labels.

| **Table 39.2** Sites where lignocaine with adrenaline should not be used |

- Digits
- Tip of nose
- Pinna of ear
- Shaft of penis

Reactions to Lignocaine

A fatal anaphylactoid reaction is very rare and most of the so-called reactions to lignocaine are in fact due to large doses used or large amounts gaining access into the circulation. This catastrophe can be avoided by aspirating prior to injecting. Also the needle is kept moving forward or backward constantly while injecting, so that even if the needle enters a blood vessel only a small amount enters the circulation. Lignocaine poisoning produces cardiac depression, in the form of hypotension, bradycardia and heart block. It also produces cerebral stimulation, in the form of excitement followed by convulsions and death.

LOCAL ANAESTHETIC TECHNIQUES

For minor surgical procedures, local anaesthetics can be used either by applying it to the surface of the skin or mucous membrane (surface anaesthesia) or by infiltrating it into the skin (infiltration anaesthesia) or by anaesthetizing a particular part of the body (regional anaesthesia).

Surface Anaesthesia

By this method, anaesthesia is obtained by applying a local anaesthetic to the surface of the skin or mucous membrane. *EMLA skin cream* is now available, which consists of a mixture of lignocaine and prilocaine. Also available is tetralid cream which is a combination of tetracaine and lidocaine. Only a superficial anaesthesia is produced after about 1 hr of application of a thick layer of the cream. Hence, the usefulness for cautery or minor surgical procedures is doubtful. However, *mucous membrane* can be easily anaesthetized in the form of eye–ear drops, throat lozenges or rectal jelly.

For anaesthetizing the nasal mucosa (prior to cautery for the treatment of epistaxis), a ribbon gauze soaked in lignocaine and adrenaline is packed in the nose. 4% Lignocaine solution is available to anaesthetise the cornea or conjunctiva before removal of a foreign body. 5% Lignocaine ointment is available to anaesthetize the oral mucosa.

Local Infiltration Anaesthesia

In this method, the anaesthetic is infiltrated into the tissues to be operated upon. It is suitable for small skin lesions and for suturing small lacerations. Lignocaine with adrenaline is usually preferred for routine surgical procedures, which do not require prolonged anaesthesia. If longer duration of action is required, bupivacaine is used.

First, a small intradermal wheal is raised by injecting a small amount of anaesthetic superficially. The needle is then introduced through this wheal and passed through the subcutaneous tissue along the planned line of incision or laceration. Small amount of the anaesthetic is continuously injected as the needle is advanced to the end point. If the total area is not covered, the needle should be reinserted through a previously anaesthetised area only, in order to minimise the pain.

Certain special situations deserve comment. In case of a *lacerated wound*, the injection can be given from inside the margin of the wound. In the *scalp*, if during infiltration no resistance is felt, the needle is probably below the aponeurosis and not in the subcutaneous tissue. This will result in an incomplete block. In the *palms*, *soles* or *nose* where the skin is tightly bound down, infiltration is difficult. While infiltrating the *dome of an abscess*, a small quantity is given by an insulin syringe very superficially. Blanching is seen as evidence that the correct plane has been infiltrated.

Regional Anaesthesia

The particular region in question can be anaesthetised by a field or a nerve block. In the removal of a sebaceous cyst on the back for example, a *field block* is used, where local anaesthetic is infiltrated on the skin of the back in the area encircling the cyst. In a *nerve block*, the anaesthetic is deposited near the nerve. The area supplied by this nerve will be thus anaesthetized and minor procedures can be performed. There are slight anatomical variations in the localization of the nerves and hence a large volume of the anaesthetic given in a wider area is advised (flooding technique). The injection should never be made into the substance of the nerve. This can be recognized by the occurrence of paraesthesia during infiltration.

- ***Supraorbital nerve block***: The supraorbital nerve emerges from the supraorbital notch, which can be felt at about two fingers breadth from the median plane. 5 mL is injected just above and parallel to the eyebrow at this site. This will anaesthetise the skin of the forehead.
- ***Digital nerve block*** (Figs. 39.1 & 39.2): It is a very useful block and a safe one if not more than 4 mL of *plain lignocaine* (*i.e., without adrenaline*) is injected. Approximately

1 mL is injected subcutaneously on one side of the base of the finger on the dorsal aspect, to block the dorsal digital nerve. The needle is then advanced until it is palpable on the palmar surface and further 1 mL is injected, to block the palmar digital nerve. Similar procedure is repeated on the other side of the base of the finger. The whole finger is thus anaesthetised.

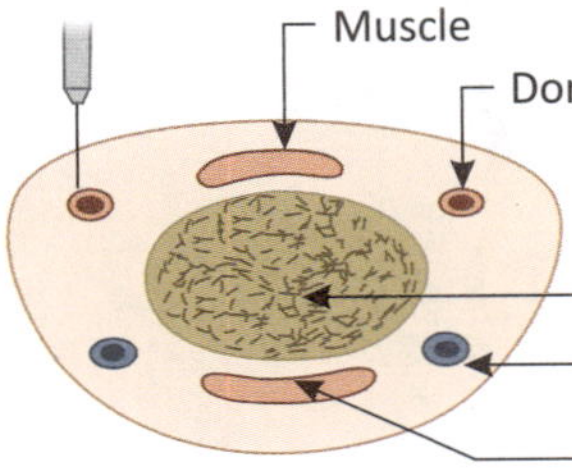

| **Fig. 39.1** Digital nerve block |

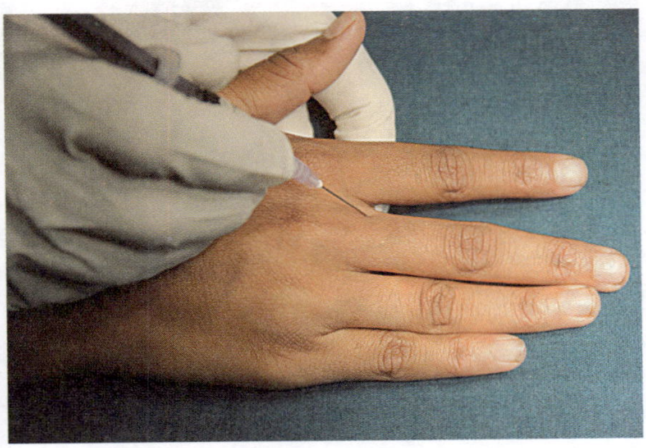

| **Fig. 39.2** Digital nerve block |

- ***Median nerve block***: This nerve lies behind the palmaris longus tendon at the wrist (Fig. 39.3). 5 mL of lignocaine is injected between the two most prominent tendons in the middle of the wrist (palmaris longus and flexor carpi radialis) about 2 cm proximal to the distal wrist crease and at a depth of 1 cm. This will anaesthetize the thumb, index finger, middle finger, half of the ring finger and the corresponding area of the palm (both on the dorsum and the palmar aspect) (Fig. 39.4).

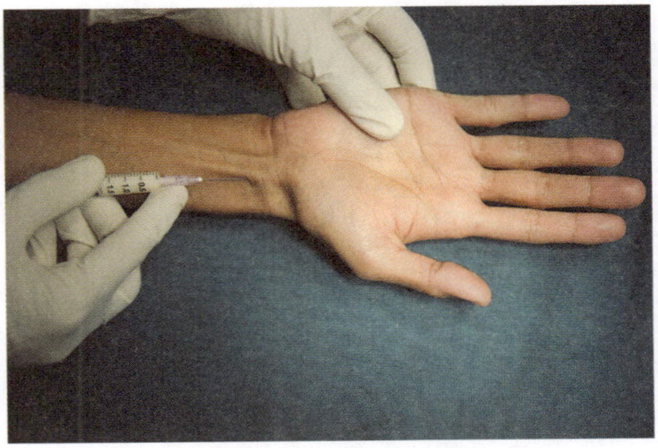

| **Fig. 39.3** Median nerve block |

- ***Ulnar nerve block*** (Fig. 39.5): 5 mL of lignocaine is injected on the radial border of the prominent tendon (flexor carpi ulnaris) seen near the lower end of the ulna at the wrist, at the same level and at the same depth as the median nerve block. This will block the little finger and the medial half of the ring finger. A combined median and ulnar block will anaesthetise the whole hand.
- ***Posterior tibial nerve block***: About 5 mL of lignocaine is injected just anterior to the Achilles tendon at the level of the medial malleolus. This block is useful for dealing with injuries and lesions on the plantar aspect of the foot (Fig. 39.6).
- ***Calcaneal nerve block***: If 5 mL lignocaine is injected as a band into the skin below the level of the medial malleolus, the skin of the heel is anaesthetised. A combined posterior tibial and calcaneal nerve block will anaesthetise the whole sole. This block is useful for removing corns or giving a steroid injection to a tense patient suffering from plantar fasciitis or for suturing lacerations in the plantar skin.

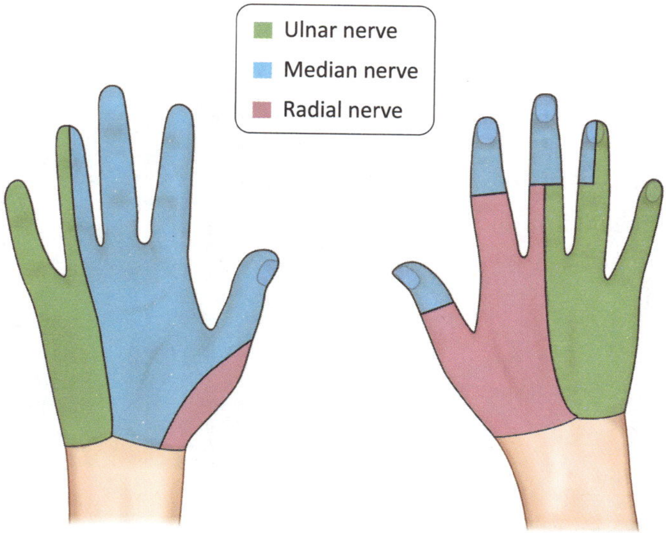

| **Fig. 39.4** Sensory innervation of hand |

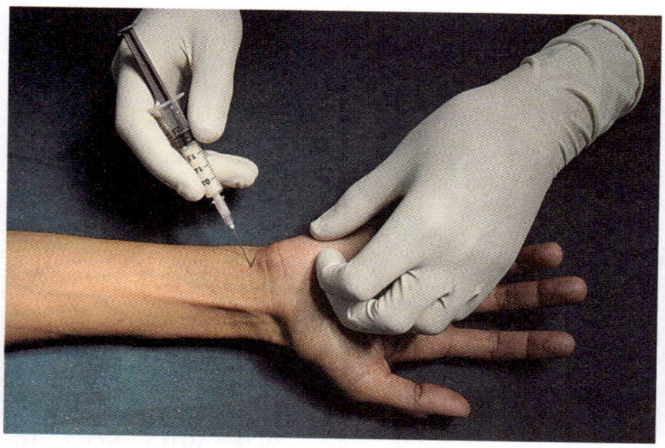

| **Fig. 39.5** Ulnar nerve block |

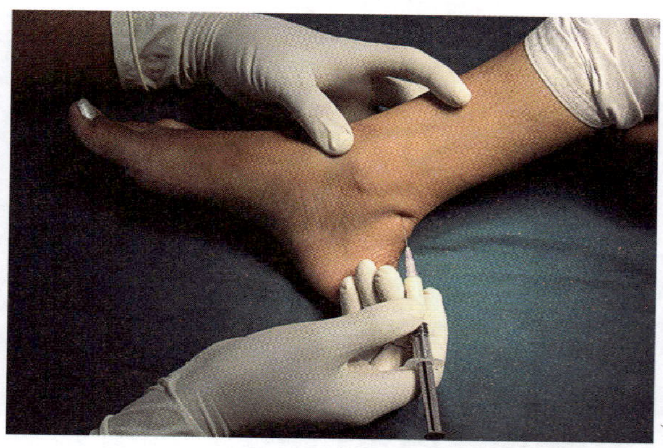

| **Fig. 39.6** Posterior tibial nerve block |

- ***Ankle block***: This block will anaesthetise the whole foot, but this is hardly ever required for minor surgical procedures done by a general practitioner. The sole can be independently anaesthetised as described above. Some such conditions on the dorsum of the foot like a ganglion, can be easily removed by using a field block.
- ***Penile block***: The physician's index finger is placed on the pubic symphysis, the needle and the syringe containing 5 mL of lignocaine is directed past the finger tip at an angle of 15° towards the root of the penis. 2.5 mL is then injected at the root of penis on each side. Additional ½ mL may be required at the frenulum. *Lignocaine with adrenaline should never be used.* A complete ring block is unnecessary, as the nerve enters only along the dorsal aspect. This block is useful for circumcision and for correcting paraphimosis.

CHAPTER 40

Minor Procedures in General Practice

- Catheterization of the Bladder
- Tapping Ascitic Fluid
- IUCD Insertion
- Cervical Pap Smear
- Tapping Pleural Fluid
- Enema
- Cautery
- Electrosurgery
- Gastric Lavage
- Proctoscopy
- Removal of Wax from Ear
- Anterior Rhinoscopy

CATHETERIZATION OF THE BLADDER

Acute retention of the urine is not a dire emergency so that two common complications, i.e., creating a false passage and introducing infection are inexcusable. The second complication can largely be reduced, by using plastic disposable catheters, which are packed in a series of sealed envelopes and are gamma irradiated. There is no handling, as the outer envelope is cut by an assistant and the inner envelope is then opened by the operator. The catheter is then introduced in the urethra from within the envelope without anytime touching it. The first complication can largely be reduced by following the instructions given below.

The patient is made to relax and lie down. After scrubbing the genitalia with 1% chlorhexidine, the anterior urethra is anaesthetised by instilling 2% lignocaine gel inside the urethra. After waiting for 2–3 min for the anaesthesia to act, the penis is wrapped in sterile gauze and pulled vertically upwards by the left hand, to the make urethra straight. The tip of the catheter, lubricated with lignocaine jelly is gently introduced down the urethra. As the bulb of the urethra is reached, the penis is now taken down parallel to the body and the catheter is gently pushed further up into the bladder. Once the catheter enters the bladder, urine flows out of the other end of the catheter.

The procedure, simple as it may sound, may at times be difficult.

1. It can get obstructed somewhere in the mucosal pockets in the urethra. Withdraw slightly and then again proceed further.
2. The catheter stops at the junction of the scrotum and the penis. Thus, is a common site for stricture. Do not use force. Try using a smaller sized catheter.
3. If the catheter stops further down at the external sphincter, the patient is probably tensed causing the sphincter to contract. Reassure the patient, ask him to relax by taking deep breaths, tell him to imagine that he is passing urine, etc. If everything else fails give IV

diazepam 10 mg slowly and the catheter usually slips in.

4. If there is obstruction at the posterior urethra, he probably has an enlarged prostate. Put your finger in the rectum and press it. The catheter can then be manipulated inside the bladder.
5. If the catheter still fails to pass, try a sterile infant feeding tube.

If in spite of the above measures, if the catheter cannot be passed, give up gracefully and don't force. Remember, creating a false passage is inexcusable.

Technique of Suprapubic Puncture

If catheterization of the bladder fails and immediate referral to a hospital is not possible, there is one alternative which can be utilized, viz., drainage by a suprapubic puncture.

After painting the suprapubic region with povidone iodine and spirit, infiltrate 3–4 mL of lignocaine in the pelvic abdominal wall, two fingers above the pubic symphysis in the midline. The urine can now be aspirated with a 20-mL syringe attached to a No.20 needle and a 3-way, entering the bladder vertically. The urgency over, the patient should now be referred to a hospital. This is necessary because when the bladder fills up again, the urine will start leaking into the abdominal cavity through the punctured site. Do not send the patient home. Also the patient has to be investigated for the cause of retention.

Method of Inserting and Removing a Foley's Catheter

In a general practice setting, removal of the catheter probably is more often required than inserting it. This catheter is used for chronic retention of urine when the catheter has to be left in place till definitive measures are taken.

The distal end of the Foley's catheter (Fig. 40.1) has two tubes, one to drain the urine and the other to inject water, so that the balloon at the proximal end will inflate. The proximal end with a single tube is inserted into the bladder through the urethral opening. Once the catheter is inside the bladder, as evidenced by the urine coming out, it is advanced by a few centimetres. 15–20 mL of water is injected through the second tube to inflate the balloon. The catheter is gently pulled so that now the balloon sits snugly on the internal sphincter and the catheter does not slip out. While removing the catheter, the water has to be aspirated through the second tube by a syringe. The balloon deflates and the catheter can be taken out by simple pulling.

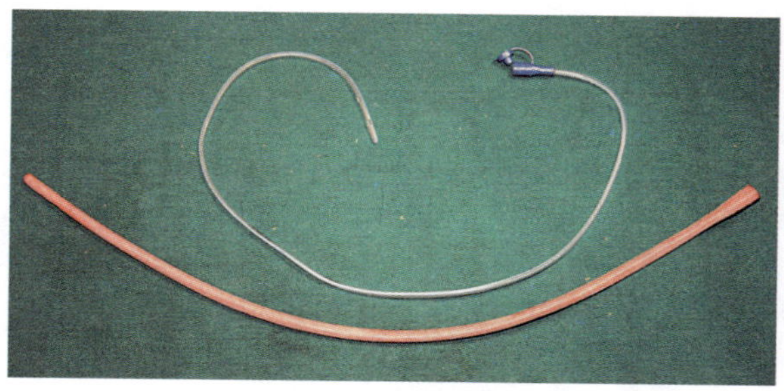

| **Fig. 40.1** **(a)** Infant feeding tube; **(b)** Simple rubber catheter |

TAPPING OF ASCITIC FLUID

Tapping is required for diagnostic purposes, when only a small amount of the fluid needs to be removed. Sometimes however, optimal level of diuretics may fail to relieve the marked abdominal discomfort or breathlessness, when 2–3L of fluid is required to be removed. In most patients, the fluid reaccumulates in a few days and hence the aim should be to remove only that much amount of fluid necessary to alleviate symptoms.

The patient is asked to evacuate the bladder and then lie down comfortably in a supine or semi-reclining position with a backrest. The actual *puncture site* is selected and marked. This is usually on either side of lower abdominal wall, midway between the anterior superior iliac spine and the umbilicus. Another site commonly selected is in the flank midway between the costal margin and the iliac crest.

Lignocaine is then injected through the skin and down to the peritoneum. After waiting for the area to get anaesthetised, an 18-no. bore needle about 3½ inch in length connected to a long rubber tubing, is inserted at the site perpendicular to the abdominal wall.

The ascitic fluid will be seen coming out of the other side of the tube, which can be collected in a bottle. The rubber tube is held in place on the abdominal wall by adhesive tape. Once sufficient fluid is drained, the needle is removed and the site of puncture sealed with tincture benzoin.

'**Abdominal paracentesis**' as it is called, is a very simple procedure, which does not require any sophisticated equipments. It is also a safe procedure and can be done even at the patient's home. A rare complication is fainting, if large amounts (more than 5 L) are removed very rapidly and should be treated by giving rapid IV fluids. Perforation of the bowel loop and peritonitis are very rare complications indeed.

INTRAUTERINE CONTRACEPTIVE DEVICE (IUCD) INSERTION

Types of IUCDs: Many varieties are available but most widely used are copper based 'T' shaped devices available in three different sizes.

Instruments required: IUCD (sterilized) with plunger, Cusco's speculum or Sim's speculum with anterior vaginal wall retractor and 'sound' to measure the uterine height.

Choice of Patient

- Ideally for birth spacing in women having normal menstrual cycles.
- Contraindicated if having any pelvic pathology like fibroids, PID, bicornuate uterus, etc.
- Avoided if there is h/o menorrhagia or dysmenorrhoea.
- Caesarean section is a relative contraindication—IUCD not to be inserted before 3 months.
- To be delayed if there is vaginitis, cervicitis, erosion, etc.

Method

Give the patient lithotomy or left lateral position after assuring an empty bladder. Do bimanual pelvic examination to r/o uterine or ovarian pathology (see above) and for judging uterine size and height.

R/o obvious vaginal or cervical pathology by doing per speculum examination. With the speculum in place, pass a uterine sound to measure the height of the uterus. Choose a proper size IUCD according to the size of the uterus. The introducer of the IUCD is passed through the cervical canal after adjusting the 'stop' of the introducer to the length of the uterus. Don't force the sound or the introducer—it may cause a false tract and hence uterine perforation. The plunger is pressed so that the device uncoils within the uterine cavity. The procedure should be abandoned immediately if the woman has pain. The introducer with the plunger is then removed and threads of the IUCD are cut with scissors. The speculum is removed and the threads are confirmed to be easily palpable in the vagina. The patient is instructed to feel for the threads. The patient should be aware of the shape of the IUCD inserted.

Follow-up after her next menstrual period is a must to confirm the presence of the IUCD.

After that, a visit after 3 months and then yearly is advised.

Possible Complications

Though seemingly a simple procedure, it is not devoid of complications. Intermenstrual spotting, menorrhagia, dysmenorrhoea and intermenstrual pain are fairly common and patient should be warned about them. These symptoms may last for first few cycles. Acute and chronic salphingo-oophritis occurs in 1–2% cases. Perforation of the uterus may occur at the time of insertion or later. It is to be suspected if the threads are not felt in the vagina. USG and X-ray examination will be required to locate the position of the device in the peritoneal cavity. It need not be removed as T-shaped open devices are not likely to cause intestinal obstruction. Spontaneous extrusion of IUCD in 1st year of insertion is seen in 2–10% of cases. Pregnancy in spite of the presence of the device, is observed in 2–5% cases. Fracture of the arms of IUCD can occur if it is left in the uterus for more than the recommended period (2–3 years for copper based and 8–10 years for progesterone-based devices).

CERVICAL PAP (PAPANICOLAOU) SMEAR

Pap smear is a simple procedure that can be done easily in a GP's OPD. The purpose of a cervical smear is not to diagnose cancer of the cervix but to detect premalignant lesions that can be treated in time, before they progress to invasive carcinoma.

When to Advise Pap Smear?

High risk factors for Ca. cervix are multiple pregnancies, early age of first intercourse, multiple sexual partners, HPV infection, HIV infection, smoking and OC pills. These women should undergo yearly Pap smear examination after the age of 40 years. Others need the same after the age of 45 years.

Instruments

Cusco's or Sim's speculum, Ayre's spatula, spirit and glass slides.

Method

The patient is given a lithotomy position. After P/V examination, closed Cusco's speculum is inserted in the vagina fully. The blades are then gently opened to expose the cervix. The Ayre's spatula is then inserted into the os and it is turned through 360° with gentle pressure on cervix. The sample on the spatula is now applied on glass slides as thin layers. The fixing of the slides is done by immersing them in spirit for an hour. After drying, these are sent to the pathological laboratory experienced in doing Pap smear examination.

The following details of the patient are sent along with the slide to the laboratory.

- *Name of the patient*
- *Age*
- *LMP*
- *Condition*:
  - Pregnant—yes/no;
  - Postnatal—yes/no;
  - IUCD fitted—yes/no;
  - On OC pills—yes/no.

Results

These are classified into 5 groups from normal to that of positive for malignancy. Further investigations and management depend on this cytological report. But it should be remembered that 8–10% results can be false negative, so regular repeat testing is advised.

TAPPING OF PLEURAL FLUID

See Chapter 23.

ENEMA

The term enema is used to refer to the process of instilling fluid through the anal sphincter into the rectum and lower intestine for a therapeutic purpose. Occasionally, the general practitioner is called upon to give enema to one of his patients. The usual situation is either an old man who is bed ridden and therefore is constipated or a post-operative patient who has been discharged from the hospital and gets constipation or faecal impaction. There are other indications for giving enema in medical practice like cleaning the bowel before a procedure such as sigmoidoscopy/colonoscopy, or giving a contrast substance for radiological imaging of the lower bowel, or giving intrarectal medications. However, the general practitioner is hardly ever called upon to give enema in such a situation.

The patient is usually embarrassed, if this is the first time an enema is being administered to him.

You should respect his modesty throughout the procedure. Words of encouragement to the patient during the administration of the enema will be of great benefit for a positive outcome of the procedure.

An enema administration is performed using a flexible plastic rectal tube with several large holes in the tip. This is connected to the tubing from a solution bag or container. An enema can also be performed using a prepackaged solution that comes in a soft plastic bottle with a rectal tip attached. Enema solutions are prepared using plain tap water, saline, soap solutions or oil solutions.

Precautions

Enemas should not be used as a first-line treatment for constipation. Always give a fair trial to medicines to relieve constipation before using enema. Frequent use of enemas can lead to fluid overload, bowel irritation and loss of muscle tone of the bowel and anal sphincter. Never deliver more than three consecutive enemas to treat a patient.

Enema administration must be used with caution in *cardiac patients* who have arrhythmias or have had a recent myocardial infarction. Insertion of the enema tube and solution can stimulate the vagus nerve which may trigger an arrhythmia such as bradycardia. Enemas should not be given to patients with *undiagnosed abdominal pain* because the peristalsis of the bowel can cause an inflamed appendix to rupture or perforate a bowel in intestinal obstruction. Enemas should be used cautiously in patients who have had *recent surgery* on the rectum, bowel or prostate gland. Do not force the enema catheter into the rectum against resistance. This can cause trauma to the rectal tissue. Use only mild soap for soap enemas.

There are various types of enemas available, the common ones being the ready to use enemas like Neotonic Enema, the traditional soap water enema and the glycerin enema. The procedure for administering them is described below.

Readymade Enema (like Neotonic Enema)

These are very convenient as they can be prescribed and the patient can administer the enema himself, which saves the general practitioner a visit to the patient's home. The patient should be given proper instructions as to its proper method of use. Instruct the patient to first open the lid, lubricate the tip with Vaseline and then introduce the whole contents from the plastic bag deep into the rectum.

The enema solution should be introduced lying in bed in the left lateral position and when the whole contents have been instilled, the patient can go to the toilet or is given a bed pan.

Soap Water Enema

- ***Anal lubrication***: The patient's anal area needs lubrication to ease insertion of the nozzle of the tube. A gloved finger is excellent for this purpose. It allows easier entrance to the rectum. Apply a liberal amount of Vaseline to your finger tip and to the outside of the patient's anus. Next, press the tip of your finger into the centre of the patient's anus. Applying constant pressure for several seconds will usually allow the anus to relax allowing you to insert a lubricated finger. Apply lubricant liberally around and inside the anus and into the rectum.
- ***Suspend the enema bag*** on an IV stand about 1 foot to 18 inches above the anus. Suspending an enema container higher than 18 in. produces a faster flow and will increase the chance of cramping. Always open clamp and allow any air to escape tubing before inserting the nozzle or rectal tube.
- ***Inserting the nozzle/rectal tube***: The nozzle should slide in easily, if proper and sustained pressure is applied. Never force an enema nozzle into the rectum.
- ***Next open the clamp slowly***: Don't try to give the entire amount of solution at once. It can take as much as 15 min to administer the whole enema. If the recipient has a full colon he may not be able to take the full amount of solution at one time. Ask him to evacuate and then refill the container and administer another enema.
- If the fluid will not flow in, gently rotate the tubing within the rectum to clear the holes of the tubing from the wall of the bowel or the impacted stool that may be occluding the flow.
- ***Watch for signs of cramping***: If this occurs you should slow or stop the flow until the patient can relax.
- Request the patient to ***massage his abdomen*** in anti-clockwise direction. This will help move the solution higher into the colon. Start on the lower left side and slowly and deeply massage up and across just below the ribs and down the right side.
- Encourage the recipient to ***retain the enema*** solution for 5 or 10 min before evacuating to achieve good results. If he finds it difficult, he can press a wet towel against his anus. Ask the patient to breathe only through the mouth while retaining the enema solution.
- ***When expelling the enema***, massage abdomen in a clockwise direction. This will help move the solution back towards the rectum and anus. The best position for evacuation is squatting over the toilet like in Indian toilet and not sitting down on it like in a western commode. The squatting position puts pressure on the abdomen from the thighs and brings about an easier bowel evacuation.

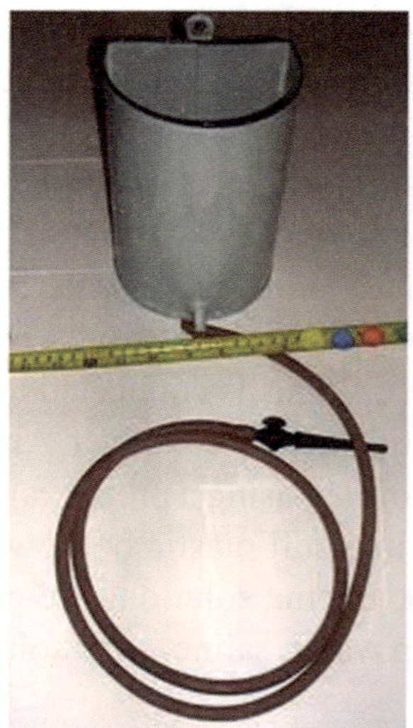

| **Fig. 40.2** Soap water enema instruments |

Glycerin Syringe Enema

Instead of soap water, glycerin is used which lubricates the faeces. This helps in gently expelling the faeces without causing contractions and cramps in the abdomen. About 30 mL of glycerin is poured in the funnel which is connected to the enema catheter put in the rectum.

After the evacuation is complete, watch the expression of the patient. You will see a sigh of relief, a sense of satisfaction and a feeling of euphoria on the face of your patient! And the patient will ever be so thankful!

CHEMICAL CAUTERY

Many general practitioners do not own an electrosurgery machine. Using acids or cytotoxic drugs to burn of these lesions is a good alternative available to them. To chemically cauterize warts, many chemicals are available. For lesions on the skin, the most common agents used are trichloroacetic acid and salicylic acid paint, while the most common cytotoxic agent used to cauterize lesions on the mucous membrane is podophyllin.

Trichloroacetic Acid

Trichloroacetic acid (TCI) (50–60%) can be used to treat superficial skin lesions like warts, molluscum contagiosum, xanthelesma, solar lentigo, etc., on the skin. TCI which is highly corrosive, can cause burns if spilled over to the normal skin. Hence before applying TCI, the normal skin surrounding the lesion to be cauterized should be covered by white petroleum jelly. An accidental spill on to the normal skin can be neutralized by a crushed sodium bicarbonate tablet.

In case of warts, epidermal naevi, skin tags, xanthelesma, etc., TCI should be applied to the lesion with the tip of a match stick. In case of mollusum contagiosum, it is essential to cauterize the molluscum body which lies *inside* each individual lesion. This should be done with a sharp tip of a diamond shaped needle. The molluscum body is pierced and the needle rotated. If this needle is not available, a hypodermic needle can be used instead.

Salicylic Acid Paint (Salactin)

Paints are available as salicylic acid and lactic acid in flexible collodium. The flexible collodium keeps the acids in place avoiding spilling over onto the normal skin. It should be applied to the wart accurately usually with a plastic applicator provided.

Podophyllin

Podophyllin is a cytotoxic drug which destroys cells by arresting mitosis. It is mainly used to treat genital warts on the mucous membrane of the glans of the penis or the vaginal mucous membrane. It should not be used in pregnancy as it can get absorbed and cause abortion. It is available as 'podowart' solution or if not available, can be ordered from a dispensing chemist as 25% podophyllin in tincture benzoin.

After applying white petroleum jelly to the surrounding area (as it is irritant to the normal skin), it is applied to the wart with a cotton swab rolled on to a tip of a match stick, allowed to dry and washed off after 4 hrs. The application can be repeated after 1 week. It is best applied by the doctor himself calling him in the clinic weekly, as the patient may over-apply the solution and blame the doctor for the severe local reaction that the patient gets.

Liquid Nitrogen

This is usually an effective treatment although the application can cause pain. Liquid nitrogen causes an inflammatory response after application for 15 sec. This consists of erythema around the wart and oedema underneath. A painful blister results and the wart usually falls off within 2 weeks as the blister breaks. A single application is usually successful but the application may have to be repeated after 2–3 weeks. Unfortunately liquid nitrogen is not freely available.

ELECTROSURGERY

In this procedure, there is destruction or removal of tissue using electrical energy supplied through a machine. It provides rapid and cost effective treatment for many skin lesions encountered in general practice like warts, molluscum contagiosum, epidermal naevi, skin tags (which are seen around the neck of many obese adults), pyogenic granuloma, xanthelesma, etc. There are now many different electrosurgery machines available in India which can be brought in any surgical store.

Electrosurgery comprises of:

- *Electrocautery*: In electrocautery machines, metal is heated by electric current from a battery. The tip of the unit consists of a wire with a high electrical resistance.

  First, the lesion to be cauterized is anaesthetized by infiltrating local xylocaine. Then current is turned on and the wire starts glowing. The tip of the wire is then touched to the lesion which bubbles and burns. A crust forms, which falls off in a few days.

  Since the heat does not penetrate deeper than the dermis, this method is used to treat superficial lesions like small skin tags or seborrheic keratosis. This method has the advantage that it achieves haemostasis and gives a bloodless field. The disadvantage is that the lesion is destroyed and is not available for histopathological examination.
- *Electrofulguration & Electrodesiccation*: A single machine can be used for electrofulguration and electrodesiccation. If the electrode is held at a slight distance from the lesion, an electrical spark is created causing very superficial destruction to the tissue. This is called electrofulguration. If the electrode is held in direct contact with the lesion this is called electrodesiccation. These techniques are used to treat small superficial lesions, and require local anaesthesia. It should be remembered that spirit should not be used to clean the lesion prior to surgery as the spark may ignite the area.

The following three modalities are usually not required in general practice.

- In electrocoagulation, the current penetrates deeper causing more tissue destruction and is used in surgery.
- In electrosection, current is used to cut tissue during surgery.
- Electroepilation is used to remove unwanted hair.

Most of the lesions mentioned above can be destroyed by either electrocautery or by a combination of electrofulguration or electrodesiccation.

If the lesion is solitary or only 3–4 lesions are present, the base of the lesion/s should be infiltrated by 2% xylocaine with or without adrenaline depending on the location. Xylocaine *with adrenaline* should not be used on the tip of the nose, fingers and penis. For small lesions, insulin syringe can be conveniently used. If there are many lesions as it often occurs in molluscum contagiosum infection, it is very inconvenient to give local anaesthesia to each and every lesion. The lesions can be anaesthetized alternatively by applying topical anaesthesia which is available as a combination of tetracaine and lidocaine

(Tetralid ointment). This has to be applied to the lesions and kept for at least 30 min for adequate anaesthesia. General anaesthesia is hardly ever required.

The steel pad supplied by the manufacturer along with the machine is placed in contact with the patient's skin after applying jelly to it. The tip of the electrodes is available in different shapes and can be used judiciously as per convenience. Once the procedure is completed, large lesions can be dressed up while for smaller lesions an antibiotic ointment can be prescribed. Healing usually occurs in a few days.

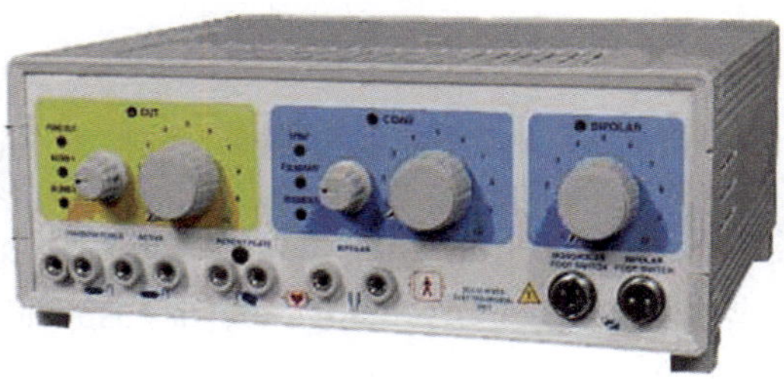

| **Fig. 40.3** Electrosurgery machine |

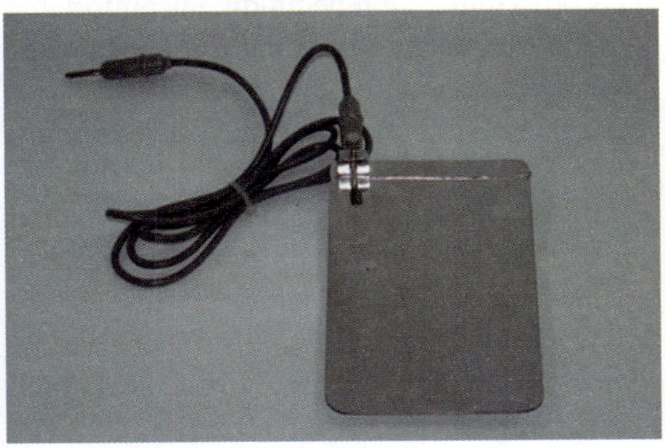

| **Fig. 40.4** Pad to be kept with patient's skin for earthing |

GASTRIC LAVAGE

The general practitioner may be called upon to perform this procedure mainly in rural areas to give stomach wash in case of poisoning, before facilities to shift the patient to a hospital are made available. Another situation is when the general practitioner may be called upon to put in the naso-gastric tube (Ryle's tube) in case of a semi-conscious terminally ill patient as a palliative measure.

Method

The procedure involves the passing of Ryle's tube into the stomach through the nostril.

- The patient should be sitting upright.
- Select the proper size of the Ryle's tube depending on the indication. In case of gastric lavage done for removal of poison from the stomach, a large size like numbers 22 or 24 is selected so that the poison is removed rapidly. For feeding purpose, number 16 should suffice.
- First examine both the nostrils of the patient to identify the roomier nostril. Lubricate this nostril with xylocaine jelly.
- Apply xylocaine jelly to the tip of the tube and pass into the nostril. Push it along the floor of the nostril till it reaches the posterior pharyngeal wall.
- There will be some resistance felt when the tip of the tube reaches the posterior pharyngeal wall. Push the tube further gently for about 1″ more when it will come to lie at the upper end of the oesophagus. If there is excessive gagging, the tube may have curled up in the throat which can be seen by a torch through the mouth. If so, withdraw and restart the procedure.
- If the patient coughs violently, the tip may have entered the trachea. Remove the tube, wait for the cough to stop, soothe the patient, give the patient xylocaine to swallow and reintroduce the tube after 5–10 min.
- Once the tube reaches the upper end of the oesophagus, ask the patient to swallow. The

larynx (Adam's apple) will move up. With the larynx in this position, push the tube into the oesophagus. Now, it will pass down the oesophagus without resistance.

- Advance the tube into the stomach till the first black mark on the tube.
- Confirm that the tube is in the stomach by aspirating with a 20-cc syringe (when stomach contents will be aspirated), and by pushing 10–20 cc of air through the outer end of the tube and listening to the bubbling sound in the epigastrium with the stethoscope.
- Fix the outer end of the tube to the nostril by an adhesive tape.
- To give gastric lavage in case of poisoning, push clear water by means of a 20-cc or 50-cc syringe rapidly and aspirate, collect the first sample and send to the laboratory for examination. Continue this procedure till the fluid aspirated is clear.
- In case this procedure is done to feed a patient, liquid feeds like milk, curds, electrolytes, water, soups, fruit juices, can be pushed every 2–3 hrs. Before pushing every time, aspirate to confirm that the previous feeds have passed into the intestine. End each feed by flushing the tube with water to prevent blocking of the tube.

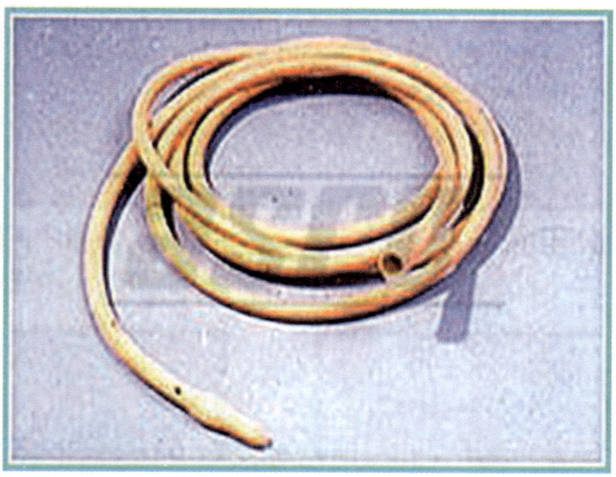

| **Fig. 40.5** Ryle's tube |

PROCTOSCOPY

Proctoscopy is a common medical procedure in which an instrument called a proctoscope is used to examine the anal cavity, rectum or sigmoid colon. A proctoscope is a short, straight, rigid, hollow metal tube, in which an obturator can be passed. It usually has a small light bulb mounted at the end. It is approximately 15 cm long. The proctoscope also has a hollow channel through which other instruments may be inserted. For example, another instrument may be inserted to take a biopsy of a small amount of tissue for examination under a microscope.

Indications

- Examination of the anal canal and the rectum to inspect for suspected haemorrhoids or rectal polyps or malignancy.
- Biopsy of a lesion if malignancy is suspected.

Procedure

This procedure might be mildly uncomfortable as the proctoscope is inserted further into the rectum. Modern fibre-optic proctoscopes allow more extensive observation with less discomfort. Disposable proctoscopes are also available.

- Place the patient in the left lateral position with the knees drawn up and the buttocks at the edge of the examination table.
- Warn the patient that an instrument will be passed into his anal canal by the doctor and this might cause some discomfort.
- Lubricate the instrument with white petroleum jelly.
- Slide the instrument into the anus with a steady pressure directed towards the symphysis pubis.
- Remove the obturator which then allows an unobstructed view of the interior of the rectal cavity.

- Examine the anal canal and the rectum with a torch or any other source as you gradually withdraw the proctoscope while asking the patient to bear down on the anus.

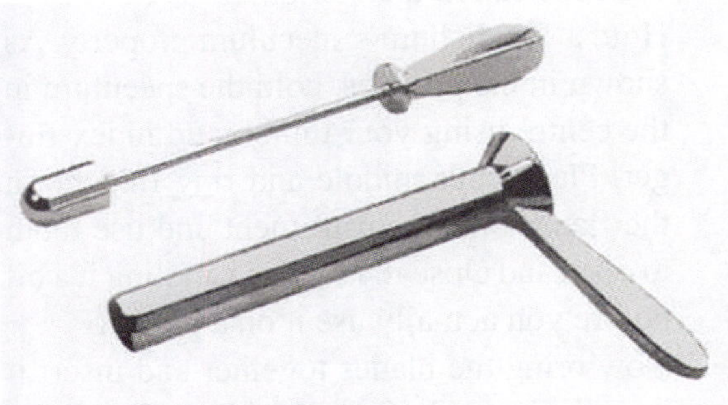

| **Fig. 40.6** Proctoscope with obturator |

REMOVAL OF WAX FROM EAR

Wax or cerumen is normally formed in the external auditory canal. When small in amount, it does not cause any symptoms. When excessive in amount and impacted, it can cause pain, tinnitus and hearing loss. The presence of wax in the auditory canal is diagnosed by direct visualization with an otoscope. Foreign bodies and otitis media should be ruled out before wax removal. Removal has been associated with complications including pain, otitis externa, dizziness, syncope, tinnitus, tympanic membrane perforation and even cardiac arrest.

Wax removal may be attempted by either manual removal by using a curette or a loop, or by irrigation of external auditory canal with lukewarm water.

Manual Removal by a Loop or a Curette

It is quicker, can be done under direct vision and does not expose the canal to moisture and therefore may lessen the risk of infection. In the ENT consultation room, it can be done under a microscope, which gives much safety and comfort. A cooperative patient and the skill of the clinician are more important than a particular method of removal. The hook is passed beyond the wax and the wax is pulled out by gentle but firm traction along the canal.

Irrigation with an Ear Syringe

If the wax is hard, prior use of wax softeners for 1–2 weeks to soften the wax always helps.

Ear syringes are inexpensive and readily available but some can be large, cumbersome, difficult to balance in hand, and can cause minor trauma to external auditory canal or tympanic membrane. To prevent a vasovagal syncope, the water should be at body temperature. Put towel on the shoulder of the patient. Ask an assistant to hold a bowl or a kidney tray below the ear of the patient for the water to flow into.

Now, apply gentle traction to the pinna in the upwards and backwards direction to straighten the canal. A jet of lukewarm water should then be directed towards the superior and posterior wall of the canal by the ear syringe. In case of impacted wax, a chink is made along the posterior wall of the meatus behind the wax. Water is now directed in the chink so that it enters behind the wax and pushes it out.

The clinician after the removal of the wax should always discuss with the patient the causes of wax formation, their normal protective role, and the dangers of using cotton buds or match sticks to remove wax.

Refer the patient to an ENT specialist, if:

- Removal fails
- Severe pain is present and if
- Vertigo develops during irrigation even with lukewarm water, as this could be perilymphatic fistula or perforation of oval window.

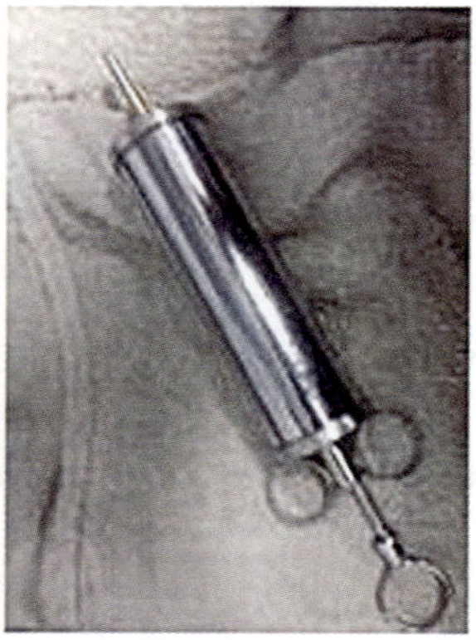

| Fig. 40.7 Ear syringe |

ANTERIOR RHINOSCOPY

Examination of the nasal cavity using a speculum is called 'anterior' rhinoscopy because you look into the nose from anterior, through the nostrils (*rhino* – nose and *scopy* – to see). Also, 'anterior' as against 'posterior' rhinoscopy which consists of examining the nose from behind, through the nasopharynx. It uses a nasal speculum—a Thudichum's or a Killian's nasal speculum, which is an inverted 'U' shaped instrument (Fig. 40.8). It has two blades at the lower end.

Procedure

- Lift up the tip of the patient's nose with your thumb. This allows you to examine the skin-lined, hair-bearing part of the nasal cavity which is called the *vestibule.*
- Hold a Thudichum's speculum properly. As shown in the pictures, hold the speculum in the centre using your thumb and index finger. Place your middle and ring fingers on the flanges of the instrument and use them to open and close it. Practise handling it a bit before you actually use it on a patient.
- Now bring the blades together and insert it into the nostril. Once inside, release the blades slowly. As they widen, you will be able to see all the structures inside the nasal cavity (see below). In a normal subject you will see:
  - Medial aspect: The nasal septum
  - Lateral wall: Inferior and middle turbinates/inferior and middle meati
  - Floor of the nasal cavity.
  - The roof of the nasal cavity cannot be seen unless there is severe atrophy as in atrophic rhinitis.
- Repeat the procedure on the other side.

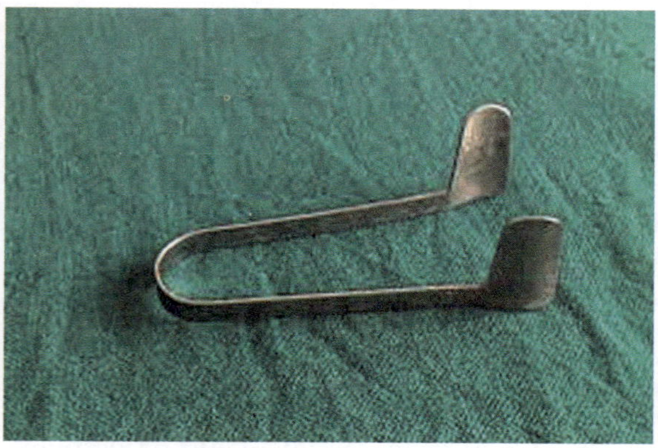

| Fig. 40.8 Thudichum's speculum |

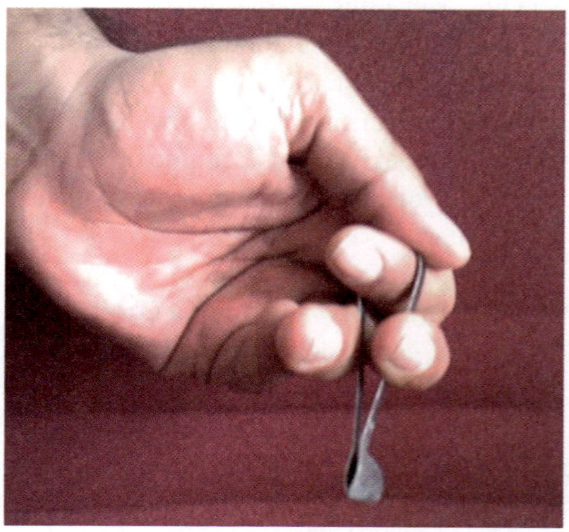

| Fig. 40.9 Method of holding speculum |

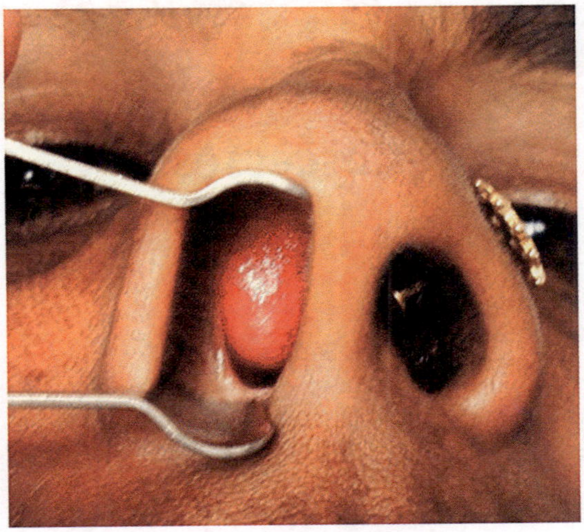

| **Fig. 40.10** A polyp seen with help of nasal speculum |

CHAPTER 41

Abscesses

- Anaesthesia
- Boil
- Acute Paronychia
- Pulp Space Abscess
- Stye
- Infected Sebaceous Cyst
- Carbuncle
- Tooth Abscess
- Breast Abscess
- Perianal & Ischiorectal Abscess
- Axillary Abscess
- Inguinal Bubo
- Abscess of Neck
- Injection Abscess
- Difficult Abscesses

Infections of the soft tissue (cellulitis) may proceed to the formation of an abscess, when the surgical management is incision and drainage. In the early stages, if proper antibiotics are instituted, the process may be aborted and suppuration does not occur. Incision during the stage of active cellulitis is highly mischievous. It is a mistake to incise too early. The presence of pus can be detected clinically by eliciting fluctuations. Fluctuations however may be absent in abscesses which are deep seated, e.g., breast abscess or ischiorectal abscess. In these situations, the diagnosis of a '*formed abscess*' is made by the patient's complaint of a change in character of pain—the dull aching pain of cellulitis is replaced by a throbbing pain, causing a sleepless night. In addition, swelling, induration and localized tenderness indicate that the abscess is ripe and that the time is also ripe for incision. In case of doubt, it is safer to aspirate the pus with a wide-bore needle before incising.

Incision and Dainage

The incision and drainage (I & D) is done by a *free incision* or by *de-roofing* or by *Hilton's method.*

Methods

1. ***Free incision*** should be used in cases of superficial abscesses. The incision is made on the point of maximum tenderness. It should be large enough to empty the pus completely. (It is better to over-incise than to under-incise.) Also, it should be made parallel to any important structure to avoid their damage and in the direction of the muscle fibres, if the muscle is to be cut.
2. ***De-roofing*** should be done if the skin overlying a large abscess is necrotic **(Fig. 41.1)**. A large cruciate incision is taken extending on to the periphery of the lesion and the edges of the resulting flaps are excised, e.g., in case of a carbuncle.
3. ***Hilton's method*** should be used, if there are important structures in the neighbourhood of a large abscess, e.g., in the neck, axilla or popliteal fossa. An incision is made into the skin and deep fascia. A sinus forceps is

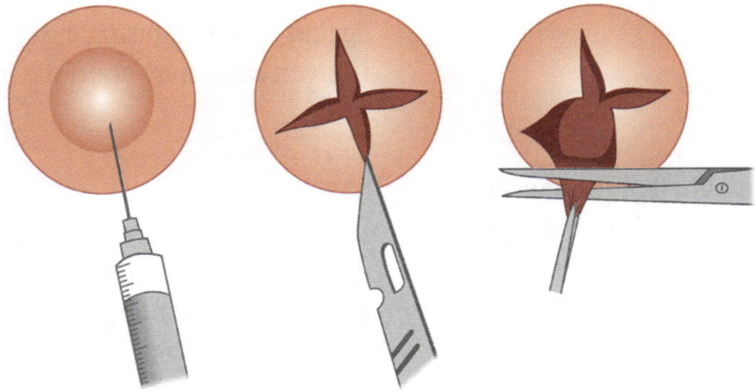

| Fig. 41.1 De-roofing |

passed through the opening in the deep fascia towards the site of the suspected abscess. Once the pus is seen coming out, the blunt sinus forceps is opened to enlarge the opening. Thus, injury to the surrounding tissues by the use of a sharp instrument like the scalpel blade is avoided. A glowed finger is then introduced into the cavity, the loculi are broken and drainage achieved. Once the pus is drained, the bleeding from the granulation tissue is stopped by a tight pack of roller gauze soaked in povidone iodine ointment. The two ends of the roller gauze are kept out of the cavity before dressing so that the whole pack is subsequently taken out and nothing is left inside. The pack is removed after 48 hrs and repeat packing may be done with the roller gauze soaked in xylocaine jelly to minimise pain. No further tight packing is necessary. In fact, a tight pack can prevent the growth of granulation tissue. Hence subsequent packs must be inserted more and more loosely to allow the granulation tissue to fill up the floor of the cavity.

ANAESTHESIA

Deep and large abscesses require general anaesthesia for which the patient should be referred to a hospital. Superficial abscesses like pyoderma can be drained without any anaesthesia by a quick stab with a scalpel at the site where the abscess is pointing. Medium sized abscesses can be drained by a GP in his clinic, using the following local anaesthetic methods.

- ***Ethyl chloride spray*** which numbs the skin by cooling is not very effective and is not used commonly these days.
- ***Dome infiltration***, where a small amount of xylocaine is infiltrated superficially in the overlying skin till blanching is seen, is much more effective. Almost immediately the skin can be punctured with a scalpel blade and the pus drained. Dome infiltration is used where the overlying skin is thin.
- ***A field block*** is used where overlying skin is thick. The normal un-inflamed skin surrounding the abscess is infiltrated with xylocaine. A period of about 5 min is required for the skin over the abscess to get anaesthetized.

Xylocaine should not be infiltrated into an inflamed area as this is extremely painful. Also, the anaesthesia is incomplete and short lasting.

COMMENTS ON ABSCESSES IN DIFFERENT LOCATIONS

BOIL (FURUNCLE)

This staphylococcal infection of the hair follicles, can be simply drained by stabbing the point of maximum fluctuations by a scalpel blade with or without anaesthesia.

ACUTE PARONYCHIA

It is an infection of the area surrounding the nail, usually by *Staphylococci*. It begins as a cellulitis but soon pus forms, which is seen on the lateral side of the nail. Without treatment, the pus may spontaneously discharge outside or may extend beneath the nail, so that a lusterless nail will be felt floating on a pool of a pus. In the stage of cellulitis, cloxacillin or amoxiclav, if given early may abort the infection. Once the pus is formed however, drainage is required, not antibiotics. This is done under digital block anaesthesia. If the pus is present below the nail, it is proper to remove the nail also.

Chronic paronychia is usually due to *Candida albicans*. It is treated conservatively with fluconazole and by keeping the fingers dry and not by incision and drainage. The results in a chronic case are not gratifying.

PULP SPACE ABSCESS (FELON)

The skin over the pulp space is attached to the periosteum by firm fibrotic strands, dividing the space into compartments. Hence, pockets of pus may remain inside after the superficial pus is removed. This may ultimately lead to osteomyelitis. Hence, proper evacuation with the help of a sinus forceps under a digital nerve block is indicated. Incision should be made directly over the abscess. This infection is usually due to *Streptococci* and hence antibiotics effective against these organisms, e.g., penicillin, amoxicillin, if given early may abort the infection.

STYE (HORDELEUM)

It is a staphylococcal infection of the glands of the hair follicle at the eyelid margins. If the pus points to the lid margin, pulling out one or more of the eyelash hair will evacuate the pus. If the pus points on the skin of the eyelid, it is incised. Local anaesthesia is not necessary. Antibiotic eye ointment like chloramphenicol applicap should be used for a few days to prevent conjunctivitis.

INFECTED SEBACEOUS CYST

Ideally, a sebaceous cyst should be removed electively and *in toto*, electively to prevent recurrences. If the patient presents with an infected sebaceous cyst with an abscess formation, removal is deferred until the infection subsides. Instead, incision and drainage with or without dome anaesthesia is done. Pus as well as the cheesy material of the cyst is evacuated. Curettage of the cavity at this juncture is painful and is not advised.

CARBUNCLE

A carbuncle is an infective gangrene of the subcutaneous tissue which is seen very commonly on the nape of the neck and upper body and in uncontrolled diabetics. It is a specific form of staphylococcal infection of the skin that is characterized by multiple loculations of pus, which open on the skin with multiple sieve-like openings. Carbuncles may abort if high dose penicillin or cloxacillin or cephalosporins are given early enough. If not, multiple pus pockets may form which require drainage using field block anaesthesia. The pus in the carbuncle is usually not liquid but thick globules which can be removed by a forceps, which speeds up the healing. If the overlying skin is necrotic and if toxaemia is present, de-roofing should be done. Although antibiotics are generally not required once the abscess is drained, anti-staphylococcal antibiotics are usually prescribed in practice.

TOOTH ABSCESS (ALVEOLAR ABSCESS)

Swelling of the cheek along with erythema and tenderness of the gums in the neighbourhood of a bad tooth, is diagnostic of a tooth abscess. The 'bad tooth' could be a caries tooth, an impacted molar, broken-off tooth with retained roots or a dead tooth. Penicillin or amoxicillin along with metronidazole to cover anaerobes, if given early and in high doses may lead to resolution. If not, the patient should be referred to a dentist for incision and drainage and extraction of the bad tooth under general anaesthesia.

BREAST ABSCESS

A lactating patient may present to a GP, sometime in the postpartum period with the signs of acute inflammation in the breast. If seen during the stage of mastitis, conservative management should be tried by giving broad-spectrum antibiotics, breast support and temporary discontinuation of breastfeeding from the affected side. If in spite of these measures, the mastitis does not resolve and an abscess forms, the patient should be referred to a surgeon for incision and drainage as a general anaesthetic is necessary. If the abscess is not drained but treated by antibiotics alone, an antibioma or a sterile abscess is formed, which in any case ultimately requires drainage.

Small superficial abscess in a non-lactating woman can be dealt with like any other abscess by the general practitioner, taking care that the incision near the nipple or the areola should be radial (and not circumferential) in order to minimize trauma to the ducts.

PERIANAL AND ISCHIORECTAL ABSCESS

In perianal abscess, an acute tender rounded swelling is present at the anal margin. It can be drained using dome anaesthesia. If the abscess is anterior to the anal margin, care should be taken to avoid injury to the urethra. An ischiorectal abscess, which is in comparison larger and deeper, should be referred to a surgeon immediately. No time should be lost in draining the pus, as the abscess may open in the rectum leading to a permanent fistula-in-ano. This then requires 'major' surgery.

AXILLARY ABSCESS

Axillary abscess is commonly due to infection of the hair follicles but may also be due to suppurative lymphadenitis. Infection of the hair follicles (furunculosis) is often recurrent and has to be treated vigorously with long-term antibiotics and repeated incision and drainage. The incision is made directly over the abscess using dome anaesthesia and the pus drained. Whenever there is a chronic discharging sinus, tuberculosis lymphadenitis should be suspected and the patient referred to a surgeon for excision biopsy under general anaesthesia.

INGUINAL BUBO OR LYMPHADENITIS

Bubo is the suppuration of the inguinal lymph nodes, following a sexually transmitted disease like soft sore, lymphogranuloma venereum or syphilis. Here mainly the horizontal chain of lymph nodes is involved. An incision into the inguinal bubo should be avoided as a chronic discharging sinus may result. Rather, the lymph nodes should be repeatedly aspirated from a non-dependent site in the normal skin. The vertical chain of lymph nodes below the inguinal ligament is involved as a result of infection in the lower limb. If suppuration occurs, a vertical incision at a dependent site is taken, since a horizontal incision in this situation is likely to gape when the thigh is flexed.

ABSCESS OF THE NECK

Although suppuration of the lymph nodes is the commonest cause in this area, a '**cold abscess**' or an extension of an alveolar abscess or a simple furuncle are other possibilities. Suppuration might start in a deep lymph node; the fascia is breached following which a superficial collection of pus is formed. This is called a '**collar stud abscess**' (Fig. 41.2). Hence, while draining an abscess in the neck, first the superficial pocket of pus is drained and then the fascia incised to drain a lurking deeper abscess. If the deeper abscess is not drained then chronic discharging sinus will ultimately result. Pus should be sent for culture-sensitivity and for the presence of tuberculous bacilli. In addition, the abscess wall should be sent for histopathological examination. The incision should be horizontal and along the skin crease for better cosmetic results.

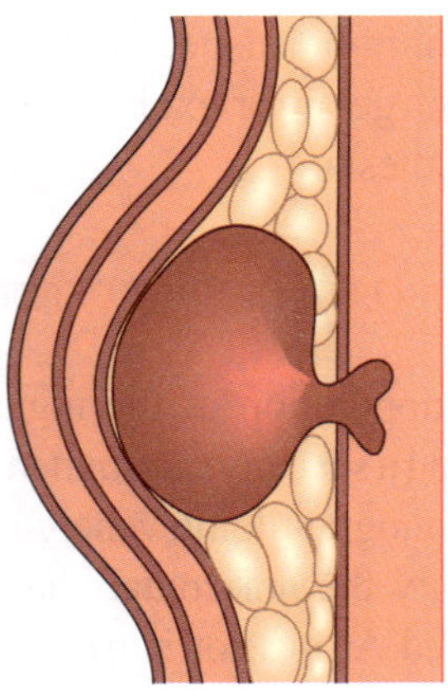

| **Fig. 41.2** Collar stud abscess |

INJECTION ABSCESS

This usually follows an injection given with less than adequate aseptic precautions. Local infiltration anaesthesia is usually adequate. General anaesthesia is required only when the abscess is deep and long standing enough to develop multiple fibrous septa.

Injection abscesses are usually encountered in the deltoid and the gluteal region. In case of a deltoid abscess, the incision is made vertically along the direction of the fibres of the deltoid at the point of maximum fluctuations. Similarly, in case of a gluteal abscess, the incision is made along the fibres of the gluteal muscle to avoid damage to that muscle. The pus is then drained using Hilton's method.

DIFFICULT ABSCESSES

The following abscesses should be preferably dealt with by a qualified surgeon in an operation theatre, under general anaesthesia for the reasons stated alongside:

- ***Palmar abscess***: The pus may not localize and may remain widespread in the palm.
  - There are no standard incisions in the surgery of the infected hand.
  - Important structures like nerves, vessels, tendons may get damaged during surgery.
- ***Breast abscess***: A dependent drain may be required, utilizing a counter incision in the lower part of the breast.
- ***Ischiorectal abscess***: Delayed or incomplete drainage leads to fistula-in-ano.
- ***Tooth abscess***: Requires extraction of the bad tooth.
  - Pus may spread deep to the deep fascia causing life-threatening '*Ludwig's angina*'.

- If not drained properly, osteomyelitis of the jaw may result.

- ***Parotid abscess***: Skin is to be incised vertically and the capsule transversely. This requires some experience.
  - Facial nerve may get damaged.
  - May leave a bad scar on the face.
- ***Thigh abscess***: Pus is deep seated and diffuse. Counter incisions may be required at the most dependent part.

Note: *These abscesses can be dealt with by a general practitioner when he gradually graduates from a 'minor surgeon' to a 'major surgeon'.*

CHAPTER 42

Surgical Casualties

- Foreign Body in Eye
- Foreign Body in Ear
- Foreign Body in Nose
- Foreign Body in Tissues
- Subungual Splinter
- Epistaxis
- Paraphimosis
- Bleeding from Tooth Socket
- Subungual Haematoma
- Perianal Haematoma
- Dislocated TM Joint

REMOVING A FOREIGN BODY FROM THE EYE

Most of the foreign bodies seen in practice will be particles of dust, small pieces of coal, insects or metal pieces getting into the eye during welding. The patient will complain of a foreign body in the eye in addition to pain, redness and watering.

Most of the foreign bodies in the eye can be identified by a powerful torch. What if the patient insists that there is a foreign body but you cannot see it? The possibility is that it is too small to be visualized by the naked eye or it might be lodged on the inside of the lid (sub-tarsal). Also a high velocity metal particle can penetrate the eye (intraocular) without causing tell-tale signs on the superficial surface. If the history is even remotely suggestive of an intraocular foreign body, refer immediately to an ophthalmologist. In other cases "*fluorescein staining*" is very useful to detect a foreign body.

Fluorescein is a yellow dye which when instilled into the eye, stains any damage to the surface of the eye as bright green. The patient is asked to look up. The lower eyelid is pulled down and a dry paper strip of fluorescein is placed inside the lower eyelid. Tears will wet the paper when the patient blinks and the dye will spread on the surface, staining any abrasion on the conjunctiva or cornea. If the paper strip is not available, use drops. But, these are too concentrated to stain the abrasions. Hence, the eye will have to be washed with saline before staining is apparent. It is always better to keep a few fluorescein strips in stock.

Once the foreign body is identified, the method of removal will depend on whether it is embedded beneath the eyelid or on the cornea. Instill one drop of 4% lignocaine. This immediately causes stinging pain and watering, which partially washes off the lignocaine. Put one more drop after 10–15 sec, which completes the anaesthesia.

Under the Upper Eyelid

To locate the foreign body, the lid must be everted. The technique of lid eversion must be known to all the general practitioners. Ask the patient to look down and keep looking down during the procedure. Then, pull the eyelid outward and gently push down the eyelid from outside either with the finger or a cotton bud. The foreign body seen after eversion can be easily wiped away with cotton.

Cornea

First, try to remove it with a piece of cotton. If the foreign body is firmly embedded in the cornea, it will not come off and you will have to use a needle. Gently brush the edge of the needle (and not the tip) against the foreign body and loosen it. The loosened foreign body can then be removed with cotton. If it does not come out, admit defeat and refer instead of using force and causing trauma. Once the foreign body has been removed, pad the eye after putting chloramphenicol applicap for at least 12 hrs.

REMOVING A FOREIGN BODY FROM THE EAR

A wide variety of materials are encountered in the external ear by general practitioners in their clinical practice. These include living insects, cockroaches, etc., to non-living household materials like buttons, plastic pieces in addition to vegetable foreign bodies like seeds, peas, etc. The patient is usually a naughty adventurous child. The first task is to identify the nature of the foreign body and then proceed accordingly.

- If it is a *living* foreign body, first kill it by filling the canal with oil, water or spirit, so that the insect suffocates. Then, remove it by syringing.
- If it is a *non-living* object, either you can remove it by hooking it out directly or by syringing.
- If it is a *vegetable matter*, never syringe as these can absorb water, swell and make removal more difficult.

For *hooking* it out, a vectis or a foreign body hook or a wax hook is used. Never use forceps as the foreign body may slip and go deeper into the canal. First straighten the ear canal to get a good view of the object by pulling the pinna. Then, carefully pass the hook along the wall of the canal and rotate it to bring the hook behind the foreign body. Now by giving gentle traction, pull it out. If there is bleeding, it is better to abandon the procedure and refer the patient to an ENT specialist.

Syringing is used for removing small smooth non-living objects and dead insects. It should be avoided in case of large pointed objects or if a tear of the drum is suspected or if the foreign body is a vegetable matter. Luke warm water is filled in the aural syringe, the pinna pulled to reveal the foreign body and a jet of water from the syringe is directed on the wall of the canal. The foreign body usually comes out along with the gush of water.

REMOVAL OF A FOREIGN BODY FROM THE NOSE

Again, the patient is usually a child who has deliberately inserted a foreign body up the nose. The foreign body is many times forgotten or its presence deliberately not told to the parents. The child is brought after a few days with a foul smelling bloody discharge from one nostril only. Examination reveals the foreign body hidden behind the discharge.

Hold the child properly and firmly either lying down on the examination table or upright on the lap of the mother. Visualize with a powerful torch. Put the foreign body hook or vectis behind the foreign body and gently drag it out. Again do not use forceps as this may accidentally push the foreign body back, probably in the larynx causing respiratory embarrassment.

REMOVAL OF 'RETAINED' FOREIGN BODIES IN THE TISSUES

A common scenario in a general practitioner's clinic is when the patient insists that there is a foreign body and the doctor is unsure about its presence. A lady gives a history that her bangles were broken a few days back and she feels that a piece is lying inside the arm or a thorn is in the sole of the foot or a wood splinter in the hand, etc. The problem needs to be dealt with along three lines.

- Is the foreign body really present? If in doubt, it is better to believe the patient and probe further. An X-ray will settle the issue if the foreign body is radiopaque, but thorns and wood splinters are not visualized.
- Does it require to be removed? Some materials like a piece of glass are inert substances and need not be removed, if it is not near a joint, nerve or other important structures.
- Do you have the experience and the set up necessary for the removal of the foreign body in question?

It is many times difficult to accurately localize the foreign body even with two X-rays taken in two different planes. Also the foreign body should be removed immediately after the X-rays have been taken and not after a few days when the foreign body may have shifted its position. In certain situations like the palms and soles, important structures like nerves, vessels and tendons lie and the foreign body lies somewhere in their midst. These should not be accidentally cut during the attempted removal of the foreign body, which requires a thorough knowledge of anatomy. If the general practitioner decides to operate, explores, but cannot find the foreign body, he should give up the procedure at the proper time and ask for help, rather than going on digging further.

REMOVAL OF SUBUNGUAL SPLINTER

A piece of bamboo or wood commonly gets embedded underneath the nail. If the tip is projecting out, it can be held by an artery forceps and pulled out. Many times it gets broken midway. Under the circumstances, the tip of a No.23 needle can be bent, put beneath the nail and the subungual splinter is hooked out. Failing this, the overlying portion of the nail is incised and removed, and the splinter exposed. It now can be easily removed by an artery forceps.

EPISTAXIS—STOPPING THE BLEEDING

Bleeding from the nose occurs in children from the lower anterior part of the nasal septum called the Little's area. This can be easily managed at general practice level by local measures. In older patients, the bleeding usually occurs from a higher inaccessible region in the nose and hence should be referred to an ENT specialist.

The first step in controlling the bleeding is to pinch the patient's nostrils together with your fingers for about 5 min. This will keep pressure on the Little's area and may arrest the bleeding. If after removal of the pressure, the bleeding reoccurs, a small gauze soaked in lignocaine with adrenaline is inserted in the anterior part of the nose and again the nostrils are pinched for five minutes. After this period, the pack is removed.

If the bleeding has stopped, anterior packing of the nose is done to prevent recurrence when the patient is sent back home. A roller gauze impregnated with a lubricant like liquid paraffin or white petroleum jelly is used, which is removed after 48 hrs. If the bleeding has not stopped with the gauze soaked in lignocaine with adrenaline, this means that the bleeding is either from a higher inaccessible area or the anterior bleeds require cautery. Posterior nasal bleeds can be stopped, as an emergency measure by the use of a Foley's catheter. Put the catheter through the bleeding nostril and inflate the balloon. This causes pressure on the bleeding vessels and stops the bleeding temporarily, tiding away the crisis. The patient should then be referred to an ENT specialist (along with the Foley's catheter in the nose!) for postnasal packing or endoscopic cautery under general anaesthesia. If the anterior bleeding has not stopped with the lignocaine plus adrenaline swab, electrocautery is required. Chemical cautery with silver nitrate or trichloroacetic acid is not effective if bleeding is continuing, but can be used to prevent further episodes once the bleeding has stopped.

EMERGENCY REDUCTION OF PARAPHIMOSIS

A very common scenario (Fig. 42.1) with a general practitioner is when a newly married man comes to his clinic with a swollen oedematous penis. What has happened is that a partially phimotic prepuce has been forcibly retracted and trapped in the coronal sulcus after sexual intercourse. The tight prepuce is constricting the glans which becomes swollen and oedematous. The diagnosis is apparent at a glance at the glans!

The constricting tight ring makes reduction of the prepuce by the patient himself impossible. Paraphimosis is also seen at other age groups, e.g., in a curious teenaged boy experimenting with the mechanism of his foreskin retraction. It also occurs in an elderly man when a young unmarried nurse pulls the prepuce back for catheterization and does not then know what to do with the stuck prepuce!

When the prepuce becomes trapped in the coronal sulcus for a long time, a tight ring of fibrous tissue of the prepuce forms which impedes blood and lymphatic flow. This results in swelling of the glans which might eventually lead to gangrene of the penis.

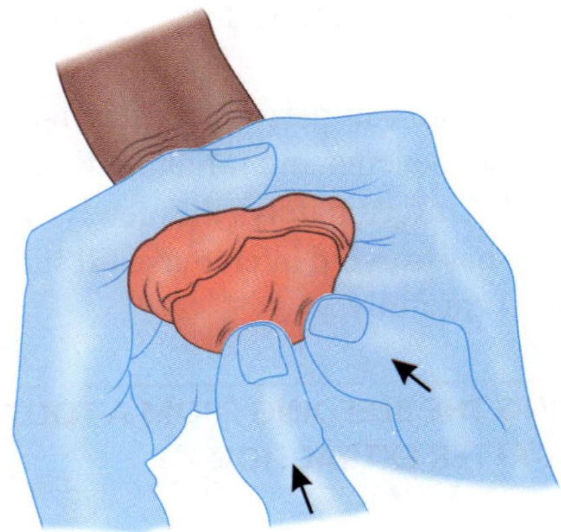

| Fig. 42.1 Reducing paraphimosis |

What to do?

- Never postpone manual reduction as the glans will become more oedematous with the passage of time.
- Try manipulative reduction under penile block anaesthesia, by pushing the glans with both the thumbs while at the same time pulling the retracted prepuce over the glans. The constricting ring should come completely over the glans along with the prepuce.
- If this fails, inject hyaluronidase into the sides of the constricting ring. After 15 min, the swelling is much reduced and manipulative reduction is possible.

- If hyaluronidase is not available, try the '*multiple puncture technique*'. Pierce the oedematous glans at 10–15 places with a no.21 needle and squeeze, so that the watery fluid comes out, reducing the swelling. Now, reduce the paraphimosis as described above.
- As a last resort, if the above manoeuvre fails, divide the constricting ring longitudinally on the dorsal aspect. The foreskin now is easily taken forward. The wound is then sutured with linen no. 60. (See dorsal slit of prepuce Chapter 42.)
- Circumcision is performed at a later date when the oedema and inflammation has resolved. Unfortunately, the newly married couple has to avoid intercourse till such time or do it carefully.

STOPPING THE BLEEDING FROM A TOOTH SOCKET AFTER EXTRACTION

The patient usually presents with slow oozing from the site of an extracted tooth, 2–3 hrs after extraction. The dentist after extracting the tooth has gone home and is untraceable.

Now what to do?

- Ask the patient to rinse the mouth thoroughly to remove all clots so that the bleeding can be localized.
- Infiltrate 2% lignocaine with adrenaline in and around the socket. Take a gauze piece twice the size of the bleeding socket and pack it in the cavity. Ask the patient to bite on it for 20 min. Twenty minutes is a long period to keep anybody's mouth shut. So, make him comfortable by making him sit on a chair, elbow on a table and the chin cupped in the hand.
- If after removing the gauze, the bleeding continues, you will have to suture the socket with 3/0 catgut. Before suturing, it is convenient to place a big piece of gauze on the buccal side of the gum inside the cheek, so that there is a room for suturing. The suturing can be done over the piece of gauze packed in the bleeding cavity, tightly till the gums blanch.
- Refer back the patient to the dentist as soon as he is available. It is his job to investigate the patient for blood dyscrasias and your job to accept a 'thank you' from the extremely relieved relatives.

DRAINING A SUBUNGUAL HAEMATOMA

This usually follows accidental crushing of the tip of the finger (Fig. 42.2). If the injury is severe and fracture is suspected, send the patient for an X-ray. If not, this very painful condition can easily be dealt with by drilling two holes on the nail with a no.21 needle and draining the trapped blood. Local anaesthesia is not necessary.

If the patient who is already in agony gets more frightened after seeing the needle, reassure him that the procedure is painless and you intend to drill through the insensitive nail and not through his fingers!

Drilling is continued till the blood comes out or the tip of the needle touches the nail bed as evidenced by the wincing seen on the patient's face. If the needle is removed, the oozing stops. Hence, the needle should be kept in place and turned from time to time till most of the blood is drained. Usually, this gives immediate relief from pain.

If the haematoma is large, the nail will separate in a week or so and can be easily taken out without anaesthesia. If the nail does not separate and the pain continues, the nail has to be removed after giving ring block.

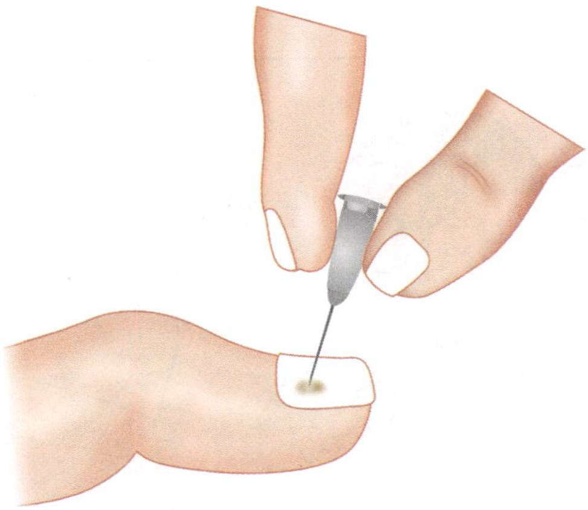

| **Fig. 42.2** Draining a subungual haematoma |

DRAINING A PERIANAL HAEMATOMA

This is an extremely painful condition, which appears all of a sudden and is due to bursting of an anal venule upon straining at stool, coughing or lifting heavy weights. The pain becomes more severe if the patient sits and hence the patient declines to take a seat in your clinic.

Keeping in mind the severity of pain, the patient should be treated immediately in your own clinic. The patient is given the left lateral position and your compounder or assistant is asked to retract the upper buttock in order to give a clear view. The dome and the surrounding area is infiltrated with lignocaine. The haematoma is bisected and the two halves are then excised along with some normal adjacent skin. The wound is then allowed to heal by secondary intention over a period of 8–10 days.

The pain relief is immediate; the cure is permanent and the patient grateful.

REDUCING THE DISLOCATED TEMPOROMANDIBULAR JOINT

Sometimes the GP is faced with a patient who has dislocated his jaw after sudden laughter (or overenthusiastic kissing probably under the influence of alcohol!). There is severe pain at the temporomandibular joint and the patient is unable to close his mouth. If it is unilateral dislocation, the patient has an asymmetric look with his chin deviated to one side. If it is a bilateral dislocation, the jaw is thrust forward and the patient looks like having a large jaw.

In order to relocate the jaw, there are two methods to be tried, sequentially. Try the second manoeuvre only if the first one fails. Essentially first make the patient sit on a chair resting his head on the back of chair. Give diazepam IV slowly. (This is not necessary if patient is already under the influence of alcohol.)

Step I

Tickle the uvula with a tongue depressor and remove it immediately. The gag that results should relocate the jaw.

Step II

If the above manoeuvre fails, put on gloves, wrap a clean handkerchief around your thumbs. Stand in front of the patient. Put your thumbs on his lower molars inside the mouth, your index fingers behind his jaw, and your middle and ring fingers beneath the mandible. Push downwards and backwards with your fingers, holding the jaw firmly in your hand. If properly performed, the jaw should relocate, to the great sigh of relief for the patient and his relative.

GP Tip

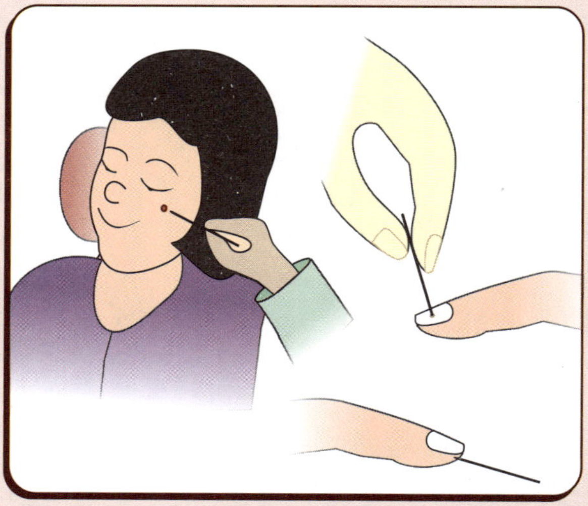

Uses of the humble hypodermic needle other than for giving an injection:

- Enucleate a molluscum
- Drain a subungual haematoma
- Remove a splinter below a nail

GP Tip

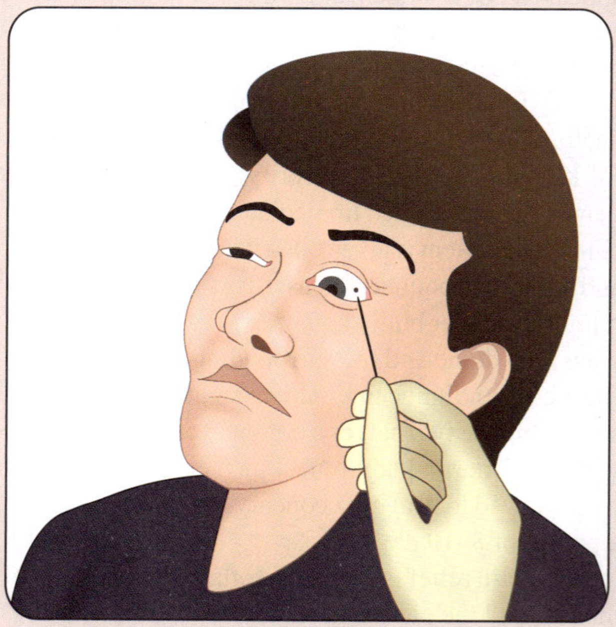

Afraid of using the tip of the needle to remove the foreign body in the cornea or conjunctiva?

- Here's a safer option—Take 20 no. intracath. Draw out the stilett and use its plastic tip to remove the foreign body. This will not harm the cornea.

GP Tip

Noninvasive and safe technique to remove foreign body from nose in a child:

- Instill Nasivion nasal drops in the nostril which contains the foreign body. Occlude the other nostril with your fingers. Then ask the patient to exhale (blow) through his nose forcefully. The foreign body will be pushed out by the blow of air.

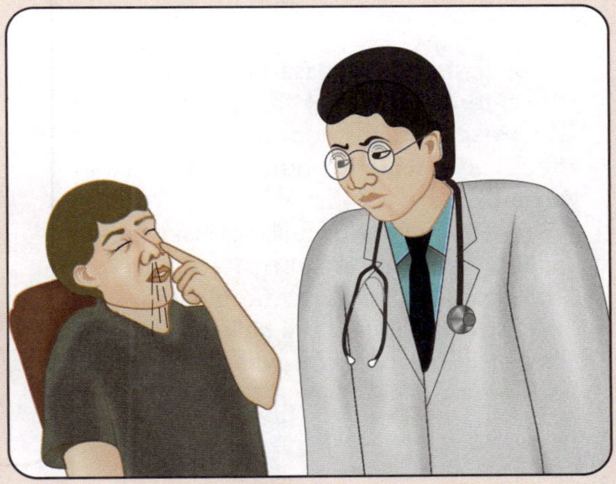

GP Tip

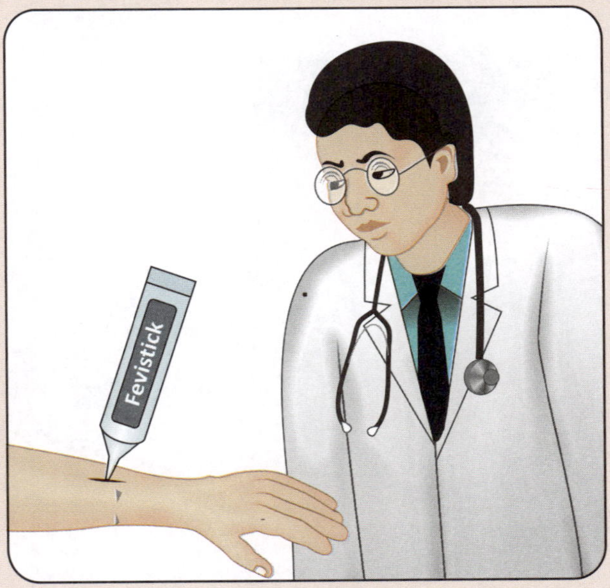

In case of a small cut injury, to suture or not to suture that is the question.

- Don't suture. Approximate the edges with your fingers, apply 'Fevistick' and bandage the wound firmly!

GP Tip

Stopping a posterior nasal bleed. When the anterior nasal pack fails to control the bleeding, a posterior nasal pack is necessary, which requires GA in a hospital.

- Try this in your own clinic. Insert a Foley's catheter lubricated with Lignocaine, through the bleeding nostril and inflate the balloon with water. The pressure will stop the bleeding.

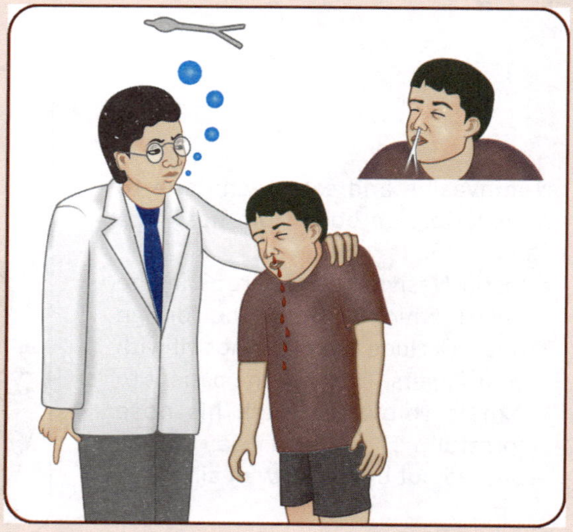

CHAPTER 43

Suturing Techniques

- Needle
- Suturing Material
- Simple Interrupted Sutures
- Knot
- Dog Ears
- Excessive Tension in the Wound
- Suturing Methods
- Suturing at Different Sites
- Suture Removal
- Other Methods of Skin Closure

Every general practitioner should master the technique of suturing wounds, as he is the first to be approached immediately after the injury. Approximation of skin edges is required in many other situations in minor surgery and hence learning this technique becomes the bare-essential-minimum for minor surgery in general practice. It can be easily learnt by reading this chapter and under the guidance of your surgeon friend.

SELECT THE PROPER NEEDLE

A curved needle has 3 parts. The *point* is the sharp tip that penetrates the tissue. The *eye* is the other end where the suture material is inserted or is already attached. The *body* is the mid-portion, which is either round or triangular in shape. Round-bodied needles have no role in suturing skin. Use triangular bodied needles, which are of two types. The *cutting needle* has a sharp edge on the inner curve of the needle while the *reverse cutting needle* has a sharp edge on the outer curve of the needle, which reduces the risk of pulling through and cutting the tissue while suturing. Hence, *the reverse cutting needle is preferred in suturing wounds* and in approximating skin edges.

Select the proper size as per requirement. Do not select too small a needle, as then only a small portion of the tip will emerge from the wound edge leading to unnecessary pulling and pushing.

SELECT THE PROPER SUTURING MATERIAL

Although there is a large choice of suture materials available for suturing wounds, for minor surgery only three types will suffice: 4/0 plain catgut (for suturing mucous membrane like lips and for subcuticular approximation); 4/0 ethilon (for wounds on face); 4/0 or 6/0 linen (for rest of the body). The costlier and superior 'Vicryl' can be used instead of catgut, and 'Prolene' instead of ethilon or linen, if cost is no consideration (see Chapter 36).

CURVED NEEDLE (SIMPLE INTERRUPTED SUTURES) (Fig. 43.1)

1. Mount the needle with the thread in the jaws of a needle holder so that the point is on the left and the eye is on the right of the operator.
2. Hold the needle holder in the right hand (in a right handed GP) and grip the needle at the junction of the middle 3rd and outer 3rd by squeezing the handle of the needle holder and locking it in the ratchet.
3. Hold the needle holder by placing the thumb and the ring finger into the loops and by placing the index finger on the fulcrum of the needle holder to stabilize it (Fig. 43.2).
4. Hold the toothed or un-toothed forceps in the left hand. Lift the skin edge of the right flap of skin with the forceps at the centre of the wound.
5. Pierce the skin with the needle a little distance from the wound edge entering at 90° to the skin surface (Fig. 43.1a). Push the needle downwards into the tissues in a curved path by progressively supinating the wrist. The needle will emerge through the wound, which should be pulled out with the needle holder.
6. Now evert the opposing left side flap of the skin and penetrate the wound at exactly the same depth (Fig. 43.1b). Again push the needle through the tissue by progressively supinating the wrist so that the needle emerges out of the skin at the same distance from the wound edge as it had entered.
7. Finally, pull the needle out of tissue by the needle holder or by the gloved fingers.
8. In case of small wounds, the needle can be driven through both the edges in one movement instead of taking each side separately, by approximating both the skin edges with forceps or fingers and by using a slightly large size needle.

| Box 1 |

The suture should be flask shaped in configuration, i.e., the stitch should be wider at its base (Fig. 43.3). This ensures *slight eversion* of the wound edges, which is necessary for proper healing (Fig. 43.4a). If the wound edges are markedly everted, a raw surface is exposed to infection and trauma. If the wound edges are markedly inverted (Fig. 43.4b), the final result will be an ugly depressed scar, as healing cannot take place between uncut skin edges.

| Box 2 |

1. Place the stitch hole as close as possible to the edge of the wound, so that ultimately a "ladder scar" or 'train-tracks' are not produced.
2. If approximation is difficult, avoid the temptation to suture under tension. You can reduce the skin tension by giving relaxing incisions or by undercutting (Fig. 43.5a & b).

HOW TO TIE THE KNOT (Fig. 43.6)

Once the suture is placed properly, the next step is to tie the knot correctly.

First, rotate the needle holder clockwise around the long end of the suture material for two complete turns. Then, grasp the free short end of the thread with the tip of the holder and pull it through the loops of the long end of the thread.

Next, rotate the needle holder anticlockwise along the long end of the thread, grasp the short free end with the tip of the needle holder and pull it through the loops (reverse loop).

One or two additional knots may be added. Finally, cut both the ends of the thread about 1–

2 cm away from the knot and proceed to the next suture.

The first suture is taken in the centre of the wound. The next sutures are midway between the first suture and end of the wound on either side. The subsequent sutures are placed midway between these sutures; so on and so forth. By this method, "**dog ears**" (i.e., puckering of the skin on either side of the wound after suturing is completed) are avoided.

WHAT IF "DOG EARS" FORM? (Fig. 43.7)

If dog ears do form, mark their bases elliptically as shown and excise the area. Elliptical defects will be produced, which are then closed producing a flat linear scar. Small dog-ears will however settle with time without correction and hence may be left alone.

WHAT IF THERE IS EXCESSIVE TENSION IN THE WOUND?

Always avoid closing skin under excessive tension. This will produce blanching of the skin; the stitches will form grooves and might give way. The final result may be ladder like scars. The tension may be reduced by:

1. 'Undercutting' the edges (Fig. 43.5a), by means of forceps, fingers or scalpel blade; or by
2. Giving a 'relaxing incision' parallel to the wound (Fig. 43.5b), which allows the skin near the wound to relax; or by
3. Giving 'guide stitches', which partially appose the edges. The definitive stitches can then be put and the stitches which have now become loose, removed.

OTHER TYPES OF SUTURING METHODS

Simple interrupted sutures (Fig. 43.8a) are the only type of sutures required for minor surgery suggested in this book. Occasionally however, the gaping of wound is so marked that by using simple interrupted sutures, a closed cavity will remain inside. In such cases, *deep buried sutures* with catgut No. 3 can be used. Very occasionally the tendency to invert is so marked that *interrupted mattress sutures* (horizontal or vertical) may be required. A *simple running suture* (Fig. 43.8b & c) is quick to apply and saves time, but does not give good cosmetic results and if one stitch is opened up the whole wound is likely to gape. It can be used in circumcision operation to tie the two layers of mucous membrane with catgut.

SUTURING AT DIFFERENT SITES

- ***Wounds on the scalp*** always bleed profusely, frightening the patients and the relatives. Many times after the hair is cut, everybody is surprised to find only a small nick. If the wound is large enough to require suturing the bleeding should first be stopped by applying pressure or by applying artery clips to bleeding points if necessary. Infiltration with lignocaine plus adrenaline usually solves the problem. If the wound is not very large, a 'trick' is to twist a bunch of hair on either side of the wound and tie them together across the wound!
- ***Wound on the face*** should be sutured with fine 5/0 prolene or 4/0 ethilon sutures for good cosmetic results. Wounds on the *eyebrows* obviously require accurate approximation and wounds on the *eyelids* are best sutured by a plastic surgeon. Wounds below the chin, commonly seen in children, can be left alone if the gaping is not too large.

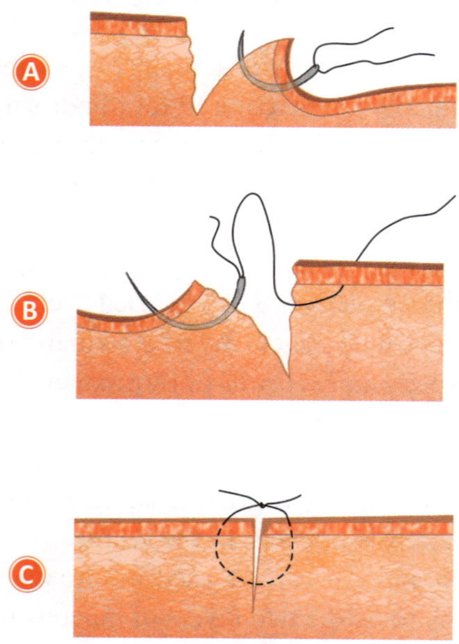

| Fig. 43.1 Suturing technique. Simple interrupted sutures (see text) |

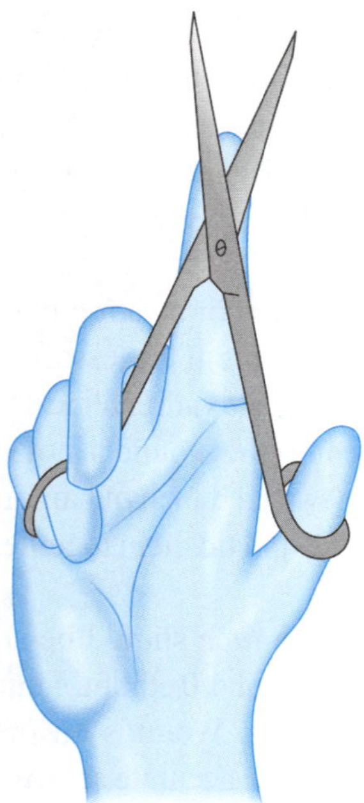

| Fig. 43.2 Correct way to hold scissors or needle holder |

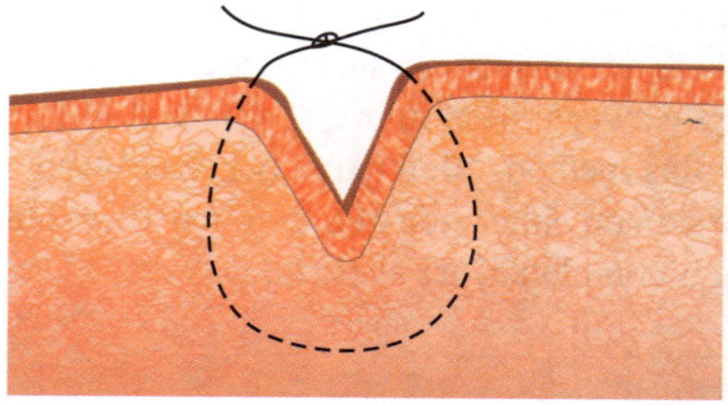

| Fig. 43.3 Flasked shaped suture |

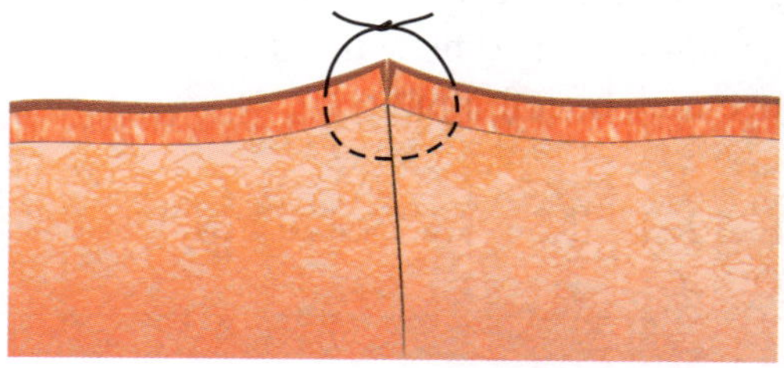

| Fig. 43.4a Slight everted edges: Good cosmetic result |

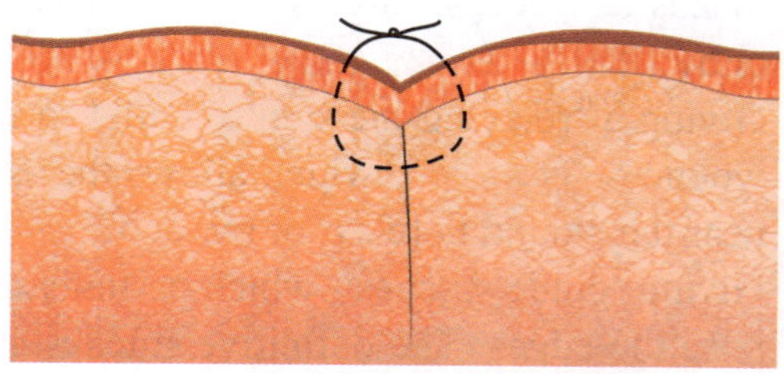

| Fig. 43.4b Inverted edges: Depressed ugly scar |

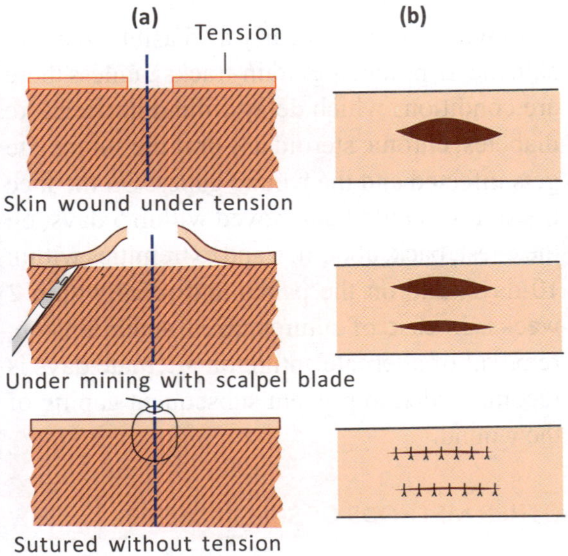

| **Fig. 43.5** a) Undercutting to relieve tension; b) Relieving the tension by giving a parallel incision |

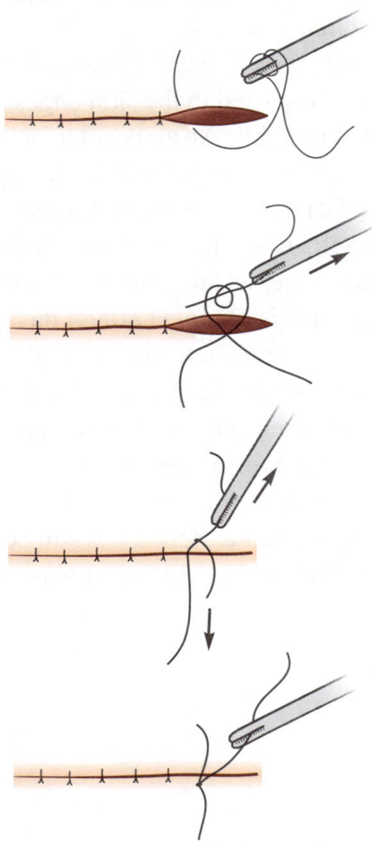

| **Fig. 43.6** Tying a knot |

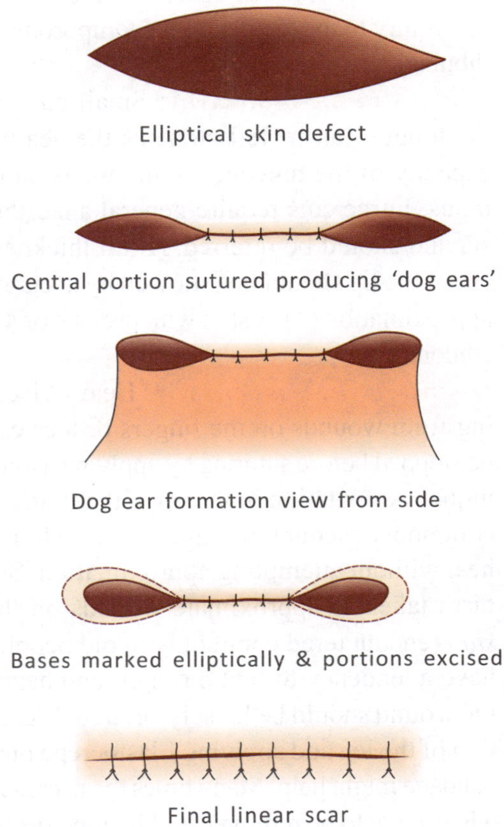

| **Fig. 43.7** Dog ears |

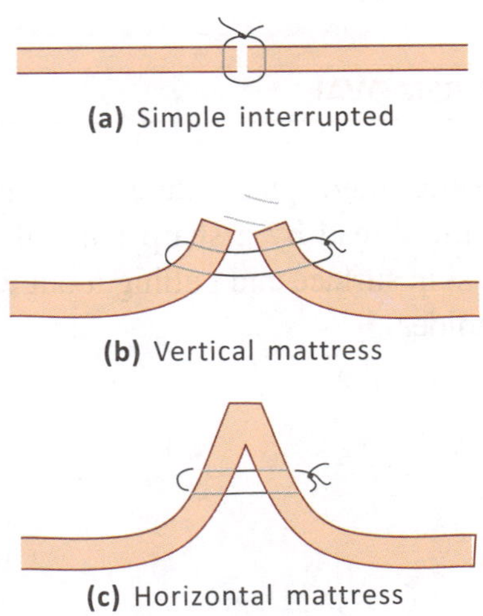

| **Fig. 43.8** Simple interrupted and mattress sutures |

Remember to rule out fracture of the mandible, injury to the teeth or to the temporomandibular joints.

- *Wounds in the oral cavity*: Small cuts on the tongue can be left alone as the healing capacity of the mucous membrane is enormous. Large cuts require general anaesthesia and should be referred. A full thickness cut of the lip should be followed by accurate approximation of the skin with prolene or 4/0 ethilon.
- *Wounds on the arms and legs*: Heavy bleeding from wounds on the fingers or toes can be stopped before suturing by applying a tourniquet. Amputation of the tip of the finger is commonly encountered and should be left to heal without attempting approximation. Sutures taken to approximate wounds on the *shin* (encountered commonly in old people) have a tendency to 'cut through' and hence the wound should be loosely sutured. Elevation of the leg and applying Elastocrepe plus bandage might help. Many times the necrosed edges have to be removed and later on grafting may be required. Finally, a general practitioner should never suture dog bites, however severe.

SUTURE REMOVAL

Remove the interrupted suture by cutting the base of the thread by a sharp pointed scissor near the skin surface and pulling it out with the needle holder.

Remove the suture as early as feasible to avoid skin marks producing 'train-tracks', unless there are conditions which delay wound healing like diabetes, chronic steroid use or if the suture site gets infected and the wound gapes. On the face the suture should be removed within 5 days; on the chest, back, abdomen and extremities within 10 days; and on the palms and soles within 2 weeks. In case of sutures taken under tension, removal of alternate suture on alternate days is recommended to prevent subsequent gaping of the wound.

OTHER METHODS OF SKIN CLOSURE

1. *Dermal adhesives* can be used in areas of low tension and in uncooperative children. The results are equivalent to sutures, under these circumstances.
2. *Adhesive paper strips (Steri-strip)*: Tinc. benzoin is applied to the skin edges and left to dry thoroughly. An assistant then approximates the skin edges while the operator places the paper strips across the wound. The strip itself should never be used to approximate the edges as this can lead to a bad scar. Usually, this is removed after 4 days.
3. *Staples* are quick and easy to apply. An assistant is usually required to hold the skin edges together and still the alignment may not be accurate. A special extractor is required to remove the staples, which may not be freely available. Hence, it is still not a routine method of skin closure in general practice.

CHAPTER 44

Simple Minor Surgery

- Aspiration Techniques
- Taking a Skin Biopsy
- Excision of Sebaceous Cyst
- Excising a Lipoma
- Excising a Corn
- Treating Recurrent Epistaxis
- Frenuloplasty
- Phenolising a Pilonidal Sinus
- Excising an Ingrowing Toe Nail
- Onychogryphosis
- Dorsal Slit of Prepuce
- Excising a Chalazion

ASPIRATION TECHNIQUES

This is one of the simplest and one of the most rewarding procedures and should be undertaken by every general practitioner aspiring to do minor surgery. It does not require anaesthesia or an operation theatre and is very safe, provided secondary infection is prevented by strict aseptic no-touch technique. An 18-G needle with a 10-mL syringe is all that is required.

Aspiration of a Breast Cyst

Usually, it is easy to diagnose this condition by the feel itself. If your diagnosis is wrong and it turns out to be a solid lump, no harm can be done by a 'trial' aspiration even if the lump is malignant. An attempted aspiration cannot spread malignancy. After observing the usual aseptic precautions, the cyst should be steadied between your two fingers as a breast cyst is quite mobile. The needle should then be introduced perpendicularly into the cyst and the contents aspirated fully in one quick movement. The fluid obtained should be sent for cytological examination to rule out malignancy. The procedure is so quick that local anaesthesia is not required.

Aspiration of a Ganglion

A ganglion is a cystic lesion connected and arising from the tendon sheath or the joint capsule. It is commonly seen on the dorsum of the wrist. Other common sites are ventral aspect of the wrist, the dorsum of the foot and the distal interphalangeal joints. Sometimes, the cyst ruptures (with or without trauma) and then disappears only to recur spontaneously after a few weeks. Even after meticulous surgery, the ganglion sometimes recurs. Hence, simple aspiration of the ganglion with phenolization should be given a trial before advising surgical excision. Extra care should be taken while aspirating the ganglion on the ventral aspect of the wrist because of proximity of the median and ulnar nerves.

The contents of the ganglion are thick and viscous which cannot be aspirated in one quick movement, as in the case of a breast cyst. Hence, a small amount of 2% lignocaine is first infiltrated on the overlying skin. A wide bore needle (no.18 G) & a large syringe (10 mL) is used in order to generate maximum suction. The ganglion is then steadied with your left hand fingers, the needle inserted directly into the ganglion and the fluid aspirated. The syringe is removed with the needle still in place and 1 mL of a sclerosant solution (80% phenol) is injected. A tight Elastocrepe bandage is applied. If the ganglion recurs, then surgical excision is the only option.

Tapping a Hydrocele

Whenever surgery for hydrocele is contraindicated, like in an elderly or in a medically unfit patient, repeated aspirations of the hydrocele fluid with instillation of 10% phenol is quite a satisfactory procedure. Before embarking upon such a procedure, it is essential to be absolutely sure about the diagnosis. See that the swelling transilluminates, you can close your fingers above the swelling and that the swelling is not solid. An ultrasonography will easily confirm the diagnosis in case of doubt.

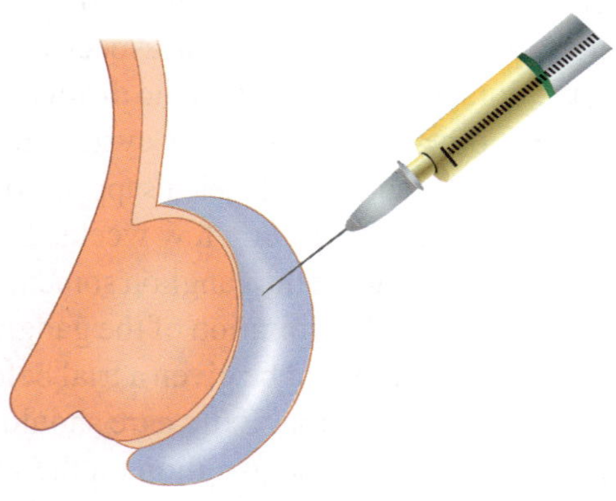

| **Fig. 44.1** Tapping a hydrocele |

Tapping is made from the lower and anterior aspect of the sac. This part is made tense by holding the upper part of the scrotum in your left hand. A small amount of lignocaine is infiltrated in the scrotal skin. An 18-G needle attached to a 20-mL syringe is now inserted and the straw coloured fluid aspirated and discarded, with the needle still in position. This way, about 100–150 mL can be removed. A 50-mL syringe or a three-way tap is more convenient but general practitioners usually do not stock these very occasionally used items in their clinics. Again, if available, an IV cannula can be used instead of a needle to prevent trauma to the testis, which can occur when the hydrocele is almost empty. This can lead to bleeding and formation of a scrotal haematoma which itself then requires drainage. Perfectionist advocates sending the fluid for cytological examination, which in my opinion really is not necessary. To avoid recurrence, 10% phenol (and not the 80% phenol used in chemical cautery or in a ganglion) is instilled into the hydrocele sac after the hydrocele has been tapped completely. In order to minimise the pain caused by phenol, about 5–10 mL of lignocaine can be instilled in the sac prior to phenol instillation.

TAKING A SKIN BIOPSY

Skin biopsy is done in practice either for diagnosis of skin lesions like suspected psoriasis, lichen planus or Hansen's disease, or for removal of superficial skin lesions like naevi. Biopsies on the face should be avoided as far as possible because of cosmetic considerations. There are two types of skin biopsies.

Excision Biopsy

Here, the whole lesion is excised with a margin of normal skin around it and hence is suitable for small lesions only (<1 cm). An elliptical incision is planned around the lesion with a margin of at least 3 mm of normal skin. The incision should always be made along Langer's lines. These are shown in detail in standard textbooks on surgery, but in practice it is useful to remember that they approximately correspond to the creases and wrinkles in the skin. The length of the ellipse should be at least four times its width; otherwise, dog ears will form at the end of the wound after skin closure. This area is infiltrated with lignocaine. The lesion itself is not infiltrated as this will disrupt the histology. The elliptical incision is now taken with a scalpel blade. One end of the incised skin is picked up with a fine-toothed forceps, the incision taken down to the subcutaneous fat and the excision of the lesion is completed by fine dissection. The specimen is placed in a bottle containing formalin and sent to the laboratory for histopathological examination. The skin is closed with 3/0 nylon or with linen No. 60. The laboratory should be given full information about the site from which the skin has been removed & the probable clinical diagnosis.

Incision Biopsy

Incision biopsy is done for larger lesions and for diagnostic purposes only. The procedure is as described above. Only a part of the lesion is taken but an area of normal skin should preferably be included in the specimen for the pathologist to compare. Incisional biopsy can be done more easily by using a '**biopsy punch**' (Fig. 44.1). The blades of this instrument are placed vertically on the anaesthetic lesion. Using a twisting motion, it is pushed into the depth of the skin. The punch is then removed. The incised tissue is picked up with a forceps and the base is cut with scissors.

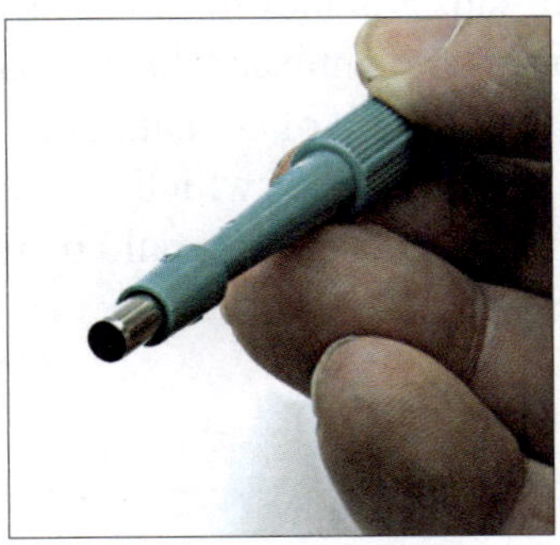

| Fig. 44.2 Incision biopsy |

The piece of skin is transferred into a formalin containing bottle and sent to the laboratory.

EXCISION OF SEBACEOUS CYST

Sebaceous cyst is a very common tumour seen mainly on the face, scalp and back. The presence of a punctum on the summit of the cyst is diagnostic. Two methods are employed for its removal.

Incision-Avulsion Method

Dome infiltration anaesthesia is used. The incision is made on the cyst and the cyst wall incised. The contents are squeezed out. The cyst wall is grasped by an artery forceps and pulled out by continuous traction.

This method is very simple, but the temptation to use this method should be avoided for two reasons. Firstly, the cyst wall is often firmly attached to the deep layers, especially if it has been infected before. Some part of the cyst wall is invariably left behind during avulsion leading to its recurrence. Secondly, this method leaves redundant skin leading to a dead space. Hence, the dissection method is recommended.

Dissection Method

An elliptical incision (Fig. 44.3) is made around the punctum with a scalpel blade taking care not to puncture the cyst. Starting at one end of the incision, a mixture of blunt and sharp dissection is done at the plane between the cyst wall and the underlying tissue again taking care not to puncture the cyst. The cyst is then removed in *toto*. If the cyst is accidentally punctured, mosquito forceps is applied to seal the punctured site and dissection is then completed.

Some cysts are best operated upon by surgeons, e.g., on the face (because of cosmetic reasons and the possibility of damage to the

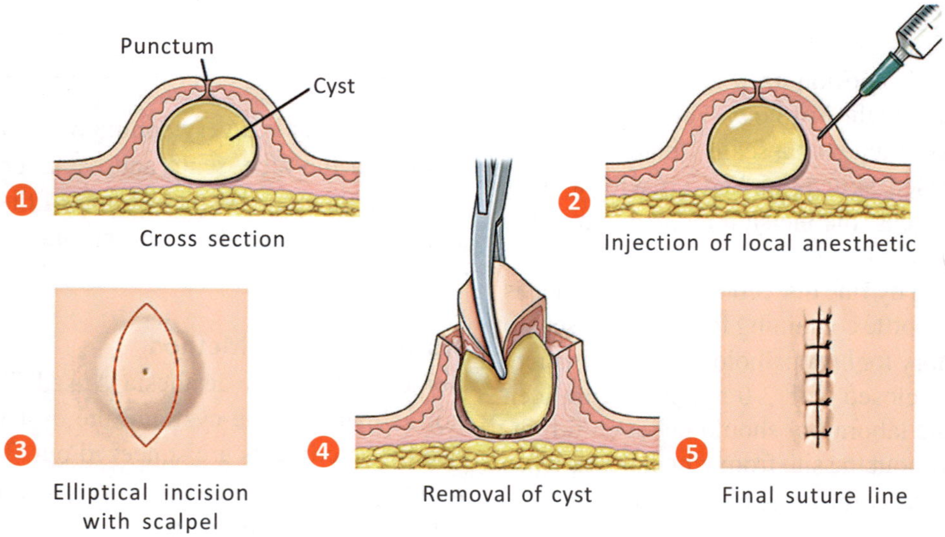

| **Fig. 44.3** Excision of a sebaceous cyst |

facial nerve), on the nape of neck (because of thick skin approximation is difficult) and the anterior triangle of the neck (because of the risk of damage to the important structures). If the patient presents with an infected cyst, it is better to give antibiotics, incise and drain it and then remove it at a later period electively.

EXCISING A LIPOMA

For the removal of a *small lipoma*, the squeeze method is employed. Here, a small incision is made in the centre of the swelling, the base of the lipoma is squeezed with the operator's fingers and the lipoma is forced out through the small opening.

In *medium sized lipomas*, an incision is made over the centre of the lipoma measuring about 2/3rd of its diameter. The incision is carefully deepened till the lipoma with its thin capsule is seen. The plane between the lipoma and the subcutaneous tissue is identified. The lipoma is separated from the attachments either by blunt dissection or by a finger. Finally, it is taken out as a whole.

In a *large lipoma*, so that a dead space should not remain, a portion of the skin needs to be excised. This is achieved by taking an elliptical incision on the centre and the lipoma removed in *toto* with an island of skin attached to it.

Very large lipomas, which are commonly seen on the back however should be referred to a surgeon as they can be surprisingly deep. Similarly, excision of a lipoma on the face can give bad cosmetic result and excision of a lipoma in the axilla may damage underlying important structures and hence should also be referred.

EXCISING A CORN

A corn is a '**pressure sore**' on the foot caused by an undue pressure from outside by ill-fitting footwear. It can also be caused by undue pressure from inside by a prominent metatarsal head.

Hence, the logical treatment is using well fitting footwear. Application of salicylic acid in flexible collodion (Salactin liquid) or the use of plasters containing salicylic acid (corn caps) is helpful at times.

If this fails, surgical treatment is advised after having informed the patient about the chances of recurrence. This consists of complete removal of the corn along with a little surrounding normal skin and tissue. A large gaping wound results, which can be closed with 3/0 nylon. A complete approximation of the wound is difficult but is not necessary, as the wound will anyway heal from beneath in a month or so.

TREATING RECURRENT EPISTAXIS WITH CHEMICAL CAUTERY

The most logical thing to do in such cases is to rule out any specific cause for the bleeding like a bleeding diathesis in children and hypertension or malignancy in adults. Having done that, it is useful to remember that 90% of the idiopathic cases are due to bleeding from the blood vessels from the Little's area, on the distal part of the nasal septum. If this area is chemically cauterized with 50% phenol, bleeding usually stops permanently. If it fails, the patient should be referred to an ENT surgeon for electrocautery or further work up.

Soak cotton with 4% lignocaine solution to which ½ mL of adrenaline is added and pack the anterior part of nose with it. Keep this in place for at least 10 min for a proper anaesthetic effect to take place. Then, remove the cotton pack and apply 50% phenol with a cotton swab to the area for about 10 sec, when blanching will be seen.

Nothing more needs to be done. Send the patient home with instructions that healing may take about 6 weeks. Nasal cautery should always be done in between bleeding episodes. Active bleeding is unlikely to stop with chemical cautery and may in fact increase. Never cauterize both the sides of the septum at one sitting, as perforation may occur. Nasal cautery is employed only for anterior bleeds. Posterior bleeds are inaccessible without endoscopes.

DIVIDING A PENILE FRENULUM (FRENULOPLASTY)

This surgery is indicated when the patient complains that there is cracking of the frenulum during intercourse resulting in pain and bleeding. The condition may be a congenitally short frenulum or may be acquired because of repeated trauma during sexual intercourse leading to fibrosis and loss of elasticity. When the prepuce is retracted, the shaft of the penis curves ventrally.

A small quantity of plain 2% lignocaine (i.e., without adrenaline) is injected directly into the frenulum. The two ends of the frenulum are tied with catgut to prevent postoperative bleeding. The frenulum is divided by a horizontal incision with a scalpel blade. Due to traction, the horizontal incision elongates into a diamond shaped area. The diamond area is converted into a vertical line by suturing with catgut or simply left alone to heal by secondary intention. Less trauma, more pleasure!

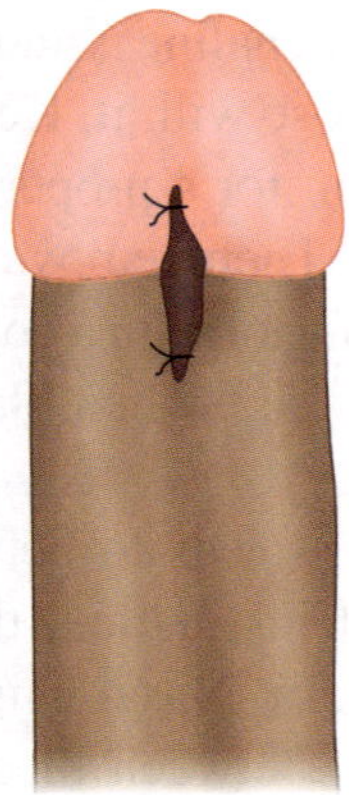

| **Fig. 44.4** Dividing a penile frenulum |

PHENOLISING A PILONIDAL SINUS

A *pilonidal sinus* is a sinus containing a tuft of hair. It is seen commonly in young 'hairy' individuals whose occupation demands sitting for prolonged periods. The most common site is in the upper end of the natal cleft. The hairs incite a foreign body reaction, resulting in a chronic discharging sinus and recurrent secondary infections. The definitive surgery, which can prevent a relapse is quite radical in the sense that all the tracts and debris have to be removed. In practice, this is difficult to achieve.

A very simple alternative is phenolization of the sinus. The skin surrounding the sinus is shaved and local anaesthetic infiltrated around the sinus. The sinus is curetted thoroughly and filled with 80% phenol for 2–3 min, after the surrounding area has been protected with petroleum jelly. Phenol causes a raw surface lining the walls of the sinus. The walls approximate and heal, leading to closure of the cavity.

EXCISING AN INGROWING TOE NAIL

The condition is caused by the edge of the toe nail curling in and digging into the adjacent tissues, inciting an inflammatory reaction. It is an extremely painful condition and usually treated by general practitioners with antibiotics and pain killers, which are not adequate as the primary cause is not removed. The condition is to be treated aggressively by surgery. There is hardly any role for the conservative management, as suggested by chiropodists because everything depends on the willingness of the patient to help himself permanently, which is rare. More than a dozen procedures have been described in literature ranging from just cutting the nail straight to a mutilating surgery nothing short of amputation. The most feasible ones in a general practitioner's setup are described here.

- ***Simple cutting down***: Simply cutting down and removing the side of the nail which is ingrowing by a pair of scissors is often effective. The patient is shown the procedure and directed to do this permanently. This will work however, only in the absence of significant inflammation.
- ***Removal of the nail segment under local anaesthesia* (Wedge resection)**: Any patient with the symptoms of short duration and presence of significant inflammation should be offered this simple procedure after informing him about the possibility of recurrence. The toe is anaesthetised by a digital nerve block and a tourniquet applied at the base. Two parallel incisions are made; one on the nail and the other on the affected nail fold as shown in Fig. 44.5. They are then joined on both the ends. The nail tissues and the nail matrix in the intervening area are excised and the toe dressed up with sofratulle or with petroleum jelly. Do not forget to

remove the tourniquet at the end of the surgery before bandaging.

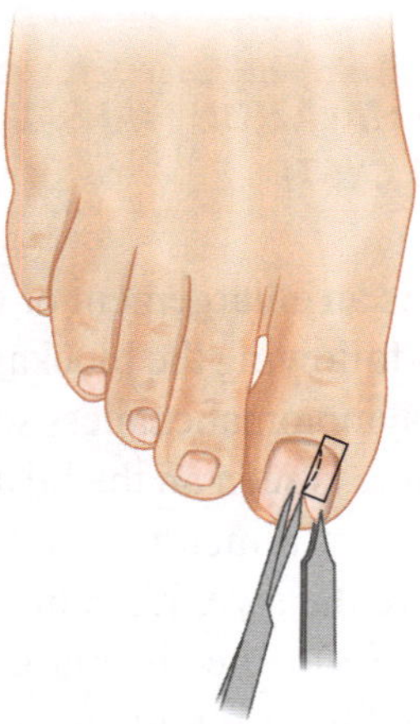

| **Fig. 44.5** Excising an ingrowing toe nail segment |

- ***Segment nail bed ablation with phenol* (SNBAP)**: This is a very easy procedure (never mind the big name) with more than 90% success rate and can be very conveniently done at a GP's clinic. It is less painful than wedge resection as destruction of the tissue is less. This treatment of choice – simple surgery – should be learnt by all GPs aspiring to do minor surgery. The principle is to destroy the nail matrix by means of a chemical cautery using 80% phenol (and not the 5% phenol in water used for injecting piles). After giving digital nerve block and applying a tourniquet, the part of the nail adjoining the inflamed tissue is cut and removed taking care that no fragments of nail are remaining (wedge resection). The resulting gutter is cleaned of the redundant tissue. Petroleum jelly is applied to the surrounding area. 80% phenol dipped in cotton is then placed in this gutter for 3–5 min. After this period, the cotton is removed, the excess phenol is wiped away by spirit and the part bandaged. It is as simple as that! Throughout the procedure, the doctor should wear protective gloves and avoid spilling phenol. Dressing is continued till complete healing has taken place, which is about 1–2 weeks.
- ***Segmental or total nail bed excision* (Zadek's procedure)**: These are the procedures undertaken only if SNBAP or wedge resection fails. Here, the part or whole of the nail, nail bed and the germinal epithelium is removed fully, so that the nail never regrows. The surgery is quite mutilating and should be considered 'major', to be done by 'major' surgeons. It cures but leaves nice and beautiful scars!

ONYCHOGRYPHOSIS

This is a condition where a few or all the toe nails are curved, thickened and distorted. It is commonly seen in the elderly, who have developed this condition over a period of years. Occasionally, it is seen in young individuals following trauma.

Simple removal of the nail will result in recurrence. The procedure for treating onychogryphosis is SNBAP with a slight modification. Instead of removing part of the nail, the whole nail is removed under ring block and the raw surface is then phenolised. Thus, it is 'total' nail bed ablation as opposed to 'segmental' ablation done for in-growing toe nail. Two or three toe nails can be subjected to this form of treatment at one sitting. Zadek's procedure is too radical for more than a few toe nails and that too in an elderly individual.

DORSAL SLIT OF THE PREPUCE

This is required to be done under three situations. A patient with a tight congenital phimosis has to be catheterized urgently. The tight phimosis does not allow the catheter in. Circumcision can correct the phimosis, but is a time consuming procedure and is not practical under the situation. The second situation is a case of acute balanoposthitis (infection of both the glans and prepuce)—the prepuce cannot be retracted and hence, the pus trapped inside cannot be drained. Lastly, dorsal slit of the constricting ring of a tight paraphimosis is at times required.

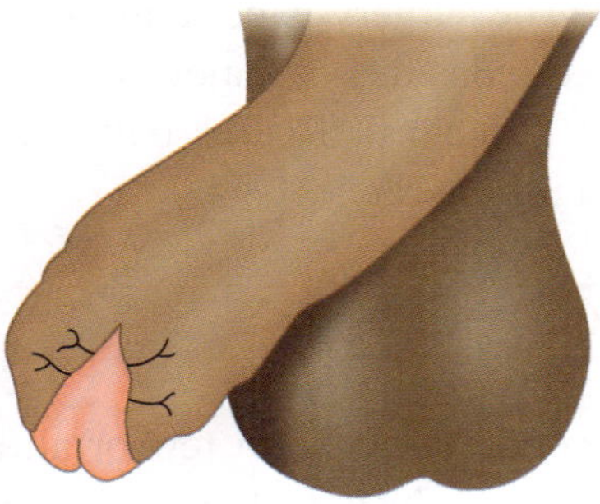

| Fig. 44.6 Dorsal slit of the prepuce |

The penis is anaesthetised using a penile block (lignocaine without adrenaline). Two artery clips are then applied lightly to the prepuce at 11'o clock and 1'o clock position. The prepuce is then cut at 12'o clock position by a pair of fine scissors for about 1–2 cm. (Don't put the blade of the scissors inside the urethra!) Bleeders are tied by No. 4 catgut. The inner and outer layers of the prepuce are sutured with No. 3 catgut. The tip of the prepuce has now a 'V' shaped 'defect,' which allows the retraction of the prepuce over the glans.

EXCISING A CHALAZION (TARSAL CYST OR MEIBOMIAN CYST)

A **chalazion** is an enlargement of a tarsal gland in the eyelids following the blockage of its duct. It is usually asymptomatic unless secondarily infected. A nodule is seen on the lid about the size of a pea a few millimetres away from the lid margin. Unlike the stye, it is non-painful, non-tender, away from the lid margin and takes weeks or months to attain the size of a pea. Thereafter, the size remains the same.

On everting the eyelid, the conjunctiva over the swelling is seen discoloured. It may spontaneously disappear or remain permanent without treatment.

Treatment consists of incision and curettage through the palpebral conjunctiva under local anaesthesia. An inexpensive chalazion forceps (Fig. 44.8) and a chalazion spoon is all that is required, which can be purchased from any corner surgical store. 2% lignocaine with adrenaline is instilled in the eye every 2 min for two or three times. 2% plain lignocaine is then infiltrated in the lid surrounding the chalazion with a 26 no. insulin syringe till a swelling is seen.

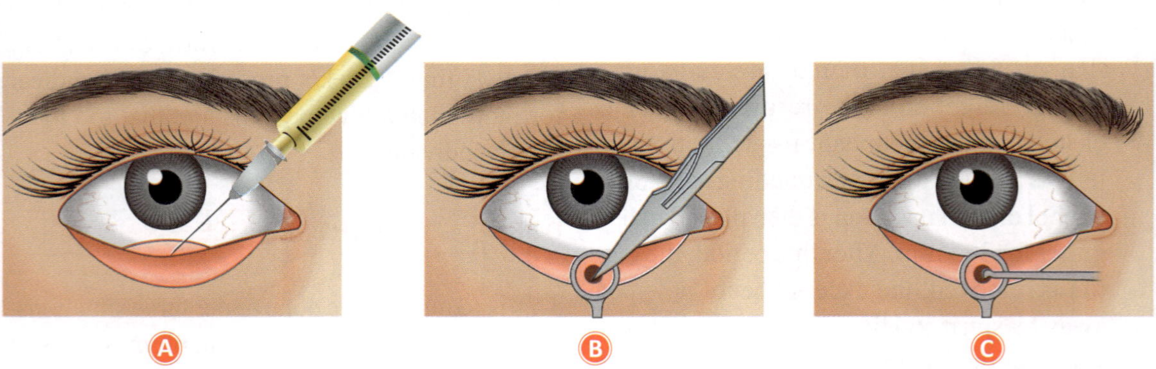

| Fig. 44.7 Excising a chalazion |

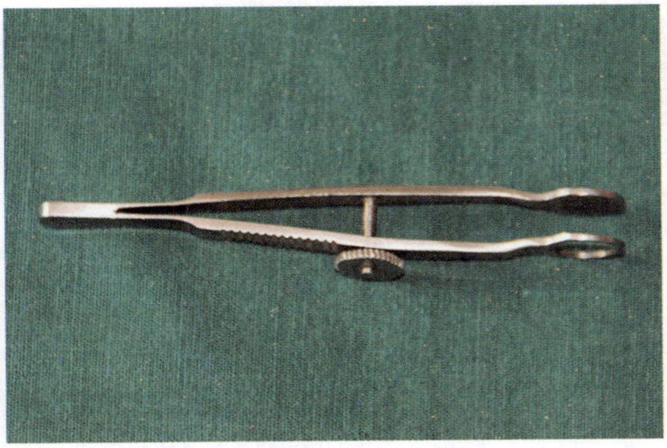

| Fig. 44.8 Chalazion forceps |

The chalazion is fixed with the chalazion forceps by putting the flat disc on the outer surface of the lid and the hollow ring on the inner surface, so that the chalazion lies in the centre of the ring. This holds the lid steady and also prevents bleeding, which will otherwise interfere with the procedure. The eyelid is then everted so that the inner surface is exposed. A vertical incision is made with a scalpel at the centre of the cyst and the contents curetted with the chalazion spoon.

After putting chloramphenicol eye ointment, the eye is padded for 24 hrs. The patient must be warned that after the procedure blood fills up the empty cavity and the swelling may be seen for a few days. Otherwise, the patient declares that the operation has failed!

GP Tip

What do you do if a patient with a scalp injury is bleeding profusely and refuses stitches to stop the bleeding?
Simple: Take bunch of hair on either side of the wound and tie them across the wound!

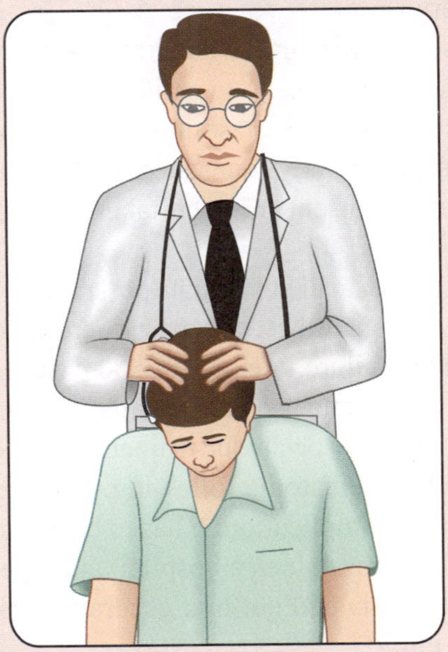

CHAPTER 45

Advanced Minor Surgery

- Vasectomy
- Excising a Ganglion
- Circumcision
- Removing Cervical Lymph Node
- Managing Piles

VASECTOMY

Under no circumstances the procedure should be undertaken lightly and without proper training. The procedure itself though simple is not without complications—medical, surgical, social or otherwise.

- Vasectomy is virtually an irreversible procedure, as there is no guarantee that it can be successfully re-anastamosed. The patient must be correctly counselled on this issue and written consent must be taken before surgery.
- There is a small but definite possibility of failure even in the best of hands. There is a documented failure rate of 1 in 500 cases.
- Vasovagal attacks, bradycardia or even convulsions may occur due to traction on the vas.
- Scrotal haematoma following vasectomy is a major complication. It has to be drained as early as possible in a hospital under general anaesthesia and not in a general practitioner's clinic.
- Finally, it has to be remembered that spermatozoa remain in the proximal vas for several months after vasectomy. Hence, it is essential to warn the patient to avoid unprotected intercourse till the sperm count becomes zero, which takes about two months. Otherwise, you may have to deal with an unwanted pregnancy.

Palpate the vas which is felt like a thick cord like structure near the neck of the scrotum. Bring it as close to the scrotal skin as possible with the grip of your left hand thumb and index finger. While still holding the vas near the surface, infiltrate the tissue around the vas with 2% lignocaine. Still holding the vas, take a small vertical incision on the skin with a scalpel blade (Fig. 45.1a–c). Gradually, dee-pen the incision till the vas is visualized as a dense white structure. By gentle dissection, the vas is separated from the spermatic cord. By holding it with an Allis forceps, a 5-mm loop is pulled out and artery forceps are placed on the proximal and distal

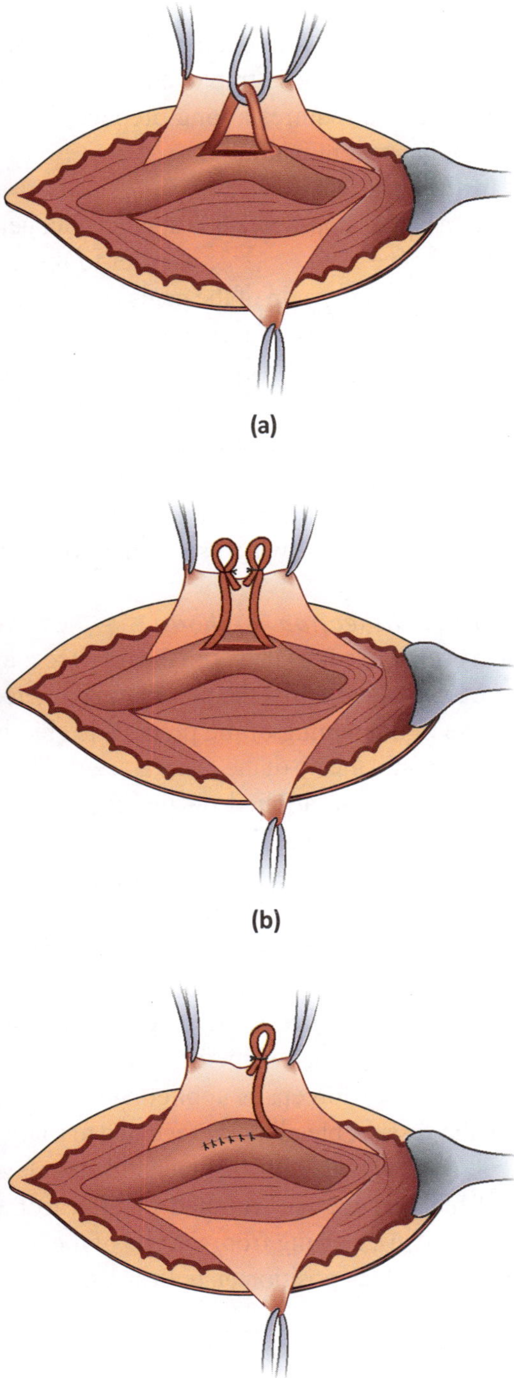

(a)

(b)

(c)

| **Fig. 45.1** Vasectomy |

ends of the loop. A short segment of the loop is cut.

One end is ligated and then turned back on itself and ligated again. This end is kept outside the spermatic cord. The other end is ligated and pushed inside the spermatic cord. Thus, the two ends are separated in an effort to prevent the recanalization of the vas. No skin sutures are usually necessary on the loose skin of the scrotum.

EXCISING A GANGLION

Ganglia are innocent tumours. They do not cause any significant symptoms except mild pain. They may disappear spontaneously and many times a surgery planned well in advance gets cancelled because at the appointment date the ganglion is nowhere to be seen! Aspiration and injecting a sclerosant is worth a trial though more than half will recur. Ganglia on the dorsum of the hand or foot can be easily excised by a GP. Ganglia at the other sites, like the ventral aspect of the forearm are in close proximity to important structures (nerves, vessels, tendons, etc.) and are best dealt with by a competent surgeon.

It is important to remember that the jelly like fluid inside the ganglion is in communication with a tendon sheath or a joint capsule. This anatomical fact has two surgical implications. First, aspiration will usually result in a recurrence, as the cyst will refill from below. Secondly, surgical excision is not that simple, as it involves removing the cyst *in toto* as well as closing the communication securely.

A transverse incision is made over the ganglion and the ganglion visualized by pulling the skin edges by retractors. The overlying fascia is stripped-off by using blunt dissection taking care not to cut open the wall of the cyst. Dissection is facilitated by flexion of the wrist as it makes the ganglion more prominent. If the cyst wall is accidentally opened, the dissection is difficult and the recurrence rate is high. The dissection is further carried down to the origin at the tendon sheath. The ganglion is held by a non-toothed forceps and excised. The skin is sutured with nylon.

CIRCUMCISION

This surgery assumes that you have been adequately trained by a competent surgeon, before operating independently. It is done for phimosis, either congenital or acquired. In children, it is important to remember that the foreskin normally cannot be retracted easily till the age of 3 years and circumcision should not be hurriedly advised. Surgery is indicated only if there is recurrent balanitis because of phimosis or for religious reasons or because the phimosis is very tight (as indicated by ballooning of the prepuce seen during the act of micturition). In the adults, it is usually indicated because phimosis is causing pain during intercourse or because of recurrent paraphimosis or because of the presence of exuberant prepusal warts.

It is a safe surgery if two aspects are taken care of. Firstly, during surgery the bleeders must be securely ligated, so that there is no heavy bleeding once the patient is sent back home. Secondly, during surgery enough skin of the prepuce is preserved for the purpose of erection. This will be explained in detail below.

A general anaesthesia is required in children but a local anaesthesia is adequate in adults. It is very important not to use lignocaine *with adrenaline* even by mistake in a penile block as this can result in gangrene of the penis, a disastrous condition. Plain 2% lignocaine is infiltrated at the base of the penis as described under 'local anaesthetic techniques'.

Technique of Operation

In children, the guillotine method is used while the dissection method is employed in adults. The former method requires a long prepuce, which may not be present in adults.

In the classical *guillotine method*, used in infants, a pair of sinus forceps is applied obliquely to the prepuce **(Fig. 45.2a)**, parallel to the corona, just beyond the tip of the penis and the skin distal to the forceps is excised (chopped off) with scissors. The sinus forceps are then removed. The outer layer of the skin retracts leaving the glans covered by the inner layer. After securing all bleeders with No. 4 catgut, the cut edges of the inner and outer layers are approximated with No. 3 catgut sutures, which spontaneously dissolve in 7–10 days.

In the *dissection method* **(Fig. 45.2b)**, which is used in adults in whom the prepuce may not be long enough, first the prepuce is retracted until the tight opening of the prepuce is clearly visible (or until the tip of the glans is seen). Three artery forceps are applied on the edge of the prepuce, one on the midline ventrally (6'o clock position) and two on either side of the midline dorsally (11'o clock and 1'o clock positions). The prepuce is then slit with a pair of fine scissors in the midline dorsally in between the two forceps (12'o clock position), reaching about 1½ cm distal to the coronal sulcus. If, before the incision is taken, an artery forceps is applied vertically to crush the vessels, bleeding is prevented to a large extent. At this level, both the inner and outer layers of the prepuce are trimmed parallel to the coronal sulcus, starting from the end of the incision at 12'o clock position on both sides, to meet at the frenulum.

The area between the glans and the overlying skin is cleaned and the smegma removed. Small oozers are stopped by pressure with a gauze piece while bigger bleeders are tied with

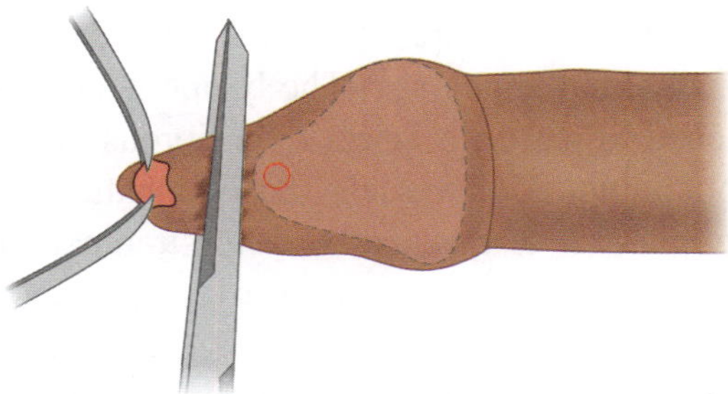

| **Fig. 45.2a** Circumcision: Guillotine method |

No.4 catgut. The inner and outer edges are then sutured with No.3 catgut. The ends of the ventral and the dorsal sutures should be kept long for the final dressings (all other methods of dressings are notoriously difficult to keep in place). Either sofratulle or a roll of gauze impregnated in povidone iodine is rolled around the sutures and held in place by the long ventral and dorsal sutures. The sutures need not be removed as they will fall off spontaneously in 7–10 days.

How to Tie the Bleeders?

A very important step, if an acute embarrassment to the doctor is to be prevented. A not so uncommon situation is when the patient is discharged and goes home, he starts bleeding from the operated site, probably after an erection. Some surgeons as a precautionary measure, give oestrogens to prevent erection.

You will require two tiny curved artery forceps and No.4 catgut. Hold the bleeder with an artery forceps with its tip pointing downwards. Once the bleeding has stopped, take the other artery forceps and with its tip pointing upwards, hold it transversely below the first to catch the bleeder. Remove the first forceps slowly. Now wind the catgut below the artery forceps and tie a knot. Once the bleeder is securely ligated, remove the second artery forceps. Repeat the procedure with other bleeders before proceeding to the next step, i.e., approximation of the inner and outer layers of the skin of the prepuce.

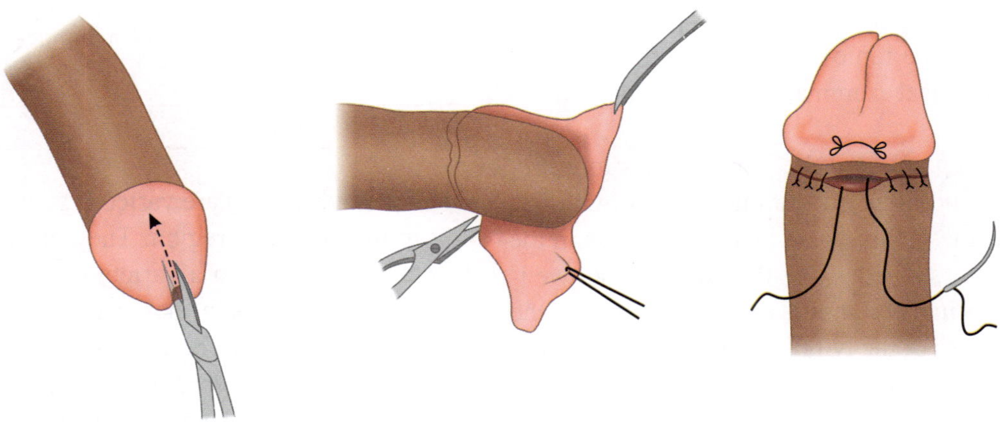

| **Fig. 45.2b** Circumcision: Dissection method |

Note: It is better to preserve a little extra preputial skin to prevent painful erection later on because of too little skin. Shorter skin gives better cosmetic results in a non-erect penis, while a longer skin gives better sexual performance in an erect penis (and that matters!).

REMOVING A CERVICAL LYMPH NODE FOR BIOPSY

Cervical lymphadenopathy is an extremely common condition. There are approximately 800 lymph nodes in the body, out which about 300 lie in the neck. The enlargement of these lymph nodes could be because of diverse aetiology like tuberculous lymphadenitis, chronic non-tuberculous lymphadenitis, subacute bacterial lymphadenitis or Hodgkin's disease. Ideally, lymph nodes in the neck should be removed under general anaesthesia by a competent surgeon, as there are important structures underneath.

However, if the GP is experienced, one or two of these lymph nodes which are easily palpable, and which mainly lie in the poste-rior triangle, can be removed for the purpose of histopathological examination by using local anaesthesia.

Having selected the lymph nodes to be removed and after infiltrating the skin with 2% lignocaine, a transverse incision is made in the line of the skin crease on the centre of the swelling. This incision should extend well beyond the boundaries of the lymph node so that the whole dissection is carried out with a good view of the surrounding important structures.

The fat and superficial fascia is cut by a No.15 scalpel blade and the area properly exposed by means of retractors. The further isolation of the lymph node is carried out by blunt dissection. If the external jugular vein or any other small vessels cannot be freed from the lymph node, they can be safely ligated at two points and cut in the centre, without untoward effects of any kind at any age. The lymph node is attached to the deep fascia by a fibrous pedicle containing blood vessels and lymphatics. The lymph node is grasped by a non-traumatizing Babcock's forceps, and an artery forceps is placed on the pedicle (Fig. 45.3). A ligature is placed below the artery forceps and the pedicle divided in between the forceps and the ligature. The lymph node is taken out along with the artery forceps and sent for histopathology. The subcutaneous tissue is closed by 3/0 catgut and the skin by 3/0 nylon.

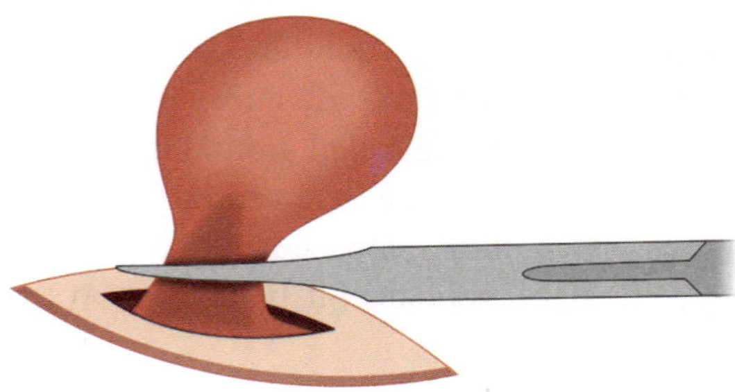

| Fig. 45.3 Removal of a lymph node |

MANAGING PILES

Haemorrhoids (piles) are varicose veins occurring in the anorectal region. They present to a general practitioner in a variety of ways, e.g., bleeding, perianal pain, perianal pruritus, etc. Conditions which can be confused with a pile mass include anal polyp, rectal prolapse or even a simple skin tag. Fissures and fistulas are usually readily diagnosed. Piles are either internal or external to the anal orifice.

The external variety is covered by skin while the internal variety is covered by mucous membrane. Another way in which piles can be classified is as follows:

First degree piles are restricted to the lower rectum and the upper anal canal. They cause painless per rectal bleeding. They are not seen perianally on inspection and cannot be palpated on per rectal examination unless thrombosed. They can however, be seen through a proctoscope.

Second degree piles are internally located. They prolapse during defaecation, get spontaneously reduced or can be reduced manually.

Third degree piles are permanently prolapsed outside and cannot be reduced manually.

First and second degree piles can be adequately treated by either a sclerosant injection or by rubber band ligation. Both are simple-to-learn procedures, do not require a general anaesthetic and can be easily dealt with by a general practitioner after a minimal training. *Third degree piles* require surgery.

Injection of Haemorrhoids

The idea of this treatment is to produce fibrosis of the submucosa of the rectum above the pile mass by injecting a small quantity of a sclerosant like 5% phenol in almond oil. The fibrosis stops bleeding from the piles by obliterating the vessels and also prevents prolapse by fixing the loose mucous membrane. Note that 80% phenol should never be used as it can cause severe necrosis of the rectal wall.

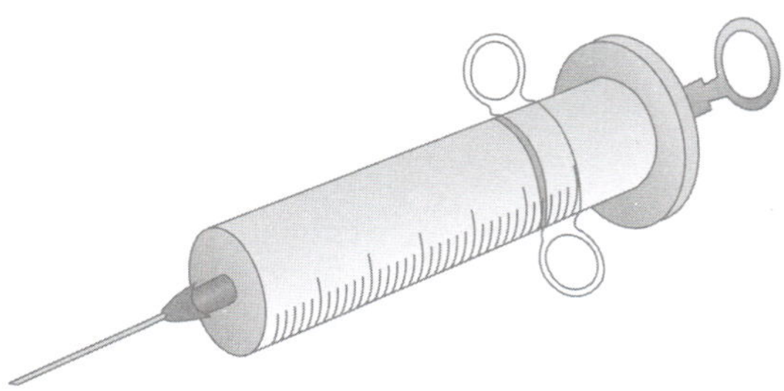

Fig. 45.4 Gabriel's syringe

The patient is made to lie down in the left lateral position. A proctoscope is fully introduced after lubricating with lignocaine jelly, so that the end of the instrument is beyond the pile mass. Now the proctoscope is gradually withdrawn. The piles will be seen to prolapse into the top of instrument generally at 3, 7 and 11'o clock positions. Using Gabriel's syringe (Fig. 45.4), with the bevel of the needle directed towards the rectal wall, 3–5 mL of 5% phenol is injected just above the pile mass. *The tip of the needle should be in the submucous layer.* This is confirmed by first moving the needle towards the centre of the proctoscope which is not possible if the tip is deep in the muscles of the rectum. If it is very superficial in the mucous membrane, then a white spot will immediately be seen after the injection is commenced. If it is rightly placed in the submucous layer, it makes a pale swelling over which fine capillaries are visible. The injection is repeated in the other piles. The procedure is painless as the rectal wall above the dentate line is insensitive. In mild cases a single injection is usually sufficient. In severe cases this may be repeated after 6 weeks. There are hardly ever any complications of the procedure except failure to achieve the desired results.

Banding of Haemorrhoids

Again this is a fairly simple procedure producing equally good results without the use of hazardous chemicals. The idea here is to apply one or preferably two rubber bands at the base of the pile mass, thus cutting off its blood supply and introducing ischaemic necrosis of the pile mass, which then sloughs off in 7–10 days.

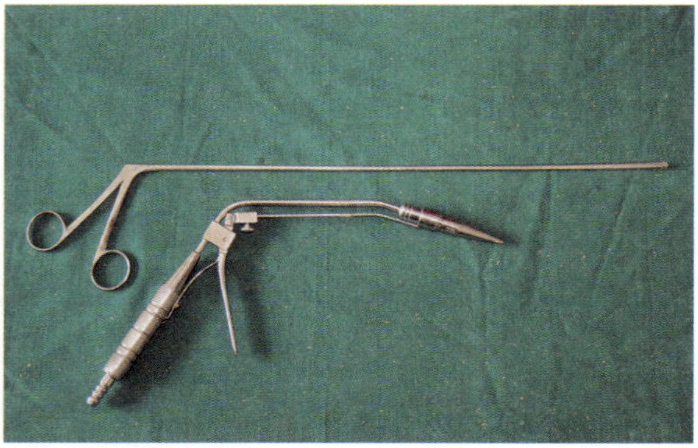

| **Fig. 45.5** Instruments used for banding of haemorrhoids |

Exactly the same procedure described above is followed but instead of the phenol injection, rubber band ligation is done at the base of the pile mass by a rubber band applicator. The pile mass is grasped with a forceps and pulled gently through the ring of the applicator. The band is then released and applied to the base of the pile.

The pile mass strangulates, which is seen to immediately change its colour to white. The same procedure is repeated in the other piles.

Again, there is hardly any major complication except pain, discharge or bleeding. Give pain-killers, warn the patient about the discharge and give cotton-wool pads underneath the undergarments to prevent staining by blood. Following both the procedures, the patient is instructed to eat a high roughage diet and is prescribed a laxative for a week or so.

CHAPTER 46

Intralesional Steroid Injections

- Indications
- Precautions
- Side Effects
- Types of Steroid Injections Used
- Method of Injecting and the Doses of Triamcinolone

Systemic steroids are the mainstay of treatment of many acute and chronic skin diseases where the response is often dramatic. The only inhibition to use them is their side effect profile. Of course, they are definitely indicated and are to be used in high doses without reservations in life threatening skin diseases like pemphigus vulgaris or Stevens-Johnson syndrome. They can also be very freely used in acute dermatosis like drug reactions where they are required to be given only for short periods. In chronic generalized dermatosis like lichen planus or nummular eczema, they may have to be given for prolonged periods. The side effects can be minimized by giving the whole dose in morning or as pulse therapy. However, in chronic localized psoriasis, their prolonged use is unwarranted and local therapy indicated.

Local steroidal therapy is given in the form of topical steroid ointments. Because of its amazing effectiveness, a big range of steroid ointments are available for more than half a century. However, even topical steroids are not devoid of side effects and number of adverse side effects have been documented after their prolonged and excessive use. Local side effects include atrophy, straie formation, delayed healing, purpura, de-pigmentation, etc. Systemic absorption is another hazard that can suppress the HPA axis, more so in infants and young children. Another limitation of topical steroid ointments is their restricted ability to cross the epidermal barrier giving rise to partial and at best a temporary response.

In specialized circumstances therefore *intradermal* (intralesional) injections of high concentrations of steroids is injected at the site of the lesion so that the drug acts at a place where it is required to act. This in addition prevents exposure of the rest of the body to a drug whose action is really required only in a particular part of the diseased skin. Adrenal suppression here too is always possible, but is rarely if ever encountered in clinical practice.

INDICATIONS

This modality of treatment is very useful in chronic localized dermatosis where there are a few lesions only. There is no role of intralesional steroid injections in acute oozing dermatosis. There are many indications for its use, but in general practice there are six common conditions, which can be easily diagnosed and treated.

1. Chronic lichenified (thickened) eczema of the ankle
2. Two to three chronic localized stable plaques of psoriasis
3. Alopecia areata
4. Keloids and hypertrophic scars
5. Lichen simplex chronicus (neurodermatitis) of the nape of the neck
6. Cystic acne
7. Chalazion

There are other indications for its use. But these are best dealt with by qualified dermatalogists, as diagnosis can be difficult for a general practitioner, e.g., discoid lupus erythematosis (DLE), hydradenitis suppurativa, certain nail dystrophies, etc.

PRECAUTIONS

- Be absolutely sure of the diagnosis before injecting (confidently diagnosing six dermatogical conditions is no big deal). Don't commit the mistake of giving intralesional steroid in a patch of fungal infection!
- Observe strict aseptic precautions. Prepare the area with povidone-iodine and spirit. Use disposable syringes only. See that there is no secondary infection present. This will exacerbate if injected with high dose steroid and the lesion will not heal for months and may even ulcerate. Postpone injection till the infection is totally eradicated with proper antibiotics.
- Rule out diabetes (uncontrolled) before injecting.

SIDE EFFECTS

In spite of the above precautions, the following mild and temporary side effects can occur.

- ***Temporary local atrophy***: This can occur if higher than recommended doses are used or if the injection is made at deeper levels. Some individuals are predisposed to development of atrophy, when this can develop at normal doses. This atrophy is however temporary and the skin reverts back to normal in a few weeks.
- ***Temporary depigmentation of the skin***: Again with higher doses or deep seated injections. The 'leucoderma' patch might be alarming to the patient. Assure the patient that this is temporary.
- ***Secondary infection***: This is rare if proper aseptic precautions are taken.
- Theoretical possibility of ***adrenal suppression***.

TYPES OF STEROID INJECTIONS USED

Although hydrocortisone and methyl prednisolone (Depo-medrol) have been used, the most popular steroid for intralesional therapy is triamcinolone- acetonide (Kenacort, Tricort, etc.). Unlike methyl prednisolone, triamcinolone has small particle size and forms a homogeneous suspension after a little shaking. This property decreases the rare possibility of small vessel blockage. (A few patients of alopecia areata on the scalp near the forehead developed blindness a few years back after they were treated with larger particulate suspension of ethyl prednisolone.) This possibility is further diminished as commercially available triamcinolone is to be diluted before use.

Triamcinolone is available as 10 mg/mL and 40 mg/mL vials. For all the above indications, 10 mg/mL vial is recommended, except in case of keloids where 40 mg/mL vial is used.

METHOD OF INJECTING AND THE DOSES OF TRIAMCINOLONE TO BE USED

This will vary with the site and the indication of intralesional therapy.

1. Lichenified Eczema, Neurodermatitis, Psoriasis

Usually an area of about 10 sq cm will require 10 mg of triamcinolone. The calculated dose is then taken in a disposable syringe and diluted approximately four times (i.e., 2.5 mg/mL) with plain lignocaine 2%. This dilution provides enough steroid to reduce inflammation and at the same time reducing the above side effects.

The injection is to be made within the lesion using a small bore needle like No. 24 or No. 26. In a small patch, a single prick should suffice. In a larger patch, injections at multiple sites will be required, in which case it is less painful to give the second injection through the previously anaesthetized area. An attempt should be made to deposit the drug as uniformly in the lesion as possible.

The injection can be repeated after 2 weeks or so till the desired effect has been achieved. The drug remains in the tissue for 6 months or 1 year in decreasing concentrations. After this period the lesion might relapse. This can then be safely re-injected.

2. Alopecia Areata

The aim is to inject adequate amounts of steroid near the root of the hair follicles where the inflammatory cells lie.

Take 5 mg of triamcinolone (1/2 mL of 10 mg/mL vial) in an insulin syringe. Dilute to 1 mL with lignocaine and inject this solution in 1–2 cm of the alopecia areata patch. More amounts will be required in a larger patch and the whole patch should be covered with multiple injections as above.

Some growth of hair (thin villous hair) should be evident after 4–6 weeks. If not, the injection should be repeated. If no growth is seen after 6 months, re-growth of hair is unlikely and it is then not worth repeating the injection.

3. Cystic Acne

Take 2.5 mg of triamcinolone in an insulin syringe and dilute it to 1 mL with lignocaine. Inject into this sterile, nonpyogenic but inflammatory lesion so that the cyst just distends slightly. Ideally the injection should be given into unruptured or unincised cyst. The response is often dramatic, the acne regressing rapidly in 48 hrs.

4. Keloids and Hypertrophic Scars

There is excessive connective tissue response to injury and hence there is hypertrophy. High dose local steroids cause atrophy and this side effect is then utilized to treat keloids.

Obviously high doses of *undiluted* triamcinolone are to be used.

Give a field block anaesthesia below and surrounding the keloid. Wait for about 5 min. Fill 20 mg, i.e., 0.5 mL of triamcinolone of 40 mg/mL vial in an insulin syringe and deposit this undiluted in the substance of the keloid. It is difficult to force the solution in the tough keloid mass and having forcibly achieved this, once the insulin syringe needle is withdrawn the solution may trickle out.

Hence, immediate pressure with a cotton wool should be applied. The lesion is reassessed after a month and if necessary the injection can be repeated every month for 2 or 3 months.

5. Chalazion

A moderate sized chalazion can be injected with local steroid with good result (see Chapter 8).

Conclusion: This is an easily mastered result oriented therapy and gives dramatic results in the indications described above.

CHAPTER 47

Steroid Injection Techniques in and around Joints

- Injections into Soft Tissues
- Intra-articular Injections

I find no reason why a good aspiring general practitioner should not use this modality of treatment very freely and very effectively in his day-to-day practice.

Advantages

It does not require any sophisticated instruments and can be easily carried out as an office procedure in one's own clinic. A set up of an operation theatre is not required. It is easy to learn. Many techniques like injecting the tennis elbow or the plantar fascia are simple and can be learned simply by reading this chapter or other similar articles on the subject. A few techniques which are difficult like injecting the shoulder joint or the wrist joint in case of the carpal tunnel syndrome, can be learned under the guidance of your orthopaedic friend or from an experienced "injector". A basic knowledge of anatomy is sufficient. Complications are rare if sound technique is practised, good aseptic precautions taken and the do's and don'ts given in Table 47.1 are adhered to. Septic arthritis which the GP fears is very rare. Steroids have excellent anti-inflammatory and fibrinolytic activity. The drug is delivered at the site of pathology in excellent concentration. It is thus result oriented, which is an important feature for any general practice to flourish.

Disadvantages

Steroids reduce immunity at a local level far greater than the generalised immunity. This may predispose to sepsis, which may be difficult to treat and may have medicolegal implications. Steroids cause local osteoporosis and should be avoided in and around osteoporotic bones.

General Guidelines

Every precaution must be taken to avoid introducing infection. A strict no-touch technique, using disposable needles and syringes, avoiding multidose vials and instead using single dose ampoules, all reduce the risk of infection. Sterile gloves are highly recommended.

| **Table 47.1** Do's and don'ts of local steroid injections |

Do's
▪ Always take strict aseptic precautions. ▪ Always use a local anaesthetic except when injecting near a nerve, as this may mask an intraneural injection. ▪ Always warn patient of post injection flare up.
Don'ts
▪ Do not inject in the presence of infection (either septic arthritis or overlying cellulitis). ▪ Do not inject in the presence of uncontrolled diabetes. ▪ Do not inject into a tendon (can lead to rupture). ▪ Do not inject into a nerve (can lead to permanent damage). ▪ Do not inject very superficially in the skin (can lead to atrophy & depigmentation). ▪ Do not inject into unstable joint. ▪ Do not inject into the joint when there is intra-articular fracture. ▪ Do not inject in patients with coagulation disorders.

The injection site should be identified and marked by a ball pen. The area should be cleaned by spirit-povidone iodine-spirit. Injection lignocaine 2% is infiltrated at this site as local anaesthesia. A 25-gauge needle is used for small joints and a 21 gauge needle for the large joints. An 18-gauge needle is necessary for aspirating a thick viscous synovial fluid.

Many depot preparations are available (Table 47.2). The long acting preparations like methyl prednisolone (Depo-Medrol or Solu-Medrol) and triamcinolone (Kenacort or Tricort) can cause serious soft tissue atrophy, fat necrosis and depigmentation of the skin. These are hence best avoided for soft tissue injections and for small joints, where hydrocostisone (Wycort) is recommended. The long acting steroids are recommended only for large joints. The dose of the steroid used will depend on the size of the joint.

A small joint like interphalangeal joint will require only 10–15 mg of hydrocortisone, while a large joint like the knee joint will require as much as 40–80 mg of methyl prednisolone or triamcinolone.

The patient must be warned that the pain might increase the following day and that the maximum effect requires 1–2 weeks. After the intra-articular injection, the patient is advised bed rest for a minimum of 2 days. This helps in retaining the steroid in the joint for a longer period and hence gives a maximum prolonged action. If there is relapse of the pain, the injection can be repeated. Intra-articular injections in large weight bearing joints should not be repeated within 2 months and not more than 3 injections should be given in a year. Injections into small joints and soft tissues may be repeated after 1 month.

| **Table 47.2** Commonly used steroid injections |

Preparation	Concentration (mg/mL)
Short acting	
▪ Hydrocortisone	25
Long acting	
▪ Methyl prednisolone	40
▪ Triamcinolone	10, 40

INJECTIONS INTO SOFT TISSUES

Local steroid injection therapy can be used effectively for the treatment of inflammatory conditions affecting tendons and ligaments. Enthesopathies (e.g., epicondylitis), entrapment neuropathies (e.g., carpal tunnel syndrome), tenosynovitis (e.g., De Quervain's) and bursitis (e.g., infrapatellar) can be easily treated by this modality, possibly avoiding the need for surgery.

Before we discuss the common soft tissue conditions amenable to this therapy, a few points need to be stressed.

The injection should not be made into the substance of the tendon or ligament as this may cause rupture. It should be placed in the area surrounding the inflamed tissue. Similarly, an injection into the substance of a nerve may cause permanent damage to the nerve. A very superficially placed injection may cause skin atrophy and depigmentation.

Always be sure of the exact site of the original pain and the correct diagnosis of the soft tissue lesion. Point tenderness is the most important and simple physical sign while determining the site. Localised tenderness excludes referred pain. Pain and restriction of movements of the inflamed soft tissue lesion again excludes referred pain. This is particularly important in treating shoulder lesions. The shoulder pain may originate from the cervical spine or may be projected from the tennis elbow.

In most of the soft tissue lesions, there will be a point of maximum tenderness and in addition there may be distinct satellite tender spots in the surrounding area. The principle is to infiltrate all these tender spots. It is a good idea to give half the volume of the steroid plus local anaesthetic into the primary site and the remaining half into the secondary tender points. A 23-G needle with a 2-mL syringe is appropriate.

Tennis Elbow (Lateral Epicondylitis)

In this condition, there is pain at the elbow, which may be referred along the back of the forearm as far as the wrist and dorsum of the hand. The point of maximum tenderness is over or just distal to the lateral epicondyle, which rules out referred pain from the neck or the wrist.

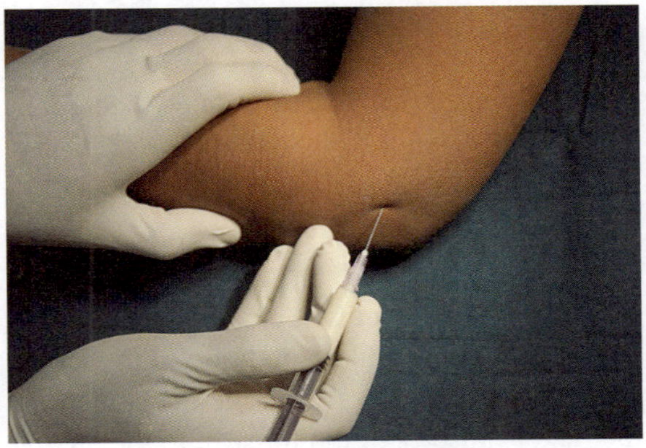

| **Fig. 47.1** Tennis elbow—injection site |

In tennis elbow, the attachment of the extensor muscles of the forearm to the lateral epicondyle is tender. This is caused by repeated, protracted or forcible wrist extension as in tennis players, though only 1% of cases actually involve tennis players.

In order to identify the point of maximum tenderness, ask the patient to pronate the forearm and extend the wrist against resistance. This point should be injected with a few droplets of a mixture of 1 mL of 2% lignocaine and 1 mL of hydrocortisone. (Avoid long acting steroids.) The needle is then inserted down until it touches the bone. A droplet is injected here and then a wide surrounding area infiltrated, with a series of half insertions and half withdrawals. Often a single injection is curative. If not, a second injection can be repeated after 6 weeks.

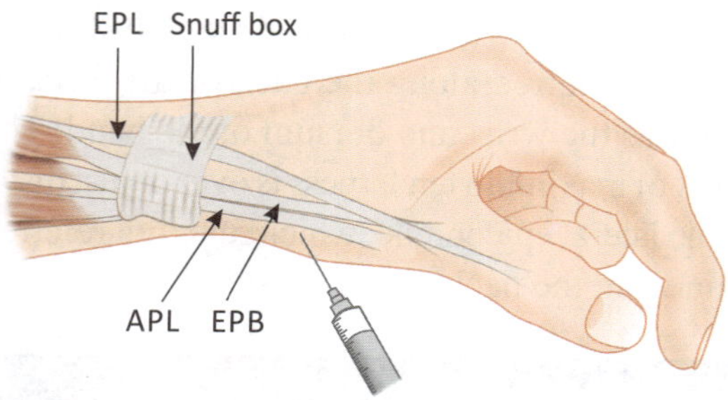

EPL—Extensor pollicis longus; EPB—Extensor pollicis brevis; APL—Abductor pollicis longus.

| **Fig. 47.2** Site for injection in De Quervain's tenosynovitis |

Golfer's Elbow (Medial Epicondylitis)

This is almost a similar condition to the tennis elbow, except that it affects the attachment of the flexor muscles of the forearm to the medial epicondyle. Resisted wrist flexion is painful and the point of maximum tenderness can be identified by this manoeuvre. The procedure for injecting hydrocortisone is similar to that in tennis elbow. Care should be taken to avoid trauma to the ulnar nerve which lies just behind the medical epicondyle.

De Quervain's Tenosynovitis

In this condition the common sheath of the tendons of the abductor pollicis longus (APL) and extensor pollicis brevis (EPB) become inflamed, thickened and finally stenosed, due to excessive and repetitive activity of the thumb. Clinically there is pain, tenderness, swelling and crepitus at the radial styloid process. If the fingers are wrapped around the thumb and the wrist gently put into ulnar deviation, the patient winces with pain (Finkelstein's test) (Figs. 47.2 & 47.3).

The tendons of APL and EPB form the palmar or radial border of the anatomical snuff box and can be identified by abducting the extended thumb. The steroid should be deposited into the sheath of the tendons and not subcutaneously or into the substance of the tendons.

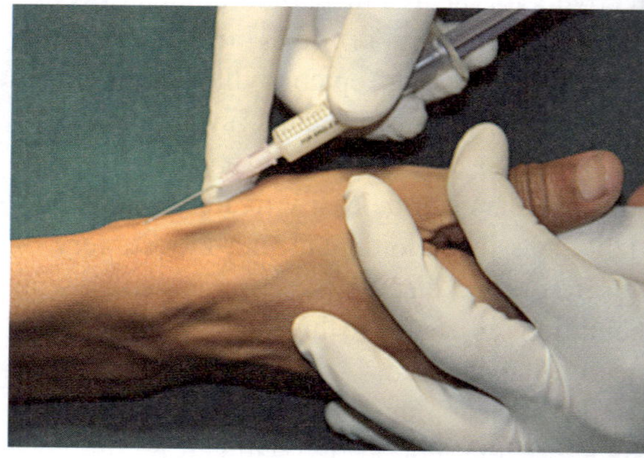

| **Fig. 47.3** De Quervain's tenosynovitis—injection site |

The needle is inserted at a point 1 cm distal to the radial styloid, advanced till it touches the tendons and then slightly withdrawn prior to injection. If the injection is deposited correctly inside the sheath, it will give rise to a sausage shaped swelling. If subcutaneous, the swelling is diffuse. If in the substance of the tendon, resistance will be felt on pushing the injection. 30–40 mg of methyl prednisolone in 1 mL of lignocaine is used. An Elastocrepe bandage is applied for 2–3 days to give rest to the part.

Trigger Finger

In this condition, which affects mainly middle aged women, the movements of the flexor tendon inside the fibrous flexor sheath is hampered and painful. This is either because the fibrous sheath is thickened and narrowed or there is a nodule formation on the tendon just distal to the constricted sheath. The tendon with the nodule can be forced down through the narrowed sheath by the powerful flexor muscles, but the patient finds it difficult to extend the finger with the rather weak extensor muscles. Hence, the finger gets locked in flexion. If the finger now is extended forcibly, the nodule enters the fibrous sheath with a click like a trigger of a pistol, hence the nomenclature.

It is usually possible to locate this nodule on the distal palm by firm palpation, when the patient's finger is passively flexed and extended. The aim is to inject 15–20 mg of methyl prednisolone or triamcinolone near the nodule inside the flexor sheath. A local anaesthetic like lignocaine is required. It can be directly infiltrated around the nodule, but the injection into the skin of the palm can be very painful.

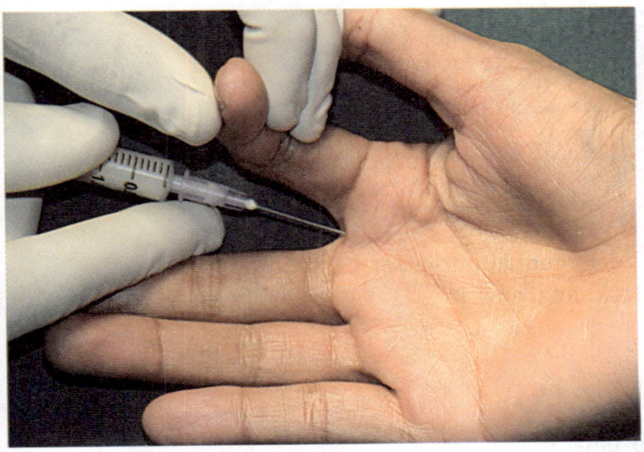

| Fig. 47.4 Local anaesthesia for trigger finger |

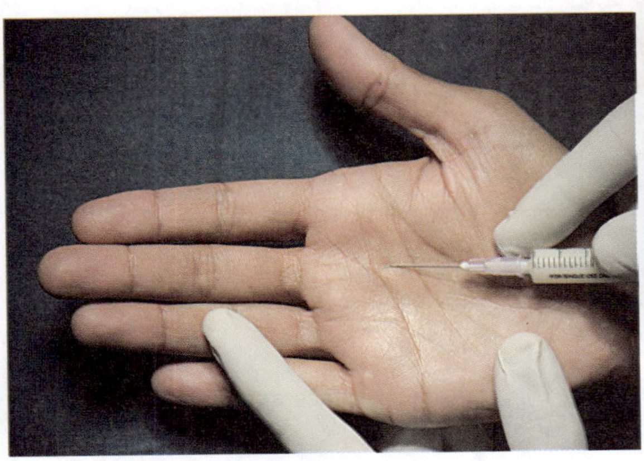

| Fig. 47.5 Trigger finger—injection site |

Alternatively, the skin can be entered through the soft dorsal skin of the web-space and lignocaine placed below the nodule. Once the palmar skin is anaesthetised, the steroid injection is made through the palm. The needle is inserted into the skin of the palm at 30° just distal to the distal palmar crease. The needle is slid into the flexor sheath and the steroid is injected. Before injecting the steroid make sure the needle is not in the substance of the tendon, by asking the patient to flex and extend the digit. If the needle moves with this movement then it is in the tendon and should be repositioned. If the sheath cannot be entered, the injection is given partly into the nodule and partly on either side.

Carpal Tunnel Syndrome

The carpal tunnel is bounded anteriorly by the flexor retinaculum and posteriorly by the carpal bones. The median nerve and the flexor tendons pass through this tunnel. If the contents of the tunnel increase in bulk (because of pregnancy, rheumatoid arthritis, myxoedema, etc.), the median nerve will get compressed, giving rise to the carpal tunnel syndrome (Figs. 47.6–47.8).

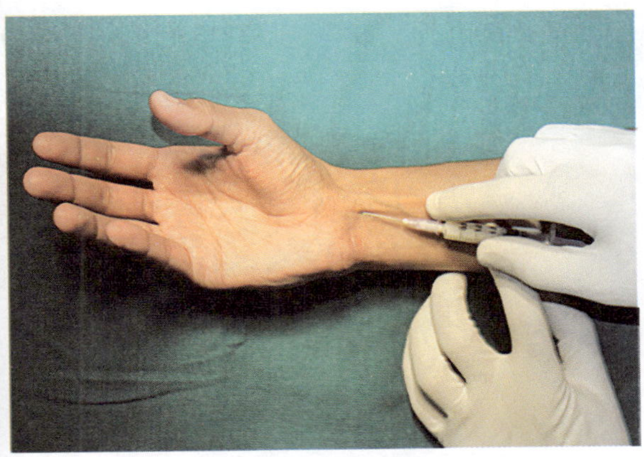

| Fig. 47.6 Injection into carpal tunnel |

In a classical case, the patient complains of pain and tingling numbness localised to the distribution of the median nerve in the hand, i.e., the

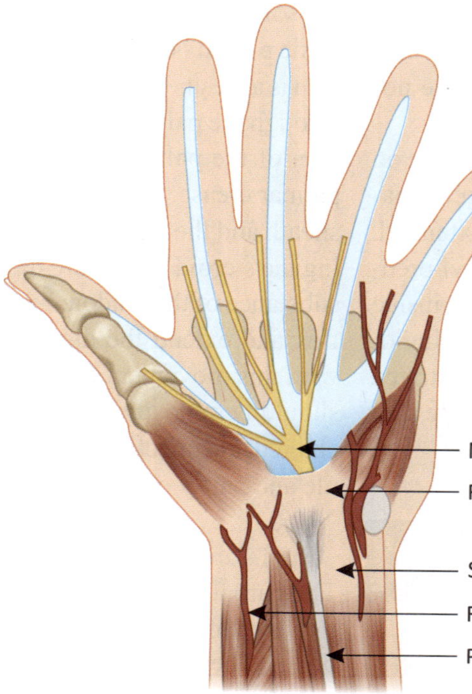

| **Fig. 47.7** Site for injection (dark spot) near median nerve for CT syndrome shown by arrow. Basic anatomy |

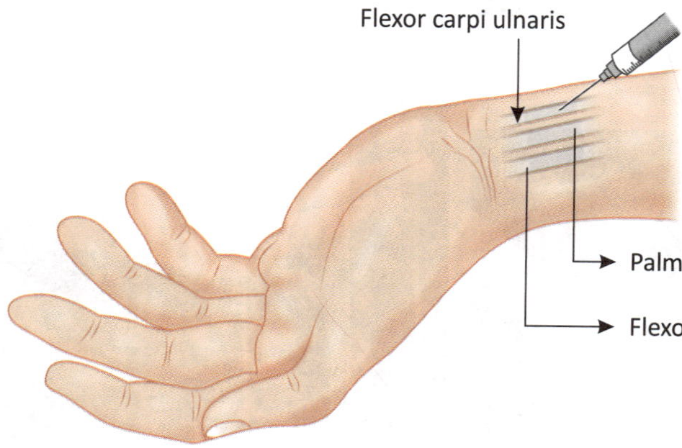

| **Fig. 47.8** Site for injection near median nerve for CT syndrome. Surface anatomy |

radial 3½ fingers on the palmar aspect of the hand. The little finger is spared and the middle finger is maximally involved. Typically the pain is worse at night waking up the patient and is relieved by hanging the hand over the edge of the bed. In an advanced case, there may be wasting of the thenar muscles. However, the pain may not be localized but shoots upwards making it difficult for the physician to differentiate it from tennis elbow or even cervical spondylosis. In case of doubt, the symptoms can be reproduced by keeping the wrist fully flexed for 2 min (Phalen's test).

About 30–40 mg of methyl prednisolone is to be injected into the carpal tunnel, taking care not to pierce the median nerve. This nerve lies in the middle of the wrist beneath the palmaris longus tendon, which can be identified by asking the patient to pinch the thumb and the little finger together or by active wrist flexion against resistance.

The forearm is supported in full supination and the wrist extended. The point of entry into the skin is identified, marked and anaesthetised about 1 cm proximal to the line of the joint on the *ulnar side of the palmaris longus tendon*. In 15% of the people, this tendon is absent and then the point is identified 1/2 cm to the ulnar side of the midline.

The skin is punctured at this point by a needle attached to a syringe filled with the steroid and advanced gradually. Resistance is felt as the carpal tunnel is pierced if the syringe is held lightly. In order to avoid the median nerve, it is important to penetrate the flexor retinaculum and no further. The steroid is then injected. In case the median nerve is pierced, there will be tingling numbness and the needle should be repositioned. In case a tendon has been pierced there will be resistance to the injection and the needle again should be repositioned.

Improvement is expected in 1–3 weeks. Surgical decompression should be advised if there is no improvement or in an advanced stage where there is wasting of thenar muscles.

Bursae

Bursae may become inflamed following unaccustomed exercise, e.g., tendo-achilles bursitis following a prolonged run. It may also result from repeated blunt trauma or constant friction, e.g., prepatellar or infrapatellar bursae on the knee (housemaid's knee) or the olecranon bursa near the elbow (student's elbow). Baker's cyst is a bursa which is seen as a swelling in the popliteal fossa and is associated with osteoarthrosis with effusion in the knee joint.

These bursae are usually painless and settle down without treatment in a month or so. If they do not, aspiration with steriod injections is indicated. The bursa should be aspirated by a wide bore needle. If the aspirate from the bursa is clear and not cloudy, indicative of infection, 20 mg of methyl prednisolone should be injected along with 2% lignocaine. The elbow or the knee should be supported by an Elastocrepe bandage for 1–2 days.

Painful Ligaments

Sometimes following a ligamentous injury or sprain, the pain does not settle down but persists for weeks or months together. Diagnosis is made by the presence of tenderness on the ligament particularly at its bony attachment. Also passive stretching of the ligament will cause excruciating pain. The attachments of the upper and lower ends of the medial and lateral collateral ligaments of the knee to the underlying bones are extremely common sites of pain. An injection of 10–20 mg of methyl prednisolone with lignocaine at these tender spots and the surrounding area will give good results (Fig. 47.9).

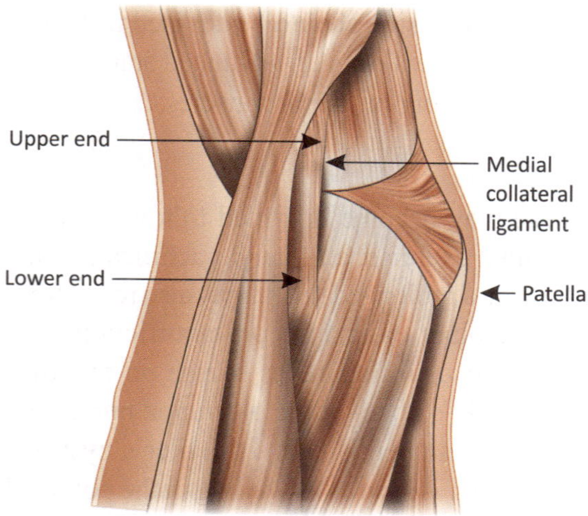

| Fig. 47.9 Site for injection at upper and lower ends of medial collateral ligament |

Fibromyalgia or Fibromyositis

Fibromyalgia is a commonly encountered disorder in general practice. Patient complains of generalized bodyache, joint pains, muscle weakness and other depressive symptoms. They feel that the joints are swollen; however, joint examination is normal. Polyarthralgia is maximum in the mornings and is made worse by cold damp weather, overexertion or stress.

The characteristic feature is the presence of tender spots at specific sites (18 such tender spots have been described by the American College of Rheumatology). The common spots are at the suboccipital muscle insertion at the base of the skull, the paravertebral area, the 2nd costochondral junction, the lateral epicondyle and around the shoulder, knee and hip joints. These tender spots can be usefully injected with 10–20 mg of methyl prednisolone plus lignocaine. This is followed by stretching of the affected muscles.

Anti-inflammatory drugs, regular aerobic exercises, antidepressants and acupuncture are advocated additionally.

Plantar Fasciitis

In this condition, the pain is felt under the heel at the attachment of plantar fascia to the calcaneus. A sharp pain in the heel on the first few steps after sitting for a prolonged period, is highly suggestive. The diagnosis is clinical and there is no need to X-ray the foot. The X-ray might show a calcaneal spur, which need not necessarily be responsible for the pain. It is thought to result from prolonged strain during standing by patients with an over-arched foot ('pes plantaris'). Hence, pain relief can be obtained by giving arch support in the footwear.

Alternatively, a steroid injection in and around the site of maximum tenderness can rapidly relieve the pain (Figs. 47.10 & 47.11).

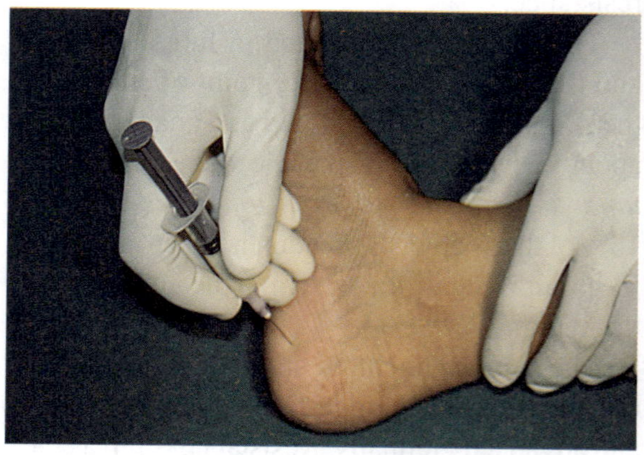

| Fig. 47.10 Injection site for plantar fasciitis |

The foot is dorsiflexed to make the plantar fascia taut. The site of maximum tenderness is identified, which is usually in the middle of the heel. 20–30 mg of methyl prednisolone mixed with 1 ml of 2% lignocaine is injected through the thick skin of the heel up to the calcaneus by a series of minor withdrawals and insertions. The patient

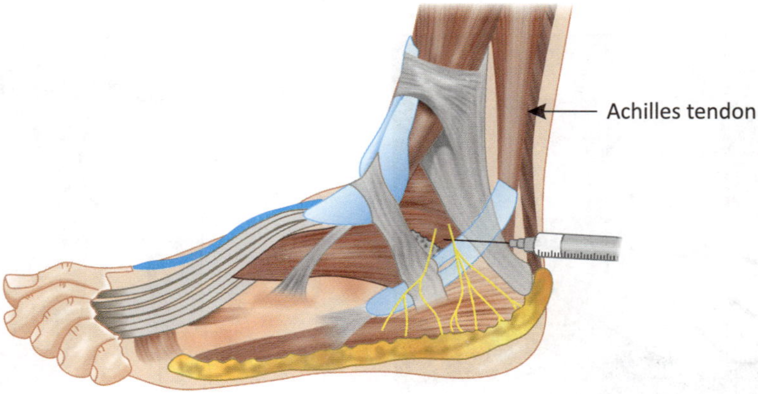

| **Fig. 47.11** Injection into painful heel |

should be warned about the painful nature of the injection, otherwise the patient will suddenly jerk the foot away.

Soft Tissues Around the Shoulder

a) ***Frozen shoulder (Adhesive capsulitis)***: There is pain and restricted movements of the shoulder usually in people above the age of 50 yr. The majority of the patients improve spontaneously within 12–18 months. In a few, permanant restriction of movements remain. Local steroid injections should be given along with physiotherapy and exercises. About 40 mg of methyl prednisolone with lignocaine should be injected over the supraspinatus tendon (Fig. 47.12) and another 40 mg in the shoulder joint cavity itself (Fig. 47.20).

b) ***Supraspinatus tendonitis*** **(Figs. 47.12 & 47.13)**: Pain occurs on abducting the arm as the inflamed portion of the supraspinatus tendon passes between the head of the humerus and the acromion. This occurs in the middle third of the abduction arc, hence called the painful arc syndrome. However, more often the pain is difficult to localize. About 20–40 mg of methyl prednisolone along with xylocaine should be injected in between the head of the humerus and the undersurface of the acromion where the tendon lies. The needle entry is just below the tip of the acromion, being directed medially and slightly downwards.

c) ***Bicipital tendonitis*** **(Figs. 47.14 & 47.15)**: It is produced by friction of the tendon of the long head of the biceps as it passes the bicipital groove. The patient has anterior shoulder pain which radiates down the forearm. Abduction and external rotation of the arm is painful. Methyl prednisolone 20–30 mg along with xylocaine is injected.

Meralgia Paraesthetica

There is pain or paraesthesia radiating down the anterolateral side of the thigh. This is due to compression of the lateral cutaneous nerve of the thigh as it passes behind the inguinal ligament about 1–2 cm from the anterior superior iliac spine. About 20–30 mg of methyl prednisolone with xylocaine is deposited at this site.

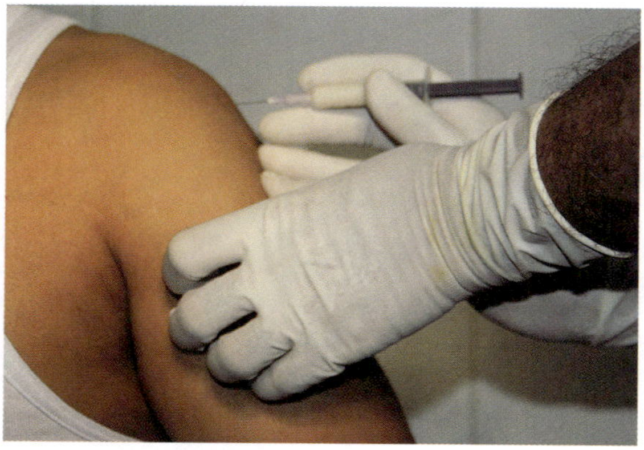

| **Fig. 47.12** Injection site for supraspinatus tendonitis |

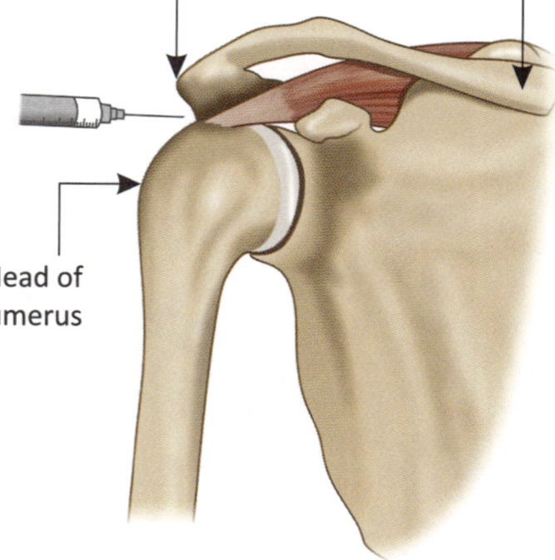

| **Fig. 47.13** Site for injection for supraspinatus tendonitis |

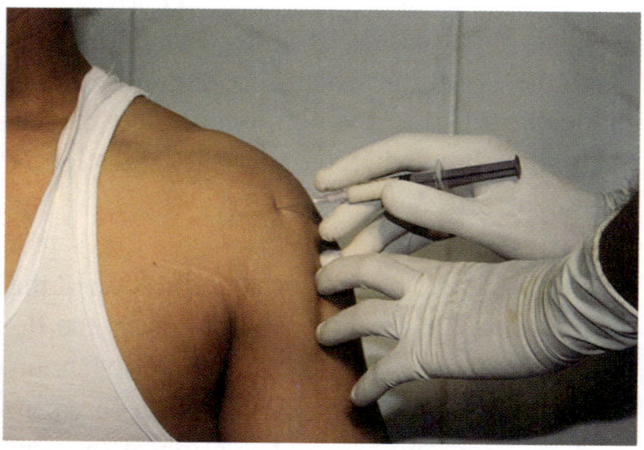

| **Fig. 47.14** Injection on the coracoid process at the origin of the short head of the biceps |

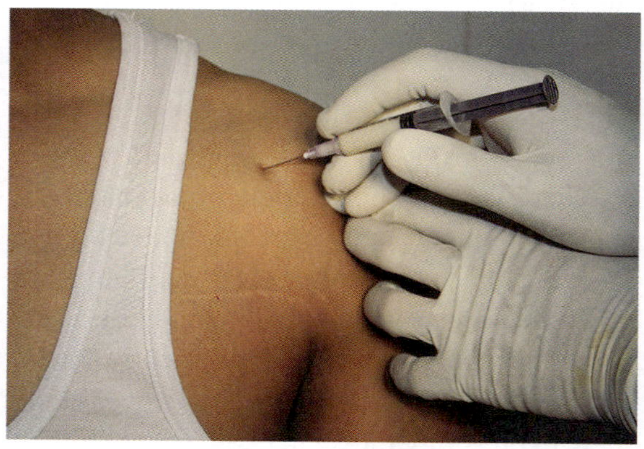

| **Fig. 47.15** Injection into the sheath of the long head of the biceps |

INTRA-ARTICULAR INJECTIONS

Finger and Toe Joints

For all these small joints, insulin syringe is preferred. A dorsolateral approach is used, as this area is devoid of nerves and tendons. The joint is flexed to open up the joint space and approximately 5 mg of hydrocortisone with a small amount of lignocaine is injected.

The carpometacarpal joint of the thumb is often involved in osteoarthritis. It is very close to the radial artery which can be avoided if the needle should enter from the dorsal side of the extensor pollicis brevis tendon.

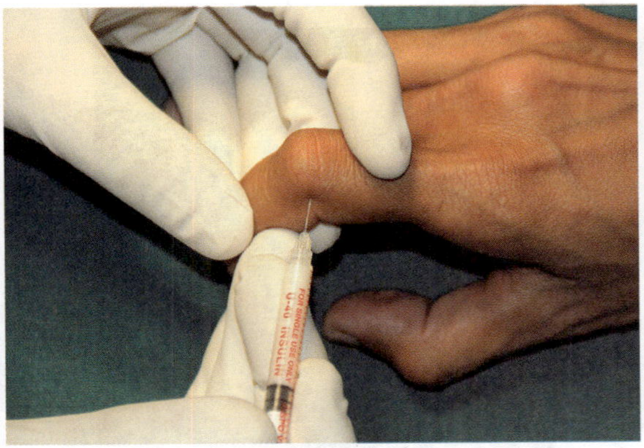

| **Fig. 47.16** Injection into interphalangeal joint |

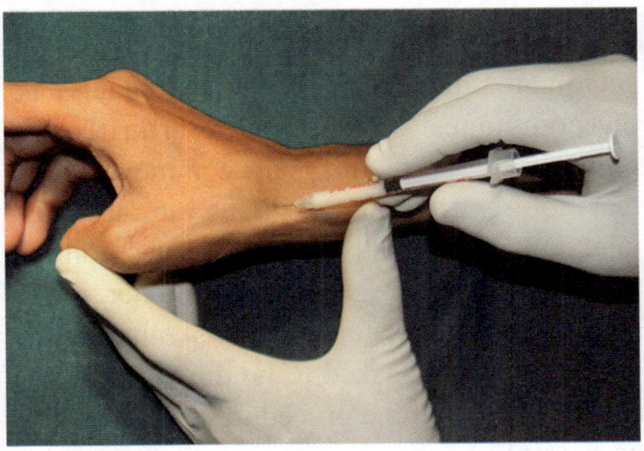

| **Fig. 47.17** Injection into thumb carpometacarpal joint |

Wrist Joint

The wrist joint is best approached through the dorsal aspect as this area is free from any important structures. The palmar aspect contains important structures like the radial artery and the median and the ulnar nerves.

The tendon of the extensor pollicis longus can be easily palpated at the lateral aspect of the anatomical snuff box if the hand is made into a fist. The wrist should be flexed and the needle directed into the joint cavity lateral to the extensor pollicis longus tendon. 20–30 mg of methyl prednisolone or triamcinolone is injected.

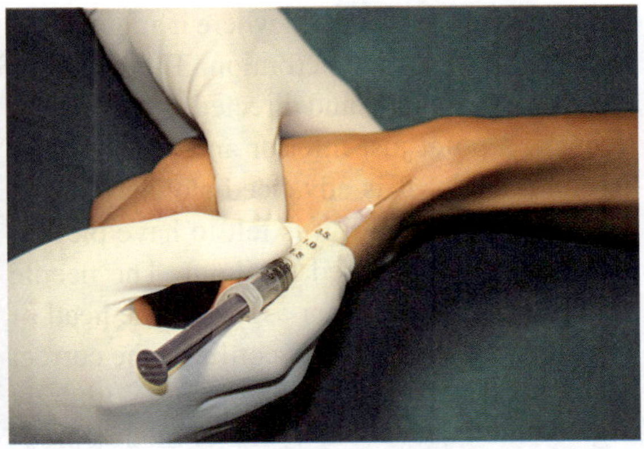

| **Fig. 47.18** Injection into wrist joint—dorsal approach in between extensor tendons |

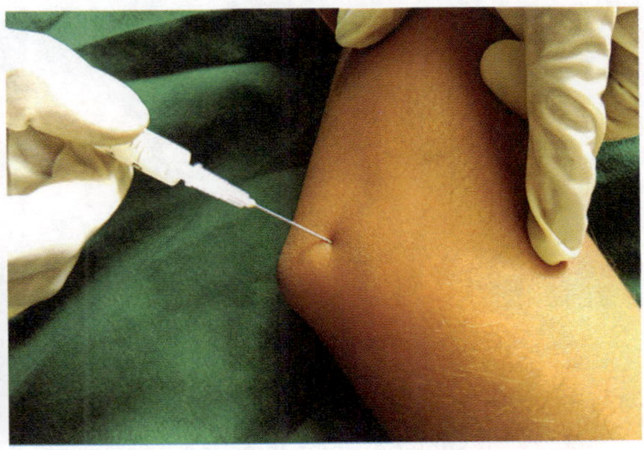

| **Fig. 47.19** Injection into elbow joint from lateral aspect of triceps tendon |

Elbow Joint

The ulnar nerve lies medial to the triceps tendon behind the medial epicondyle. Hence, in order to avoid this nerve, the needle is entered into the joint just lateral to the triceps tendon through the posterior aspect. About 40 mg of methyl prednisolone with xylocaine is required (Fig. 47.19).

Shoulder Joint

The shoulder joint can be approached either from the front, back or sideways. The posterior approach is preferable as there are no important structures which can be damaged. The patient is seated with the arm resting across the lap.

The spine of the scapula is identified and followed laterally to the point where it angulates to form the angle of the acromion. The needle is inserted horizontally and directed anteriorly entering at a point just inferior and lateral to the acromial angle. It is advanced slowly through the infraspinatus until it is felt to have pierced the capsule and entered the joint. The needle might touch the posterior aspect of the head of the humerus, which in fact confirms the correct position of the needle in the joint. Withdraw slightly and inject about 40 mg of methyl prednisolone with lignocaine.

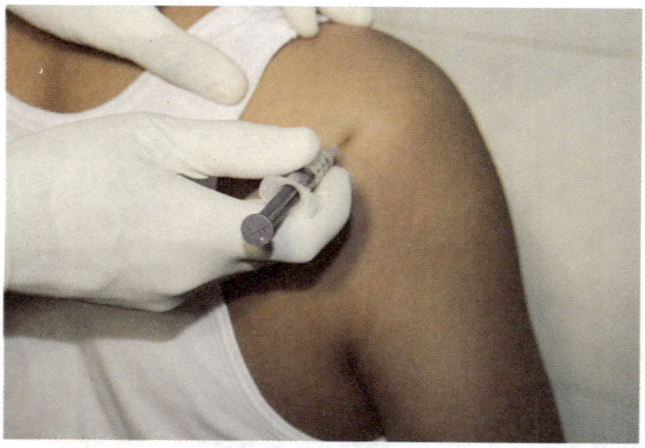

| **Fig. 47.20** Shoulder joint injection—posterior approach |

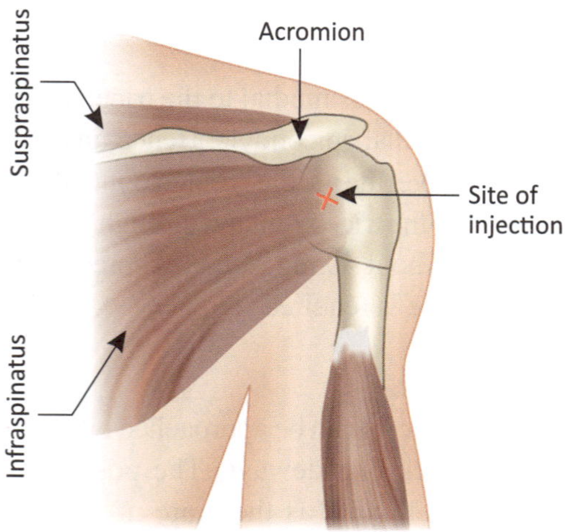

| **Fig. 47.21** Posterior approach for injection into shoulder joint |

Knee Joint

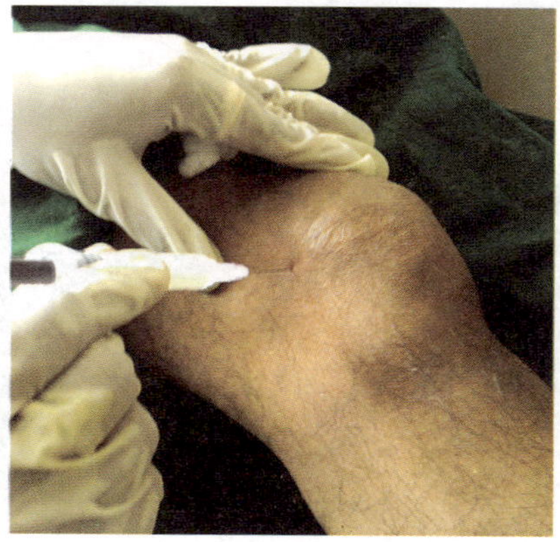

| **Fig. 47.22** Injection into the knee joint |

The knee is the largest synovial joint. It is a target joint for all major arthropathies and it is also the commonest site for septic arthritis and pseudogout. Hence, this is the commonest joint that requires aspiration or giving intra-articular injections. Fortunately, it is the easiest joint to inject or aspirate. A general practitioner, I feel, should start giving steroid injections with this joint.

The patient is asked to lie down and relax, assuring him that the procedure is not going to be painful. A tense person often contracts his quadriceps unconsciously, which makes an easy procedure difficult. The point of entry is the middle of the sulcus located between the side of the patella and the femoral condyle beneath, preferably on the lateral side of the knee. This can be located by firm palpation of upper and lateral margins of the patella. Another convenient entry site is the junction of the superior and lateral border of patella. The needle is directed inferiorly and medially, sliding just beneath the patella. If the injector is new and the patient nervous, it is better to give a local anaesthetic prior to the injection. If the joint contains effusion, this has to be removed by aspiration before the steroid injection is given. Then, methyl prednisolone 40 mg is injected with a separate syringe.

CHAPTER 48

Bandages and Plasters

- The Art of Applying Bandages
- How to Apply the Elastoplast Bandage
- Fractures and Plastering Techniques

THE ART OF APPLYING BANDAGES

Bandaging of wounds is an essential component of general practice. Hardly a day passes without a dressing being done. However, it is hardly ever taught to the medical student in his curriculum or taken as 'too trivial a matter' by the student himself while graduating. As a consequence, doctors are unable to apply a bandage that will remain in place till at least the next day.

Good bandaging can be learnt only by regular practice. It is a technique worth mastering by the GP. This is so, as apart from the therapeutic advantages, the patient goes out in the community inadvertently showing off his bandage and indirectly advertising (or maligning) his clinic. Also a nicely applied bandage is greatly appreciated by the patients and his relatives.

The ideal way to apply bandages to individual parts of the body, the types of bandages available in the market and the method of applying bandages in general is given below.

Types of Bandages

1. ***Roller bandages***: These are so-called because the bandaging material is packed and available as rolled up strips of cotton wool mesh. The open end of the bandage is called the *tail*, while the rolled portion is called the *head*. It is the most commonly used bandage as it is cheap enough to be disposed off after single use.
2. ***Adhesive bandages***: These are either inelastic rolls (e.g., Leuco-plasts) or elastic rolls (e.g., Elastoplast). They are also available as small ready-to-use dressings (e.g., Band-aid) which are available in wide range of shapes and sizes.
3. ***Cotton crepe bandages*** (*i.e.*, ***Elastocrepe***): These can stretch to almost twice their length and hence provide greater support and pressure to the part applied; for example, to treat a recently sprained ankle. Always apply them from distal to proximal.
4. ***Plaster of Paris bandages***: They are used to immobilize fractures.

5. ***Special types of bandages***: They are available or can be prepared in the clinic. For example, the triangular bandage can be used for slinging the forearm, or the T-bandage can be used for the perineum, or the suspensory bandage can be used for the scrotum, etc.

Method of Applying Bandages

First, select the proper size of the bandage required (see **Box 1**). Place the limb in the position in which it is to remain after bandaging, i.e., in functional position (e.g., the elbow should be flexed to the degree to which it will be subsequently required to be kept). Place cotton wool on the wound or between the surfaces that require bandaging and also on all bony prominences to avoid friction and ulceration.

Now, hold the head of the roll in one hand and the tail in the other. Place the outer side of roll just below the skin surface of the part being bandaged. Firmly anchor the bandage by taking two initial turns at the same level. These are called *fixation turns*. Unroll the bandage as you go on bandaging. For a limb, work from within outwards and from below upwards. Cover at least 2/3rd of the preceding turn by the succeeding turn, keeping the margins parallel as far as possible.

Finally, finish off tying the bandage by two or three complete turns at the same level. This end should be firmly secured either by a strip of adhesive plaster or by splitting the end of bandage and tying a knot.

Do not

1. Apply a wet bandage as it will become too tight when dry.
2. Tie the knot over a bony prominence.
3. Use too much bandage. This is both uncomfortable and expensive.
4. Unroll before bandaging. It is impossible to apply even pressure by a previously unrolled bandage.
5. Bandage two skin surfaces together without putting talcum powder and cotton wool. Otherwise chaffing and blister formation will take place.

| **Box 1** Choose the correct size of the bandage |

▪ Top or finger	1″
▪ Upper limb and head	2″–3″
▪ Lower limb	3″–4″
▪ Trunk	4″–6″

Basic Turns of Applying Bandages

There are 6 commonly used turns in bandaging.

1. ***The circular bandage***: The bandage is carried horizontally around the part to be bandaged, e.g., on the forehead. Circular turns are used at the beginning and at the end of bandage around a limb. Ideally, these turns should not be used all along the length around a limb as this may interfere with the circulation.

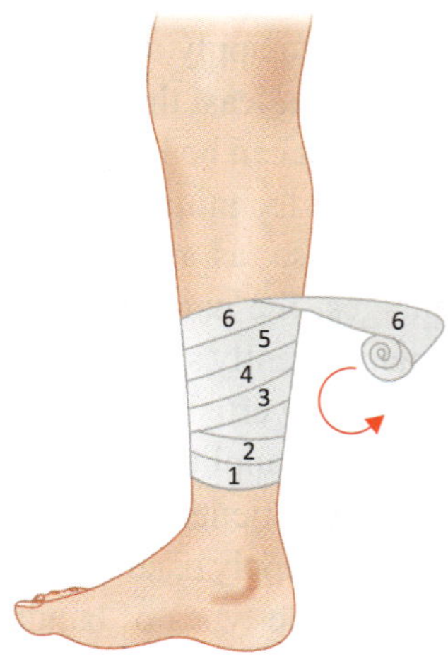

1–2: Circular fixation turns; **3–5**: Spiral turns; **6**: Reverse spiral turn

| **Fig. 48.1** Bandaging a limb |

2. ***The spiral bandage***: The bandage is carried spirally up the limb. It is applied over the parts which are of uniform thickness, e.g., finger, upper-arm, etc. (Figs. 48.1 & 48.2)

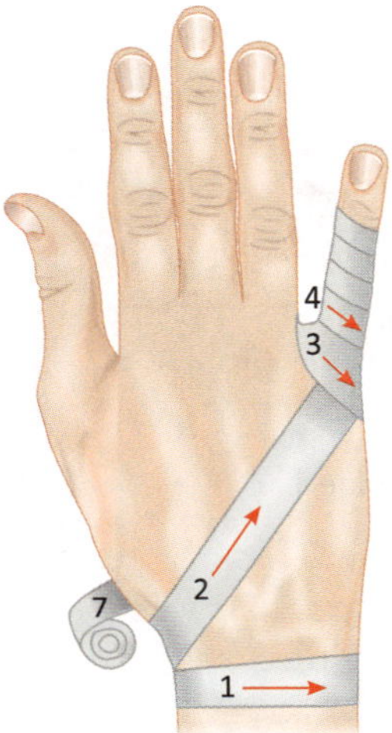

| **Fig. 48.2** Spiral bandage of the little finger |

3. ***The reverse spiral bandage*** (Fig. 48.1): This turn is applied when the bandage is applied to parts of a limb of unequal thickness, e.g., the forearm. When spiral turns are continually applied over the forearm, after a few turns, a part of the bandage gets a "kink". To make up for this, the turn is 'reversed".
4. ***The figure-of-eight bandage*** (Figs. 48.3 & 48.4): This is used when a joint has to be bandaged, e.g., bandaging the shoulder in case of fracture clavicle. The turns are carried alternately forward and backward on both the shoulders, so that a complete horizontal turn forms the figure-of-eight. This bandage can also be used for other joints like the ankle or the knee.
5. ***The spica bandage***: This is used when a joint has to be bandaged but the upper and lower parts forming the joint are of unequal dimensions, e.g., the hip or the thumb. The final appearance of the bandage looks like the ear of a corn, hence the name. This is a modified figure-of-eight bandage where one loop is wider than the other loop. Spica is of three types:

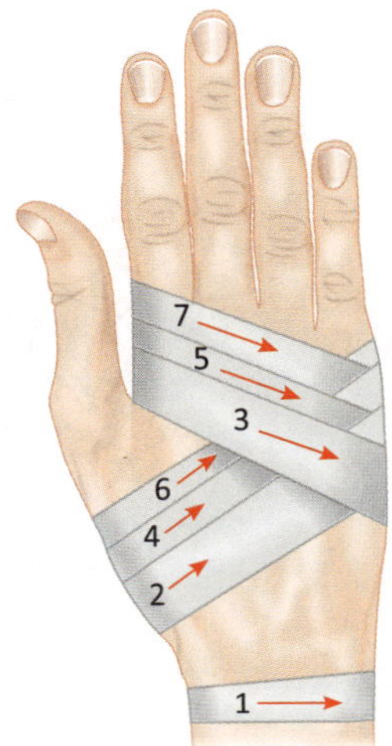

| **Fig. 48.3** Figure-of-eight bandage to hand |

   a) **Ascending spica** (Fig. 48.5): While bandaging the shoulder for example, the spiral turns start at the upper part of the arm and gradually climb up the axilla and the shoulder.
   b) **Descending spica**: Here, the spiral turns start at the upper part of the shoulder below the neck and climb down the axilla and the arm.
   c) **Divergent spica** (Fig. 48.6a & b): While bandaging the elbow or the ankle for example, the spiral turns start at the level of the joint. Then, the figure-of-eight turns are applied working alternately above and below the elbow or ankle.
6. ***The recurrent bandage*** (Fig. 48.7): This is used for tip of a finger or to the end of an amputed limb. First one or two basic turns are taken at the base of the finger. Then, the bandage is passed over the tip of the finger (or over the stump) to and fro, till the whole tip is covered. Finally, the bandage is

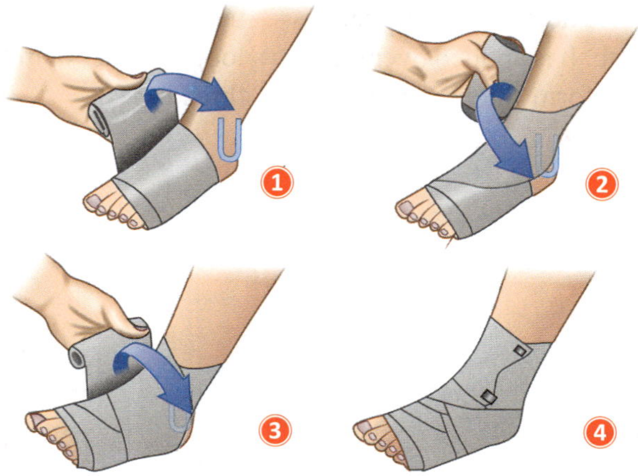

| Fig. 48.4 Figure-of-eight bandage to ankle |

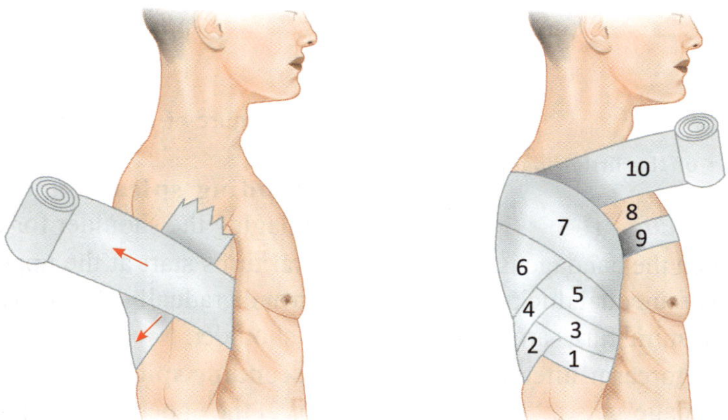

| Fig. 48.5 Ascending spica for shoulder |

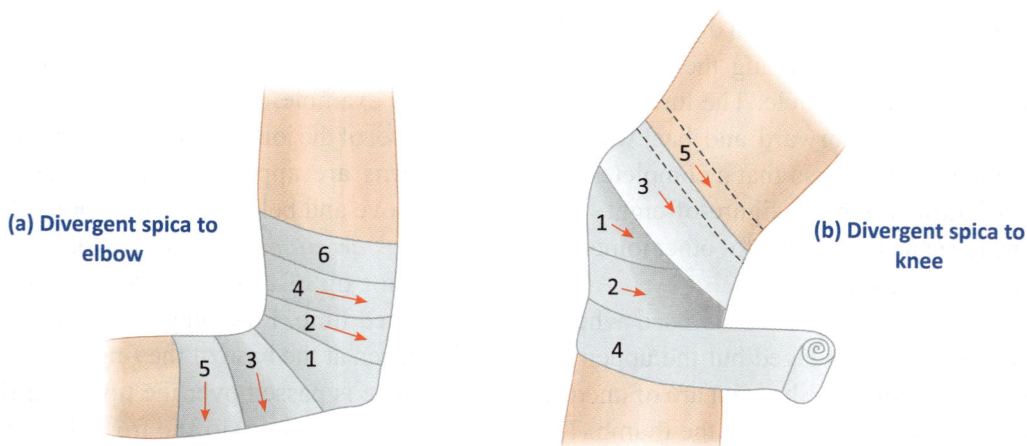

| Fig. 48.6 Examples of divergent spica to elbow and knee |

completed with one or two spiral turns at the base of the finger (or the stump).

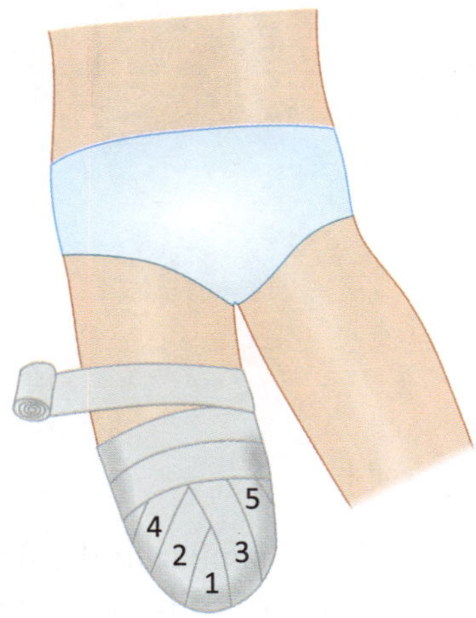

| **Fig. 48.7** Recurrent bandage to a stump |

How to Apply the Roller Bandage to Particular Areas

While reading the following description of the method of application of bandages, it is suggested to the reader that he should hold a roller bandage in his hands and follow the instruction by tying the bandage on his own self whenever possible, all the time referring to the figure alongside.

1. *Finger* (Fig. 48.2): First take a few fixation turns at the wrist. Bring the bandage round the palm to the base of the finger. Take the bandage towards the tip of the finger and back to the base by spiral turns. Finally bring the bandage back to the wrist and secure it after 2 or 3 circular turns. If the tip of the finger is to be bandaged, use recurrent turns.
2. *Thumb*: First fix the bandage at the wrist and then carry it to the base of the thumb as above. Now use the figure-of-eight turns or the spica.
3. *Hand and palm* (Fig. 48.3): Similar to the bandage of the thumb. Initial fixation turns at the wrist followed by figure-of-eight bandage running from dorsal and palmar aspect alternatingly.
4. *Forearm and upper arm* (Fig. 48.1): Start bandaging distally and continue proximally using the reverse spiral turns. Never use circular turns (except initially and at completion), as this may compromise circulation.
5. *Elbow* (Fig. 48.6a): Place the elbow at 90° flexion. Initially fix the bandage at the middle of the elbow by two circular turns. Then use the figure-of-eight bandage alternating above and below the elbow. This is divergent spica. If the whole upper limb is to be bandaged, as in case of extensive burns, the above mentioned turns are combined. The wrist and hand are bandaged with figure-of-eight, the forearm by the reverse spiral, the flexed elbow by the divergent spica and finally the upper arm by the reverse spiral turns.
6. *Shoulder* (Fig. 48.5): An ascending spica preferred. Put cotton pads in both the armpits. Take a few circular fixation turns at the upper part of the arm. Continue upwards with reverse spiral turns till the axilla is reached. Now take bandage behind the back to the opposite axilla and then across the chest to the top of the bandage above the arm. Apply a complete turn to the upper part of the arm around the shoulder. Again take the bandage behind the back, opposite axilla, chest and repeat the procedure till shoulder is covered. Finally fix the tail of the bandage to the chest.
7. *Figure-of-eight bandage for fractured clavicle*: Put large cotton pads in both the axillae to prevent compression of important structures by the bandage. Start bandaging under the axilla on the fractured side, coming up anteriorly in front of the shoulder. Then take the bandage across the back to the opposite axilla. Come up anteriorly in front of

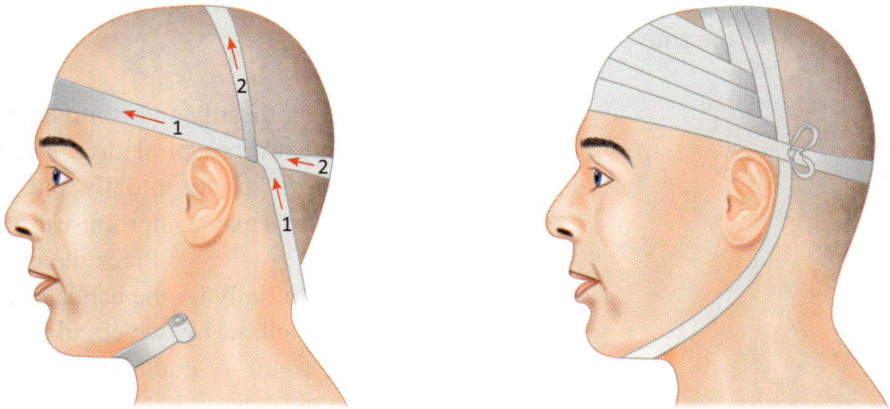

| **Fig. 48.8** Twisted bandage to the head |

the shoulder on the sound side. Take the bandage behind the back, thus completing the figure-of-eight. Repeat these turns till the shoulder is pulled back. Reapply the bandage every 4–5 days for 3 weeks. Keep the arm on the fractured side in a sling.

8. ***Head* (Fig. 48.8)**: For general practitioners, a head bandage is required to keep the dressing in position after scalp injury as an adhesive plaster is useless because of the presence of hair. Leave about 12″ of the tail of the bandage free and take the initial fixation turn starting from below the left ear. Wind round the forehead, then above right ear, going below the occipital protuberance and back above the left ear. The bandage is then twisted at this place and passed over the dressing on the scalp → right side of the face → under the mandible → back to the starting point. This process of passing below the occipital protuberance and winding around the forehead is repeated till the dressing is fully covered. The two free ends are then tied together. The popular 'Capeline bandage' is a pressure bandage meant to control excessive bleeding from the scalp and is usually not required by GPs.
9. ***Great toe***: This is similar to the figure-of-eight bandage described for the thumb.
10. ***Foot***: This is similar to the figure-of-eight bandage described for the palm.
11. ***Heel or ankle* (Fig. 48.4)**: Use figure-of-eight bandage. Start with initial fixation turns across the foot just behind the toes. Take turns from across the foot to behind the ankle alternating, each turn 1/3rd of the width higher than the previous one, until the whole part is covered.
12. ***Leg* (Fig. 48.1)**: Apply spiral turns at the lower part of the leg and reverse spiral turns for the upper part of the leg, the reverse being done at the anterolateral aspect of the leg.
13. ***Knee* (Fig. 48.6b)**: Use either a figure-of-eight or a divergent spica bandage. The former restricts the movement at the knee, gives rest to the part and hence reduces the swelling. The latter allows some degree of movement to the knee.
14. ***Thigh***: After the initial circular fixation turns at the lower part of the thigh, go on winding upwards by reverse spiral turns, taking the twists at the anterolateral aspect of the thigh.

15. *Scrotum*: A scrotal support is required in general practice to relieve pain in case of trauma to the testis or in case of acute epididymoorchits. Take a few fixation turns around the waist at the level of the iliac crest and tie the knot anteriorly. Bring the bandage on one side of the scrotum and then beneath the scrotum, finally on the other side to reach the initial fixation bandage around the waist. Hook the bandage here just above the pubic symphysis and repeat the turn to suspend the scrotum, forming a firm scrotal support. Finally, tie the tail of the bandage to the bandage around the waist.
16. *Eye*: Take the initial fixation turn around the forehead above the ears. Then, take a few turns obliquely over the affected eye below the ear, going back of the head and again over the eye, bringing the bandage a little lower each turn. Finish it with a horizontal turn around the forehead. The ear is bandaged in a similar fashion.

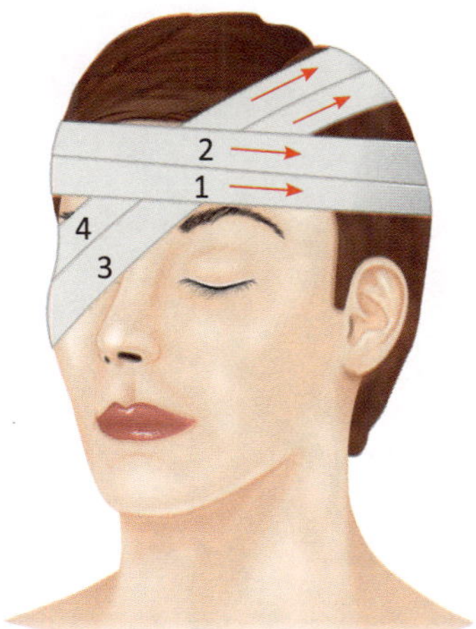

| **Fig. 48.9** Eye bandage |

HOW TO APPLY THE ELASTOCREPE BANDAGE

The Elastocrepe bandage can be usefully applied to the following common conditions:

1. Sprained ankle
2. Fractured ribs
3. Fracture of phalanges of the thumb and fingers

The elastic and adhesive nature gives a firm support for sprains and small undisplaced fractures. Irritation of the skin is a potential hazard, which can be minimized by applying tincture Benzoin to the skin prior to application of the Elastocrepe bandage. This can be removed gently using spirit.

1. ***Ankle strapping*** **(Fig. 48.10)**: The foot is held dorsiflexed and everted for a lateral sprain of the ankle, which is more common than the medial sprain. You will have to wrap the bandage from outside to the inside in order to keep the foot everted. Take two fixation turns at the base of the toe around the foot. Then, use the figure-of-eight turns to wrap the heel and the ankle. Finally, continue upwards using spiral turns till half way up the leg.
2. ***Thumb strapping***: Apply two fixation turns just proximal to the distal interphalangeal joint of the thumb. Then, use figure-of-eight turns to wrap round the base of the thumb and hand. Finish by two circular turns around the wrist.
3. ***Finger strapping (Buddy strapping)***: This is used for undisplaced fracture of the phalanges. Put a pad of cotton in between the fractured finger and the adjacent finger, to prevent pressure sores from developing because of friction. Then, apply Elastocrepe bandage around both the fingers leaving the interphalangeal joint free.

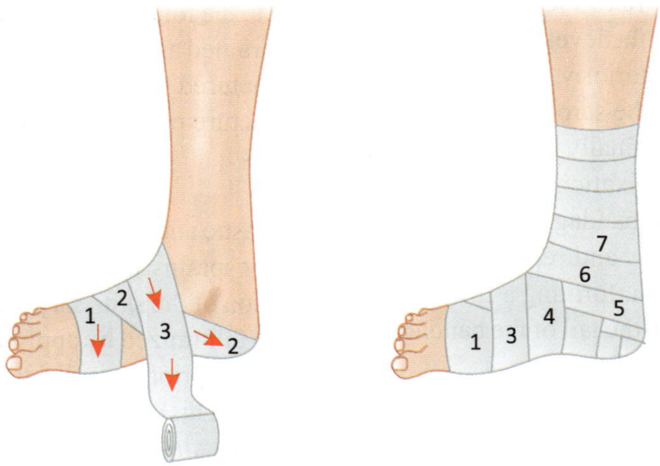

| Fig. 48.10 Elastocrepe bandage to ankle |

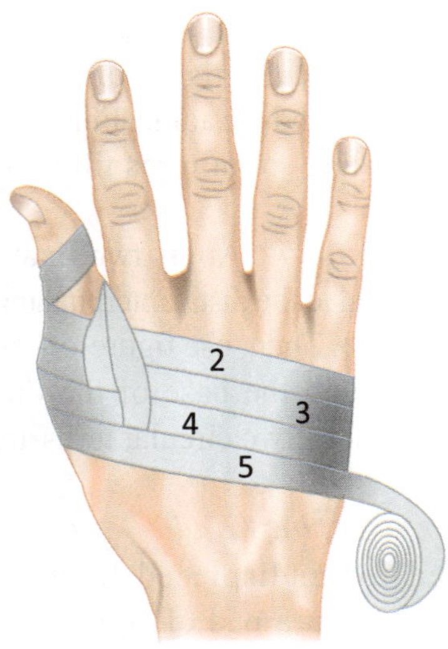

| Fig. 48.11 Elastocrepe strapping for thumb |

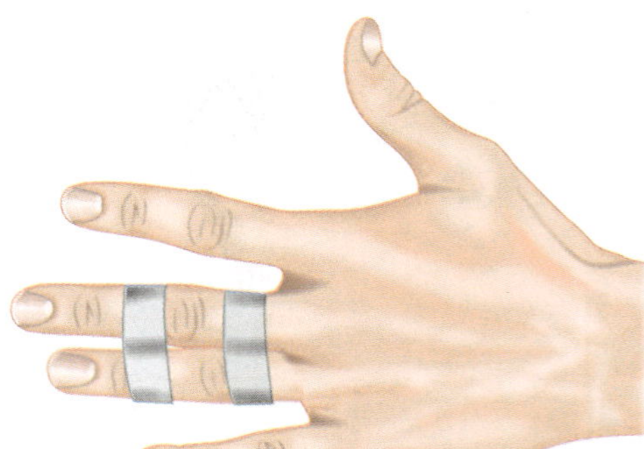

| Fig. 48.12 Buddy strapping for finger |

4. ***Strapping for fractured ribs***: See 'Rib fracture' later in the Chapter.

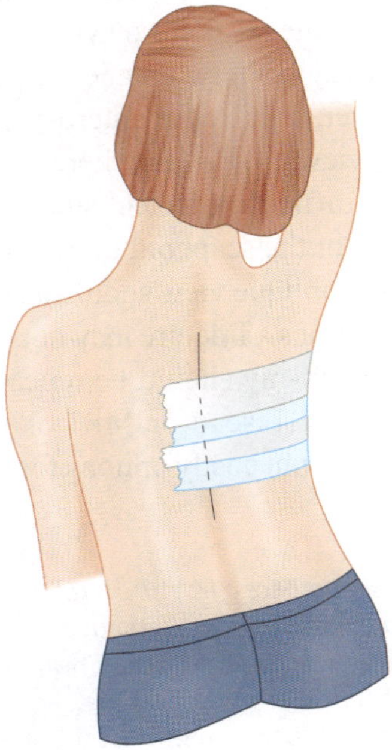

| **Fig. 48.13** Strapping for fractured ribs |

FRACTURES AND PLASTERING TECHNIQUES

Applying Plaster of Paris is a shot in the biceps for a general practitioner and his practice. Common fractures which can be dealt with by the GP in his own clinic have been described here. The method of putting Plaster of Paris slab or a cast is also described. Go through this section, request your orthopaedic friend to guide you initially in putting one or two plaster bandages and then make this a routine procedure in your clinic.

Common Terms

- A *fracture* is a break in continuity of a bone.
- In a *closed* fracture, the overlying skin is intact while in an *open* fracture there is a wound overlying the fracture site, predisposing the fractured bone to infection.
- A joint is said to be *dislocated* when its articular surfaces are wholly displaced from each other. A joint is said to be *subluxated* when they are only partly displaced.
- A *sprain* is an incomplete tear of a ligament supporting a joint.
- A fracture is *impacted* when the broken fragments are driven into one another firmly and are therefore also called *stable*. A fracture is *unstable* when these fragments are displaced.
- A *fatigue* or a *stress* fracture is an incomplete fracture resulting from repeated episodes of trauma and not from a single violent injury. These usually occur in the metatarsals in athletes or in army personnel.
- A *pathological* fracture is one which occurs in a bone weakened by a pre-existing disease. This can occur spontaneously or with trival injury. The commonest predisposing causes are osteoporosis and metastatic carcinoma.

Diagnosis

Usually, a fracture is suspected by history and clinical examination and finally confirmed by a radiological examination.

History

Ask about the details about the *nature of the fall* or accident. As a general rule, the chances of a person sustaining a fracture increases with the severity of the injury. But, this is not always so. We have seen a child falling from the second floor of a building and not sustaining any fracture. We have also seen a young person falling due to a banana peel and sustaining a fracture tibia.

Enquire about the *severity of the pain*. More severe the pain, more the possibility of a fracture. Individuals vary greatly in their response to pain. Also, a few fractures like the fractures of the scaphoid bone at the wrist give rise to minimal pain.

Ask whether the patient is able to move the limb freely. Inability or *difficulty in moving* the limb (loss of function) is an important symptom, although some degree of movement may be possible. For example, following fracture neck femur, the patient may be able to walk, but with a limp.

Clinical Examination

The so-called classical signs of a fracture may or may not be present, but watch out for the following:

- *Tenderness* is almost always present.
- *Deformity* may or may not be present.
- *Swelling* is usually seen after a few hours and is due to inflammatory exudates and haematoma.
- *Local temperature* may be raised on account of inflammation.
- *Loss of function* as elicited by pain on passive movements, is almost always present.
- *Abnormal mobility or crepitus* may by elicited at the fractured site, but this is best avoided.

For the radius, metacarpals, metatarsals or phalanges, a simple test for the diagnosis of a fracture is to apply *axial compression* from end to end, when patient will wince with pain. For example, for a suspected fracture of the shaft of the radius, grasp the wrist and the elbow with your hands and compress in the long axis towards the suspected fracture site. The patient then may localise accurately the site of fracture.

Radiological Examination

Having suspected a fracture on history and examination, an X-ray is mandatory. Although in high proportion of cases the fracture will be 'ruled out', this is largely unavoidable, as failing to diagnose a fracture is disastrous both from the clinical and medicolegal point of view. Always request for X-ray from two planes at right angles to one another, usually the antero-posterior and the lateral views. At sites where a fracture is notoriously difficult to detect such as the head of the radius or the scaphoid bone, a request for an additional oblique view should also be made. In these situations a fracture may not be still visible, when an X-ray should be repeated after a few weeks. A CT scan or MRI or bone scan are other useful but costly options for immediate diagnosis.

Common sites where a fracture is missed because reasonable function is preserved:

- Impacted fractures—neck of humerus, neck of femur, lower end of radius.
- Fatigue fractures—metatarsal bones, fibula
- Scaphoid fractures
- Rib fractures
- Greenstick fractures—in the forearms of children.

Request X-ray from a different angle and/or follow-up X-ray after a few days.

Principles of Management

Having now diagnosed the fracture accurately, a number of key decisions will have to be made by the GP.

1. ***Does the patient require hospitalization?*** The decision is usually easy, being dictated by the seriousness of the injury.
2. ***Is the fracture open or closed?*** All open fractures should be considered as emergencies and immediately referred to a competent orthopaedic surgeon. The main danger here is the risk of infection, which if occurs may lead to chronic osteomyelitis requiring months or even years of treatment and even

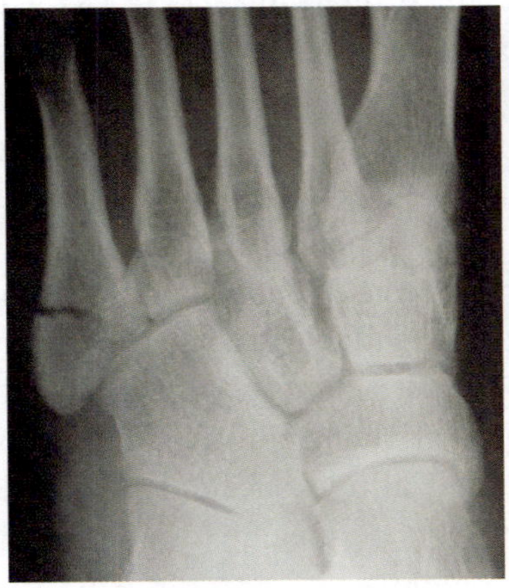

(a) Crack fracture of base of 5th metatarsal

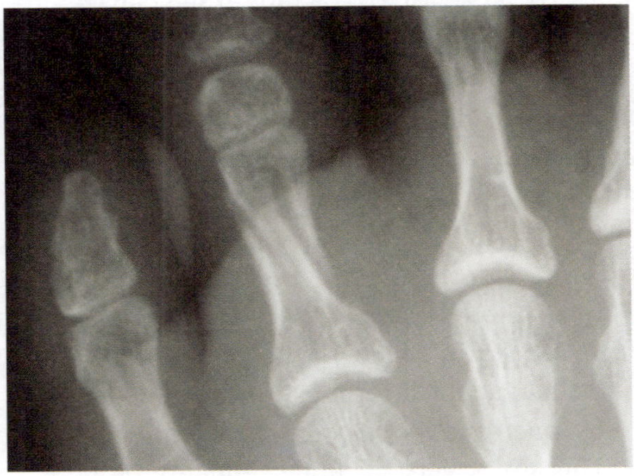

(b) Fracture phalanx

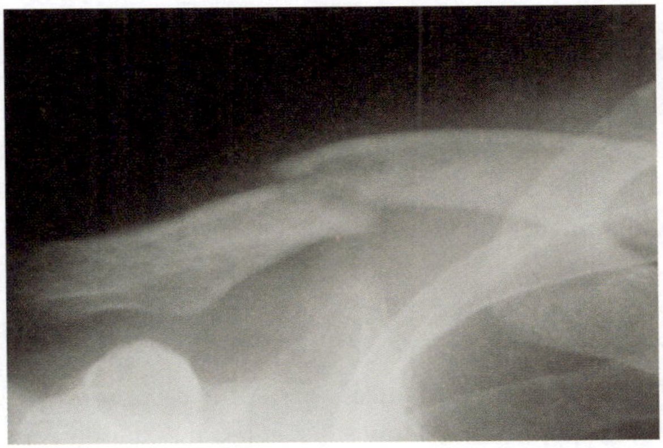

(c) Fracture clavicle

| Fig. 48.14 |

then ultimately leading to loss of the limb. Uncomplicated closed fracture not requiring reduction under general anaesthesia in a hospital can be managed in a GP's clinic.

3. ***Which fractures require reduction and should be referred?***
   - Highly displaced fracture of the limbs always requires reduction under general anaesthesia to prevent deformity and loss of function. Always refer.
   - Fractures of the radius and ulna, even if slightly displaced require accurate reduction as even a slight mal-alignment may lead to difficultly in pronation and supination. Always refer.
   - Again fractures near the ankle joint even if slightly displaced may require reduction, as even a slight deformity may lead to osteoarthritis. Always refer.

In other situations, some displacement is often acceptable. In old people when the risk of anaesthesia outweighs the benefits and the result of conservative treatment is as good as operative treatment, there is nothing to be gained in trying to achieve perfect reduction.

Similarly, in a case of fracture of the clavicle, especially in children and young adults, normal function can be restored even without accurate alignment. These and other select fractures can be easily managed in a GP's clinic.

4. ***If the fracture requires reduction, how does the orthopaedic surgeon achieve this?***
   - *By closed reduction under general anaeathesia*: This is the commonest method adopted for most fractures.
   - *By open reduction under anaesthesia*: This gives very accurate reduction but carries the risk of infection. This method is therefore reserved for cases when closed reduction has failed or accurate reduction by internal fixation with screws, plates or intramedullary nails is required.
   - *By applying continuous traction for several weeks*, e.g., fracture femoral shaft or the cervical spine in the elderly.
5. ***To immobilize or not immobilize?*** Not all fractures need to be immobilized. The scaphoid fracture, fracture of the neck of femur and fracture for the shaft ulna require rigid immobilization for proper healing. However, there are other fractures which heal without immobilization, viz., clavicle, ribs, scapula, stable fracture of the pelvic rim, metacarpals, metatarsals and phalanges. In some fractures, immobilization may result in more harm than good. The wrist may be immobilized for months without any problems but if the fingers are immobilized for more than a few weeks, this will almost certainly result in permanent joint stiffness.
6. ***If then the GP has decided to immobilize the uncomplicated closed fracture, how can he achieve this?*** This is most easily achieved by plaster of Paris (POP) bandage. There are newer materials like fibreglass available for plastering. These are stronger than POP casts, lighter in weight and are in addition, waterproof. However, their main disadvantage is that they are difficult to apply and are more expensive and hence will not be described here. Plaster of Paris remains the most widely used material because of its obvious advantages. It is easily available, easy to use and reasonably cheap. It is light and comfortable if properly applied. Being porous, it absorbs perspiration and allows the underlying skin to breathe. It is permeable to radiography and easy to remove.

Method of Applying POP Cast or Slab

Plaster of Paris is made from gypsum. The POP bandages were earlier made in the hospital itself by impregnating this powder into ordinary cotton bandages. Now almost all plaster bandages are available as ready to use proprietary bandages (Gypsona, Rapidur) in various sizes (6″, 4″, 3″, etc.). This makes application of POP bandages much easier. The application is done in one of the two forms:

- As a *complete plaster cast*, which encircles the whole circumference of the limb. As a general rule, the joints above and below need to be incorporated in the plaster. It is used as a definitive form of fracture treatment.
- As a *plaster slab* (or splint), which encircles only part of circumference of the limb. A cast is fashioned by laying longitudinal strips of wet plaster and then enclosing the limb partially, to form a gutter. This is used when swelling of the limb is expected or is already present and is held in place by wet gauze bandage. It is a temporary splint used in the initial stage of fracture treatment till the swelling has subsided.

Everything required should be assembled before starting to apply the plaster, viz., a bucket of tepid water, a soft roll of cotton or a stockinet and the selected size of POP rolls. Make use of 15 cm (6″) for the forearm, the ankle or foot; 10 cm (4″) for the wrist and 7.5 cm (3″) for the thumb and fingers. The limb is covered by a layer of stockinet, easily available in the market. This prevents the plaster from sticking to the hairs. Alternatively, a layer of soft cotton bandage is rolled on to the limb. In addition, a layer of cotton is applied to the bony prominences to prevent friction.

For the application of a plaster cast, the end of the POP roll is slightly unrolled and held in a bucket of tepid water for a few seconds until bubbles cease to rise. The POP roll is then lifted out of the water and gently squeezed to take out the surplus water. This can now be wrapped round the part of the limb to be plastered. The wet plaster rolls are applied distally and proceeded proximally layer by layer, overlapping half the proximal layer every time.

After an acute injury, if much swelling is anticipated, use a plaster slab in preference to a complete plaster cast. A POP roll is unrolled on a flat dry surface to its required length and doubled backwards and forwards on itself. This is then dipped in tepid water as described above, and laid on the affected limb. It is held in place by a wet cotton bandage, which is applied with even tension, working distally to proximally. After a few days when the swelling has subsided, the slab should be removed and the full plaster cast applied.

The procedure for applying the cast and the slab and their removal by special heavy scissors or an electric saw can be easily learnt under the initial guidance of an orthopaedic surgeon. Never forget to instruct the patient to report back immediately if there is intense pain, swelling, paraesthesia or change in colour of the fingers or toes. This could be circulatory embarrassment or pressure on a nerve, which demands immediate removal of the plaster.

Five Fractures which can be Treated by the GP in his Clinic

Fracture of the Clavicle

This is one of the commonest fractures seen in childhood and early adult life and is usually caused by a fall on the outstretched arm. In children, the fracture is usually of the greenstick variety. The clavicle typically breaks in the middle of the shaft or at the junction of the middle and outer one third. The weight of the arm pulls the outer fragment downwards and forwards. The patient presents to you supporting the weight of the injured arm with the other arm. The diagnosis is easily confirmed by an X-ray.

Treatment: The clavicle usually unites rapidly and minimal intervention is called for. This essentially consists of putting the injured arm in a broad sling for 2–3 weeks and giving analgesics for a few days.

Complications are rare. If there is marked displacement of the fractured ends, the time honoured method of bringing the fragments into apposition is to apply the figure-of-eight bandage or clavicular rings (Fig. 48.15) to the two shoulders. The 'calvicular rings' can be created by stuffing two stockinets with cotton wool in the central portion. This central padded portion is placed in front of the shoulders and the free ends are tied behind. The patient is then asked to brace the shoulders back and the free ends of the calvicular rings are tied behind. If stockinet is not available, roller gauze can be used instead to tie a figure-of-eight bandage.

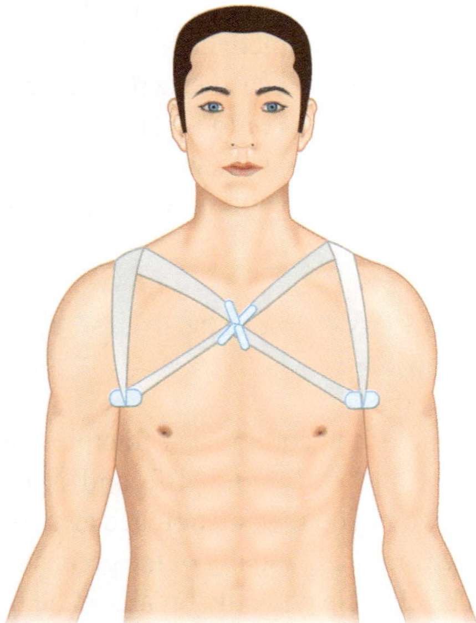

| **Fig. 48.15** Clavicular rings for fracture clavicle |

Both the clavicular rings and the figure-of-eight bandages are invariably uncomfortable and are of doubtful value. Apposition is hardly ever achieved and instead there is danger of important nerves and vessels getting compressed.

Hence, many surgeons these days rely only on a sling for the injured limb even when there is marked displacement. The fracture almost always unites and non-union is seen in less than 1% of cases, which is again usually symptomless. Non-union is more common with fracture of lateral end of the clavicle and these patients may be referred to an orthopaedic surgeon for opinion.

Fracture of the Scaphoid

Injuries of the wrist are frequently dismissed as 'sprains' and are not X-rayed or even treated, as the pain is mild and the patient continues to use the hand. Consequently, the fracture of the scaphoid is missed with disastrous consequences. The diagnosis 'sprain of the wrist' is a dangerous one.

The fracture nearly always occurs transversely through the middle (waist) so that the proximal and distal fragments are about equal size. The blood supply enters the scaphoid through the distal portion and hence the proximal portion may be deprived of blood supply leading to avascular necrosis of the proximal part and permanent osteoarthritis. Hence, it is important not to miss these fractures. This is not so easy as this fracture does not produce substantial clinical and radiological signs. Characteristically, there is tenderness in the anatomical snuff box and longitudinal pressure applied on the thumb in the direction of the scaphoid bone causes pain.

Management: Under the slightest suspicion always order an X-ray, the standard AP and lateral views and an additional oblique 'scaphoid' view. The fracture is usually hairline and hard to visualize on X-ray.

Therefore, even if the X-ray is normal, put the patient on a 'scaphoid plaster' under clinical suspicion alone. After 2 weeks, remove the plaster and repeat the X-ray. If now the X-ray does not reveal a fracture and there is clinical improvement, the wrist may be left free and no harm has been done. If the fracture is now apparent on the X-ray, apply a fresh scaphoid cast. Repeat the X-ray after 8 weeks. If the X-ray reveals evidence of union, remove the cast. If non-union is seen, refer to orthopaedic surgeon for internal fixation.

The classical scaphoid plaster: The plaster used is slightly more extensive than that for Colles' fracture. The wrist is placed in a neutral position and the hand as if holding a glass, i.e., with the forearm in the neutral position, the wrist in slight dorsiflexion and the thumb semiopposed. The plaster cast is then put below elbow up to the knuckles (leaving the interphalangeal joint free to move) and on the thumb up to the first metacarpal bone (leaving the distal interphalangeal joint free). If the patient cannot perform a pinch, the plaster has been wrongly applied.

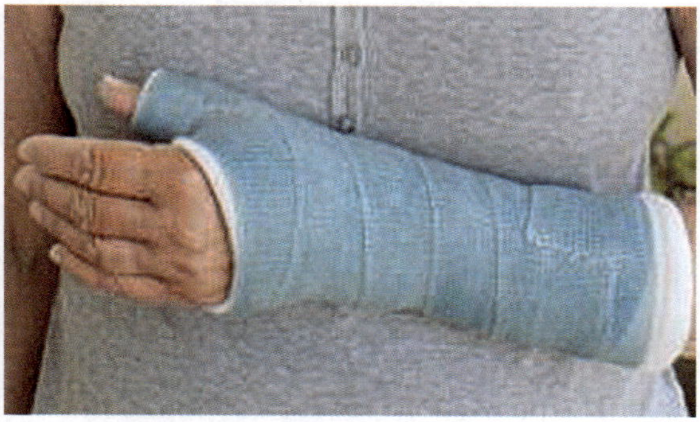

| **Fig. 48.16** Plaster cast for scaphoid fracture |

Rib Fracture

Most fractures of the ribs usually occur at the angle of the rib following direct injury. A simple rib fracture can be extremely painful. Inspiration and coughing increase this pain further. There is localized tenderness at the site of the fracture. An X-ray confirms the diagnosis and excludes underlying lung injury like pneumothorax and haemothorax, caused by a fragment penetrating the pleura.

Try anti-inflammatory analgesics. If there is no pain relief, about 5 mL of 2% xylocaine can be infiltrated at the site of maximum tenderness, which gives instant relief. This can be repeated everyday for 3–4 days.

Another alternative is to do strapping of the chest wall by an Elastocrepe adhesive bandage (Fig. 48.13). Make the patient sit on a chair with the arm on the side of the fractured rib raised and resting on the head. Apply the end of a strip of Elastoplast bandage about 5 cm below the nipple anteriorly on the normal side. Ask the patient to breathe out completely and then run the bandage towards the fractured side, encircling the chest wall, crossing the vertebral column and finally fixing the ends of the strip at a point on the unaffected side, behind the original point, posteriorly. It is essential that the bandage crosses the midline both anteriorly and posteriorly, for proper immobilization.

Apply 3 or 4 strips after full expiration, in a similar way so that each one covers the previous one by 1/3rd of its width. The bandage can be removed after a week or so.

Fracture of the Metatarsals

- ***Fracture of the base of the 5th metatarsal***: This is the commonest fracture of the lower limb. Following sudden inversion of the foot, the base of the 5th metatarsal is torn off by the tendon attached to it (avulsion fracture). There is pain, tenderness and swelling on the outer border of the foot with difficulty in walking. The patient complains of having sprained his ankle and is often reluctant to get his foot X-rayed. If only the ankle is X-rayed, the fracture will be missed. An X-ray of the foot confirms the diagnosis (Fig. 48.14a).

  Most of these fractures are undisplaced, but even the markedly displaced fractures do not require reduction. Immobilization is required mainly for the relief of pain and not for the union. If the pain is mild, give Elastocrepe bandage for 2–3 weeks. If the pain is severe, give a standard below-knee walking plaster cast (Fig. 48.17) for 3 weeks, followed by active exercises.
- ***Fracture of the metatarsal shafts*** (Fig. 48.17): This usually occurs following a heavy object falling on the foot. Commonly 1 or 2 metatarsal shafts are fractured and the

displacement is slight. Here, again immobilization is required for pain relief only and treatment is as above.

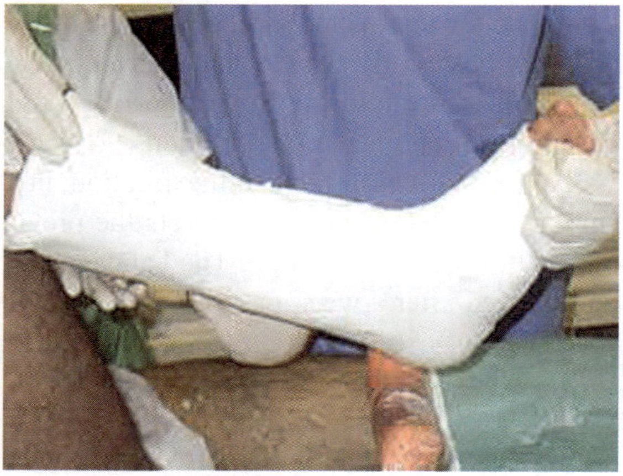

| **Fig. 48.17** Below-knee plaster cast |

- ***Multiple displaced fractures of the shaft and fracture of the 1st metatarsal***: These require reduction under general anaesthesia and possibly internal fixation and hence should be referred.
- ***The below-knee plaster cast* (Fig. 48.17)**: The plaster extends from just below knee, down to the ankle and then up to a position well proximal to the toes, so that the toes are free for active movements. The ankle is held at right angle and foot is placed in a neutral position (i.e., neither inverted or everted).

Fractures of the Phalanx of the Toes

These fractures occur because of a heavy object falling on the toes. The phalanx is usually severely communited but hardly displaced. There is severe pain and swelling. Minimal treatment is required for these fractures. The swelling can be reduced by elevation of the foot for a few days. The pain can be reduced by immobilizing the toe by 'buddy strapping', i.e., the fractured toe is strapped to the adjacent toes by buddy strapping (Fig. 48.12). Wearing of shoes will protect the toes further.

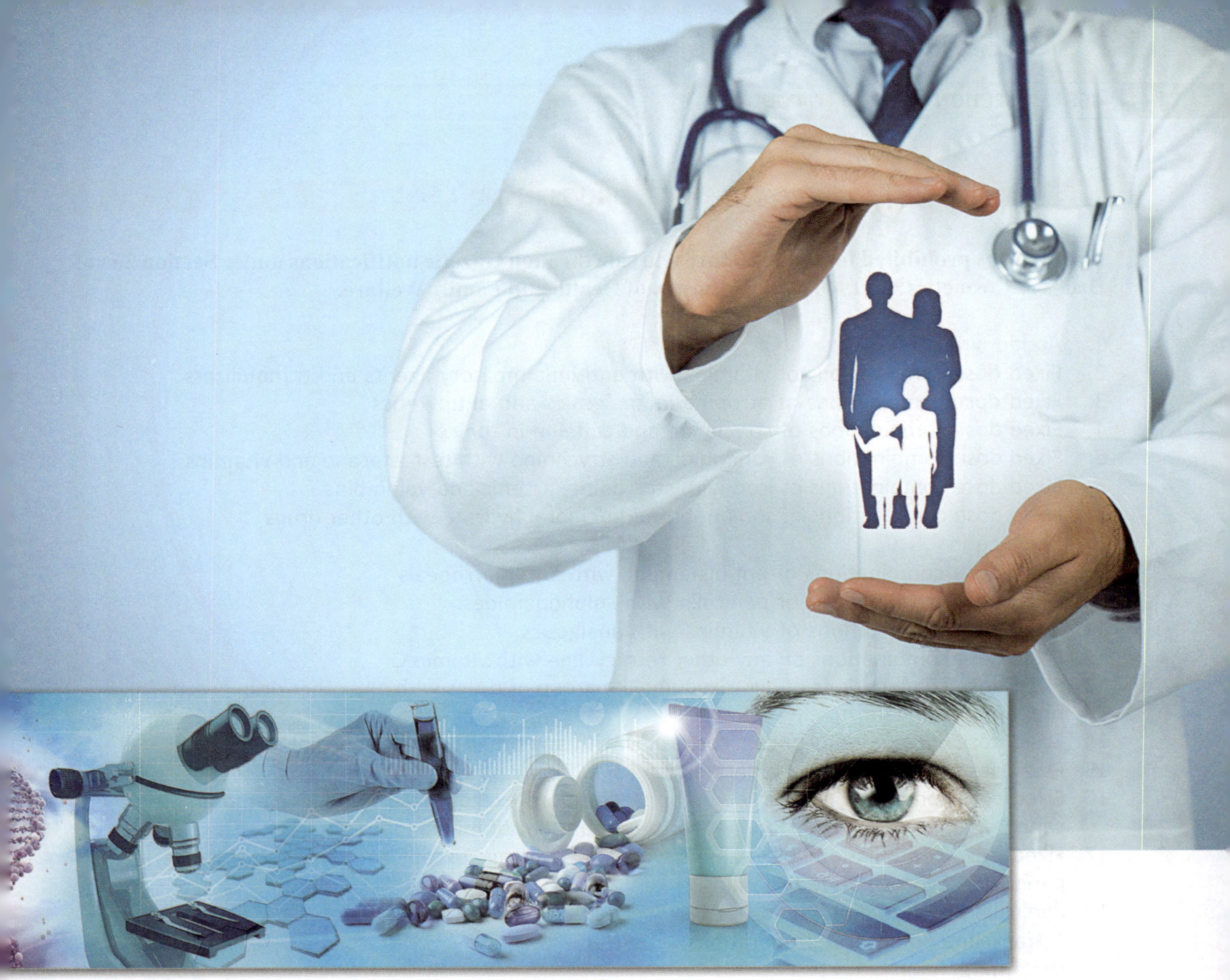

SECTION 4

DRUG FORMULARY

BANNED DRUGS IN INDIA

List of drugs prohibited for manufacture and sale through Gazette notifications under Section 26a of Drugs & Cosmetics Act 1940 by the Ministry of Health and Family Welfare.

1. Amidopyrine
2. Fixed dose combinations of vitamins with anti-inflammatory agents and tranquilizers
3. Fixed dose combinations of atropine in analgesics and antipyretics
4. Fixed dose combinations of strychnine and caffeine in tonics
5. Fixed dose combinations of yohimbine and strychnine with testosterone and vitamins
6. Fixed dose combinations of iron with strychnine, arsenic and yohimbine
7. Fixed dose combinations of sodium bromide/chloral hydrate with other drugs
8. Phenacetin
9. Fixed dose combinations of antihistaminic with anti-diarrhoeals
10. Fixed dose combinations of penicillin with sulphonamides.
11. Fixed dose combinations of vitamins with analgesics
12. Fixed dose combinations of any other tetracycline with vitamin C
13. Fixed dose combinations of hydroxyquinoline group of drugs with any other drug except for preparations meant for external use
14. Fixed dose combinations of corticosteroids with any other drug for internal use
15. Fixed dose combinations of chloramphenicol with any other drug for internal use
16. Fixed dose combinations of crude ergot preparations except those containing ergotamine, caffeine, analgesics, antihistamines for the treatment of migraine, headaches
17. Fixed dose combinations of vitamins with anti-TB drugs except combination of isoniazid with pyridoxine hydrochloride (Vitamin B_6)
18. Penicillin skin/eye ointment
19. Tetracycline liquid oral preparations
20. Nialamide
21. Practolol
22. Methapyrilene, its salts
23. Methaqualone
24. Oxytetracycline liquid oral preparations
25. Demeclocycline liquid oral preparations
26. Combination of anabolic steroids with other drugs
27. Fixed dose combination of oestrogen and progestin (other than oral contraceptives) containing per tablet oestrogen content of more than 50 µg (equivalent to ethinyl estradiol) and progestin content of more than 3 mg (equivalent to norethisterone acetate) and all fixed dose combination injectable preparations containing synthetic oestrogen and progesterone.
28. Fixed dose combination of sedatives/hypnotics/anxiolytics with analgesics-antipyretics.
29. Fixed dose combination of rifampicin, isoniazid and pyrazinamide, except those which provide daily adult dose given below:

Drugs	Minimum	Maximum
Rifampicin	450 mg	600 mg
Isoniazid	300 mg	400 mg
Pyrazinamide	1000 mg	1500 mg

30. Fixed dose combination of histamine H_2 receptor antagonists with antacids except for those combinations approved by Drugs Controller, India*
31. The patent and proprietary medicines of fixed dose combinations of essential oils with alcohol having percentage higher than 20% proof except preparations given in the Indian Pharmacopoeia
32. All pharmaceutical preparations containing chloroform exceeding 0.5% (w/w or v/v), whichever is appropriate
33. Fixed dose combination of ethambutol with INH other than the following: INH ethambutol 200 mg, 600 mg, 300 mg, 800 mg
34. Fixed dose combination containing more than one antihistamine
35. Fixed dose combination of any anthelmintic with cathartic/purgative except for piperazine/santonim
36. Fixed dose combination of salbutamol or any other drug having primarily bronchodilatory activity with centrally acting anti-tussive and/or antihistamine
37. Fixed dose combination of laxatives and/or anti-spasmodic drugs in enzyme preparations
38. Fixed dose combination of metoclopramide with systemically absorbed drugs except fixed dose combination of metoclopramide with aspirin/paracetamol
39. Fixed dose combination of centrally acting, antitussive with antihistamine, having high atropine like activity in expectorants
40. Preparations claiming to combat cough associated with asthma containing centrally acting anti-tussive and/or an antihistamine
41. Liquid oral tonic preparations containing glycerophosphates and/or other phosphates and/or central nervous system stimulant and such preparations containing alcohol more than 20% proof
42. Fixed dose combination containing pectin and/or kaolin with any drug which is systemically absorbed from GI tract except for combinations of pectin and/or kaolin with drugs not systemically absorbed
43. Chloral hydrate as a drug
44. Dovers powder I.P
45. Dover's powder tablets I.P
46. Antidiarrhoeal formulations containing kaolin or pectin or attapulgite or activated charcoal
47. Antidiarrhoeal formulations containing neomycin or streptomycin or dihydrostreptomycin including their respective salts or esters
48. Liquid oral antidiarrhoeals or any other dosage form for paediatric use containing diphenoxylate loperamide or atropine or belladona including their salts or esters or metabolites, hyoscyamine or their extracts or their alkaloids
49. Liquid oral antidiarrhoeals or any other dosage form for paediatric use containing halogenated hydroxyquinolines
50. Fixed dose combination of antidiarrhoeals with electrolytes
51. Patent & proprietary oral rehydration salts other than those conforming to standard formulations
52. Fixed dose combination of oxyphenbutazone or phenylbutazone with any other drug
53. Fixed dose combination of analgin with any other drug
54. Fixed dose combination of dextropropoxyphene with any other drug other than anti-spasmodics and/or non-steriodal anti-inflammatory drugs (NSAIDS)
55. Fixed dose combination of a drug, standards of which are prescribed in the second schedule to the said act with an ayurvedic, siddha or unani drug
56. Mepacrine hydrochloride (Quinacrine and its salts) in any dosage form for use for female sterilization or contraception
57. Fenfluramine and dexfenfluramine

58. Fixed dose combination of diazepam and diphenhydramine hydrochloride
59. Rimonabant
60. Rosiglitazone
61. Nimesulide formulations for human use in children below 12 years of age
62. Cisapride and its formulations for human use
63. Phenylpropanolamine and its formulation for human use
64. Human placental extract and its formulations for human use
65. Sibutramine and its formulations for human use
66. R-Sibutramine and its formulations for human use
67. Gatifloxacin formulation for systemic use in human by any route including oral and injectable
68. Tegaserod and its formulation for human use
69. Cosmetics licensed as toothpaste/tooth powder containing tobacco
70. Parenteral preparations fixed dose combination of streptomycin with pencillin
71. Fixed dose combination of vitamin B_1, vitamin B_6 and vitamin B_{12} for human use
72. Fixed dose combination of haemoglobin in any form (natural or synthetic)
73. Fixed dose combination of pancreatin or pancrelipase containing amylase, protease and lipase with any other enzyme
74. Fixed dose combination of nitrofurantoin and trimethoprim
75. Fixed dose combination of phenobarbitone with any anti-asthmatic drugs
76. Fixed dose combination of phenobarbitone with hyoscin and/or hyoscyamine
77. Fixed dose combination of phenobarbitone with ergotamine and/or belladona
78. Fixed dose combination of haloperidol with any anti-cholinergic agent including propantheline bromide
79. Fixed dose combination of nalidixic acid with any anti-amoebic including metronidazole
80. Fixed dose combination of loperamide hydrochloride with furazolidone
81. Fixed dose combination of cyproheptadine with lysine or peptone
82. Astemizole
83. Terfinadine
84. Fenformin
85. Rafecoxib
86. Valdecoxib and its formulation
87. Diclofenac and its formulations for animal use

DRUG FORMULARY

— Madhu Oswal

Opioid Analgesics

Drug	Available form	Dose	Side effects	Indications
Morphine (*Morcortin, Rilimorf S.R., inj. Morphine*)	10 mg, 30 mg, 60 mg tab, inj. 15 mg/mL im, sc	2.5–5 mg oral or im or sc	Constipation, respiratory depression, hypotension. Urinary retention. Dependency and tolerance. Dryness of mouth	Severe and intractable pain, anti-tussive, LVF, severe diarrhoea, MI
Pethidine (*Pethidine HCl*)	50–100 mg tab inj. 100 mg/2 mL	50–100 mg im, sc or oral	Similar to morphine	Preferred in biliary colic Same as morphine
Pentazocine (*Fortwin*) **with paracetamol** (*Fortagesic*)	Inj. 30 mg/mL 25 mg tab	25 mg tds-qid, inj. 1–2 mL can be repeated 4 hourly im or iv	Local fibrosis at injection site. Others same as morphine	Same as morphine
Tramazac (*Tramadol*)	50 mg cap, inj. 50 mg/mL, 100 mg/mL	50–100 mg tds	Low addiction. No drug dependency Not given < 16 yrs	Moderate to severe pain
Buprenorphine (*Tidegesic, Norphin*)	0.2 mg tab Inj. 0.3 mg/mL	1–2 tab sublingual tds 1–2 mL im or slow iv tds	Not to use in <16 yrs	Postoperative pain, MI, cancer pain
Dextropropoxy-phene (*Parvodex*) **with paracetamol** (*Spasmovon*) **with acetaminophen** (*Proxyvon*)	65 mg cap 33 + 300 mg tab 65 + 400 mg tab	60–120 mg bd or tds	CI in < 12 yrs Same as morphine but lesser	Muscular pain. Toothache, neuralgias, headache

Analgesics and Anti-Inflammatory Drugs

Drug	Available form	Dose	Side effects	Indications
Aspirin (*Ecosprin, Disprin, Colsprin*)	150, 325 m tab 350 mg tab 100, 325, 600 mg tab	0.3–0.6 gm tab for analgesic and antipyretic effect. 4–6 g/day in acute rheumatic fever	Nausea, vomiting, epigastric pain, peptic ulcer. Hypersensitivity, asthma, rash. In high dose—salicylism. Avoid in children below 6 yrs. Stop 1 wk before surgery	Analgesic, antipyretic, anti-rheumatic, prevents platelet aggregation in low dose, post MI, stroke
Paracetamol (*Calpol, Crocin, inj. Febrinil*)	500 mg, 125 mg/ml syrup, 150 mg/ml drops	15 mg/hr tds or qid	Nephropathy, hepatotoxicity. Less gastric irritation	Antipyretic, analgesic but poor anti-inflammatory
Nimesulide (*Nise, Nimegesic*) **with paracetamol** (*Nimsaid P, Sumo*) **with betacyclo-dextrin** (*Denim juicy*)	100 mg tab 100, 200 mg tab	100 mg bd	Rash, hepatotoxicity in children Not to give in children	Antipyretic and analgesic
Ibuprofen *(Brufen, Ibugesic, Febrilix)* **with paracetamol** (*Combiflam)*	200, 400, 600 mg tab, 100 mg/5 mL susp	200–600 mg	Mild gastric discomfort. Headache, dizziness, asthma, dysmenorrhoea	Antipyretic, analgesic for RA, OA, muscular pain
Indomethacin (*Indocap, Indoflam)* *Mederheumol suppository*	25, 75 mg tab 100 mg	25, 50 mg tds	Gastric irritation, headache, psychosis, rash, asthma CI in epilepsy, renal disease, psychotic patient	Potent anti-inflammatory for RA, gout, OA, sprain, fractures

contd.

Diclofenac sodium (*Jonac, Voveran*)	75, 50, 100 mg tab inj. 75 mg/3 mL Supp 12.5 mg, 100 mg	50 mg tds or 100 mg bd	Epigastric pain, headache, rash, oedema, asthma CI: Peptic ulcer, asthma	Potent anti-inflammatory and analgesic. RA, OA Postoperative pain, trauma
Diclofenac with paracetamol (*Diclonac-P*) **Diclofenac with serratiopeptidase** (*Diclosar*)	Same as above	Same as above	Same as above	Same as above
Aceclofenac (*Hinac, Aceclo*)	100 mg tab	100 mg bd	Same as diclofenac but better tolerated	Used in RA, OA, acute sprain
Ketorolac tromethamine (*Ketanov, Ketarol*)	10 mg tab inj 30 mg/mL	10–30 mg tds	Nausea, epigastric pain, gastric ulcer, not to give to patients on anticoagulants. Bronchospasm, angioedema	Potent analgesic. Post operative pain, musculo-skeletal pain
Mephenamic acid (*Dysmen, Meftal*)	500 mg tab 250 mg tab	250–500 mg tds	Diarrhoea, epigastric pain, rash, dizziness	Moderate muscular skeletal pain, dysmenorrhoea Prostaglandin inhibitor
Etoricoxib (*Nucoxia, Etody*)	90 mg tab 120 mg tab	1 tab od	No cardiac side effects	Cox II inhibitor OA, RA, acute gout
Propyphenazole with paracetamol	150 mg tab	1–2 tabs tds	Rash	Potent antipyretic and analgesic

contd.

(Saridon, DART) **Drotaverine** *(Drotin)*	40, 80 mg tab	40–80 mg tds	None		Does not mask signs and symptoms of a serious illness when given in acute abdomen
Glucosamine sulphate *(Cartigen, Cartriz)*	250 mg tab	500 mg tds	Rare		Helps in re-synthesis of cartilage. Used in OA, RA
Sulphasalazine *(Sazo-EN)*	500 mg tab	1 g/day up to 3–5 gm/day	Rash, hepatotoxicity, renal toxicity, tinnitus		RA
Chlorzoxazone with paracetamol and diclofenac *(Diclonac MR Flamar MR)*	250 mg tab	250, 500 mg tds	GI irritation, headache		Muscular spasm
Tizanidine *(Sirdalud, Tizan)*	2 mg	2 mg tds	Dry mouth, GI irritation		Muscular spasm
Baclofen *(Liofen)*	10 mg, 25 mg	15–75 mg/day	Rare		Biliary, renal colic, peptic ulcer. Does not mask signs and symptoms of acute abdomen
Valdecoxib (Valdone, Valus)	10 mg, 20 mg tab	10–12 mg od	Peripheral oedema		Cox II inhibitor OA, RA, post-operative pain

Drugs Used in Gout

Drug	Available	Dose form	Side effects	Indications
Colchicine	0.5 mg tab (*Goutnil*)	1 mg followed by 0.5 mg	Diarrhoea, till pain subsides. Max 8 mg/day	Acute gout anaemia, myopathy
Allopurinol (*Zyloric, Allgoric*)	100 mg, 300 mg tab	Initially 100–200 mg daily followed by 200–600 mg as maintenance dose	Rash, nausea, leucopenia, LFT ↑	Chronic gout, prevention of uric acid nephropathy
Probenecid	500 mg tab (*Benamcid*)	250–500 mg bd	Rash	Chronic gout–promotes excretion of uric acid

Drugs for Migraine

Drug	Available	Dose form	Side effects	Indications
Ergotamine with caffeine (*Migranil*) **with caffeine, cyclizine** (*Migril*)	1 mg tab 2 mg tab	1 mg every ½ hr till relief. Max 6 mg/day	Nausea, vomiting, TNs of extremities. CI: coronary, peripheral vascular disease, pregnancy, lactation	Migraine, cluster headache
Sumatriptan (*Sumitrex*)	25, 50, 100 mg tab 6 mg/mL SC	50–300 mg/day	Sudden wheezing, rash, angioedema, coronary ischaemia	Same as above
Flunarizine (*Flunarin, Sibelium*)	5 mg, 10 mg tab	10 mg hs > 40 kg 5 mg hs < 40 kg	Drowsiness, wt gain, extrapyramidal symptoms	Prophylaxis of classical and common migraine
Propranolol				See beta blockers

Anti-Epileptic Drugs and Drugs for Neuropathy

Phenytoin *(Eptoin, Dilanhin)*	50, 100 mg tab, syp, inj.	Loading dose 20 mg/kg 5–10 mg/kg/day in 2 dd	Gingival hyperplasia	Generalised, tonic clonic, partial, status epilepticus
Carbamazepine (*Mazetol, Zen)*	200 mg, 300 mg 100 mg, 100 mg/ 5 mL tab, syp	Start with 10 mg/kg and increase to 20–30 mg/kg/day in 2 dd	Hepatitis	Generalised, tonic-clonic, partial seizures
Phenobarbitone *(Gardenal)*	30, 60 mg tab, syp	Loading dose 20 mg/kg 5–10 mg/ kg/day od	Drowsiness, hyperkinesias	Tonic-clonic seizures, partial seizures, febrile seizures
Sodium valproate (*Valparin)*	100, 200 mg tab. Syp 200 mg/5 mL	20–30 mg/kg/day in 2 dd	Nausea, tremors, wt gain	Generalized seizures, temporal lobe epilepsy
Clobazam (*Frisium, Lobazam*)	5 mg, 10 mg 20 mg tab	5–80 mg	Sedation, dizziness	Refractory epilepsy. Partial seizure
Gabapentin (*Gabapin*) *with* **Mecobalamin** (*Nervimax g*)	100 mg, 300 mg, 400 mg, cap 600 mg, 800 mg, tab	900–1800 in 3 dd/day	Drowsiness, ataxia, fatigue, dizziness, diplopia	Seizures, peripheral neuropathy
Lamotrigine (*Lametec*)	25 mg, 50 mg, 100 mg, 200 mg	50 mg od slowly titrated to max 200–400 mg 1 day in 2 dd	Rash, diplopia, drowsiness, tremor, haematological, disturbance	Epilepsy, sec convulsions
Topiramate (*Topirol*)	25 mg, 50 mg 100 mg	25 mg od, slowly titrated to max 800 mg 1 day in 2 dd	Confusion, mood, disorders. Dizziness, diplopia, leucopenia	Epilepsy sec convulsions
Pregabalin (*Maxgalin*) **mecobalamin with** (*PGM*)		70–150 mg bd max 300 mg	Dizziness, drowsiness, blurred vision ataxia, tremor weight gain	Neuropathic pain

Anti-Parkinsonism Drugs

Drug	Available form	Dose	Side effects	Indications
Levodopa *(Levopa, Bidopal)*	500 mg tab	Start with 0.25 g and maintain at 2–3 g/day	Nausea, vomiting, postural hypotension, angina, facial tics, choreoathetoid movements	Parkinsonism—reduces hypokinesia and rigidity
Carbidopa + Levodopa *(Syndopa 110* *Tidoma LS* *Tidomet Plus* *Syndopa 275)*	 10 + 100 mg 10 + 100 mg 25 + 100 mg 25 + 250 mg tab	Start 1 tab bd, increase by 1 tab every 3rd–4th day to 4–8 tabs daily	Postural hypotension, involuntary movements, behavioural problems	Combination reduces dose of levodopa and also the side effects
Bromocryptine *(Proctinal, Brom)*	2.5 mg tab	Start with ½ tab, increase by 1 tab every fortnight till response is seen	Nausea, vomiting, hypotension, nasal stuffiness	Used with levodopa in late cases. Used to reduce lactation, prolactinoma
Amantidine *(Amantrel)*	100 mg tab	100 mg od or bd	Insomnia, dizziness, nightmares	Used in mild cases, has rapid action but low efficiency
Selegiline *(Selgin, Selmax)*	5 mg tab	10 mg od or in dd	Involuntary movements, postural hypotension. CI in convulsive disorders	Reduces dose of levodopa in early cases. Believed to halt the process of Parkinsonism
Trihexyphenidyl *(Pacitane, Triphen)*	2 mg tab	2–10 mg in dd	Confusion, delusion, dryness of mouth, blurring of vision, dizziness	Most useful for tremors, trigeminal neuralgia

Sedatives and Tranquilizers

Drug	Available form	Dose	Side effects	Indications
Diazepam (*Calmpose, Valium*)	5, 10 mg tab 2 mg/5 mL susp 10 mg/2 mL inj.	5–30 mg in dd	Dizziness, ataxia, amnesia, dependence, tolerance, synergistic action with alcohol	Used in anxiety disorders, insomnia, as a muscle relaxant, in alcohol withdrawal, as an anticonvulsant esp. in status epilepticus
Alprazolam (*Alprax, Trika*)	0.25, 0.5, 1 mg tab	0.25–5 mg in dd	Same as above	Anxiety neurosis, mild antidepressant
Chlordiazepoxide (*Librium, Equicalm*)	5, 10 mg tab	10 mg 2–4 times/day	Same as above	Same as diazepam
Lorazepam (*Ativan, Calmese*)	1, 2 mg tab inj. 2 mg/mL	1–6 mg/day	Same as above	Used in anxiety with depression, obsessive compulsive neurosis
Chlorpromazine (*Chlorpromazine, Relitil*)	10, 25, 50, 100 mg tab, inj 25 mg/mL	10–25 mg tds	Drowsiness, confusion, insomnia, postural hypotension, acute dystonia, jaundice, skin rash	Psychosis, hypomania, intractable hiccup, nausea, vomiting
Nitrazepam (*Nirven, Nitravet*)	5, 10 mg tab	5–10 mg hs	Same as diazepam	Insomnia, infantile spasm, myoclonus, insomnia
Buspirone (*Anxipar, Buspin*)	1, 5 mg tab	5–10 mg/day	Dizziness, headache	Anxiolytic without sedation. Used for aggressive behaviour

contd.

Haloperidol *(Serenace, Depidol)*	0.5, 1.5, 5, 10, 20 mg tab 2 mg/1 mL liquid inj 5 mg/mL	10–15 mg/day, then maintain at 1–10 mg/day	Extrapyramidal symptoms. Less sedation and anticholinergic side effects	Acute and chronic schizophrenia, agitated and manic patients, psychosis, severe anxiety
Trifluperazine *(Relicalm, Trinicalm)* **with chlorpromazine** (*Trinicalm forte, Relicalm SF)* **with trihexi-phenidyl** *(Trinicalm plus)*	1, 5 mg tab	1–2 tabs tds	Anticholinergic side effects like dry mouth, constipation, urinary retention, etc.	Same as above
Fluphenazine decanoate (*Anatensol*)	1 mg tab. inj. 25 mg/mL	2.5–10 mg/ day oral inj. every 2–4 wks	Same as above	Same as above
Risperidone (*Risdone, Zepid*)	1, 2, 3, 4 mg tab	1–3 mg/day in 2 dd	Dyskinesia, akathesia, insomnia	Atypical antipsychotic drug
Olanzapine (*Oleanz,Joyzol*)	2.5, 5, 7.5 mg tab	5–20 mg/day	Agranulocytosis. Less extrapyramidal symptoms	Major psychosis. Chronic schizophrenia
Trichlofos *(Pedichlor)*	500 mg/ 5 mL soln.	10 mL in adults, 2.5 mL, in children	Rash. No major side-effects	Insomnia, recurrent colic with persistent crying in children
Zolpidem (*Nitrest, Zoldem*)	5, 10 mg tab	5–10 mg hs	Same as above but no dependence or tolerance	All types of insomnia
Melatonin *(Meloset)*	3 mg	1–5 mg	Drowsiness, fatigue, headache	Disturbed biorhythms, insomnia

Tricyclic Antidepressants

Drug	Available form	Dose	Side effects	Indications
Imipramine (*Depsonil, Depsol*)	25, 75 mg tab	25–50 mg tds	Anticholinergic side effects, arrhythmias, sedation, tremors, hypotension, cholestasis	Antidepressant, nocturnal enuresis, migraine, acute panic attack
Amitriptyline (*Tryptomer, Relidep*)	10, 25, 75 mg tab	25–100 mg/day	Same as above	Depression with anxiety, agitation, neuropathy
Amoxapine (*Demolox*)	50, 100 mg tab	50–200 mg/day	Same as above	Psychotic depression
Nortriptyline (*Sensvral, Primox*)	25 mg tab	50–200 mg/day	Same as above	Masked depression
Trazodone (*Trazonil, Trazodep*)	25, 50, 100 mg tab	50–200 mg/day	Less anticholinergic action	Atypical, obsessive compulsive disorder
Clomipramine (*Clofranil*)	25, 50 mg tab	25–100 mg/day	Anticholinergic side effects	Obsessive compulsive disorder, panic disorder, depression with anxiety
Fluoxetine (*Fludac, Prodep*)	10, 20, 60 mg tab Susp 20 mg/5 mL	20–80 mg/day	No anticholinergic side effects Nervousness, anxiety insomnia	Depression, obsessive compulsive disorder
Doxepin (*Doxin, Spectra*)	10, 25, 75 mg tab	10–75 mg/day	Headache, less cardiovascular side effects	Preferred in elderly
Sertraline hydrochloride (*Serlift, Serta*)	50, 100 mg tab	50–100 mg/day	Anxiety, headache	Depression OCD, panic disorder

contd.

Venlafaxine (*Venlor*)	25, 37.5, 75 mg tab	25–75 mg od	Same as fluoxetine	Depression generalised anxiety disorder
Citalopram (*Citara*)	10, 20, 40 mg tab	10–40 mg/day	Increased sweating, insomnia, agitation	Major depression, panic disorder
Duloxetine *(Duzela)*	20 mg, 30 mg, 40 mg	40–60 mg	Anorexia, constipation, insomnia, fatigue, rash	Major depressive disorder, diabetic neuropathic pain
Escitalopram *(Nexito)*	5 mg, 10 mg, 20 mg	10–20 mg	Insomnia, ejaculation disorder, fatigue	Major depressive disorder

Antiemetics

Drug	Available form	Dose	Side effects	Indications
Metochlopramide *(Maxeron, Perinorm)*	5 ,10 mg tab Liquid 5 mg/mL inj 10 mg/mL	0.25–0.5 mg/mL	Sedation, dizziness, diarrhoea, extra-pyramidal symptoms, tardive dyskinesia	Vomiting, GERD, gastritis, hiccups
Domperidone *(Domperon, Domstal)*	10 mg tab Susp. 1 mg/mL	0.3–0.6 mL	None	Vomiting, GERD
Ondansetron *(Emeset, Vomiset)*	4, 8 mg tab inj 2 mg/mL Syr 2 mg/5 mL	8 mg bd	Headache	Potent anti-emetic
Prochlorperazine (*Stemetil, Vertex*)	5, 12.5, 25 mg tab inj 12.5 mg/mL	5 –25 mg tds	Sedation, dry mouth	Vertigo with vomiting
Promethazine theochate *(Avomine)*	25 mg tab	25 mg half an hour before travel	Sedation, dry mouth	Motion sickness
Meclizine (*Pregnidoxin*)	25 mg tab	25–50 mg daily in dd	Anticholinergic side effects	Motion sickness, morning sickness
Doxylamine (*Doxinate, Vomitex*)	10 mg tab	2 tab at bedtime	Drowsiness, dizziness	Morning sickness

Drugs Used in Vertigo				
Prochlorperazine (*Stemetil*)	5 mg tab	5 mg tds	Drowsiness, dry mouth	Vertigo, Meniere's disease, migraine, vomiting, labryinthitis
Cinnarazine (*Vertigon, Stugeron, Stugeron forte*)	25 mg tab 75 mg forte	25–50 mg tds	Sedation, GI upset	Vertigo, tinnitus, Meniere's disease, motion sickness
Dimenhydrinate (*Gravol, Draminamine*)	50 mg tab	50 mg tds	Drowsiness, dry mouth	Nausea, vomiting, vertigo, motion sickness
Beta-histine (*Vertin*)	8 mg, 16 mg tab	1 tab tds	GI upset	Vertigo, Meniere's disease

Anti-Allergics

Drug	Available form	Dose	Side effects	Indications
Diphenhydramine (*Benadryl*)	25–75 mg tab 12.5 mg/mL syrup	25 mg tds	SI-Sedation, fatigue, tinnitus, diplopia, anticholinergic side effects	Allergic diseases, urticaria, hay fever, rhinitis, anaphylaxis, angioedema
Pheniramine maleate (*Avil*)	25, 50, 75 mg R 22.75 mg/mL inj.	25 mg tds or 75 mg retard hs	Same as above	Same as above
Chlorpheniramine maleate (*Piriton*)	5–20 mg tab	5–20 mg tds	Same as above	Same as above
Promethazine (*Phenargan*)	10, 25 mg tab 25 mg/mL inj. 5 mg/mL elixir	25–50 mg oral, im tds	Drug induced extrapyramidal symptoms	Same as above
Astemizole (*Astalong*)	10 mg, 5 mg/ 5 mL tab	10–30 mg od	Dry mouth, weight gain, and diarrhoea. Less sedation	Same as above
Terfenadine (*Terf, Terin*)	60, 120 mg, tab, 30 mg/ 5 mL	60 mg bd or 120 mg od	Same as above Cardiotoxicity	Same as above
Cetrizine (*Cetri, Cetzine*)	10 mg, 5 mg/ mL tab	10 mg od	Drowsiness in few	Same as above

contd.

Levocetrizine (*Levocet*)	5 mg tab	5 mg od	Less sedative	Same as above
Hydroxyzine (*Atarax*)	10, 25 mg 10 mg/5 mL syrup inj 25 mg/mL	25–50 mg oral, im tds	Sedation, anticholinergic side effects	Same as above
Fenofexadine (*Allegra*)	120, 80 mg tab	120–80 mg od	Not to give in <12 yrs	Same as above
Loratidine (*Lorfast, Loridine*)	10 mg tab	5, 10 mg od	None	Allergic conditions
Desloratidine (*Delotid, Dazit*)	5 mg tab	5 mg od	Dry mouth, fatigue	Same as above

Drugs for Cough				
Drug	**Available form**	**Dose**	**Side effects**	**Indications**
Antitussive **Codeine** (*Coxex, Ephredex, Lin. Codeine)*	Liquid	1–2 tsf tds	Constipation	For nonproductive cough
Noscapine (*Coscopine, Ephredex*)			Nausea	
Dextromethorphan (*Alex cough formula, Zedek)*			Less constipation than codeine	
Expectorants *(Avil expectorant, Phensedyl expectorant, Zeet expectorant)*	Liquid	1–2 tsf tds	Sedation	For productive cough
Bromhexine *(Pulmorest, Bromhexine)* with combination (*Chestor, Cosome, Zedex*)	8 mg tab syrup	1–2 tsf tds	Insignificant	Mucolytic for sticky, difficult secretions
Ambroxol *(Mycolite)* **Carbocisterne** *(Mucodyn*)	Liqiud	1–2 tsf tds	Insignificant	In bronchitis, bronchiectasis, sinusitis

Drugs Used in Asthma/COPD

Drug	Available form	Dose	Side effects	Indications
Adrenaline *(Adrenaline)*	0.5 and 1 mL ampoules	0–2–0.5 mL sc/IM	Palpitation, headache. Use withcaution in elderly, IHD, HT	Status asthmatics or acute asthma not responding to other treatment
Salbutamol *(Asthalin)*	2 –4 mg tab 2 mg/5 mL susp, rotacaps, inhaler, respirator soln.	2–4 mg tds	Nervousness, drowsiness, tremors	Bronchial asthma. To delay delivery in premature labour
Salmeterol *(Serobid)*	25 μg/metered dose inhaler, rotacaps	Metered dose inhaler 1–2 puffs, rotacaps (50 μg)	Same as above, but lesser	Long-acting
Aminophylline	0.25 g ampoule	0.25 g in 20 mL of 10% glucose	Nausea, vomiting, hypotension, cardiac arrhythmia, twitching of mouth	Bronchial asthma, esp. in status asthmaticus. Cardiac asthma
Theophylline + Etophyline *(Deriphyllin, Theobid SR)*	200, 300, 400 mg tab retard, syrup, inj.	1–2 tabs tds or bd if retard tab	Same as above	Same as above
Terbutaline *(Bricanil)*	2.5 mg, 5 mg inj, 0.5 mg/mL	5 mg tds, 0.5 mL sc. 0.01 mg/kg	Same as above	Status asthmaticus
Sodium cromoglycate *(Fintal inhaler)*	1 mg MDI	2 puffs tds–qid	Rare	Exercise induced asthma, allergic rhinitis. Prevent attacks of asthma

contd.

Ipratropium bromide *(Ipravent)*	Inhaler, respiratory soln.	40–80 mg tds	Dry mouth	Perennial rhinitis, chronic bronchitis
Ketotifen *(Kitofen)*	1 mg tab, syrup 1 mg/5 mL	1 mg bd	Drowsiness, dry mouth, wt gain	Prophylaxis in childhood asthma, allergic rhinitis, conjunctivitis
Budesonide *(Budecort)*	Resp. soln, inhaler.	100 mg bd	Oral candidiasis	To prevent asthma attacks
Beclomethasone dipropionate *(Beclate)*	Inhaler	100 mg tds	Same as above	Same as above
Fluticasone *(Flohale)*	25–125 μg MDI, rotacaps 50–250 μg	100–1000 μg/day in 2 dd	Same as above	Same as above
Montelukast sodium *(Montair)*	5, 10 mg tab	5–10 mg od	None	Prophylaxis and treatment of asthma
Bambuterol *(Bambudil)*	10, 20 mg tab	10–20 mg od	Same as salbutamol	Maintenance treatment of asthma, nocturnal attacks—long acting
Tiotropium bromide *(Tiova)*	18 μg rotacaps	1 rotacap 1 day	Dry mouth, glaucoma, urinary retention	COPD
Doxoffylline *(Doxobid)*	400 mg	400 mg 1 day		Asthma, COPD
Acebrophylline *(A B Phylline)*	100 mg cap	100 mg 1 day	Epigastric pain	Bronchitis, asthma, sinusitis

Drugs for Constipation

Drug	Available as	Dose	Side effects	Note/Important information
Isabghula *(Igol, Naturolax, Softovac)*	*Powder 100 g, 150 g*	*1–2 tsf in 100 mL of water bd or tds*	*Flatulence. All laxatives are contraindicated in constipation with abdominal pain or vomiting, constipation due to stricture, obstruction of bowel, malignancy*	*Bulk forming laxative. Takes 1–3 days for action. 1st choice in functional constipation*
Docusates (*Laxicon, Cellubril)*	100 mg tab, syrup, enema, Cap 100 mg	1–2 tabs 2–3 times a day	Intestinal cramps	Stool softener. Used when straining has to be avoided as in recent MI, pregnancy, postoperative
Liquid paraffin (*Cremaffin, Stuflow)*	Emulsion	15–30 mL at bedtime	Unpleasant taste	Lubricant. Not recommended in children < 3 yrs
Bisacodyl (*Dulcolax, Bidlax)*	5, 10 mg tab suppositories	1–3 tabs at bedtime	Abdominal cramps	Action in 6–8 hrs. Used for preparation of bowel for radiological exam
Senna (*Sofsena, Laxena)*	12 mg tab	2–4 tabs at bedtime	Cramps	Stimulant. Not recommended in children and pregnancy
Lactulose *(Dulphalac, Laxose)*	Liquid, syrup	15–30 mL tds with plenty of water	Intestinal cramps, flatulence in hepatic encephalopathy	Osmotic laxative. Costly. Used
Castor oil	Liquid	15–30 mL	Gripping pain, fluid loss, nauseating after taste	Purgative, rapid evacuation time 1–3 hrs

contd.

Mosapride (*Moza*)	2.5 mg, 5 mg	5 mg tds	Diarrhoea, dry mouth	Gastro-esophageal reflux, chronic gastritis
Itopride Hcl (*It pride*)	50 mg	50 mg	Diarrhoea, dizziness	Abdominal pain, nausea, vomiting, bloating
Tegaserod	2 mg , 6 mg	2–6 mg bd	Abdominal pain, diarrhoea, dizziness	Constipation, bloating, IBS

Drugs Used for Treatment of Acid Peptic Disease

Drug	Available form	Dose	Side effects	Indications
Plain antacid (*Digene, Gelusil MPS)*	Tab, liquid	1–2 tabs or 3 tsf qid (3 hrs after each meal and at bed time)	Constipation or diarrhoea. Interferes with absorption of drugs like tetracycline, steroids	Interferes with absorption of iron, steroids, tetracycline. Magnesium based antacids contra indicated in renal failure
Antacid with anaesthetic oxethazine *(Mucaine Gel, Tricaine MPS*)	Liquid	5–10 mL before meals 10–20 mL tds	Same as above	Useful for heartburn, oesophagitis, hiatus hernia
Antacid with alginic acid (*Acigon, Riflux*)	Liquid, tab	1–2 tabs or 10–20 mL tds	Same as above	Reflux oesophagitis, sour eructations
Magaldrate with simethicone *(Maggel, Alcaine MPS)*	Liquid, tab	1–2 tabs or 10–20 mL tds	Same as above	Sustained action as acid neutralizer
H_2-blockers				
Cimetidine (*Ulciban, Taximet)*	200, 400 800 mg tabs inj 200 mg/mL	400 mg bd or 800 mg hs (4 wks for DU, 8 wks for GU)	Headache, GI upset, dizziness. Should not be given with antacids. Delays absorption of diazepam, phenytoin, theophylline	DU, GU, GERD, oesophagitis
Ranitidine *(Aciloc, Histac, Rantac, Zinetac*)	150, 300 mg tab inj 25 mg/mL	150 mg bd or 300 mg hs × 4–8 weeks	Rare	Same as above Long acting, therefore od dose
Famotidine *(Famtac, Famocid)*	20 mg, 40 mg 20 mg/mL	20 mg bd or 40 mg hs × 4–8 weeks	Rare	Same as above

contd.

Proton-pump inhibitiors				
Omeprazole (*Lomac, Omez*)	10 mg, 20 mg cap	20, 40 mg od × 4–8 weeks before meals	Minimal nausea, headache, GI upset. Slow elimination of diazepam, phenytoin, aminophylline	DU, GU, GERD, oesophagitis
Lansoprazole *(Lan-15, Lanzap)*	15, 30 mg cap	15 mg bd or 30 mg od	Same as above	Same as above
Pantaprazole *(Pantocid, Pantodac)*	40 mg tab	40 mg od before break fast for 2–4 weeks	Same as above	Same as above
Rabiprazole *(Rabeloc, Rablet)*	10, 20 mg tab	20 mg od before breakfast	Same as above	Same as above
Esomepra-zole *(Esoz, Sompraz)*	20, 40 mg tab	20–40 mg od before breakfast	Same as above	Same as above

Other Anti-Ulcer Drugs

Drug	Available form	Dose	Side effects	Indications
Sucralfate *(Mucoguard, Sucrase)*	1 g tab, susp.	1 g qid before meals × 4 weeks	Constipation, dry mouth	Not to be given along with antacid or H_2 blocker
Colloidal bismuth *(Pylocid, Trymo)*	120 mg tab	1 tab bd × 4–8 weeks	Blackening of stools, nausea,	Same as above Vomiting
Drugs for treatment of *H pylori* infection				
Omeprazole + Amoxicillin + Tinidazole (*Helipac, Helikit*)	20 mg + 750 mg + 500 mg tabs in kit	1 kit bd × 7 days	Headache, diarrhoea	Recurrent ulcers not responding to usual treatment for eradication
Lansaprazole + Amoxicillin + Tinidazole (*Pylomox*)	15 mg + 750 mg + 1000 mg tabs in kit	1 kit bd × 7 days	Same as above	Same as above

Drugs for Diarrhoea

Drug	Available form	Dose	Side effects	Indications
Loperamide (*Imodium, Andial*)	2 mg cap, tab Liquid (1 mg/5 mL)	2 stat, followed by 1 tab after each stool	Cramps, rashes Paralytic ileus in children	Not to be given in children < 4 yrs
Diphenoxylate + Atropine (*Lomotil, Lomofen*)	2.5 mg + 0.025 mg tab	1–2 tabs 6 hrly	Same as above	Contraindicated in children < 6 yrs of age
Racecadotrel (*Enuff*)	100 mg tab 10, 30 mg sachets	1 tab tds	Drowsiness, nausea	Antisecretory action
Mebeverine (*Colospa*)	135 mg tab	1–2 tabs 3–4 times a day, 15 min before food	Heartburn, dizziness	Irritable bowel syndrome
Sulphasalazine (*Salazopyrin*)	500 mg tab	2–4 tabs 3–4 times a day for 2–3 weeks Maintenance 3–4 tabs daily	Oligospermia, rash, fever, nausea	Ulcerative colitis Contraindicated in those hypersensitive to sulphonamides or salicylates
5-Aminosalicylic acid (*Masacol, Tidcol*)	400 mg tab	6 tabs daily in dd Maintenance 3–6 tabs daily	Headache, GI upset	Ulcerative colitis
Digestive enzymes preparations				
Fungal diastase + Pepsin-based (*Digeplex, Aristozyme, Bestozyme, Unienzyme*)	Liquid, drops Cap, drops Cap, syrup Syr, drops, tab	1–2 tabs bd after food 5–100 mL bd	Rare	Dyspepsia, antiflatulant Enzyme deficiency
Pancreatic based (*Pankreatoflat, Panzynorm*)	Tab	2–4 tabs daily		Chronic pancreatitis (costly)

contd.

Hepatobiliary drugs				
Phospholipid *(Essentiale)*	Cap	2–3 caps tds	Insignificant	Helps regenerate liver cells in alcoholic and drug induced hepatitis Contraindicated in hepatic encephalopathy
Silymarin (*Silybon, Sirylar*)	70, 140 mg tab	140 mg tds × 1 month infective hepatitis. 140 mg tds × 3–6 mon for alcoholic hepatitis	Safe and well tolerated	Same as above
L-ornithine-L aspartate (*Hepamerz, Livogard*)	Tab, granule, syrup	1–2 tab tds 5–10 mL tds	Transient nausea, vomiting	Acute and chronic liver disease. Contraindicated in renal insufficiency

Antibiotics

Drug	Available form	Dose	Side effects	Indications
Penicillins				
Fortified procaine penicillin G inj.	0.5, 1 MU dry powder in vial	8–10 lac IM OD	Pain at IM injection site. Anaphylaxis. Rash	Streptococcal infections like pharyngitis, otitis media, scarlet fever, rheumatic fever. Pneumococcal infections like otitis media, meningitis, osteomyelitis. Gonorrhoea. Syphilis, diphtheria, tetanus, rat bite fever
Penidure (Benzathine penicillin)	Inj 6, 12, 24 lacs units	6–12 lacs every 3 weeks in rheumatic fever	Same as above	Same as above
Pentids (Penicillin G)	200, 400, 600 tab	Pot penicillin-G oral use: 2–8 lac U qid 1 hr before or 2 hrs after food	Same as above	Same as above
Cloxacillin *(Klox, Clopen) inj. Klox*	250, 500 mg cap 125 mg/5 mL	250–500 mg tds or qid	Rash, GI upset	Furuncle, abscesses, carbuncle, impetigo, osteomyelitis, etc.
Ampi + cloxacillin *(Ampilox, Baxin)*	Cap 250, 500 inj. 125, 250, 1 g dry. Syr 125 + 125	250–500 mg tds	Same as above	Same as above

contd.

Amoxicillin *(Biomox, Mox)*	Cap 250, 500 mg KT – 125 mg inj. 250 mg/mL 500 mg/mL	250–500 mg tds	Same as above	URTI, LRTI; ENT, GUT infections due to Gram +ve and Gram -ve organisms
Amox + clox *(Novaclox)*	Cap 250, 500 mg Paed tab	250–500 mg tds	Same as above	Furuncle, abscesses, carbuncle, impetigo, osteomyelitis, etc.
Amox + Bromhexine (*Bromoxyl forte)*	Cap 250, 500 mg	250–500 mg tds	Same as above	URTI, LRTI
Mox + clavulanic acid (*Augmentin Clavum)*	625 mg tab 375 mg tab	1–2 tab 6 hourly	Same as above	Active against β-lactamase producing organisms. RTI, UTI, skin and soft tissue infections

Cephalosporins

Drug	Available form	Dose	Side effects	Indications
Cefazolin sodium *(inj Reflin, inj Cezolin)*	250, 500, 1000 mg inj.	500 mg to 1 g im or iv qid	Rash, GI upsets pain at inj site, thrombophlebitis	1st generation. RTI, UTI, skin and soft tissue infections, GUT infections, bone and joint infections
Cefixime trihydrate *(Ceftas, Taxim O)*	200 mg tab, dry syp 100 mg/mL 200, 100 mg tab, DT 50, 100 mg dry syr 50 mg/5 mL	200–400 mg daily od or in 2 dd	Phlebitis, anaphylaxis, nephrotoxicity	3rd generation RTI, UTI, biliary tract infections
Ceftazidime *(Inj Fortum, inj Tazid)*	250, 500 mg, 1 g	1–6 g daily in dd	Same as above	3rd generation. Serious infections of RT, GIT, ENT, skin and soft tissue. Septicaemia, meningitis
Cephalexin *(Ceft, Cephaxin, Blucef)* **Cephalexin + probenecid** (*Cefalong*)	Cap 250, 500 mg 125 mg, DT 250 mg syp 125 mg/5 mL 100 mg/5 mL drops 250 + 250 mg tab 500 + 500 mg tab	1–4 g daily in 3–4 dd	Same as above	1st generation RTI, UTI, skin and soft tissue infections, GUT infections, biliary tract, bone and joint infections
Cefadroxil (*Bludrox, Cefadrox*)	DT 250, tab 500 mg Dry syrup 250 mg/ 5 mL 125 mg DT inj. 125 mg/5 mL Drop 100 mg/1 mL	1–2 g daily in 2 dd	Same as above	Same as above
Cefotaxime *(C-Tax, Taxim)*	125, 250, 500 mg, 1, 1.5 g 125, 250, 500, 1, 2 g	2–4 g daily in 2–3 dd	Same as above	3rd generation. Serious infections of RT, GIT, ENT, skin and soft tissue. Septicaemia, meningitis, gonorrhoea, typhoid

contd.

Ceftriaxone (*Monocef, Powercef)*	125, 500 mg, 1 g, 2 g inj 125, 250, 500, 1 g inj.	1–4 g daily od or in dd	Same as above	Same as above
Cefaclor *(Keflor, Vercef)*	Cap 250 DT 125, 250 mg Dry syr 125 mg/5 mL		Same as above	2nd generation RTI, UTI, skin and soft tissue infections, GUT biliary tract, bone and joint infections
Cefuroxime *(Forcef, Zocef)*	125, 250, 500 mg tab inj 250, 750, 1.5 g	250, 500 mg tds	Same as above	3rd generation. As above plus meningitis
Cefoperazone sodium (*Magnamycin, Magacef*)	inj 250, 1 g, 2 g	1–2 gm bd	Same as above	Same as above
Cefoperazone + sulbactum *(Cefactum inj)*	0.5 + 0.5 g inj. 1 g + 1 g inj.	1–2 gm bd	Same as above	Same as above
Cefpodoxime proxetil *(Cepodem, Monocef O)*	100, 200 mg tab Dry syrup 50–100 mg/5 mL	100–200 mg bd	Diarrhoea, pain in abdomen	Same as above
Cefpirome (*Cefrom, Forgen)*	Inj. 250 mg, 500 mg, 1 g	1–2 g daily in dd	Same as above	Same as above
Cefdinir (*Adcef Sefdin)*	Cap 300 mg, 125 mg/5 mL	300 mg bd	Same as above	Same as above
Cefepime *(Megapime, Cepime)*	500 mg, 1 g inj. 1 gm inj.	1–2 gm bd	Same as above	Same as above

Macrolides

Erythromycin (*Althrocin, Erythrocin*)	250, 500 mg, DT 250 tab KT 125 mg syrup 125 mg/5 mL paed drops 100 mg/mL	250–500 mg tds or qid 30–60 mg/kg in dd	Epigastric pain, diarrhoea, allergy	URTI, pneumonia, skin infection, acne
Polymyxin B and colistin (*Walamycin*)	25 mg/5 mL susp	25–100 mg tds 5–15 mg/kg 3 dd	Same as above	GI infections
Azithromycin (*Aziwok, Azee*)	100 mg kid tab, 250, 500, 1000 mg, susp 100 mg/5 mL	500 mg od × 3 days 1 hr before meal	Same as above	Same as Erythromycin. Once a day therapy and long acting, therefore requires short treatment period
Roxithromycin (*Roxem, Roxid*)	50 mg kid tab, 150 mg liquid 50 mg/5 mL	150 mg bd	Same as above	URTI, pneumonia, acute bronchitis, sinusitis
Clarithromycin (*Clarithro, Crixan*)	250, 500 mg tab, 125 mg/5 mL	250–500 mg bd	Same as above	All above plus skin and soft tissue infection
Clindamycin (*Clincin, Dalacin*)	150, 300 mg cap, inj 300 and 600 mg vials	150–300 mg 6 hrly oral 600 mg IM or IV bd	Same as above	Same as above
Lincomycin (*Lincin, Lynx*)	250, 500 mg cap 300 mg/mL inj susp 125 mg/5 mL	500 mg tds or qid 600 mg im or iv bd or tds. Child 10 mg/kg iv bd or tds and 30–60 mg/kg in dd orally	Same as above	All above plus otitis media, osteomyelitis, septic arthritis, endocarditis
Spiramycin (*Rovamycin*)	Tab 1.5 MIU susp 0.325 MIU/5 mL Tab forte 3 MIU	0.1–0.15 MIU/kg in 2 dd	Same as above	All above plus toxoplasmosis

Quinolones

Drug	Available form	Dose	Side effects	Indications
Ciprofloxacin *(Ciplox, Baycip)* Ciplox with ornidazole *(Ocimix)*	100, 250, 500, 750, 1000 mg tab 100 mg/ 50 mL infusion	250–500 mg bd	Diarrhoea, vomiting, rash	UTI, GIT infections, gonorrhoea, enteric fever, tuberculosis
Gatifloxacin *(Gatiquin, Gator)* **with ornidazole** *(Gatimore OZ)*	200, 400 mg tab	200–400 mg od	Seizures, tachycardia, confusion, hallucination, rash	All above plus acute bronchitis, CAP, sinusitis
Sparfloxacin *(Bluspar, Genspar)*	100, 200 mg tab	400 mg on 1st day then 200 mg od	Allergy, photosensitivity, diarrhoea	Same as above
Norfloxacin *(Norflox, Norbid)*	100, 200, 400, 800 mg tab DT 100 mg	400 mg bd	Nausea, vomiting, rash	UTI, gonorrhoea, GI infection
Morifloxacin *(Moxif)*	400 mg tab	400 mg od	Same as above	Same as ciplox
Nalidixic acid *(Gramoneg, Ulin P, Ulix)*	150, 250 mg syr 300 mg/ 5 mL	1 g 6 hourly, 55 mg/kg in dd	Same as above	GIT infections, UTI
Ofloxacin *(Ofler, Tarivid)*	200, 400 mg tab, sus 50 mg/5 mL	200–400 mg bd	Same as above	Same as above
Of + TZ *(Oflin TZ, Tin-off)*	200 + 600 mg tab 50 + 100 mg sup	Same as above	Same as above	Same as above
Of + Met *(Zenotin sup, Zenol M sup)*	50 mg + 100 mg/5 mL	Same as above	Same as above	Same as above
Of + Orn *(Zenflox OZ)*	Tab 20 + 500 mg Sup 50 + 125 mg/5 mL	Same as above	Same as above	Same as above

contd.

Aminoglycosides				
Amikacin (*Amikef, Mikacin)*	Inj. 100, 250, 500 mg/vial	15 mg/kg body wt/day in 2 or 3 divided doses	Ototoxicity, nephrotoxicity, skin rash, tremors	Bacteraemias, septicaemias, respiratory tract, bones and joint, CNS (including meningitis), skin and soft tissue, intraabdominal infections
Tobramycin sulphate, *(Tobcin, Tobramycin)*	Inj. 60, 80 mg/vial	3–5 mg/kg/ day in 3 dd	Ototoxicity, nephrotoxicity, skin rash, tremors	Same as above
Gentamicin *(Garamycin, Genticyn)*	Inj. 20, 80 mg/2 mL 60 mg/1.5 mL	3–5 mg/kg/ day in 2–3 dd	Same as above	Same as above

Sulphonamides

Drug	Available form	Dose	Side effects	Indications
Cotrimoxazole TMP + SMX (*Bactrim, Bactrim DS*)	80 + 400 mg tab 160 + 800 mg tab paed 20 +100 mg susp 40 + 120/5 mL	2 bd for 2 days then 1 tab od or 1 DS tab bd	Rash, nausea	UTI, URTI, skin infections, PCP
Tetracyclines/Chloramphenicol				
Tetracycline (*Hostacyclin, Resteclin)*	250, 500 mg cap	250–500 mg 6 hourly	GI disturbance, tooth discolou-ration. CI in pregnancy	URTI, RTI, UTI, ENT, GUT infections, STDs, acne
Oxytetracycline (*Terramycin, Tetramac)*	250, 500 mg cap	250–500 mg 6 hourly	Same as above	Same as above
Doxycycline *(Doly-1, Biodoxy)*	100 mg tab	100 mg bd followed by 1 od	Same as above	Same as above
Minocycline *(Cynomycin)*	50, 100 mg cap	1–2 tabs daily	Same as above	Not recommen ded < 8 yrs
Chloramphenicol (*Chlormycetin, Paraxin)*	Cap 250, 500 mg susp 125 mg/mL	250–500 mg tds	GI upset, allergic rash, anaemia, bone marrow suppression in high doses. Avoid in pregnancy and lactation	H influenza meningitis, UTI, enteric fever
Linezolid *(Linospan)*	600 mg, 2 mg/mL/ inj 200/100 mL infusion	600 mg bd	Dyspepsia, rash, dizziness, constipation	Skin and soft tissue infections, pneumonia, osteomyelitis

Antileprotics

Dapsone *(Dapsone)*	100 mg tab	100 mg od	Haemolysis in G6PD def., nausea, vomiting, headache, rash, FDE, hyper-pigmentation, phototoxicity	Leprosy, dermatitis hepatiformis, malaria, pneumocystis pneumonia, cutaneous leishmaniasis
Clofazimine (*Hansepran Clofozine*)	50, 100 mg cap	300–600 weeks or 50 mg od	Reddish-brown discolouration of skin	Leprosy, lepra reaction (ENL), MDR TB, DLE
Rifampicin (*R-cin)*	150, 300, 600 mg tab	600 mg single dose once a month	Flu like syndrome	Leprosy, tuberculosis

Antimalarials

Drug	Available form	Dose	Side effects	Indications
Chloroquine (*Clokit, Clokit-P, Lariago, Lariago DS*)	250 mg tab 500 mg tab syrup 160 mg/ 10 mL Inj. 64.5 mg/mL	1 g stat followed by 500 mg after 6 hrs and then 500 mg daily for 2 days	Nausea, vomiting, headache, itching, hypotension, cardiac depression, convulsion on iv use. Prolonged use can cause retinal damage and loss of hearing	Malaria, extraintestinal amoebiasis. Giardiasis. RA, SLE, DLE, lepra-reaction
Mefloquine *(Meflam, MQF)*	250 mg tab	15–25 mg/kg	Bitter taste, nausea, bradycardia, vertigo	Chloroquine resistant falciparum malaria
Quinine sulphate *(Falciquin, Quininga)*	300 mg tab 100, 300, 600 mg tab, inj 300 mg/mL	25 mg/kg or 300–600 mg tds for 5 days	Cinchonism if taken in large doses. Nausea, ringing in ears, headache, confusion, hearing and vision difficulty. Rash, purpura, haemolysis	Avoid in pregnancy. Resistant *P. falciparum* malaria. Nocturnal cramps

contd.

Artemether *(Larither, Marither)* Artesunate (*Falcigo*)	40 mg cap Inj 80 mg/mL 50 mg tab inj. 60 mg	80 mg bd or 1.6 mg/kg bd for 3 days 100 mg bd on 1st day, then 50 mg bd × 4 days Total dose 480 mg	Bradycardia, fever, neurotoxicity Same as above	Resistant or complicated falciparum malaria Same as above
Primaquine (*Malarid, MQ-Inga*)	2.5 mg tab 7.5 mg tab	15 mg/day × 14 days 0.3 mg/kg/day	Abdominal pain, anaemia	Radical cure of malaria
Sulphadoxine + Pyrimethamine *(Rimodar, Reziz)* *(Rimodar Forte, Reziz forte)* *(Reziz syrup)*	500 + 25 mg tab 750 + 37.5 mg tab 250 + 12.5 mg syrup	2–3 tabs as a single dose	Rash, GI upset	Prophylactic or suppressive therapy of malaria

Anti-Tubercular Drugs

Drug	Available form	Dose	Side effects	Indications
Isoniazid (INH) (*Isonex forte, Isonex)*	300 mg tab 100 mg tab	450 mg if wt > 50 kg 300 mg od < 50 kg 10 mg/kg/dose od	Peripheral neuropathy, hepatitis, rash. Rare—optic neuritis, acne	Kills fast multiplying organisms. No action against atypical tubercular micro. Crosses BBB
Rifampicin (*Rimactane, R-cin)*	150, 300, 450 mg cap, syrup 100 mg/mL	450 mg if wt < 50 kg 600 mg if wt > 50 kg 10–15 mg/kg od	Hepatitis, nausea, vomiting, flu-like syndrome, orange coloured urine, faeces. Contraception failure	Acts on slowly and intermittently growing tubercular bacilli. Acts against atypical organisms. Also used for leprosy, meningococcal carriers, staphylococcal infections
Ethambutol (*Combutol, Koxi)*	200, 400, 600, 800, 1000 mg tab	25 mg/kg < 50 kg 800 mg > 50 mg 1200 mg	Optic neuritis, nausea, vomiting. Reduce dose in renal insufficiency	Not given in child < 6 yrs. Bacteriostatic. Crosses BBB, acts on atypical organisms
Pyrazinamide (*PZA)*	750, 500 mg syrup 250 mg/ 5 mL	750 mg bd, 25–35 mg/kg in 2 dd	Hepatotoxic, hyperuricaemia, rash, arthralgia	Bactericidal. Kills intracellular organisms
Streptomycin *(Ambistryn-S)*	0.75 g 1 g inj.	15–20 mg/kg od 1 g > 50 kg od 0.75 g < 50 kg od	Vestibular damage, hearing loss, nephrotoxicity	Used in relapse and failure cases of TB Also used in plague, meningitis, SBE

Combinations

INH + Rif + PZA + Etham – (Zucox E kit, AKT- 4, Forecox tab)

INH + Rif + Etham – (AKT-3, Zucox kit)

INH + Rif – (Rcinex)

Antihelmintics

Drug	Available form	Dose	Side effects	Indications
Mebendazole *(Mebex, Wormin)*	100 mg tabs, susp 100 mg/ 5 mL	100 mg bd x 3 days > 2 yrs Half dose < 2 yrs	Abdominal pain, diarrhoea	Broad spectrum antihelmintic
Albendazole *(Bendex, Noworm)*	200, 400 mg tab Susp 200 mg/5 ml	400 mg single dose > 2 yrs, 200 mg single dose < 2 yrs. For tape worm 400 mg bd × 3 days. For hydatid cyst 400 mg bd × 1 month	Same as above	Same as above. Used for hydatid cyst, neurocysticercosis, tape worm
Ivermectin (*Ivermectol, Scavista*)	3, 6 mg tab	3–12 mg single dose	Same as above	Same as above
Niclosamine (*Niclosan*)	500 mg tab	2 tabs chewed with water early in morning followed by 2 tabs after 1 hr. Then give castor oil (15–30 mL) after 2 hrs	Same as above	Tape worm, *H.nana* infection
Praziquintel *(Cysticide)*	500 mg tab	50 mg/kg/day in 3 dd for 15 days for neurocysticercosis. For tapeworms—15 mg/kg single dose	Mild headache, drowsiness, rash	Costly. Most effective drug for neurocysticercosis
Diethyl carbamazine citrate (DEC) (*Hetrazan, Banocide*)	50, 100 mg tab Syr 120 mg/ 5 mL	2–6 mg/kg × 21 days for filariasis 4 mg/kg bd or tds for tropical eosinophilia	Nausea, anorexia, dizziness, headache	Only drug for filariasis. To avoid hypotension, start with 1 mg/kg/ day and then taper up

Anti-Amoebic Drugs

Drug	Available form	Dose	Side effects	Indications
Metronidazole (*Flagyl, Metrogyl*)	200, 400 mg tab Susp 200 mg/5 mL	200–400 mg tds × 7 days	Unpleasant taste, nausea, abdominal cramps. Disulfiram like reaction to alcohol	Giardiasis, amoebiasis, trichomonal vaginitis, bacterial vaginosis, anaerobic infections, guinea worm infection
Tinidazole (*Tini, Fasigyn, Tiniba*)	300, 500 mg tab Susp 75 mg/5 ml	500 mg bd × 5 days or 2 g od × 3 days	Same as above	Same as above
Secnidazole (*Secnil, Seczole*)	500 mg tab 1000 mg tab	2 g or 30 mg/kg single dose	Headache	Same as above
Ornidazole (*Dazolic*)	500 mg tab	500 mg bd × 5 days	No nausea or altered taste	Same as above
Diloxanide furoate (DF) (*Furamide, Entamazole*)	500 mg tab	500 mg tds (20 mg/kg) 10 days	Flatulence	Luminal amoebicide used for eradication
8-Hydroxyquinoline (*Enteroquinol, Diodoquin*)	250 mg tab, 850 mg tab	1–2 tabs tds	Nausea, optic neuritis	Chronic intestinal amoebiasis. Not useful in acute amoebic dysentery

Antifungal Drugs

Drug	Available form	Dose	Side effects	Indications
Griseofulvin (*Grisovin FP, Dermonorm*)	250, 500 mg tab	250 mg bd	Headache, nausea, vomiting, peripheral neuropathy, rashes, intolerance to alcohol	Superficial fungal infections
Fluconazole (*Forcan, Syscan*)	50, 150 mg tab 50, 100, 200 mg tab Infusion 2 mg/mL–100 mL	5–6 mg/kg	Nausea, vomiting, diarrhoea, rash. Rise in LFTs	Tinea, candidiasis, tinea versicolor, cryptococal infection, histoplasmosis
Ketoconazole (*Phytoral, Ketozole*)	200 mg tab	1 tab od or bd	Nausea, vomiting, headache, rash, gynaecomastia, rise in LFTs	Indications same as above. Costly. Not to use with H_2 blocker or antacid
Itraconazole (*Sporonox, Canditral*)	100, 200 mg tab	100–200 mg od	Less toxic than ketoconazole	Same as above. Used esp. in onychomycosis
Nystanin (*Mycostatin*)	5 lac units tab	tds	Nausea, vomiting, diarrhoea, rash	Intestinal and oral candidiasis
Anti-viral agents				
Acylovir (*Lovir, Ocuvir, Zovirax*)	200, 400, 800 mg Susp 400 mg/5 mL inj 200 mg vial	200 mg 5 times for HS 800 mg 5 times for HZ	Phlebitis, twitching and hypotension on IV use. Headache, nausea	Treatment of herpes simplex and herpes zoster infection

contd.

Famcyclovir *(Famtrex, Virovir)*	250, 500 mg tab	250–500 mg tds	Headache, nausea	Same as above
Valacyclovir (*Valcivir*)	500 mg, 1g tab	1 g tds for HZ 500 mg tab HS	Haemolytic uraemic syndrome Transient LFT, anaemia	Same as above
Ribavirin *(Ribavin, Virazide)*	100, 200 mg cap 50 mg/5 mL syp	200 mg tds	Hypertension, cardiac arrest	Hep B, C, D, G, herpes simplex, herpes zoster, influenza

Anti-Retroviral Drugs

NRTI (Nucleoside reverse transcriptase inhibitors)

Drug	Available form	Dose	Side effects	Indications
Zidovudine (AZT) *(Zidovir, Zidovex)*	100, 300 mg cap 50 mg/5 mL syp	300 mg bd in combination. Monotherapy only for prevention of transmission from mother to child	Anaemia, headache Lactic acidosis	HIV + ve patients with AIDS defining illness on CD4 count < 200/dL or plasma viral load >35000 copies of HIV RNA/mL. Post-exposure prophylaxis, prevention of mother to child transmission of HIV
Didanosine (dd1) *(Dinex, Dinosin)*	100 mg tab	200 mg bd	Pancreatitis, peripheral neuropathy, LFT	Same as above
Zalcitabine (ddC)	0.75 mg tab	0.75 mg tds	Same as above	Same as above
Stavudine (d4T) *(Stavir, Stavex)*	30, 40 mg tab	30 mg if wt < 60 kg 40 mg if wt > 60 kg	Not to be used with ddc ddl and AZT	Same as above
Lamivudine (3TC) *(Lamivir, Virolam)*	100, 150 mg tab 50 mg/5 mL syp	150 mg bd 4 mg/kg	Headache, nausea	Same as above
Abacavir *(Abacir)*	600 mg tab	600–1200 mg bd tds	Rash, hypersensitivity syndrome	Same as above
Tenofovir *(Tenof)* **with emtricitabine and efavirenz** *(Trustiva)*	300 mg tab	300 mg od	Renal dysfunction, abdominal pain	Same as above

Non-Nucleoside Reverse Transcriptase Inhibitors

Drug	Available form	Dose	Side effects	Indications
Nevirapine *(Nevirex, Nevimune)*	200 mg	200 mg for 14 days, then 200 mg bd	Rash, SJ syndrome, liver toxicity	Treatment of HIV infection, PMTCT, PEP as given under AZT
Efavirenz *(Efavir, Efcure)*	200, 600 mg	200 mg tds or 600 mg od	Rash, liver toxicity, CNS side effects like psychosis, ataxia, etc.	Same as above
Protease inhibitors				
Saquinavir *(Saquin)*	200 mg cap	6 caps tds	GI disturbances, nausea	Same as above
Ritonavir *(Ritovir)*	250 mg cap	600 mg bd Lower dose with other PIs	GI disturbances, nausea	Same as above
Indinavir *(Indivan, Indivir)*	800 mg cap	800 mg tds	GI disturbances, nausea, nephrolithiasis, hepatic impairment	To be taken on empty stomach
Nelfinavir *(Nelfin)*	500 mg cap	500 mg to 1 g tds	Diarrhoea	To be taken with food
Atazanavir with Ritonavir *(Atozor–R)*	300 mg/ 100mg	300 mg/100 mg od	Indirect hyper bilirubinemia	Same as above
Lopinavir with ritonavir *(Ritomax L)*	133.3 mg/ 33.0 mg	400 mg/100 mg	Diarrhoea, nausea, hypercholeste-rolaemia	Same as above

Combinations

- AZT, 3TC, NEV—*Duovir-N*
- d4T, 3TC, NEV—*Triomune, Nevilast*
- AZT, 3TC—*Combivir, Duovir*
- d4T, 3TC—*Virolis, Lamivir S*

Anti-Hypertensive Drugs

Beta-blockers

Propranolol *(Inderal, Betabloc)*	10, 40, 80 mg tab	120–360 mg/day in 3–4 dd	Bradycardia, bronchospasm,hypoglycaemia. May mask symptoms of hypoglycaemia. Aggravates AV conduction. To be avoided in asthma, COPD, abnormal lipid profile, and elderly	Drug of choice in young hypertensive, especially with angina, anxiety or post MI. Also used for anxiety, tremors, migraine
Atenolol (*Aten, Tenolol)*	25, 50 100 mg tab	50–200 mg/day	Cardioselective, lesser side effects	Drug of choice in young hypertensive, especially with angina, anxiety or post MI
Metoprolol (*Betaloc*)	50 mg tab	50–300 mg/day	Same as above	Same as above
Carvidelol *(Carloc)*	6.25, 12.5, 25 mg tab	6.25–25 mg bd	Same as above	Same as above

Calcium Channel Blockers

Drug	Available form	Dose	Side effects	Indications
Nifedipine *(Nicardia, Cardules)*	5, 10 mg, 20 mg R cap	10–30 mg qid	Headache, flushing, tachycardia, pedal oedema. To be avoided in heart block, failure, peripheral vascular disease	Drug of choice in isolated systolic hypertension, asthma, COPD patients
Diltiazem (*Dilzem, Dilgard)*	30, 60, 90 mg tab	30–60 mg tds	Same as above, but lesser	Same as above
Amlodepin (*Amlopress, Amlocor)* **with atenolol** *(Amlo-AT, Amlopress AT)* **with enalapril** *(Amace)* **with lisonopril** *(Amlopress-L)*	2.5, 5, 10 mg tab	2.5–10 mg/day od	Same as above	Long acting, therefore once a day therapy
Verapamil *(Isoptin, Vasoptin)*	40, 80 mg tab	40–80 mg tds oral or IV	Same as above	Atrial tachycardia and other arrhythmias Angina pectoris

ACE-Inhibitors				
Captopril *(Aceten, Capotril)*	12.5, 25 mg tab	12.5–75 mg/day in 3 dd	Agranulocytosis, 1st dose hypotension, dry cough CI – pregnancy, renal artery stenosis	Drug of choice is diabetes, hyper-lipidaemia, CCF, LVF
Enalapril *(Envas, Nuril)*	2.5, 5, 10 mg tab	2.5–40 mg/day od	Same as above	Same as above
Lisinopril *(Linvas, Lipril)*	2.5, 5, 10 mg tab	10–40 mg/day od	Same as above	Same as above
Ramipril *(Ramace, Cardace)*	1.25, 2.5 mg tab	2.5–20 mg od	Same as above	Same as above
ARB				
Losartan *(Losar, Losacar)*	25, 50 mg tab	25–100 mg od or bd	Does not produce cough	Same as above
Valsartan (*Valzaar*)	40 mg, 80 mg, 160 mg	80–160 mg 1 day	Headache, dizziness, fatigue	Hypertension
Olmesartan (*Olmy*)	20 mg, 40 mg	20–40 mg 1 day	Dizziness, hypotension	Hypertension

Alpha Blockers

Drug	Available form	Dose	Side effects	Indications
Methyldopa (*Alphadopa*)	250 mg tab	0.5, 20 mg tds	Sedation, lethargy, weight gain, postural hypotension	Pregnancy with hypertension
Clonidine (*Catapress*)	100 µg tab	50–100 µg tds	Same as above	Migraine
Reserpine (*Adelphane, Serpasil*)	0.1 mg tab	Start with 0.25–0.5 mg, may increase to 1 mg	SI – Depression, impotency, nasal block, wt gain. CI – Peptic ulcer, epileptics, parkinsonism	Pregnancy with hypertension
Prazosin (*Prozopress, Minipress XL*)	1, 2 mg tab	1–10 mg in dd	Hypotension	Moderate to severe HT, BHP, bladder neck dysfunction, Raynaud's disease
Terazosin (*Hytrin*)	1, 2, 5 mg tab	2–10 mg in dd	Same as above	Same as above
Terazosin (*Hytrin*)	1 mg, 2 mg	2–10 mg 1 day start at 1 mg and increase every week	Hypotension, dizziness, oedema, blurred vision	Hypertension, BPH
Doxazosin (*Doxacard*)	1 mg, 2 mg, 8 mg	1–8 mg 1 day	Hypotension, dry mouth, blurred vision, fatigue, dyspnoea	Hypertension, BPH

Diuretics				
Hydrochlor-thiazide *(Esidrex)*	50 mg tab	12.5–100 mg	Weakness, loss of drive, impotence, hyperglycaemia, hyperuricaemia. Avoided in diabetics, gout, abnormal lipid profile, young hypertensive CI – Renal, hepatic failure.	Drug of choice in elderly. Isolated systolic hypertension. Low cost therapy.
Xipamide (*Xipamid)*	20 mg	20–40 mg	Same as above	Same as above
Frusemide *(Lasix)* **with amiloride** *(Amifru-40)* **with spironol-actone** *(Lasilactone 50, 100)*	40, 100 mg inj 20 mg/ 2 ml	20–80 mg	Same as above	Oedema in CCF, hepatic or renal disease Forced diuresis in poisoning
Spirono-lactone (*Aldactone*)	25, 100 mg tab	20–200 mg in dd	Rash, gynaecomastia, hirsutism	Hypertension, oedema Potassium sparing diuretic
Triamterene & Amiloride (*Frusemene)* **with hydro-chlorthiazide** *(Biduret)*	100 mg 200 mg	100–200 mg in dd	Same as above	Same as above
Torasemide (*Dytor*)	10 mg, 20 mg, 100 mg	5–20 mg in oedema 2.5–20 mg in hypertension	Vertigo, visual impairment, calf muscle pain, anorexia vomiting	Oedema, hypertension

Vasodilators

Drug	Available form	Dose	Side effects	Indications
Hydralazine (*Nepresol*)	25 mg	75–200 mg/day	Flushing, headache, palpitation, angina, nasal stuffiness CI: IHD	Hypertension, heart failure
Minoxidil	2.5–40 mL		Same as above	Hypertensive emergency, baldness—local application
Anti-anginal drugs				
Glyceryl trinitrate GTN, nitroglycerin *(Angised, Nitrocortin CR, Angispan TR, GTN spray, Myovin ointment)*	0.5 mg tab 2.6, 6.4 mg tab Cap SR 2.5 drops 0.4 mg 2%, 30, 60 g	For acute pain 0.5 mg tab sublingually every 3 min till pain sub-sides. Prophylaxis 1–2 cap tds	Fullness of head, throbbing headache, sweating, palpitation	Unstable angina, MI, LVF
Isosorbide dinitrate *(Isordil, Sorbitrate)*	5, 10 mg tab	5–100 mg tds	Same as above	Acute angina as well for prophylaxis
Isorsorbide mononitrate *(Imdur, Ismo)*	30, 60 mg 10, 20, 40 mg	20–30 mg bd or tds	Same as above	Prophylaxis of angina, LVF, MI. Not for acute attack of angina
Nicocardil *(Zinicor, Nicoran)*	5, 10 mg tab inj 2, 4 mg	10–20 mg bd	Same as above	Used for CAD. Costly
Beta blockers CCB				See in antihyper-tensive drugs

Antiplatelet drugs				
Aspirin (*ASA, Loprin)*	50, 75 mg tab	50–100 mg od	Gastritis, broncho-spasm	Prophylaxis in cases of increased risk if blood clotting like TIA, MI, stroke
Clopidogrel (*Clopilet, Clopigrel*)	75 mg tab	75 mg od	Neutropenia, purpura, rash	Same as above
Dipyridamole (*Cardiwell, Persantin*)	25, 50, 75 mg tab	150–225 mg/day in dd on empty stomach	Rash, worsening of angina, flushing	Same as above

Lipid Lowering Drugs

Drug	Available form	Dose	Side effects	Indications
Lovastatin *(Lovastat, Lovadac)*	10–20 mg tab	10–80 mg/ day od	Flatulence, nausea, heartburn, myopathy, transaminitis	Hypercholestero-laemia with or without mild hypertrigly-ceridaemia
Simvastatin (*Simlo, Simcard)*	10, 20 mg tab	5–40 mg/ day od	Epigastric distress, loose motions, raised BSL, rash. CI: pregnancy, lactation, active hepatitis	Same as above
Atorvastatin (*Atorva)*	5, 10 mg tab	10–40 mg od	Same as other statins	Hypercholeste-rolaemia with or without mild hypertrigly-ceridaemia
Fibrates Gemfibrozil *(Normolip, Lopid)*	300, 600 mg tab	900–1500 mg in dd	Epigastric discomfort, motions and loose motions	Hypertrigly-ceridaemia
Ezetimibe *(Ezedoc, Ezee 10)*	10 mg tab	10 mg od	CI: Pregnancy, lactation	Hypercholeste rolaemia-used alone or with statins

Drugs Used in Obstetrics & Gynaecology

OC Pills

Drug	Available form	Dose	Side effects	Indications
Ovral-G *(Norgestrel 0.5 + Ethinyl estradiol 0.05)* **Ovral-L** *(Levonorgestrel 0.15 + ethinyl estradiol 0.03)* **Ovral** *(Levonorgestrel 0.25 + ethinyl estradiol 0.05)* **Phased pills** *(Triquilar) (6 + 5 + 10)* – **esp for >35 yrs** **Injectable** **Depot medroxyprogesterone** (*DMPA*) **acetate** *(Depo provera)*	21 tabs packet Inj.	1 tab from 1st day of menstrual cycle for 21 days followed by 7 days gap 150 mg/mL in 1st 5 days of MC, once every 3 months	*Serious complications:* Leg vein thrombosis, coronary thrombosis, hypertension, gall stone. Nausea, vomiting, headache, weight gain, vaginal candidiasis, **chloasma.** *CI:* Pregnancy, hepatic dysfunction, moderate to severe HT, thromboembolic disease, impending major surgery, suspected malignancy of breast/genitals. *Relative contraindications:* → Diabetes, smoking, obesity, undiagnosed vaginal bleeding, mentally ill, age – 30 yrs, mild hypertension. Contraceptive failure may occur with anti-epileptics. Injectable form may cause disruption of menstrual cycle, amenorrhoea, sometimes permanent sterility	Contraception Dysmenorrhoea endometriosis, irregular menstrual cycles
Centchroman (*Centron, Saheli*) ***tabd***		2 tabs per week startingof on 1st day of MC × 3 mon, then once a week	CI: PCOD, lactation, recent history jaundice	Non-hormonal contraception Poor contraceptive action

Oestrogens

Drug	Available form	Dose	Side effects	Indications
Conjugated oestrogens (*Premarin*)	0.25, 1.25 mg tab, 25 mg inj.	1.25–25 mg oral or IM	See in O.C. pills Use with caution in those with migraine, epilepsy asthma, cardiac or renal disease	As contraceptive menopausal syndrome, senile vaginitis, delayed puberty in girls, postmenopausal osteoporosis, DUB, acne, carcinoma prostrate and breast
Ethinylestradiol (*Lynoral, Progynon*)	0.01, 0.05 mg tab	0.02–0.2 mg/day	See in O.C. pills	Same as above
Estriol succinate (*Evalon*)	2 mg tab	8–16 mg/day, maintenance 2–4 mg/day	Same as above	Same as above
Diethyl stilbestrol (*Stilbestrol*)	1, 5 mg tab 5 mg/mL 1 mL inj	1–5 mg tds	Same as above	Same as above
Estradiol transdermal patches (*Estraderm MX*)	25, 50, 100 mg	Once every 3–4 days. Cyclic therapy (3 weeks on, 1 week off)	Same as above	Same as above
Estradiol (*E-2, Evalon gel*)	0.06% 15 g tube	Everyday in 1st week, then 3 times a week, then weekly	Same as above	Senile vaginitis

Progestins

Drug	Available form	Dose	Side effects	Indications
Dydrogesterone (*Duphaston*)	5 mg tab	10–25 mg daily	Nausea, breast enlargement, migraine, mood swings, acne. CI → thrombo-embolism,undiagnosed vaginal bleeding, hepatic dysfunction	Pure progestin, contraceptive, DUB, endometriosis, premenstrual syndrome, threatened abortion, adjunct to estrogen replacement therapy, postponement of menses. Only pure progestins can be given during endometrial carcinoma, pregnancy
Hydroxy-progesterone (*Fetugest, Maintane, Proluton depot*)	Inj 250, 500 mg	25–500 mg weekly	Same as above	Pure progestin
Lynestrenol (*Orgametril*)	0. 5 mg tab	5–10 mg daily	Same as above	Same as above
Norethisterone (*Primolut N, Regesterone*)	1, 5 mg tab	5–20 daily	Same as above	Same as above
Allylestrenol (*Gestanin, Fetugard*)	5 mg tab	Same as above		Pure progestin
Natural micronised progesterone (*Endogestgestin*)	100 mg / 200 mg tab and inj	200–400mg 1 day in 2 dd in threaten-ed abortion or premen-strual syndrome	Weight gain, intermenstrual bleeding	Infertility, puerperal depression, threatened abortion

Ovulation Induction/Infertility Drugs

Drug	Available form	Dose	Side effects	Indications
Clomiphene (*Clomid, Fertomid*)	50 mg tab	50 mg for 5 days from 2 to 3 days of menstrual cycle	Polycystic ovaries, multiple pregnancy. Exclude ovarian enlargement or pregnancy before starting treatment *CL:* Abnormal vaginal bleeding	To induce ovulation. Stein Leventha syndrome, post-pill amenorrhoea. Male infertility, oligozoospermia
Human chorionic gonadotrophin (*Profasi, Pregnyl*)	1000, 2000 5000, 10,000 IU inj.	Threatened abortion 10,000 IU followed by 5000 IU twice week	Ovarian hyperstimulation syndrome, false positive pregnancy tests, multiple pregnancy	Habitual/Threatened abortion, anovulatory cycles, infertility
Bromocriptine *(Proctinal)*	1.25, 2.5 mg tab	2.5 mg bd 14–21 days, start soon after delivery	Nausea, vomiting, confusion, psychoses	Hyperprolactinaemia, prevention of lactation
Menotrophin (*Inj Menodac*)	75 IU, 150 IU Inj.	3 equal doses on alternate days	Polycystic ovarian disease, multiple pregnancy	Amenorrhoea, infertility

Corticosteroids

Drug	Available form	Dose	Side effects	Indications
Hydrocortisone succinate (*Efcorlin, Primacort*)	100 mg/vial 100, 200, 400 mg/vial	100–500 mg slow IV	Cushing's syndrome, hyperglycaemia, skin striae, muscle weakness, susceptibility to infection, delayed healing of wound, peptic ulcer, osteoporosis, cataract and glaucoma, suppression of HPA axis	Allergic reactions, asthma, severe shock, rheumatoid arthritis, rheumatic fever, collagen disease, autoimmune disease, eczema, pemphigus, ulcerative colitis, Crohn's disease, cerebral oedema, etc.
Prednisolone (*Wysolone, Deltacortril*) (*Depo-medrol*)	5, 10, 20, 30 40 mg inj. 40 mg/mL for intra-articular use	5–60 mg dd Preferably give single morning dose	Same as above	Same as above
Betamethasone (*Betnelan, Celestone*)	0.5 mg tab inj 4 mg/mL, Paed drops 0.5 mg/mL	0.5–5 mg/day oral 4–20 mg im, iv	Same as above	Same as above

contd.

Dexamethasone (*Decadron, Dexona*)	0.5 mg tab, Paed drops 0.5 mg/mL inj. 4 mg/mL	0.5–5 mg/day oral 4–20 mg im, iv	Same as above	Same as above
Triamcinolone (*Tricort, Kenacort*)	10 mg/mL 40 mg/mL	4–32 mg/day in dd	Same as above	Intra-articular and intralesional injection
Hydrocortisone acetate (*Wycort*)	Inj 25 mg/mL	Depends on the indication	Same as above	Same as above
Deflazacort (*Defnalon*)	1 mg, 6 mg, 24 mg, 30 mg	3–18 mg in long term use lowest possible dose	Same as above	RA, asthma, pemphigus, uveitis, nephrotic syndrome

20 mg hydrocortisone = 5 mg prednisolone = 0.75 mg dexamethasone = 0.6 mg betamethasone.

Anabolic Steroids

Drug	Available form	Dose	Side effects	Indications
Decadurabolin *(Decaneurobol)*	25, 50, 100 mg/mL	25–500 mg IM every 3 weeks	Oedema, cholestatic jaundice, gynaecomastia, rash, virilisation. Use with caution in diabetics, epileptics CI – Pregnancy, hepatic dysfunction	Osteoporosis, sub-optimal growth in children, defective protein metabolism in children, following burns, major illness
Drugs used in thyroid disorder				
Carbimazole (*Neo-mercazole, Thyrozole)*	↓ 5, 10, 20 mg 5 mg tab	Start with 15–20 mg in dd in mild cases, up to 40 mg in severe cases Maintain at 2.5–25 mg	Bone marrow depression, mouth ulcer, hepatotoxicity, alopecia	Thyrotoxicosis, hyperthyroidism
Thyroxine *(Thyronorm, Eltroxin)*	0.025, 0.05, 0.1 mg tab	Start with 0.05 tab and increase dose every 3–4 week by 0.05 mg till T3-T4 levels are stabilized	Angina, palpitations, tachycardia, loss of weight	Hypothyroidism, cretinism

Oral Hypoglycaemic Agents (OHA)

Drug	Available form	Dose	Side effects	Indications
Sulphonylureas				
Tolbutamide (*Rastinon*)	500 mg tab	2–3 times a day	GI upset, blood dyscrasias, rash	Weak, short acting
Chlorpropamide (*Diabenase*)	100 mg tab	Once a day	Same as above	Can cause dangerous hypoglycaemia & jaundice
Glybenclamide (*Daonil, Euglucon*) **with metformin** (*Diabetrol*)	5 mg tab	1–2 times a day	Same as above	Potent but slow acting
Glipizide 5 mg (*Glynase*) **with metformin** (*GlynaseMF*)	5 mg tab	1–2 times a day	Same as above	Fast acting
Glymeperide (*Glypride*) **with metformin** (*Glicomet GP*)	1, 2 mg tab	Once a day	Same as above	Longer duration of action
Gliclazide (*Diamicron*) **with metformin** (*Glicomet*)	80 mg tab	1–2 times a day	Same as above	Has in addition antiplatelet action

Biguanides

Drug	Available form	Dose	Side effects	Indications
Metphormin (*Glyciphage*)	500 mg tab	1–2 times a day	GI upset	Used in obese
Acarbose (*Glucobay*)	50 mg tab	1–2 times a day	Same as above	Blocks absorption of glucose. Used to treat post-prandial hyperglycaemia
Voglibose (*Volix*)	0.2 mg, 0.3 mg	0.2–0.3 mg 2–3 times a day	Flatulence, increased liver enzymes, diarrhoea, hypokalaemia	Postprandial hyperglycaemia

contd.

Repaglynide *(Eurepa)*	1, 2 mg tab	2 times a day	Headache	Rapid action. Acts on beta cells of the pancreas
Rosiglitazone *(Result)*	2, 4 mg tab	1–2 times a day	Increase of cholesterol, wt gain, and anaemia	Decreases insulin resistance
Pioglitazone *(Glizone)*	15–30 mg tab	Once a day	Headache	Decreases insulin resistance

Drugs Used in BPH (Benign Prostate Hypertrophy)

Drug	Available form	Dose	Side effects	Indications
Prazosin *(Prozopress)*	1, 2 mg	1–2 mg tds	Postural hypotension, weakness, dry mouth	BPH, bladder neck dysfunction, hypertension
Terazosin *(Hytrin)*	1 mg	1 mg hs. Increase every week by 1 mg up to 10 mg	Same as above	Same as above
Finasteride *(Finast, Fincar)*	5 mg tab	5 mg od	Decreased libido, gynaecomastia, impotence	BPH, alopecia
Doxazosin *(Doxacard)*	1, 2, 4 mg	1 mg hs. Increase every 2 week up to 4 mg	Same as prazosin	BPH, bladder neck dysfunction, hypertension
Tamsulosin hydrochloride *(Contiflo OD)*	0.4 mg	0.4–0.8 mg od	Headache, nausea	BPH
Drugs for erectile dysfunction				
Sildenafil citrate *(Edegra, Nyte)*	25, 50, 100 mg tab	25–100 mg before sexual activity	Headache, flushing, rash CI – Patients on nitrates	Erectile dysfunction
Tadalafil *(Tadalis)*	10, 20 mg	5–20 mg	Same as above	Same as above

Vitamins

Drug	Available form	Dose	Side effects	Indications
Vitamin A (*Adexolin, Arovit, Aquasol A)*	Tab 5000 IU Tab 50,000 IU, drop (1,50,000 IU/mL) Cap 50,000 IU inj 50,000 IU/mL	*For severe def*: 2 lac units on day 1, 2, 30 *For mild def*: 5000 IU x 15 days od *For prophylaxis*: 2 lac units every 6 months for 5 yrs	Hypervitaminosis: Nausea, vomiting, dermatitis, liver disease, teratogenecity	Prophylaxis and treatment of Vit A deficiency, xerosis, ichthyosis
Vitamin D *(ABDEC, Inj. Arachitol, Calcirol sachets*)	30,000 and 60,000 IU-inj 60,000 IU granules	*Prophylaxis* – ABDEC 0.3 mL below 1 yr, 0.6 mL above 1 yr *Mild Vit D def*—inj or granules 6 lac IU *Severe def*—Vit D-inj 6 lac IU on day 1, 15, and if required on 30	Hyper-vitaminosis—D leading to decalcification of bones, hyper calcaemia, etc.	Vit D deficiency in growing children and postmenopausal females
Vitamin E (*Evion, Tocofer, Evit)*	200, 400 mg cap	200–400 mg/day	Large doses cause abdominal cramps, loose motion	Muscle cramps, claudication, fibrocystic breast disease. As an anti-oxidant
Vitamin C *(Celin, Sukcee, Redoxon*)	100, 500 mg tab Inj. 500 mg/5 mL Drops 100 mg/mL	500–1500 mg/day inj or oral	Prolonged use causes oxalate calculi in kidney	Vit C def esp. in children, elderly, alcoholics
Vitamin B_1 *(Berin, Beneuron)*	100 mg tab 100 mg/mL inj	100 mg od	Sensitivity reaction on im use	Peripheral neuropathy, beriberi, alcohol withdrawal tremors

contd.

Vitamin B_2 (*Lipabol, Riboflavin inj*)	20 mg tab 10 mg/mL	20–40 mg/day	None	Deficiency state causing stomatitis, neuropathy, etc.
Vitamin B_3 (Niacin) (*Vibelan forte, Pilonin*)	100 mg tab	Prophylaxis 20–50 mg/day oral Treatment 200–500 mg/day in dd oral	None	Pellagra
Vitamin B_6 Pyridoxin (*Blong, Benadon*)	100 mg tab	50–100 mg/day	None	With INH therapy, morning sickness, to suppress lactation
Vitamin B_{12} Cyanocobalamin (*Inj Eldervit 12, Macraberin forte, Optineuron forte*)	1000 mg B_{12} with B_1 and B_6	500–10,000 mg im × 10 days	None	Deficiency states, pernicious anaemia, peripheral neuropathy
Multivitamin complex (*B_1, B_2, B_3, B_6, B_{12} with folic acid, Vit C*)	Polybion tab, liquid Beplex, tab, liquid ABDEC drops Visyneral liquid Cap Becosule Multivit FM tab		None	Deficiency states
Folic acid (*Folvite*)	5 mg tab	1–2 tab/day	None	In pregnancy, megaloblastic anaemia

Iron Preparations

Drug	Available form	Dose	Side effects	Indications
Ferrous sulphate (*Fesovit, Fersolate, Fefol-Z, Iberol)*	Cap, syrup	*Treatment* 200 mg/day elemental iron in 2–3 dd, i.e., 3–5 mg/kg/day × 3 months *Prophylaxis* < 1 yr 5 drops > 1 yr 10 drops Adult 1 cap od	Epigastric pain, vomiting, metallic taste, staining of teeth, constipation, diarrhoea. Use Z-technique to give iron injection. Pain at injection site. Should give after testing. Fever, headache, joint pains, palpitations, lymph node enlargement can occur after iron injection	Compounds other than sulphate, gluconate and fumarate are expensive and less efficient. Injectable iron to be given, if oral treatment is not tolerated. Rise in Hb of 1 g/week is an optimum response
Ferrous fumarate (*Autrin, Fercel 300, Vitcofol)* **Paed drops** (*Siderplex, Fezocar)*	Cap, syrup	300–600 mg/day	Same as above	Same as above
Ferrous gluconate (*Dexvita)*	Syrup	300–600 mg/day	Same as above	Same as above
Ferric ammonium citrate (*Dexorange*	Cap, syrup	Same as above	Same as above	Same as above

contd.

Plus) **Ferrous calcium citrate** (*Raricap forte)*	Tab, liquid	Same as above	Same as above	Same as above
Ferrous succinate *(Hematrene)* **Iron dextran** *(Imferon)* **Iron sorbitol citrate** *(Jectofer)*	Inj. for im use	Same as above	Same as above	Same as above

Calcium

Drug	Available form	Dose	Side effects	Indications
Calcium carbonate *(Calcium sandoz, Ossopan, Osto-calcium – tab, sy)*	Tab, syrup	500–1000 mg/day	None	Calcium def. causing cramps, tetany, osteoporosis
Organic calcium (*from oyster shell*) *(Shelcal, Trical D, Ocal)* *(Inj Mecalvit IM, Calcium sandoz IV)*	Tab, syrup 10 mL vial	Once or twice a day 10 cc slow	None	IV calcium for tetany
Appetizers				
Cyproheptadine (*Ciplactin, Practin)*	2, 4 mg 2 mg/5 mL	5 mg bd for 2–6 yrs 4 mg bd for 6–12 yrs	Sedation, dry mouth, confusion	Appetizer Antihistaminic
Buclizine (*Longiphene*)	Syrup 6 mg/ 5 mL	25 mg tds	No sedation	Same as above
Protein preparation				
Portal M powder *Prosan powder* *Alprovit powder, Liquid, drops, Proteinules, Threptin biscuit*	Tin	Protein supplement	None	For protein energy malnutrition. After trauma, burns

Topical Applications: Acne Vulgaris

Drug	Available form	Dose	Side effects	Indications
Benzoyl peroxide (*Benzac AC, Pernox Gel*)	2.5%, 5%	Slowly increase the application time from 15 min initially to overnight	Excessive dryness, scaling erythema	Acne vulgaris, acne rosacea
Retinoic acid (*Retino A cream, Eudyna cream)*	0.25%, 0.05%	Once or twice a day	Avoid in pregnancy Irritation, redness Avoid rubbing, dryness	For comedomes, acne vulgaris
Erythromycin (*Eryacne gel, Erytop lotion*)	4% gel	Once or twice a day	Nil	Acne vulgaris
Clindamyclin *(Cindac-A gel)*	1% gel	Same as above	Same as above	Same as above
Adalphane *(Adaferin)*	0.1% gel	Same as above	Same as above	Same as above
Metronidazole *(Metrogyl Gel)*	10 mg/g	Od or bd	Same as above	Inflammatory papules and pustules, acne rosacea

Antifungal Topical Drugs

Drug	Available form	Dose	Side effects	Indications
Clotrimazole (*Candid, Canesten Candid V vaginal pessaries)*	Cream, powder, lotion, gel	2–3 times a day	None	Skin and vaginal infections due to yeast, candida and dermatophytes. Also for trichomonal and Gram +ve vaginal infections
Miconazole (*Candistat, Zole)*	Oint, cream, lotion, powder, spray	2–3 times a day	Local irritation, burning	Same as above
Ketoconazole (*Phytoral ointment, Nizral shampoo)*	Oint, shampoo	Oint 2 times a day Shampoo to be applied ½ before head bath	Local irritation, hr burning	Same as above
Ciclopiroxo-lamine (*Batrafen, Laprox*)	Cream, soln, vaginal cream	2–3 times a day	Local irritation, burning	Same as above
Tolnafate *(Tinaderm, Tolsol, Tinavate)*	Soln, cream,	2–3 times a day	Local irritation, burning	Same as above
Terbinafine *(Exifine, Sebifine*)	Cream	1–2 times a day	Local irritation, burning	Tinea infections, P. versicolor
Butanafine (*Butop)*	1% cream	1–2 times a day	Local irritation, burning	Same as above

Antiscabietics

Drug	Available form	Dose	Side effects	Indications
Gamma Benzene Hexachloride (*Gama-scab, Scaboma)*	Lotion, cream	2 applications 24 hrs apart	Skin irritation Rarely vertigo, convulsions in children Not to apply on face Use in diluted form in children	Scabies, pediculosis
Permethrin (*Permite, Perlice)*	Cream, lotion	Single application	Safer in children	Same as above
Crotomiton *(Crotorax)*	Cream, lotion	2 applications 24 hrs apart	Safer in children. Not to use in fresh weeping lesions	Scabies, pediculosis Antipruritic action
Benzyl Benzoate *(Scabindon)*	Oint, lotion	2 applications 24 hrs apart		Same as above

Anti-psoriatics

Drug	Available form	Dose	Side effects	Indications
Coal tar *(Exora, Derobin)*	Cream Oint		Staining, irritation	Psoriasis
Steroids and salicylic acid preparations				See relevant sections

Antiseptic/Antibiotic Topical Preparations

Drug	Available form	Dose	Side effects	Indications
Framycetin sulphate *(Soframycin)*	Cream, powder	2–3 times a day	Local irritation, burning	Injuries, burns, bacterial skin infections
Neomycin with polymyxin *(Neosporin)*	Powder, ointment	Same as above	Local irritation, burning	Same as above
Silver sulphadiazine *(Silverex, Silvindon)*	Cream ointment	Same as above	Same as above	Same as above
Cetrimide *(Cetrimide, Endruf)*	Soln Soln, lotion	Same as above	Same as above	Dandruff, antiseptic, disinfectant
Chlorxylenol *(Dettol)*	Liquid, cream	Same as above	Same as above	Antiseptic, disinfectant
Povidone Iodine *(Betadine, Wokadine)*	Oint, soln, powder, spray, gargles	Same as above	Same as above	Antiseptic, disinfectant
Mupirocin *(Bactroban, T-bact)*	Oint	3 times day	Same as above	Bacterial skin infection
Fusidic acid *(Fusibet Fusidin)*	Cream	Same as above	Same as above	Same as above
Nadilofloxacin *(Nadoxin)*	Cream	Same as above	Same as above	Same as above, acne vulgaris

Topical Steroids

Drug	Available form	Dose	Side effects	Indications
Potent				
Beclomethasone Dipropionate *(Beclate)* **Betamethasone Valerate** *(Betnovate)* **Clobetasol propionate** *(Tenovate, Lobate)* ***Lobate G*** (*with gentamycin*) **Lobate M** (*with miconazole*) **Fluocinolone acetomine** (*Fluderm, Flucort ,Flucort N, Flucort NM)*	Cream, oint	OD or BD	Thinning of skin, telangiectasia, striae, delayed wound healing, secondary fungal and bacterial infection	Allergic contact dermatitis, lichen planus, psoriasis, seborrhoiec dermatitis and other steroid responsive conditions
Mild				
Clobetasol butyrate *(Eumosone)* **Hydrocortisone acetate 2.5%** *(Wycort)*	Cream Oint	OD or BD	Same as above	To be used on face and in children. Atopic eczema and other steroid responsive conditions
Mometasone *(Momenta, Momate Elocon)*	Oint		Potent, but devoid of side-effects	Same as above
Desonide (*Desowen*)	Cream		Same as above	Same as above
Prednicarbate *(Dermatop)*	Cream		Same as above	Same as above
Hydrocortisone acetate 1% *(Lycortin)* - Hydrocortisone-17 buturate *(Locoid)*	Cream		Same as above	Same as above

Drugs for Hyperpigmentation

Drug	Available form	Dose	Side effects	Indications
Melalite (*Hydroquinone + glyceryl monopara-aminobenzoate*)	Cream	3–6 months application	Irritation, avoid eyes	Melasma, post-inflammatory hyperpigmentation, etc. Response is slow
Melacare (*Hydroquinone + Tretinoin + Mometasone*)	Cream	Same as above	Same as above	Same as above
Eslite (*Hydroquinone 2%)*	Cream	Same as above	Same as above	Same as above

Drugs for Hypopigmentation

Drug	Available form	Dose	Side effects	Indications
Melanocyl (*Methoxsalen* 0.75% + *Para amino-benzoic acid* 2%) (*Methoxsalen 0.75%*)	Ointment Soln 10 mg tab	At bedtime or 2 hrs before sun exposure 1–2 tabs 2 hrs before exposure to sunlight —0.6–0.7 mg/kg	Irritation, burning	Vitiligo
Neosoralen (*Trimethyl psoralen*)	5, 25 mg tab, lotion	Same as above	Same as above	Same as above

Keratolytics

Drug	Available form	Dose	Side effects	Indications
Salicylic acid, benzoic acid, tar *(Exora, Whitfield SF Salicyclix SF, Salactin)*	Ointment liquid, corn cap	OD or BD application	Irritation	Corns, warts psoriasis, lichenified eczema, ringworm

Anti-Seborrheics

Drug	Available form	Dose	Side effects	Indications
Selenium sulphide, Zinc pyrithione, (*Selsun shampoo)*		Before hair bath to be applied for half an hour	None	Dandruff
Ketoconazole *(KZ Shampoo, Endruff shampoo)*		Same as above	Same as above	Dandruff

Emollients

Drug	Available form	Dose	Side effects	Indications
Cetraban cream (*White petroleum jelly, liquid paraffin*) **Silodermointment** (*Dimethicone, Zinc oxide, Calamine*)	Cream, ointment	Od or bd	None	Contact and irritant dermatitis, atopic eczema

Anti-Obesity Drug

Orlistat (*Obelit*)	120 cap	120 mg tds with meals	Fatty stool, vitamin deficiency	Obesity

Eye/Ear Drops

Drug	Available form	Dose	Side effects	Indications
Norfloxacin (*Norcid, Norflox*)	Drops 0.3% 5 mL, ointment	2–3 drops every 2–3 hrs	Irritation, burning	Conjunctivitis, keratitis, kerato-conjunctivitis, corneal ulcers, dachryocystitis, otitis externa, acute otitis media, chronic suppurative otitis media
Ofloxacin (*Zenflox*) **with dexametha-sone** (*Zenflox-D*)	Same as above	Same as above	Same as above	Same as above
Ciprofloxacin (*Ciplo, Zoxan*) **with dexametha sone** *(Ciplox-D)*	Drops 0.3% 5 mL, ointment	Same as above	Same as above	Same as above
Gentamicin *(Gentamicin, Genticyn)*	Same as above	Same as above	Same as above	Same as above
Chloramphenicol *(Chloromycetin)* **with dexametha-sone** *(Chlorodex)*	5 mL drops, applicaps	Same as above	Same as above	Same as above
Tobramycin (*Tobacin, Tobramin)*	Same as above	Same as above	Same as above	Same as above
Acyclovir *(Ocuvir, Zovirax)*	Ointment 5 g		Same as above	Herpes simplex conjunctivitis

contd.

Betamethasone *(Betnesol)*	Oint 5 g, drops 5 mL	1–2 drops 3–4 times a day	May worsen the existing infection Prolonged use may lead to perforation, cataract, glaucoma	Infection with inflammation Allergic and inflammatory conditions of eye
Dexamethasone *(Dexona)*	2.5 mL drops 3–4 times a day	1–2 drops as above	Same as above	Same
Flurbiprofen sodium *(Flur)*	Drops 0.3% 5 mL	1 drop every ½ hr	Burning, stinging inflammation	Postoperative & post laser
Diclofenac sodium (*Oxalgin, Profenac*)	0.1% 5 mL		Burning, stinging	Postoperative & post laser inflammation
Ketorolac tomethamine (*Kerol, Ketanov)*	0.5% 5 mL	1 drop 4 times a day	Burning, stinging	Itching and associated symptoms of seasonal allergic conjunctivitis
Sodium cromoglycate (*Fintal, Ifiral*)	5 mL drops	1–2 drops 4–6 times/day	Same as above	Allergic conjunctivitis,hay fever, vernal keratitis
Fluorometholone (*Flurisone*)	5 mL drops	1–2 drops 4–6 times/day	Same as above	Instill one drop into the conjunctival sac two to four times daily
Hydroxy propyl cellulose or polyvinyl alcohol *(Moisol, Tearsplus)*	Drops 10 mL	1–2 drops 4–6 times/day	None	Xerophthalmia, chronic conjunctival irritation
Atropine (*Atropine, Atrosulph*)	Drop 5 mL Ointment 5 g	1–2 drops at night	Photophobia, palpitations	Iritis, iridocystits, keratitis & corneal ulcer
Tropicamide	3 mL, 5 mL	1–2 drops as	Increased intra-	For mydriasis in

contd.

(*Tropicamet, Tropicon)*	drops	required	ocular pressure, systemic anti-cholinergic effects	diagnostic proce-dures
Pilocarpine (*Pilocar*)	1%, 2%, 4% drops	1–2 drops	Initial stinging sensation, painful spasm of accommo-dation	Open angle glaucoma
Timolol maleate (*Timolet*)	0.25, 0.5% drops	1–2 drops	Bronchospasm Reduction in resting heart rate & blood pressure	Chronic open angle glaucoma, aphakic glaucoma
Betaxolol (*Betapress*)	0.5% drops	1–2 drops	Pain, stinging	Open angle glaucoma
Clotrimazole (*Candid, Fungidrops*)	15 mL	3–4 times a day	None	Otomycosis
Chloramphenicol, dexamethaone, clotrimazole (*Candibiotic*)	5 mL			Allergic and inflammatory conditions
Paradichlo-robenzene, lignocaine (*Desol, Otoclean*)	Drops	10–15 drops	None	Ear wax, otalgia

Nasal Drops

Drug	Available form	Dose	Side effects	Indications
Xylometazoline *(Otrivin, Decon)* **Oxymetazoline** *(Nasivion, Nasivion Paed)*	0.1% 10 mL 0.05% 10 mL 0.025% 10 mL	2–3 drops into each nostril	Stinging sensation, rebound congestion	Nasal congestion
Phenylephrine *(Dristan)*	Liquid 10 mL	2–3 drops into each nostril	Stinging sensation, rebound congestion	Nasal congestion
Sodium cromoglycate *(Ifral)*	5 mL	Initially 2 drops in each nostril 4 times, then 1 drop 3–4 times	Bronchospasm	Prophylaxis of allergic rhinitis
Steroid nasal drops *(Betnesol-N, Efcorlin)*	Soln 5 mL Drops 10 mL	2–3 drops 3–4 times daily		Nasal congestion, inflammation & allergic condition of nose
Fluticasone propionate *(Flomist)*	100 mL spray	2 sprays in each nostril per day	Headache, burning of nostrils	Allergic and perennial rhinitis

Mouthwash, Gum paint, Toothpaste

Drug	Availlable form	Dose	Side effects	Indications
Betadine Gargle	50 mL, 100 mL	3–4 times a day after food	None	Oral hygiene
Gumex	Bottle 10 mL, 25 mL, 60 mL	3–4 times a day after food	None	Gingivitis
Metrogyl DG *(Metronidazol dental gel)*	1% 20 g	To be applied twice daily	None	Stomatitis, periodontitis, apthous ulcer
Sensoform, Sensolin toothpaste	50 g, 100 g		None	Sensitive teeth and gum

BEST GUESS APPROACH ANTIMICROBIAL THERAPY IN GP

- Respiratory Tract Infections
- Urinary Tract Infections
- Gastrointestinal Infections
- Obstetrics and Gynaecological Infections
- Genital Tract Infections
- Eye Infections
- Ear Infections
- Skin & Soft Tissue Infections

The aim of this article is to provide a simple, "best guess approach" to the treatment of common infections encountered in general practice in India.

Definitive therapy depends on the microbiologic diagnosis by culture and sensitivity tests. In general practice, before prescribing antibiotics resorting to culture sensitivity tests is not practically feasible. And prescribing antibiotics irrationally will promote bacterial resistance in the community.

Hence, this chapter helps in the selection of the first choice antibiotic in that particular infection without the help of culture sensitivity tests.

This chapter is based on the updated available evidence in India as to the selection of the first choice antibiotic. However, its application may be modified as per situation, keeping in mind scientific principles and professional judgement, e.g., the dose and duration of treatment suggested may be revised upwards and a longer course may be given in severe or recurrent cases.

Practice Pearls

- To minimise the emergence of bacterial resistance in the community, prescribe an antibiotic only when there is likely to be a clear clinical benefit.
- Do not (or at least delay) prescribe antibiotic in predominantly viral infections like acute sore throat, common cold, etc.
- Prophylactic antibiotics may be justified in patients with higher risk of complications (like pre-existing co morbidity, young children born prematurely, people over 65, type 1 or 2 diabetes, patients on oral corticosteroids, immunosuppression, etc.)
- Avoid broad spectrum antibiotics (e.g. amoxiclav, quinolones and cephalosporins) for a prolonged period as they increase risk of *Clostridium difficile*, MRSA and resistant UTIs.
- In pregnancy, avoid tetracyclines, aminoglycosides, and quinolones and high dose of metronidazole.

The following empirical or presumptive antibiotic therapy is based on evidence from the literature, Internet search (clinical trials and reviews) and from the experience of educated and experienced clinicians. The contents of this chapter include the commonest infections encountered in a general practitioner's practice. All the doses given below here are for oral administration and for adults.

UPPER RESPIRATORY TRACT INFECTION

- *Acute cough with upper respiratory tract infection*: No antibiotic.
- *Acute bronchitis*: No routine antibiotic.
- *Acute cough & higher risk of complications*: Immediate or back-up antibiotic.
- *Acute cough & systemically very unwell*: Immediate antibiotic.

Illness	Likely causative Organism	Key points	Best guess antibiotic	Alternative antibiotics
Common Cold	Heterogenous group of viruses	Runny nose, sneezing, nasal congestion	Antibiotics not recommended	Nil
Acute Pharyngitis	90% Viral	As most cases are viral no antimicrobial therapy required	Nil	Nil
Acute Pharyngitis	10% Bacterial Group A β-haemolytic Streptococci (GABHS), Group C, G Streptococcus	Patients with fever, exudates in tonsils, cervical adenopathy, absence of cough or otitis media benefit from antibiotics	Amoxicillin 500 mg tds for 5 days	Azithromycin 500 mg od for 5 days
Acute Tonsillitis	Group A β-haemolytic Streptococci is leading pathogen	Purulent exudates in tonsils, anterior cervical lymphadenopathy. Risk of Rheumatic disease and glomerulonephritis	Inj. Procaine Penicillin 6 lac units daily IM after sensitivity test for 7 days	Amoxicillin500 mg tds for 5 days Azithromycin 500 mg od for 5 days
Acute Laryngitis	Most are viral	Hoarsness of voice with other URT symptoms	Nil	Nil
Otitis Media	Most are viral	Resolve spontaneously within 4 days	Nil	Nil
Acute Rhinosinusitis	Many are viral. *S. pneumoniae*, *H. influenzae*, *M. catarrhalis*	Three symptoms S/O bacterial: purulent nasal discharge, unilateral maxillary tenderness,	Amoxicillin 500 mg tds for 5 days Only about 1/3rd will benefit with antibiotic. Reserve for	Co-amoxiclav 625 mg bd for 5–7 days Or Ciprofloxacin 500 bd Plus Metronidazole 400 bd

		worsening of symptoms after initial improvement	severe or symptoms more than 5 days	for 5 days
Influenza	Influenza virus A and B	Supportive treatment. Vaccination	Nil	Oseltamivir (Tamiflu) may decrease symptoms by 1 day, if started within 48 hrs of symptom onset

LOWER RESPIRATION TRACT INFECTION

Illness	Likely causative organism	Key points	Best guess antibiotics	Alternative antibiotics
Acute bronchitis	Most are viral	Antibiotics not required	Nil	Nil
		May be used in patients with higher risk of complications (see above)	Amoxicillin 500 mg tds for 5 days	Azithromycin 500 mg od for 5 days or Doxycycline 200 mg stat. Then 100 mg od for 5 days
Acute exacerbation of chronic bronchitis or bronchiectesis	*S. pneumoniae* *H. influenzae* *M. catarrhalis*	Approximately 50% are bacterial. Use antibiotics if increased dyspnoea and if sputum becomes purulent. Treatment failure is seen in patients who have taken repeated courses of antibiotics	Amoxicillin 500 mg tds for 7–10 days	Doxycycline 200 mg stat. Then 100 mg od for 7–10 days Or Levofloxacin (under guidance of a specialist) 500 mg od for 7–10 days Duration is based on severity of bronchiectesis, previous culture and sensitivity results, and response to treatment

contd.

		and a previous sputum culture with resistant bacteria.		
Community acquired pneumonia-treatment in community	*S. pneumoniae*, *H. influenzae*, *Legionella*, *E. coli*, *Klebsiella* sp., *S. aureus*	In adults hospitalize the patient based on clinical judgement and presence of **Confusion**, **Urea** > 45 mg/dL), **RR** ≥ 30/min, **Blood pressure** (<90/60 mm Hg), age > 65 yrs (Mneumonic: CURB 65) Start antibiotic immediately. If no response in 48 hrs consider admission	Amoxicillin 500 mg tds for 5–7 days Plus Inj Ceftrixone gm daily for 5 days	Add to cover Mycoplasma infection Doxycycline 200 mg od 7–10 days Or Clarithromycin 500 mg bd 7–10 days
Hospital acquired pneumonia	*P. aeruginosa*. *Staphylococcus aureus,* including methicillin-susceptible *S. aureus* (MSSA) and methicillin-resistant *S. aureus* (MRSA) *Klebsiella pneumoniae* *Escherichia coli*	In hospital acquired pneumonia, symptoms or signs of pneumonia start after 48 hrs of hospital admission.	Amoxicillin 500 mg tds for 5–7 days Plus Inj Ceftrixone 1 g daily for 7 days	Piperacillin-Tazobactam 4.5 g IV 6 hourly Or Cefoperazone-Sulbactam 3 g IV 12 hourly

URINARY TRACT INFECTIONS

- Pregnant women, men, children or young people: immediate antibiotic after confirmation of infection.
- All cases of painful or burning micturition (dysuria) may not be UTI. Always request for urine exam before starting antibiotics.
- In the elderly, do not treat presence of bacteria in routine urine examination (asymptomatic bacteriuria) with antibiotics. It occurs in 25% of women and 10% of men and is not associated with any symptoms or complications.
- Asymptomatic bacteriuria in any patient should not be treated immediately except in pregnant women and immunocompromised patients. One should monitor the patient for development of symptoms and complications.
- Antibiotics will not eradicate bacteriuria in the presence of a catheter. Only treat if pyelonephritis likely.
- In chronic UTI when considering antibiotics, take account of severity of symptoms, risk of complications, previous urine culture and susceptibility results, previous antibiotic use which may have led to resistant bacteria.

Illness	Likely causative organism	Key points	Best guess antibiotics	Alternative antibiotics
Uncomplicated UTI, i.e. Urinary tract is structurally normal (no BPH, no strictures) and no calculi	*E. coli* in about 90% In the rest: *Proteus*, *Klebsiella*, *Enterobacter*	Multi-resistant *E. coli* are increasing. So perform culture in all treatment failures	Nitrofurantoin 50 mg four times daily for 7 days	Depends on susceptibility of organism
Acute prostatitis	*E. coli*, *Klebsiella*	Get urine and prostatic massage cultures before antibiotic. Select antibiotic based on sensitivities.	Doxycline 100 mg BD Or Co-trimoxazole 960 mg BD for 3–4 weeks	In severe cases, Piperacillin-Tazobactam 4.5 g IV 6 hourly or Cefoperazone-sulbactam 3 g IV 12 hourly or Meropenem 1 g IV 8 hourly
Recurrent Urinary Tract Infection	*E. coli*, *Klebsiella pneumoniae*, *Proteus*	Daily antibiotic prophylaxis	Prophylactic Prophylactic Nitrofurantoin 50 mg od for 6 months to 1 year	Prophylactic Trimethoprim 100 mg od for 6 months to 1 year

contd.

Acute uncomplicated Pyelonephritis	*E. coli, Klebsiella pneumoniae, Proteus*	Advice mid stream urine culture and sensitivity and repeat after therapy for proof of cure	Amikacin 1 g od IM/IV for 5–7 days	In severe cases, Piperacillin-Tazobactam 4.5 g IV 6 hourly Or Cefoperazone-sulbactam 3 g IV 12 hourly for 5–7 days
Acute uncomplicated Cystitis	*E. coli, Klebsiella pneumoniae, Proteus*	Advice mid stream urine culture and sensitivity and repeat after therapy for proof of cure	Nitrofurantoin 100 mg BD for 7 days	Cefuroxime 250 mg BD for 3–5 days Or Cotrimoxazole 960 mg BD for 3–5 days Or Ciprofloxacin 500 mg BD for 3–5 days
UTI in Pregnancy	*E. coli, Klebsiella pneumoniae, Proteus*	Advice mid stream urine culture and sensitivity and repeat after therapy for proof of cure.	Nitrofurantoin 100 mg BD for 7 days	

GASTROINTESTINAL INFECTIONS: OPD TREATMENT

Illness	Likely causative organism	Key points	Best guess antibiotics	Alternative antibiotics
Acute Gastroenteritis	Viral in 90% Entero-toxigenic & Entero-pathogenic *E. coli*	Oral or IV rehydration therapy essential	None	None
Food poisoning	*Staph aureus, Bacillus cereus, Clostridium botulinum*	Oral or IV Rehydration therapy essential. Report to local authorities	None	None
Cholera	*V. cholerae*	Oral or IV Rehydration therapy essential. Report to local authorities	Doxycycline 300 mg oral stat	Azithromycin 1 g oral stat or Ciprofloxacin 500 mg BD for 3 days
Bacterial dysentery	*Shigella* sp., Campylobacter	Antibiotic therapy is not usually indicated unless patient has fever. Fluoroquino-lones are not preferred due to high level of resistance in many parts of India	Ceftriaxone 2 g IV OD for 5 days or oral Cefixime 200 mg bd × 5 days	Azithromycin 1 g OD × 3 days
Amoebic dysentery	*E. histolytica*		Metronidazole 400 mg oral TDS for 7–10 days	Tinidazole 2 g oral OD for 3 days. Add Diloxanide furoate 500 mg TDS for 7–10 days for chronic recurrent cases

contd.

Giardiasis	*Giardia lamblia*		Metronidazole 400 mg Oral TDS for 5 days	Tinidazole 2 g oral OD for 3 days
Enteric fever	*Salmonella typhi, Salmonella paratyphi A*	Ceftriaxone to be changed to oral cefixime when patient is afebrile to finish total duration of 2 weeks	*Outpatients*: Cefixime 200 mg bd for 2 weeks Plus Ciprofloxacin 500 mg bd for 2 weeks	*Inpatients*: Ceftriaxone 2 g IV BD for 2 weeks ± Azithromycin 500 mg BD for 7 days
Eradication of *Helicobacter pylori*	*Helicobacter pylori*	Usually treated with a combination of one antibiotic (amoxicillin or clarithromycin), one amoebicidal (metronidazole or tinidazole) and a proton pump blocker (omeprozole or pantoprozole)	Omeprazole 20 Plus Amoxicillin 500 And Tinidazole 750 mg (Helipac Cipla)	Tinidazole 500 Plus Clarithromycin 250 mg And Lansoprazole 30 mg (Pylokit Cipla) Box of 7 Kits × 6 tablets = 42 tablets/Box
Diverticulitis Mild- OPD treatment	*Gram-Negative bacteria Anaerobes*	Severe cases should be admitted for: Ceftriaxone 2 g IV OD + metronidazole 500 mg IV TDS	Amoxycillin-Clavulanate 625 mg tds for 7 days + Metronidazole for 7 days	Ciprofloxacin + Metronidazole for 7 days
Hospital acquired diarrhoea	*C. difficile*	Stop unnecessary antibiotics	Metronidazole 400 mg oral TDS for 10 days	*Severe disease*: Vancomycin 250 mg oral 6 h for 10 days

GENITAL TRACT INFECTIONS

Illness	Likely causative Organism	Key points	Best Guess antibiotics	Alternative antibiotics
Candidial vaginitis	Candida species	*Pregnancy*: Avoid oral azoles. Recurrent: 150 mg oral fluconazole every 72 hrs for 3 doses (induction) followed by 1 dose once a week for 6 months (maintenance).	Clotrimazole cream Or Clotrimazole 500 mg vaginal pessary	Fluconazole 400 mg mg orally single dose. For recurrent, not responding infection, higher doses and more frequent doses have been recommended
Bacterial vaginosis	Many bacteria	Treat sexual partner	Metronidazole 400 mg oral BD × 7 days Plus Metronidazole vaginal gel × 7 days	Tinidazole 2 g orally stat × 3 days Or 2% Clindamycin Vaginal cream × 7 days
Trichimonal vaginitis	Trichomonas vaginalis	Treat sexual partner with metronidazole 2 g single dose. In pregnancy or breastfeeding: avoid 2 g single dose metronidazole Topical clotrimazole gives symptomatic relief	Metronidazole 2 g single dose or 400 mg oral BD × 7 days	Tinidazole 2 g oral single dose

contd.

Cervicitis	*C. trachomatis* *N. gonorrhoeae* Herpes simplex virus (HSV)	Evaluate and treat sex partner/s	Ceftriaxone 250 mg IM single dose + Azithromycin 1 g single dose	Doxycycline 100 mg BD × 7 days
Pelvic Inflammatory Disease	*S. aureus*, *E. Coli*, Gonococci	Evaluate and treat sex partner/s Drainage of tubo-ovarian abscess, if present	*Outpatient*: Ceftriaxone 250 mg IM/IV single dose Plus Metronidazole 400 mg BD × 14 days Plus Doxycycline 100 mg BD × 14 days	*Inpatient*: Clindamycin 300–600 mg bd IM/IV Plus Ceftriaxone 250 mg IM/IV till patient admitted then change to metro + doxy for 14 days

EYE INFECTIONS

Illness	Likely causative organism	Key points	Best guess antibiotics	Alternative antibiotics
Viral conjunctivitis (*Pink eye*)	Adenoviruses	Burning sensation in eye with watery discharge	No antibiotics required	None
Bacterial conjunctivitis (*Red eye*)	*S. aureus, S. pneumoniae, H. influenzae*	Intense redness of eye Unilateral, Mucopurulent discharge Self-limiting	Chloramphenicol 0.5% drops 2 hrly reducing to 4 times a day PLUS Chloramphenicol 1% ointment or applicaps at night	Gatifloxacin 0.3%, levofloxacin 0.5%, Moxifloxacin 0.5% eye drops 2 hrly
Herpes Simplex keratitis	Herpes Simplex virus (HSV)	Fluorescein staining shows typical dendritic figures	Trifluridine ophthalmic soln 1 drop 2 hourly while awake up to maximum 9 drops/day until corneal ulcer has healed. Then 1 drop 4 hourly upto 5 drops/day for total duration of 21 days	Ganciclovir 0.15% ophthalmic gel 5 times a day (about every 3 hrs while awake) until the corneal ulcer has healed, and then 3 times a day for 7 more days
Varicella Zoster ophthalmicus	Varicella–Zoster virus	Always do HIV test	Trifluridine ophthalmic soln as above Plus Valacyclovir 1 g oral TID X 10days	Famciclovir 500 mg BD Or TID Or Acyclovir 800 mg 5 times/day x 10 days
Acute bacterial keratitis	*S. aureus, S. pneumoniae, S. pyogenes, Haemophilus* spp.	IV antibiotics will be required in MRSA	Moxifloxacin eye drops: 1 drop 1 hourly for first 48 hrs, then reduce as per response	Gatifloxacin eye drops: 1 drop 1 hourly for first 48 hrs, then reduce as per response

EAR INFECTIONS

Illness	Likely causative organism	Key points	Best guess antibiotics	Alternative antibiotics
Acute otitis media	*S. pneumoniae* *H. influenzae* *Morexella catarrahalis*	Common in children	Amoxycillin-Clavulanate 625 mg tds for 7 days	Cefuroxime axetil 250 mg BD
Acute mastoiditis	*S. pneumoniae* *S. aureus* *H. infiuenzae* *P. aeruginosa*	Select antibiotics as per culture report	Ceftriaxone 2 g IV daily od for 7–10 days	Cefotaxime 1–2 g iv 4–8 hourly for 7–10 days
Chronic mastoiditis	Polymicrobial	Select antibiotics as per culture	Piperacillin-tazobactam 4.5 g IV 8 h	Meropenem 1 g IV 8 hrly

SKIN & SOFT TISSUE INFECTIONS

Illness	Likely causative organism	Key points	Best guess antibiotics	Alternative antibiotics
Impetigo	*Streptococcus pyogenes* (common), *Staph aureus*	Infected pustule with crust is hall mark. Remove crust before applying ointment	Amoxycillin-Clavulanate 625 mg tds for 7 days Mupirocin or fusidic ointment 3 times a day	Cefuroxime, 250–500 mg twice daily for 5 days
Furunculosis (*Boils*) **Folliculitis**	*Staphylococcus aureus*	Deep infection of the hair follicles. Red painful nodules with pus of varying sizes	Amoxycillin-Clavulanate 625 mg tds for 7 days	Cefuroxime, 250–500 mg twice daily for 5–7 days
Cellulitis	*Streptococcus pyogenes* (common), *Staphylococcus aureus*	Swelling, pain and redness involving sub-cutaneous tissue	Amoxicillin-Clavulanate 1.2 g IV TDS Or	Cefuroxime, 250–500 mg twice daily for 10 days

contd.

		Borders are not well demarcated. If high grade fever and systemic symptoms, admit for IV antibiotics	Amoxycillin-Clavulanate 625 mg tds for 7 days	
Erysipelas	Streptococcus pyogenes	Fiery red patch on leg with sharp border and streak of lymphan gitis above patch, may be finely dimpled	Inj Procaine penicillin 6,00,000–1,200,000 Units IM once a day for 10 days	Linezolid 600 mg every 12 hrs for 10 days
Reccurent furunculosis	MRSA (Methicillin-resistant *Staphylococcus aureus*) MSSA (Methicillin-sensitive *Staphylococcus aureus*)	Apply Mupirocin or fusidic ointment in nose Chlorhexidine soap during bath Instructions for washing clothes	Clindamycin 300 mg every 6 hrs for 7–10 days. May be followed by 150 mg clindamycin for 3 months	Linezolid 600 mg BD for 7–10 days
Carbuncles	*Staphylococcus aureus*	Cluster of furuncles connected subcuta-neously, causing suppuration with multiple openings Common in diabetics	Amoxicillin-Clavulanate 1.2 g IV TDS Or Amoxycillin-Clavulanate 625 mg tds for 10 days	Cefuroxime, 500 mg twice daily for 10 days

CONVENTIONAL DOSAGE AND ADVERSE REACTIONS GUIDE FOR COMMONLY USED ANTIBIOTICS

Antibiotic	Paediatric dose	Adult dose	Adverse reactions
Amoxycillin	*Oral*: 20–50 mg/kg/day 3–4 doses	*Oral*: 250–500 mg 8 hourly	Rash, *diarrhoea, GI upset,* transient elevation of liver enzymes
Amikacin	15–20 mg/kg/day in 2–3 doses IV	Intravenous/IM: 15 mg/kg/day divided 8–12 hourly	*Nephrotoxicity, Ototoxicity*
Amoxycillin-clavunate (*co-amoxyclav*)	*Oral*: 25–50 mg/kg/day in 2–3 doses *Intravenous*: 50–100 mg/kg/day (amoxicillin) in 2 doses	*Oral*: (Amox 500 mg/Clav 125 mg) 625 mg 8–12 hourly	Rash, diarrhoea, GI upset, transient elevation of liver enzymes
Ampicillin	*Oral*: 100–200 mg/kg/day in 4 doses *Intravenous*: 100–400 mg/kg/day in 4 doses (IV)	*Oral*: 500 mg to 1 g 6 hourly	Hypersensitivity reaction, skin rash, *precipitates rash in infectious mononucleosis, diarrhoea, GI upsets*
Azithromycin	*Oral*: 10 mg/kg/day once daily Enteric fever 20 mg/kg/day once daily	*Oral:* 500 mg daily for 3–5 days	Leukopenia, transient elevation of liver enzymes, renal toxicity.
Benzathine penicillin IM	6 lac units (<30 kg) 12 lac units (>30 kg) IM (Inj Penidura LA 6, 12, 24 lac per vial)	12–24 lac/week. AST Deep Intramuscular	*Hypersensitivity reaction, anaphylaxis,* Jarisch Herxheimer reaction, haemolytic anaemia
Procaine penicillin	6 lac units (<30 kg) 12 lac units (>30 kg) IM (Inj PP: 4 lac units/vial)	6–12 lac units IM daily AST for 5–10 days depending on the disease	*Hypersensitivity reaction, anaphylaxis,* Jarisch Herxheimer reaction

contd.

Penicillin G aqueous IV	*IV*: 2–4 lac units/ kg/day in 4 divided doses	*Intravenous*: 2–24 million units day in divided doses q 4–6 hrs	*Hypersensitivity, anaphylaxis, serum sickness, rash*
Penicillin V oral (*Phenoxymethyl penicillin*)	*Oral*: 20–50 mg/ kg/day in 4 divided doses	*Oral*: 250–500 mg 6—8 hourly	*Hypersensitivity, rash*, haemolytic anaemia
Cephalexin	*Oral*: 30–40 mg/kg/day in 3 divided doses.	*Oral*: 250–500 mg 8 hourly	Transient elevation of liver enzymes, neutropenia, arthralgia, rash, eosinophilia
Cefixime	*Oral*: 8 mg/kg/day in 2 divided doses	*Oral*: 200–400 mg 12 hrly	Diarrhoea, leucopenia, renal toxicity, transient elevation of liver enzymes
Cefadroxil	*Oral*: 30 mg/kg/day in 2 divided doses	*Oral*: 500 mg to 1 g 8 hourly	Rash, eosinophilla
Cefotaxime sodium	*Intravenous*: 100–150 mg/kg/day in 3–4 divided doses	*Intravenous*: 1–2 g 6–8 hourly	Transient elevation of liver enzymes, renal toxicity. Arrhythmia
Ceftriaxone	*Intravenous*: 50–100 mg/kg/day in 2 divided doses	*Intravenous*: 1–2 g 12–24 hourly	Transient elevation of liver enzymes, renal toxicity
Cefuroxime axetil	*Oral*: 20–30 mg/kg/day in 2 divided doses IM/ IV: 75–100 mg/kg/day in 3 divided doses	*Oral*: 250–500 mg 12 hrly IM/IV: 750 mg to 1.5 g 8 hourly	Leukopenia, transient elevation of liver enzymes, renal toxicity
Cepodoxime proxetil	*Oral*: 10 mg/kg/day in 2 divided doses	*Oral*: 100–200 mg 12 hrly	Abdominal pain, bloating, diarroea, chest tightness, confusion
Clindamycin	*Oral*: 20–40 mg/kg/day in 3–4 divided doses	*Oral, IV*: 150–300 mg 6–8 hourly	Diarrhoea *pseudomembranous colitis*, skin rash,

contd.

			transient elevation of liver enzymes, *bone marrow depression*
Chloramphenicol	*Oral*: 50–75 mg/kg/day in 4 divided doses *IV*: 100 mg/kg/day in 4 divided doses	*Oral*: 250–500 mg 6–8 hourly	*Bone marrow suppression, aplastic anaemia, grey baby syndrome*, haemolysis in G6PD deficiency
Ciprofloxacin	*Oral*: 20–40 mg/kg/day in 2 divided doses *IV*: 10–20 mg/kg/day (Max 800 mg/day)	*Oral, IV*: 250–750 mg 12 hourly	*Nausea, abdominal discomfort,* photosensitivity, transient elevation of liver enzymes, arthralgia
Cloxacillin	*Oral*: 50–100 mg/kg/day in 3–4 divided doses *Intravenous*: 100–200 mg/kg/day divides q 6 hourly	*Oral*: 250–500 mg 6–8 hourly *Intravenous*: 1–2 g 6 hourly	*Neutropenia*, transient elevation of liver enzymes, Cholecystitis, nephritis
Cotrimoxazole (*Trimethoprim-Sulpha-methaxozole, TMP-SMZ*)	*Oral*: 5–10 mg/kg/day of TMP or 25–50 mg/kg/day of in 2 divided doses (5–10 mg trimethoprim)	*Single strength* 80 mg/400 mg 2 bid *Double strength* 160 mg/ 800 mg 1 bid	*Megaloblastic anaemia, skin rash, erythema multiforme*
Clarithromycin	*Oral*: 15 mg/kg/day in 2 divided doses	*Oral*: 250–500mg 12 hourly	Transient elevation of liver enzymes, *renal toxicity,* nausea, GI upset
Clindamycin	*Oral*: 20–40 mg/kg/day in 3–4 divided doses	*Oral*: 150–300 mg 6–8 hourly	*Diarrhoea, pseudomembranous colitis*, skin rash, Erythema multiforme, Transient elevation of liver enzymes, thrombocytopenia, leucopenia
Doxycycline	2–5 mg/kg/day in 2 divided doses	200 mg on day 1 followed by 100 mg daily	Diarrhoea, stomach upset, esophagitis, rash, avoid in

contd.

			children due to risk of staining of teeth and growth retardation
Ertapenem	*IM, IV*: 3–12 years: 15 mg/kg/day twice daily	13 years and above: *IV*: 1 g of infusion in 50 mg of 0.9% Sodium chloride *IM*: 1 g once daily in 3–5 mL of lidocaine	Vomiting, diarrhoea, *pseudo membranous colitis. Headache, hallucination seizures.* Arrhythmia
Erythromycin	*Oral*: 30–40 mg in 4 divided doses	*Oral*: 250–500 mg 6 hourly	*Hepatitis.* Arrhythmia
Gentamycin	*IM, IV*: 5–7.5 mg/kg/day in 2–3 divided doses	*IM, IV*: 250 mg/day in 3 divided doses	*Nephrotoxicity ototoxicity and optic neuritis*
Linezolid	*Oral, IV*: 10 mg/kg/dose 6–8 hourly	*Oral*: 400–600 mg 12 hourly	*Peripheral and optic neuropathy, thrombocytopenia, bone marrow suppression*, colitis
Metronidazole	*Oral, IV*: 15–20 mg/kg/day dose 3 times/day	*Oral*: 400 mg 8 hourly *IV*: 500–700 mg 8 hourly	*Nausea, metallic taste, Disulfiram like reaction with alcohol*
Nalidixic acid	*Oral*: 8 mg/kg/day in 2 divided doses	*Oral*: 1 g 4 times/day	*Hepatotoxicity, leukopenia,* vertigo, rash, pseudotumour cerebri, seizure
Norfloxacin	*Oral*: 20–30 mg/kg/day in 2 divided doses	*Oral*: 400 mg 12 hourly	Nausea, abdominal discomfort, *photosensitivity,* transient elevation of liver enzymes, arthralgia
Nitrofurantoin	*Oral*: 5–8 mg/kg/day in 2 divided doses	*Oral*: 50–100 mg 6 hourly	*Discolouration of urine, rash*, vertigo,

contd.

			methaemoglobinaemia, hepatitis and neuropathy
Ofloxacin	*Oral*: 20 mg/kg/day in 2 divided doses	*Oral*: 200–400 12 hourly	Transient elevation of liver enzymes, leukopenia, renal toxicity May precipitate psychosis/seizures
Piperacillin–Tazobactum	*IV*: 200–400 mg/kg/day in 3–4 divided doses	*IV*: 4.5 g 8 hourly	*Leukopenia,* transient elevation of liver enzymes, renal toxicity
Vancomycin	*IV*: 40–60 mg/kg/day in 3–4 divided doses	*IV*: 1 g 12 hourly	*Oto-toxicity, nephrotoxicity,* red man syndrome

INDEX

A